# THE GENERAL PRACTITIONER

# The
# General Practitioner

**A STUDY OF MEDICAL
EDUCATION AND PRACTICE
IN ONTARIO
AND NOVA SCOTIA**

by Kenneth F. Clute

B.A., M.D., F.R.C.P.(C)

UNIVERSITY OF TORONTO PRESS

# Preface

"What is this book about?" "To whom is it addressed?" These are questions that a potential reader may be expected to ask before giving any book more than a casual glance. The book is *about* general medical practice. It is neither reminiscences nor stories of dramatic cases; it is not instruction in diagnosis or treatment; it does not tell how to set up an office or how to carry out this or that procedure. It is an account of a detailed study of eighty-six general practices in Ontario and Nova Scotia, with particular attention to the quality of medical care and to problems of medical education and of the organization of medical care as these relate to quality.

The book is *addressed to* all those who are interested in the broader aspects of a question that is being debated in Canada at the present time, namely, how our people can best be provided with good medical care. This question is, naturally, of great interest to the medical profession. Interest in the matter extends far beyond the profession, however. Within the past two years, the Saskatchewan Government has fought the 1960 election primarily on the question of medical care, has had a commission consider how a comprehensive medical service should be organized, and has already passed the legislation necessary for implementing its programme. Similarly, the federal Government has appointed a Royal Commission on Health Services, which has been sitting since the autumn of 1961 to consider the whole problem of Canada's health needs.* This book is addressed, then, not only to those who have a professional interest in problems of medical

*Since this book went to press, one of the political parties in Ontario is reported to have "served notice it will make medical care insurance a major issue both at the next session of the Ontario legislature and in the next provincial general election" (*Toronto Daily Star*, August 21, 1962, p. 17).

care—practising physicians, medical educators, workers in the field of public health, and others—but quite as much to those members of the public who are interested in the provision of medical care as one of the contemporary problems of our society.

An author who ventures to write at the same time for both a professional audience and a lay audience faces the twofold problem of not boring the former by oversimplification and of making himself intelligible to the latter. So highly specialized are many fields today, including many medical fields, that it is all but impossible for those within the pale to communicate with those outside. Fortunately, I am dealing with a subject that can be discussed in terms with which the intelligent general reader may be expected to be familiar. Accordingly, I have felt it my duty to avoid medical terminology that would be meaningless to the non-medical reader, and I ask my medical readers to bear with me when, now and then, I mention "removal of the gall bladder" instead of "cholecystectomy." In certain places, however (notably chapters 16 and 17), in which quality of practice is considered, it has been essential to introduce some clinical examples and a few medical terms, in order to make clear the criteria upon which we based our assessment of quality. The few medical terms with which the general reader might not be familiar are defined in a glossary. The clinical examples cannot be evaluated without medical training, but the layman's inability to evaluate them should not interfere either with his understanding what went on in practice or with his following the development of the argument. Similarly, though statistical tests have been used and though the results of these are reported, I have assumed that some of my readers will have no knowledge at all of statistics and have explained briefly in chapter 2 the very few points that are needed for an understanding of what follows. In fact, I would say that it is no more necessary to understand statistical theory or techniques in order to read this book than it is to understand the way in which an automobile works, or the way in which electricity works, in order to drive an automobile or to turn on a light. In short, though I have presented the detailed evidence required by the critical medical reader, I have tried throughout to make the book intelligible to the non-medical reader.

Having said that this book has been written as much for the general reader as for the physician, I must explain why. During the past six years, my associates and I have been privileged to have such a view of general medical practice, at first hand, as no one in this country has ever had before or, for reasons of cost, is ever likely to have again.

When we began our work, there had for some years been demands for changes in the organization of medical care; but it appeared that many years might yet elapse before government would intervene in the affairs of the profession. Accordingly, whenever my thoughts ran ahead to the then-distant day of accounting, I thought vaguely in terms of a report to our sponsoring bodies and, if the findings should warrant it, to the medical profession. During the intervening years, however, public interest in matters of medical care has increased so rapidly and the demands for changes have become so insistent that it now appears likely that major changes will come about within the next few years. Whatever decisions are made, whether wise or foolish, will undoubtedly affect medical care in this country for many years to come. It is to be hoped, then, that they will be made, not for selfish personal, professional, or political ends, but with a view only to improving the quality of Canada's medical care. Though the quality of the care depends directly upon the individual physician who provides it, any governmental action that determines the conditions under which a physician practises can have far-reaching effects. These effects may be either good or bad. Since governments tend to be responsive to the moods of the voters, at any rate on popular issues, public pressure may well determine whether changes brought about by government will cause the quality of practice to improve or to deteriorate. The public, since it will share with government and with the medical profession the responsibility for the future of medicine, will have need of all the information that can be laid before it, if it is to choose wisely. Bearing these things in mind, I am convinced that I should be acting irresponsibly if I were to make our findings available only to the medical profession. Thus this book is addressed equally to the medical profession and to the general public, because I believe that the quality of medical care in the future depends on each group's having an understanding of the problems that are involved in the provision of medical care of high quality.

This study of general practice could not have been carried out, had it not been for the assistance that I have received from many individuals and organizations. It gives me great pleasure to be able to acknowledge in print the assistance of my principal benefactors. Some, however, must accept my thanks anonymously: those whose comments and suggestions have moulded my thoughts and become incorporated into them without my being clearly aware of their source. First of all, I must pay tribute to the College of General Practice of Canada, which first conceived of making a study of general practice in this country; to the Steering Committee for the Survey and its consultants, who largely determined the form that the study would take; and to Dr. W. Victor Johnston, who, as Executive Director of the College ever since its founding and as Chairman of the Steering Committee, probably played a larger part than any other single person in setting the plan in motion. In addition to getting the Survey started and, in collaboration with the University of Toronto, appointing me to the position that I have occupied for the past six years, the Committee has continued to give me the benefit of its advice; and its Chairman, especially in the early days of the work, was most helpful to me in many ways. Yet the Committee has at no time directed me, and it has shown a rare degree of patience in waiting for the completion of the study.

To the University of Toronto I am indebted for an appointment to its staff for the duration of the study and for giving appointments to my associates while they were working with me. I wish particularly to thank Professor Andrew J. Rhodes, Director of the School of Hygiene, and Professor Milton H. Brown, Head of the Department of Public Health, for accepting us into the Department of Public Health, for their interest, encouragement, and, when needed, active assistance during these years, and for reading and criticizing my manuscript.

The beginning of this work was made possible by a grant of the Governments of Canada and of Ontario under the National Health Grants programme and by a grant from the Canadian Life Insurance Officers Association; for the major portion of the financing we are indebted to the munificence of the Rockefeller Foundation. To each of these, I wish to express my appreciation of its assistance. I must mention specially Dr. Osler L. Peterson, of the Rockefeller Foundation's staff, who advised the Steering Committee in the planning stage of the study, made available to us the methods that he had worked out in his study of general practice in North Carolina, instructed me in the use of these methods during a most delightful three-week visit that I made to North Carolina, and visited me in Toronto on a number of occasions to advise and encourage.

My principal associate in this work was Dr. John B. Firstbrook, who was with me for four and a half years. Since leaving me a little over a year ago to become Associate Professor of Physiological Hygiene in this University, he has continued to give generously of his time. If I had not had his assistance, it is doubtful whether the study could have been carried to a successful conclusion. Though Dr. Firstbrook has not taken part in the writing of this book and is not responsible for the ideas that are set forth, he has read the entire manuscript—some parts of it more than once—and has made countless invaluable suggestions, for which I am deeply obligated. Dr. David Penman, who carried out the field work in Nova Scotia, was most faithful and meticulous in the performance of his duties. I am grateful to him for carrying the work in that province to a satisfactory completion.

For help in connection with the sampling in Ontario, I am indebted to the late Dr. Frederick W. Jackson, Director of Health Services, Department of National Health and Welfare, and to Mr. T. G. Donnelly, at that time of the Dominion Bureau of Statistics, who supervised the drawing of the sample.

Professor D. B. W. Reid, of the Department of Epidemiology and Biometrics of the School of Hygiene, has been most generous with his time and advice regarding statistical problems throughout the study. He has steered us away from many pitfalls.

I am grateful to Dean Chester B. Stewart, of the Faculty of Medicine of Dalhousie University, for his encouragement and advice and for doing all that he could to expedite our work in Nova Scotia. In particular, I appreciate his welcoming Dr. David Penman and making office space available to him during his year and a half in that province. Dr. C. J. W. Beckwith, Executive Secretary of the Medical Society of Nova Scotia, and Dr. M. R. Macdonald, Registrar of the Provincial Medical Board of Nova Scotia, also were most helpful in advising me in the planning stage of the Nova Scotia study.

To the deans of medicine at the University of Toronto, Queen's University, the University of Western Ontario, the University of Ottawa, McGill University, the University of Montreal, and Dalhousie University, I wish to express my gratitude for allowing me access, on a confidential basis, to the academic records of the physicians whose practices we studied.

The writing of a book that is not confined to the reporting of indisputable facts is a heavy responsibility for an author. For this reason, the critical reading of one's manuscript by others who are less intimately involved is an act of great kindness. Those who have done me the kindness of reading the entire manuscript, in addition to those already named, are Professor Oswald Hall, of the Department of Political Economy of the University of Toronto, who has commented from the point of view of his long-standing interest in problems of medical sociology, and Mr. Frederick B. Rainsberry, Ph.D., whose many years of experience with education at various levels and whose acute perception of social problems have fitted him to give me the reaction of the reader who has had no professional involvement in the problems of the medical profession or of medical care. Dr. R. Rolf Struthers, who has long been interested in problems of medical education and was Secretary of the Curriculum Committee of the Faculty of Medicine of McGill University that made recommendations for revision of its medical curriculum a few years ago, and Professor Alexander M. Bryans, Head of the Department of Paediatrics of Queen's University, have very kindly read, and offered valuable comments on, the chapters dealing with problems of medical education. I wish to express my deep appreciation to all those who have taken the time to read all or parts of the manuscript and give me their ideas.

Yet, in spite of all the assistance that I have acknowledged, this study could not have been carried out, had it not been for the willing co-operation of the general practitioners who participated in it. To these men and their wives, who were so generous with their time, their ideas, and their hospitality, I wish to offer the thanks of myself and my two associates. I believe that the contribution that they have made to the advancement of medical care in this country is one in which they can take pride.

I am indebted to the University of Toronto Press and especially to Miss Francess G. Halpenny, its Editor, whose gentle but apt questioning has shown me the need to amplify in some places, to condense in others, and to clear up certain obscurities. Working with Miss Halpenny has been an interesting and valuable experience for me; of more importance, she has contributed to this book much for which the reader may be grateful.

I have been so fortunate as to have the same secretary throughout the six years of this study. Mrs. Margaret E. Koster's ability as an expert typist has greatly lightened my work. I wish to thank her for her loyalty in seeing this book through to completion.

Finally, I owe most of all to my dear wife, who has read the entire manuscript a number of times, whose comments have clarified much of my thinking, who has helped with matters of grammar, punctuation, and style, who has shown unending patience during the many months when I have had almost no time for anything but this book, and whose confidence and enthusiasm have been a constant source of strength. I have been fortunate, indeed.

K.F.C.

*School of Hygiene*
*University of Toronto*
*January 31, 1962*

# Foreword

The College of General Practice of Canada was established in 1954 as a voluntary educational and standard-setting body for general practitioners. In May, 1962, its membership of 2,400 embraced about 25 per cent of all Canadian general physicians. Unique among Canadian professional associations, the College requires a minimum of 100 hours postgraduate study every two-year period for continuing active membership. This requirement stems from its basic philosophy that competence was and remains the most valuable attribute of the Canadian family doctor.

The College very early realized the need to become better informed about the whole field of general practice as quickly as possible. It resolved that an analytical survey of general practice should be one of its methods for obtaining knowledge on which to base its future educational programme. A donation from the Canadian Life Insurance Officers Association happily set in motion a chain of events culminating in this intensive study by Dr. Kenneth F. Clute. The College appreciates the financial assistance of the Canadian life insurance industry, the National Health Grants, and the Rockefeller Foundation, which made this examination of general practice possible. (These grants were: Canadian Life Insurance Officers Association, $30,000; National Health Grants, $22,500; Rockefeller Foundation, $110,000.)

The co-operation of the doctors interviewed, the organizational talent of the author and the support of his associates, Dr. John B. Firstbrook and Dr. David Penman, have resulted in the successful completion of this monumental task—an analysis of contemporary general practice which is truly both penetrating and exhaustive. This report fulfils one of the aims of the College, namely to centre attention on education and standards of practice. It does not shield poor practice and neither

should the College. It holds few surprises for those currently practising and one is quite sure that any similar analytical study applied
to other groups of the medical profession, or to another profession,
would reveal a comparable range of quality of work. It is most re-
freshing and reassuring to have definite evidence that the honourable
ideals traditionally attributed to physicians still govern most of them
in spite of the thrust of profound social changes.

To those of us in the College of General Practice interested in
improving training for general practice and developing more and
better educational opportunities for those in practice, this report will
serve as a source of factual information—a *vade mecum* or guide—
which we can use to broaden and deepen our endeavours.

Many interpretations in a book of this kind are bound to be controversial and call for deliberation. As the author points out in his report,
the conclusions arrived at are his own. They do not necessarily represent the thinking or the policy of the College of General Practice.

The survey indicates how and where practices are poor but also
reports that most practices are excellent or at least satisfactory. It
might have been supplemented by more details of good practices. It
is the able practitioner who stirs the imagination and shows the way
for others. Seeing ourselves as we should be, in itself, increases our
stature.

The College has always taken a keen interest in the role of psychiatry
in general practice. Inevitably many problems of a psychiatric nature
present themselves in the consulting office of the general practitioner
and it has been our policy to encourage our members to think seriously
about their responsibilities in this field and to seek training to meet
them. We would like to have seen more time devoted to the assessment
of psychiatric problems and of the intangibles of dealing with people
under the varied patterns of general practice. The capacity of the
general physician in the field of psychiatry could be a fruitful area for
future investigation.

There is room for disagreement with the author on the question of
hospital privileges for general practitioners. He found no evidence
that the general practitioner was being excluded from hospitals in
Ontario and Nova Scotia except from teaching hospitals. The College
has consistently maintained that the privilege of participation on the
active staff of their neighbouring general hospitals, including teaching
hospitals, is a fundamental privilege which assures able general practitioners a place on hospital committees and departments and enhances
their competence as medical practitioners. The College finds that such

active staff membership for capable general practitioners is not yet permitted in a considerable number of large city general hospitals.

Some of the author's views on the subject of solo versus group practice probably will be at variance with those of many experienced physicians.

We commend this book to all those interested in the general practice of medicine. We think that it is better read as a whole rather than in part, keeping in mind what has been pointed out by the author, that the method of assessment has some gaps with little or no appraisal of the surgical skills employed, obstetrical deliveries, and psychiatric management.

The author has had a unique view of medicine. Such matters as a doctor's preparatory training, his problems of time and finance, are thoughtfully discussed. The book contains a very revealing report on the workload of a general practitioner. The assessment of how the doctors deal with the many different facets of general practice is a major contribution.

This study shows exhaustive research in the reasons underlying various patterns of general practice. Definitions and yardsticks are carefully set forth, with an abundance of statistical tables to support the findings.

It will be of great value to all those concerned with teaching twentieth-century medicine to twentieth-century young men and women. In the words of the author, the good general practices may well be the pride of the medical profession and the poor ones its challenge.

W. VICTOR JOHNSTON, M.D.
*Executive Director*
*College of General Practice of Canada*

# Contents

# INTRODUCTION

## A NOTE ON THE ORGANIZATION OF MEDICAL PRACTICE
## IN CANADA

For the sake of any reader who may not be familiar with the relationship that exists at present between the medical profession in Canada and the people whom it serves, a brief description of the present system follows.

Most of the general practitioners and most of the specialists are in private practice. Those who are carrying on clinical work but are in salaried positions are mainly those who are employed by certain departments of the Government of Canada (the Departments of Veterans Affairs, of Indian Affairs, of Immigration, or of Defence), those employed by departments of health of the various provincial governments to care for tuberculous patients and mental patients, those employed by local departments of public health, those employed by the Workmen's Compensation Board in the various provinces, a few employed by industrial concerns to look after employees and, sometimes, their families, and a few specialists who are employed by medical schools or by teaching hospitals associated with medical schools. With such exceptions as these, it may be said that all specialists and general practitioners who are engaged in clinical practice are in private practice. These doctors, both specialists and general practitioners, see patients in their offices, sometimes in the patients' homes, and in the hospitals. A few physicians who are carrying on general practices are qualified in one or another specialty. Some of the specialists limit their practices strictly to those patients who are referred to them by colleagues, whereas other specialists, though confining their work to their specialty, see patients without requiring that they be referred by another physician. Virtually all of the practitioners in a particular area, at least in the two provinces that were studied during this survey, have privileges in one or more of the hospitals in that area, although, as will be made plain, various limitations are set to the work that a physician may undertake in a hospital.

In the teaching hospitals and in a few other large hospitals, patients on the public wards are attended by the practitioners who make use of the hospital and who constitute its staff. The physicians in many of these hospitals receive no financial remuneration for their services to these patients. In a few areas, the doctors contract to provide complete coverage for their patients on a capitation basis (i.e., at so much per person per year), but this is not common. In a few areas also, the number of which is decreasing, doctors are paid a basic salary by the municipality, which they may augment by charging the patient for certain specified services. With these exceptions, payment for the services rendered by a physician to his patient is on a fee-for-service basis. In some cases, the fee is paid by such organizations as the Department of Veterans Affairs or the Workmen's Compensation Board; in many others, the fee is paid by an insuring body (e.g., Physicians' Services Incorporated, Windsor Medical Services, Maritime Medical Care) sponsored by the medical profession itself; in the remaining cases, payment for the care rendered by a private physician, whether in hospital, in his own office, or in a patient's home, is the direct responsibility of the patient or of those who are responsible for him. Some of those in the last group carry insurance with commercial insurance companies.

# 1 / The Survey of General Practice
## *Origin and Purpose*

One late October evening, in 1955, the author, in browsing through the *Canadian Medical Association Journal*, was much surprised to come across an advertisement for a "physician to direct a 'survey of general practice of Canada' sponsored by the College of General Practice and the University of Toronto. A full time appointment for three years." The advertisement gave no clue to what the sponsors had in mind. Because he had an increasing interest in problems of medical education, the author answered the advertisement, though with no real expectation that this "survey" would have anything to do with educational problems. Both his surprise and his interest were considerably heightened when, two days later, sitting across the luncheon table from Dr. W. Victor Johnston, Executive Director of the College of General Practice of Canada, he listened to Dr. Johnston asking questions that were almost precisely the same as questions in the author's own mind. It was apparent that the group that was attempting to get the "survey" under way was indeed interested primarily in problems of medical education. The upshot of the meeting was that the author was requested, if he was seriously interested, to appear at a meeting of a Steering Committee the next day.

At this meeting the author was interviewed by the members of the Committee, and some two months later he was offered the position of Director of the Survey of General Practice. He assumed his new position in mid-January, 1956. For his qualifications and those of his associates, which are intimately connected with the methods used, the reader is referred to the next chapter.

The survey thus initiated had had its origin some months earlier in the feeling of a group within the one-year-old College of General Practice of Canada that a great deal of attention had been given to the problems of the specialists and to raising the standards of specialty practice but little or no attention to the difficulties associated with being a good general practitioner. It was to fill this need that the Survey of General Practice in Canada was conceived. The original, fairly modest plan was to send a questionnaire to all the general practitioners in the country. The Survey in its final form was something quite different, enormously more ambitious.

A Steering Committee was set up and met for the first time on June 2, 1955. Since this group was instrumental in getting the Survey under way and continued to function as an Advisory Committee throughout the course of these studies, the composition of the Committee is of more than passing interest. The chairman was Dr. W. Victor Johnston, Executive Director, College of General Practice of Canada; and the other members were Dr. Milton H. Brown, Professor of Hygiene and Preventive Medicine, University of Toronto; Dr. W. Cameron Cowan, general practitioner, Richmond Hill, Ontario; Dr. Charles D. Farquharson, Medical Officer of Health, Scarborough Township, Ontario; Dr. Jean-Baptiste Jobin, Dean of the Faculty of Medicine, Laval University; Dr. Peter A. Kinsey, general practitioner, Toronto; Dr. Joseph A. MacFarlane, Dean of the Faculty of Medicine, University of Toronto; Dr. J. Wendell Macleod, Dean of the College of Medicine, University of Saskatchewan; Dr. Arthur F. W. Peart, Assistant Secretary, Canadian Medical Association; Dr. Crawford Rose, general practitioner, Aurora, Ontario; Dr. Chester B. Stewart, Dean of the Faculty of Medicine, Dalhousie University; and Dr. Thomas Tweedie, general practitioner, Hamilton, Ontario. Acting as consultants to the Committee were Dr. Charles D. Gossage, Associate Medical Director, Confederation Life Association; Dr. Frederick W. Jackson, Director of Health Services, Department of National Health and Welfare, who was succeeded, after his retirement, by Dr. Roger B. Goyette, of the same department; Dr. W. Harding leRiche, Physicians' Services Incorporated, Toronto; and at a later date Dr. Andrew J. Rhodes, Director of the School of Hygiene, University of Toronto.

As one considers this list, one cannot help being struck by the variety of the groups represented. Striking, also, is the fact that the minutes of the first meeting of the Committee lay great emphasis on the *quality* of practice. A portion of a letter from a very prominent general practitioner is included in these minutes and states, "I hope we can make an outstanding point of this [i.e., quality of practice*] so that when the survey report is published, it will be something of a yard-stick for men in practice and going into practice and a definite leadership given away from the malignant idea of '10 patients per hour.'" The minutes go on to say: "It was generally agreed by those present that a close study should be made of the quality of general practice. It was also agreed that too many doctors are trying to see too many patients in one day and that some office set-ups are too elaborate."

The most noteworthy of the Committee's consultants was Dr. Osler L. Peterson, Staff Member of the Rockefeller Foundation and, at that time, Director of Program Planning Section, Division of Health Affairs, University of North Carolina, who had just completed a study of general practice in North Carolina. Dr. Peterson warned the Committee of the difficulties that are encountered when information is sought by mailed questionnaires and advised against such an investigation. He told the Committee of his own findings in North Carolina, the most significant of which, based on direct observation, was the great variation in quality of practice among the general practitioners whom he had visited. Though his study had not started out as a study of quality, the great difference between practices quickly obtruded itself upon his attention so markedly that he felt compelled to try to obtain quantitative results and devised a measuring scale for this purpose. In view of his experience, he recommended an intensive study of individual practices.

The Steering Committee was impressed by what Dr. Peterson reported. Whether a similar variation in quality of practice existed in Canada was not known, though the minutes of the meeting, quoted above, indicate that a variation in quality was suspected.† As it seemed desirable to obtain definite information on this point, the decision was made to repeat in Canada what Dr. Peterson had done in North Carolina.

Though the College of General Practice had taken the steps that initiated the Survey and did not lack the enthusiasm to continue on with it, it became apparent that it would be necessary to have also the sponsorship of a university. The Department of National Health and

---

*Recently, the President Elect of the College of General Practice has referred again to the College's wish to ascertain the quality of general practice. I. W. Bean: Journal of the College of General Practice of Canada, 8: 3, 13, 1961.

†That doubts about the quality of some general practices were not confined to the group that set up the Survey became apparent during the interviews with some of the physicians whose practices were studied. See pages 157 and 172.

Welfare was interested in the project and had indicated that favourable consideration would be given to a request for a National Health Grant, but such a grant could be made only to a university. Moreover, if, as was hoped, one of the foundations should prove willing to give financial assistance, this also would almost certainly have to be administered by a university.

Several universities showed an interest in being associated with the Survey. The University of Toronto was approached first, because it was obvious that its location in the same city as the headquarters of the College of General Practice would greatly facilitate the study. This University agreed to collaborate with the College of General Practice. It was decided that the personnel should be selected by the Steering Committee and the University acting in consultation and should be appointed to the staff of the Department of Hygiene and Preventive Medicine* of this University for the purpose of carrying out the study.

In the opinion of the author, the decision to have the actual work done within a university was most fortunate. Not only did the arrangement make library facilities available, but the workers were able to benefit from the discussion, the inquiry, the atmosphere of scepticism, which are part of university life. Of equal importance, the work was done in a school that has only minor contact with either general practitioners or medical students, and therefore in an organization whose policies have very little bearing on the quality of general practice. This gave the investigators greater freedom than would have been possible had they been working directly for any of the professional organizations. The author is not implying that any pressure was brought to bear on him to change either his methods or his findings to suit the interests of any particular group. The fact is—and this cannot be emphasized strongly enough—that the author was given an absolutely free rein throughout the whole course of the work. Indeed, when he asked Dr. Johnston, at an early stage of the study, whether he would like to look over some part of the work, Dr. Johnston's reply was that he did not wish to see it until the work was completed. Even though there was no interference on the part of any of the interested organizations, nevertheless to work as a staff member of a school that occupied a disinterested position was an immense advantage, as it left the workers free to pursue the truth as they saw it, without even the possibility of pressure from any interested group.

*This department, under the direction of Professor Milton H. Brown, which had previously been a part of the Faculty of Medicine, became the Department of Public Health of the School of Hygiene on July 1, 1956.

Such was the beginning of six years of fascinating adventure. Like most explorers, the author had little conception of the magnitude of the territory that he was entering nor did he foresee the obstacles that lay across his path—the need to consider, not only problems of under-graduate and postgraduate medical education, but the matter of responsibility in relation to medical practice; the interrelationships between medical education and economics at various stages of a doctor's life; the relationships between general practitioners and specialists; the effects, not only of changes in medicine, but of changes in modern living, on a doctor's practice; and many other problems. Finally, the author had no suspicion, at that time, that this journey of exploration would end by convincing him that some of the traditional concepts of medical practice should be seriously questioned and that fundamental changes were needed in the organization of medical practice.

So far, the objectives of the Survey have merely been touched upon. It is now desirable to state them fully. In a request for aid that was submitted to the Rockefeller Foundation, the following objectives were listed:

1. To determine the types and the volume of illness treated by general practitioners, under the different circumstances that obtain in different parts of Canada.

2. To determine how adequately such illnesses are being diagnosed and treated.

3. To study the factors that determine the quality of general practice. Factors that are thought to be of importance include:

(*a*) Characteristics of the doctor himself. In this regard, an attempt will be made to observe and to record in general terms the characteristics of the men whose practices are studied. Information will be collected from the doctors studied on the adequacy of the counselling that is available to medical students and to doctors taking postgraduate train-ing. It is hoped to ascertain whether adequate counsel is available to young people who are trying to decide whether to enter the medical course and to recent medical graduates who are faced with choosing between several types of medical career.

(*b*) The adequacy of the doctor's training. The study will attempt to evaluate how well present-day medical education prepares doctors for general practice. This will include an assessment of undergraduate and interneship training and of postgraduate courses and facilities for the continuing instruction of general physicians. It is hoped to recommend improvements in undergraduate and postgraduate training.

(*c*) The circumstances under which the doctor is working, with special attention to (1) the effect of office organization and management, including the effects of practising alone or as a member of a group, (2) financial aspects of practice, including the effect of voluntary and government medical and hospital care prepaid plans on general practice, (3) the effect of availability of hospital facilities and consultants, and (4) the effect of climate and geography.

4.  To determine, on the basis of the results of the objectives already listed, what kind of general practice is needed by the Canadian people—in particular: (*a*) what work the general practitioner should be trained to cope with, under average circumstances and under certain unusual circumstances (e.g., in isolated areas); (*b*) what training will best prepare doctors for such practices; (*c*) whether general practice should, ideally, be a solo, or a group, enterprise; (*d*) what hospital and consultant facilities are necessary if the general practitioner is to give the best service of which he is capable.

5.  To examine the relationship of the doctor to his family, to professional organizations, and to the community in which he lives.

It must be apparent from the breadth of these objectives that there was virtually no limit to what might be attempted. The originators of the project had some reason to suspect that the quality of some practices might not be up to acceptable standards. If this was so, they thought that both the causes and the remedies lay mainly within the field of education—undergraduate, postgraduate, or continuing education. Based on these thoughts, the one specific injunction that the Committee laid upon the author was that Dr. Peterson's method was to be used to assess the quality of practice of a randomly selected sample of general practitioners. It was agreed, also, that the major emphasis would be put on educational problems, though the Committee did not specify the approach that was to be used. Beyond these two matters, quality and education, the author was left free to pursue whatever course he thought best.

Several studies of general practice had already been made elsewhere, and these were reviewed by the author for possible help in planning his own. In 1950, J. S. Collings published the results of a study of general practice in England.* He visited 55 practices, which were carried on by 104 doctors, and sat in on each of these practices for a period varying from one to five days. His conclusions contain such statements as, "The present state of general practice is unsatisfactory. Its defects . . . arise from failure to define general practice and to establish and maintain standards" and, "the future of general practice is largely being determined without deliberate consideration of its problems . . . in terms of compensation for recognized, or half-recognized, deficiencies, instead of the correction of these deficiencies."

*J. S. Collings: The Lancet, 258: 555–85, 1950. The quotations which follow are from pages 578 and 579.

Again, he refers to "the widening schism between the specialist and the general practitioner, and inability to see beyond the practitioner's few but dramatic sins of commission (e.g., surgical) to his many more serious, if less obvious, sins of omission (e.g., missed or mistaken diagnosis)." He made two recommendations, that "an attempt should be made to define the future province and function of general practice . . ." and that "basic group-practice units . . . should be formed as soon as possible." To the latter recommendation we shall refer again in chapter 26.

In 1950, a Special Committee appointed by the Council of the British Medical Association instructed Stephen J. Hadfield, Assistant Secretary of the Association, to make a survey of a random sample of different types of practice in the United Kingdom. Hadfield picked a random sample of 200 doctors, of whom he visited 188. With each, he spent the better part of a day, in the course of which he was present at one, or sometimes more than one, office session, accompanied the practitioner as he made his round of house calls, and was invited to be present at the house calls in more than half of the practices. His findings were published in 1953.* After a general description of the practitioner's life and practice, he discusses, among other things, the adequacy of investigation and treatment, the adequacy of the premises, and the adequacy of the equipment in the practices that he visited. He concludes that 44 per cent of the practices were "good" and another 44 per cent "adequate." Unfortunately his criteria are not made clear. When he says, "In the category 'good' I placed those practitioners whose skill was evident and whom I found exercising a constant care and thoroughness with every patient, a keen appreciation of the whole man in the patient, together with a friendliness and spirit of kindness and helpfulness," one cannot but wish that he had reported in detail the evidence that proved the practitioner's "skill." Especially does one wonder about his criteria since he has previously stated that 69 per cent do satisfactory examinations, that 7 per cent show "a need for revision of the methods of diagnosis they use," and that the remainder (24 per cent) "vary over a fairly wide range. Some of these seem ready now and again to take a chance. . . ." Again, when he says, "Some of the senior practitioners, though undertaking little in the way of examination, have obviously developed an instinct or sixth sense," he does not explain how he could be sure that the doctor's diagnosis was correct, i.e. that his "sixth sense" was adequate.

A third study of general practice in the United Kingdom was

*S. J. Hadfield: British Medical Journal, 2: 683–706, 1953. The quotations which follow are from pages 687 and 705.

carried out by Stephen Taylor at the invitation of the Nuffield Provincial Hospitals Trust. His purpose was not to make a systematic
study of quality, though there are references here and there to
quality, but, as the title of his report suggests, "to find and describe
in detail the best in general practice; to analyze these findings . . . ;
and to present the results in such a way that the GP, or the young
doctor intending to become a GP, may learn something of value
about the organization and conduct of practice."[*]

Collings, in his report, makes some penetrating criticisms, but he
was not dealing with a random sample and had not evolved a method
for carrrying out a detailed assessment of his practices. Hadfield also
fails to make clear the criteria used in assessing quality; and he makes
no specific recommendations. All three of these studies, as is to be
expected, deal at great length with the British National Health Service.
To fundamental determinants of quality little reference is made,
except in some of Collings's remarks. The practitioner is pictured as
he was seen by one or another of the observers at a particular moment
in the course of his career. No description is given of the doctor's
background, either general or educational, from which one might
arrive at a better understanding of him as he manifests himself to
the observer.

The sole detailed, first-hand study of general practice in North
America was Peterson's study of 88 general practitioners in North
Carolina.[†]As has already been stated, Peterson found a great variation in quality of practice and devised a rating scale in order to facilitate
comparison of different practices. He states in his report (page 143)
that while "many physicians were performing at a high level of professional competence . . . other physicians were performing at a lower
level." From his examination of the data available to him, he was convinced of "two basic facts," that "the better medical student [i.e.,
better as judged by academic record] tends to become a better physician" and that "the more training a physician has received in internal
medicine the more likely he is to become a good physician." On the
latter fact he lays a good deal of emphasis. He feels (page 144) that
"the importance of training in internal medicine [rather than in surgery or obstetrics or other clinical fields] lies . . . in its comprehensive
viewpoint and emphasis on the basic techniques of diagnosis. These
are the core of medical practice." Peterson's beliefs have been reported

[*]Stephen Taylor: Good General Practice (Oxford University Press, 1954), p. 2.
[†]O. L. Peterson *et al.*: Journal of Medical Education, *31*, No. 12, Part 2:
1–165, 1956.

here because of the great influence that they had in the planning of this study. His other findings need not be repeated here, since reference will be made to them at various junctures in later chapters.

Peterson's report covers a great deal of ground, as a glance at its table of contents quickly makes clear. Because he was pioneering, it is not surprising that his results show certain blank spots, to two of which we draw attention. First, his report does not give a coherent picture of the background of the practitioner. He is seen as he is at the time of the study; and occasional bits of his past are glimpsed in brief flashes. Secondly, though such objective facts as time, place, and duration of medical training were ascertained, little attention was paid to the doctor's opinions and criticisms of his education, as is shown by the fact that Peterson's questionnaire lists only three questions dealing subjectively with the doctor's educational experience (see his page 152).

The planning of the present study was influenced both by what had been done previously and by what had not been done, as shown in the reports cited above. Just as their comments on quality of practice, both in Britain and in the United States, strongly suggested that a Canadian study should include an investigation of quality, so also the appearance of gaps in these previous investigations influenced the present workers to try to fill in the gaps. Thus, in the planning of the study, it was hoped to trace the lives of the practitioners from their youth up to the time of the study and to try to understand their practices in the light of their past history and of their present relationships with colleagues, hospitals, family, and community.

Something should now be said about the geographic scope of the Survey. The Steering Committee's original thought was to include in the study all the general practitioners in Canada. When the plan of collecting information by mail only was discarded in favour of studying a smaller number of practices by direct observation, it quickly became obvious that the great amount of travel and the tremendous expense of such a study would necessitate carrying out the work by stages. Because the Survey had its headquarters in Toronto, Ontario was chosen for the first stage of the study, in order to keep the difficulties to a minimum. As the detailed planning progressed—and the next chapter will make plain how much preliminary work had to be done before the actual field work could be started—the magnitude of the task raised grave doubts about the wisdom of planning a ten-province study as a single project. Therefore, the plans were modified to include only three provinces: Ontario, one of the western provinces, and one of the Atlantic provinces. If these studies were successfully completed, the Survey could later be extended to other areas if this should still be desirable.

Even this lesser goal proved unattainable. In spite of a prolonged and wide-ranging search for doctors with suitable qualifications for doing the field work, it was possible to recruit such men for two provinces only. When it became necessary to choose between using an unqualified observer in the third province or limiting the Survey to two provinces, there was no real choice. Accordingly, the following chapters will describe and discuss general practice as it has been observed in two provinces, Ontario and Nova Scotia. The field work in Ontario was done between July, 1956, and October, 1957; that in Nova Scotia between December, 1958, and February, 1960.

In the account of the origin of the Survey, the author has referred to himself in the third person. This has been done because some of the events described antedated his association with the Survey. Because he and his associates, as they were appointed, carried out the actual work of the Survey and, more particularly, because the opinions expressed in this book are those of the author, the use of the impersonal third person will now be abandoned in favour of the first person.

The origin of this study has been described at some length, because we think it important that the reader be made fully aware that this study was not conceived by university people as an interesting academic exercise but that it originated with general practitioners of medicine, members of the College of General Practice of Canada, who were genuinely concerned about the state of general practice and anxious to do something positive about it. The objectives were originally determined by the Steering Committee, composed of representatives of a number of different organizations or groups; the adoption of one of the important methods, that used to assess quality of practice, was decided upon by the Committee; and at no time has the Committee shown itself opposed to the policies being pursued in the conduct of the study. Throughout the course of the Survey, the Committee, meeting at intervals of from six to eighteen months, has been kept informed of the progress of the work and has given valuable advice. We, however, working within a university, have been completely free from interference in our work, and the conclusions arrived at are ours alone.

# 2 / Methods and Personnel

Exploration of general practice requires as careful preparation as does exploration of any other unknown ocean. Making the necessary preparations is inevitably less exhilarating than contemplating the destination. Yet some description of our methods is essential for all of our readers, in order that they may understand the following chapters. It is suggested, however, that the reader whose interest is primarily in obtaining an over-all view of the problems of general practice might read some parts of this present chapter somewhat more cursorily than the reader whose work is connected with these problems and whose more direct concern with the validity of the results may demand that he linger over the details of the methods.

Before starting on the methods, we shall try to picture the relationship that existed between the general practitioner and whichever one of us visited the particular practice. First of all, we wish to emphasize that every one of the practices with which this account deals was visited and studied on the spot and that all the observations were made by physicians. The visit lasted for a period of at least two, usually three, and occasionally more than three, days. Though some of the doctors generously invited the observer to stay in their homes, these invitations were declined, as a matter of policy, except in rare circumstances in which no other accommodation was available. We were aware that the doctor's participation in the study must cause him some inconvenience, and we did not wish to add to the imposition unnecessarily. Moreover, we believed that, if the observer was freed, for part of each day, from the pleasant but inevitable obligations of a guest, he would be able to order his thoughts and arrive at his conclusions with greater objectivity.

The usual routine was that the observer met the doctor at the beginning of the morning's work and accompanied him during his hospital rounds, his house calls, and his office work throughout the day, and throughout the evening if the doctor's work extended into the evening. Since many of the doctors and their wives were most generously insistent that the observer share their mid-day and evening meals, the result was that the observer was with some of the doctors continuously from early morning until late evening, or even until well after midnight, for two or three successive days. These physicians and their families not only made every effort to make the observer feel welcome and to provide the information that he sought, but also, by their enthusiastic discussion of the particular problems that were of concern to them, often gave him valuable insights. Other doctors, understandably, preferred to spend the mealtimes with their families, and perhaps to relax, without the presence of a stranger. These men, however, were most co-operative in giving the observer a full view of their practice. A few doctors, fortunately a very small percentage, did co-operate less than might have been expected. The occasional doctor, for example, would tell the observer that he would not be doing any work in his office that evening, though it later became known to the observer that he had, in fact, seen a significant number of patients in the course of the evening. On rare occasions, also, though the date of the observer's visit was set several weeks in advance after discussion with the doctor, the doctor would choose to go away on a pleasure trip for a whole day in the middle of the observer's visit with no apparent concern either for the observer, who was left to await his return in a small-town hotel or motel, or, more important, for the added expense to the Survey. Such occurrences were so uncommon, however, as to stand out in bold contrast with the unstinting co-operation of the vast majority of the doctors visited.

We have said that the observer accompanied the doctor as he carried on his practice. This means that, with few exceptions, the observer was present at consultations between patients and practitioner. The observer accompanied the doctor into his patient's room in the hospital and into the patient's home and was present as the doctor examined his patient and gave his instructions. In the doctor's office, the observer was assigned a place to sit, where he could listen and watch as the doctor questioned, examined, or carried out various procedures of laboratory work or treatment. Occasionally, the doctor would invite the observer to question or to examine the patient. Frequently, the doctor was interested in discussing the *particular* case or that *type* of case with the observer. This was more noticeable with the better doctors.

Some doctors wondered how their patients would react to having a strange doctor present. Initially, we also wondered about this, since the success of the study would depend upon the patients' acquiescence. The occasional patient indicated a desire to be alone with the doctor; in such circumstances, the observer immediately withdrew. Incidents of this type were rare, however, occurring probably in less than one per cent of cases. The remaining patients accepted their physician's brief introduction of the observer as an adequate guarantee. On one occasion, when the doctor and the observer had left a house, the doctor, referring to the patient whom they had just seen, said, "Mrs. —— was the second of two patients that I thought might possibly object to a stranger. The other was Mr. —— this afternoon. Neither of them seemed to give it a thought, did they?" The sequel to this was that this doctor, who had been somewhat apprehensive about taking part in the Survey, voluntarily had a medical student with him the next year for a week or two.

Repeatedly, it was apparent to the observers that it was the doctor's attitude, not his patients', that determined how much of the practice was seen by the observer. If the doctor was comfortable in the situation, patients very rarely objected. When the observer was excluded from a consultation, it was usually because the *doctor* did not wish the observer to be present. Even these occurrences were uncommon.

A few words should be said about night calls. Though we accompanied the practitioner on his evening house calls—and these occasionally went on until after midnight—we made no attempt to go with him on calls that came in after we had left him for the night. Quite apart from any personal feelings that we might have about getting out of bed, the difficulties involved in having the observer wakened in a small hotel or motel and in arranging a meeting place in dark and unfamiliar surroundings would have caused such delay, with possible danger to the patient, and such annoyance to the doctor as to outweigh by far any possible benefit to the Survey.

We are now ready to describe the three methods that were used. First of all, because we wished to know what the general practitioner's work comprised, we asked each of the physicians whom we visited to keep a list of the patients seen by him during one week, i.e. seven consecutive days. Though a longer period might have been preferable, we had to bear in mind that the practising physician is often very busy and that a request for him to do extra work for us should be kept within reasonable limits. Since most men's work is organized on a weekly basis, the week seemed a reasonable period to choose. Though the work of a particular practice might vary from season to season, our observations, which would be made over a period of more than a year in each province, could be expected to give us a good idea of the work done by general practitioners as a group. For this reason, it did not seem necessary to burden each man with listing his cases at different seasons of the year.

When the observer began his visit, he supplied the practitioner with an instruction sheet and mimeographed forms, on which the physician was asked to keep a record of all patients seen by him during the days of the observer's visit and during the remainder of that week. The information requested was such as could be supplied readily and quickly by the doctor. In fact, the data on each patient occupied only one line on the form. The items that appeared on the form will be discussed in detail in later chapters (see pages 195, 236).

In the Ontario study, the list of patients was kept, throughout the seven days, by the practitioner himself. Because this resulted in certain inaccuracies, which will be referred to when the items are being considered individually (see page 237), in Nova Scotia the list was filled in by the observer during the days that he spent with the practitioner. For the remainder of the week, of course, the doctor was asked to keep the list. When the list was being compiled by the observer, he recorded, for each patient, the information (including diagnosis) that was supplied by the doctor.

Some of the physicians failed to send in the list of patients whom they saw in the days following the observer's departure. In such instances, a letter was sent requesting the physician to send in the list for the missing days. Since we knew that some doctors were too busy to go back to their records to make up the lists and that it was impossible for others to go back because they had no records, the doctor was told in the letter that he might substitute the *same* days in a current week, if this was more convenient for him. A number of doctors responded immediately to this request. Others did not respond, and no further effort was made to obtain the lists from them.

The second of the three methods used to study general practice was direct observation of the doctor's practice. Because from the start it had been stated explicitly by the Steering Committee that one of the primary purposes of the Survey was to make an evaluation of the quality of general practice, the greatest attention was given to this aspect of the work. With certain minor modifications, the method evolved by Peterson° was used for this assessment. In order that the reader, when he comes to the description of quality of practice, may have the criteria fresh in his mind, the details of the method of scoring are deferred to chapter 16, where they will immediately precede the observations on quality. At present, therefore, we shall limit ourselves to a general description of the method.

The essence of the method is that the observer, who, we repeat, was a physician, watched the practitioner as he carried on his practice and assigned him a score according to predetermined criteria of quality. The items on which the doctor was scored fall into seven major categories: the taking of the patient's history, the physical examination of the patient, the use of laboratory work, treatment, management of obstetrical patients, preventive medicine, and the keeping of clinical records. Observations were made also of the doctor's surgical work and psychiatric work and of the use he made of consultants, though no quantitative scoring of these aspects of practice was found possible.

In carrying out the evaluation of quality, we were guided by certain principles, which we considered of fundamental importance. First of all, our concern was to find out what the practitioner was actually doing, not what he *could* do under such special circumstances as, for example, the pressure of an examination for a licence to practise. For this reason, in our scoring, we laid greater emphasis on what we saw the doctor do than on what he told us he would do in a certain situation. Occasionally, we gave credit for a particular item on the basis of what the doctor told us. More often, however, because we came across repeated instances of a doctor's saying the correct thing and later doing the opposite, we preferred to mark an item as "Not assessable" rather than to give credit for what the doctor said unless there was supporting evidence, for example, in his case records.

Because we wished to see what the physician ordinarily did rather that what he *could* do, we avoided doing anything that might induce him to try to change his procedure. For this reason, we did not tell the physicians that we were making an evaluation of quality. We made it part of our policy also to refrain from voicing adverse criticism. Common courtesy demanded this, since we were highly privileged in being allowed to observe the doctor's practice. Apart from this, however, we knew with certainty that any adverse criticism might seriously interfere with, or even make impossible, detailed evaluation of the practice. Occasionally, a situation occurred in which it was clear that

°O. L. Peterson *et al.*: Journal of Medical Education, *31*, No. 12, Part 2, 1956.

a very serious mistake was being made and that the observer's responsibility to the patient transcended all other considerations. In such circumstances, the observer's suggestions were made as tactfully as possible. In cases other than the type just described, it was our policy to confine our discussion within the limits indicated by the practitioner's own remarks and to remain silent or non-committal rather than to disagree with him. When asked to examine a patient after the practitioner, we avoided doing a more thorough examination than the physician himself had done. For example, if he listened to only one area of the lungs with his stethoscope, we would not do more than a localized examination, even though a complete examination of the chest might seem necessary.

Although we tried not to do or say anything that might cause a change in the doctor's quality of practice, we doubt very much whether any great and sustained change is possible on short notice. We were aware that some practitioners, during the first hour or two of the visit, were doing things that they did not usually do. One doctor, for example, started off by doing red blood cell counts on almost every patient—a time-consuming procedure for which there was no need with any of the patients that he saw. After the first hour or so, he abandoned this practice and did not revert to it during the remainder of the observer's visit. Probably most men, though they might change their ways for an hour or two, would find it too great an effort to keep up the change for two or three days, particularly if the demands of the practice were heavy. As the usual length of our visit was three days, we think that we saw the doctor practising as he usually did. Whatever slight change in quality there may have been would have been for the better and would have resulted in the doctor's being given a score that was a little on the high side.

This brings us to another principle to which we adhered in assigning the scores: that in deciding doubtful points we should give the benefit of the doubt to the physician. We wished, in reporting whatever deficiencies we might find, to be able to say that we were not exaggerating but, if anything, were understating.

In line with our principle of giving the practitioner the benefit of the doubt, we constantly asked ourselves (and each other, as we reviewed the data in Toronto) whether there were factors of which we were not cognizant. Was it possible that the aspects of the history that appeared to have been neglected were already known to the doctor? Could it be that the item of examination or of laboratory work that obviously should have been done but had been omitted had already been done last week or yesterday and that a change since then was so unlikely as to make unnecessary a repetition of the procedure today? These questions were continually in our minds. Whenever there was any reasonable doubt, we refused to use that particular case in arriving at the score; and, if the discarded evidence was all that we had on which to evaluate the doctor's practice in regard to a certain item, we marked that item "Not assessable." Because of these difficulties, we attached the greatest importance, in the scoring, to new illnesses or, even better, to new patients, since in these cases we were on an even footing with the doctor.

Another principle of the utmost importance was that, in the scoring, we should keep our standard as unvarying as possible. With field work extending over several years and with three different observers, we might have changed our standard without realizing it, had we not taken precautions to avoid this. The difficulty was compounded by the fact that the different doctors were being assessed on different cases. This latter difficulty, we think, was met reasonably well, in that the practitioner was assessed, not on a single case, but on the many cases that he saw in the course of three days. Thus, the score that he was assigned for a particular item of, say, physical examination or treatment would represent an estimate of his average performance in respect of that particular item and might be based on several, or many, observations.

In order to maintain the same standard of scoring, we reviewed the data after each visit. In the Ontario study, in which only two of us took part, the man who observed the practice presented his observations to his colleague within a day or two of his return from the visit. As the colleague listened to the case histories that were presented, he might challenge the decisions that had been made about this or that item. He might think that the score should be increased or decreased or perhaps that the evidence on a particular item was too uncertain to make any decision about it.

When the third member of our group joined us to carry out the field work in Nova Scotia, it was apparent that the other two of us, situated in Toronto, could not have this sort of presentation of the data week by week. Instead, the record, completely written up, was sent up to Toronto, where the two of us reviewed it separately and then went over all the difficult or doubtful points together. One or other of us went down from Toronto to Nova Scotia every two months. At these times, the records of the previous two months' work were taken back to Nova Scotia and any difficulties that had not been resolved in Toronto were gone over again with the observer and a final decision was reached. This was a cumbersome and time-consuming method. We believe, however, that it was worthwhile, since, if the scores were not based on the same standard throughout the study, no relationships between quality of practice and other factors could be looked for. Since the reader may wonder whether the observer's view of general practice in Nova Scotia was influenced beforehand by a knowledge of the findings in Ontario, we must make clear that the observer in Nova Scotia did not know what the findings had been in Ontario and that the observers in Ontario had not at that time completed the analysis of the data.

Just as we made every effort to keep the same standard before us, so, in applying our criteria and assigning a score, we did not "make allowance for" adverse factors in a particular doctor's circumstances. Since this is a matter of great importance, let us consider an example. Suppose that one agrees that the lungs should be thoroughly examined in a possible case of pneumonia and that inadequate examination may be detrimental to the patient. Since the possible detriment is the same regardless of the reason for the inadequacy, the doctor's score should be the same whether his omission of the necessary examination is due to ignorance or to lack of time or to any other cause. However, although we did not "make allowance for" individual circumstances in the sense of varying our standard of scoring, we did try to understand why a practitioner failed to come up to an acceptable standard. Was the doctor's training inadequate? Was he overworked? Was the practice poorly organized? Was the doctor's own health impaired?

Finally, what sort of standard did we set? Since it was impossible to foresee and to provide for every eventuality, our touchstone was the need of the patient in the particular situation rather than the arbitrary routine of any particular teaching hospital or medical school. Many routines of teaching centres, of course, coincide with the needs of the patient. There is general agreement, for example, that prenatal patients should have their weight and blood pressure measured at each visit and that the urine should be examined for protein. These procedures we included among our criteria of good obstetrical care, because they were necessary for the patient's protection. On the other hand, some teaching clinics have a rule that each new patient is to have a tuberculin test. Whereas we would commend the general practitioner who adhered to this routine in his practice and would consider that he showed special skill in trying to detect new cases of tuberculosis as early as possible, yet we regarded it as unrealistic to demand that every new case be tested in this way and to penalize the practitioner who did not do this. Instead, we asked ourselves whether, on the basis of the patient's history or the findings on physical examination, tuberculosis should be considered as a possible diagnosis, and, if so, whether the tuberculin test would be of help to the physician in arriving at a diagnosis. If the answers to these questions indicated that a tuberculin test should be done, then the score for this item was assigned according as the doctor did or did not do the test.

Similarly, with history-taking, we did not require that a patient who came for treatment of a sprained ankle or a cut finger or an obvious case of eczema be questioned about symptoms that have to do with heart disease or disease of the central nervous system. On the other hand, if the patient's complaint was loss of weight, poor appetite, chronic fatigue, a low-grade fever, a general feeling of not being well, or other such vague symptoms, we regarded it as reasonable to expect that the practitioner would take a thorough history, do a complete physical examination, use whatever special methods of examination might seem indicated (including referral to a specialist if necessary), in order to determine the cause of the symptoms and to exclude the numerous serious conditions whose early stages are manifested only by such general symptoms as those mentioned. To repeat, our standard of scoring was determined by the welfare of the patient, not by the dictates of academic medicine.

Having described, in general terms, the method used to assess the quality of practice, we must consider whether the method is reliable, i.e. whether it gives reproducible results. The ideal way to test this would be to have several observers make independent assessments of a practice simultaneously. Because of time and expense—to say nothing of the disruption of the practices being subjected to this procedure—this is quite obviously out of the question. However, five of the practices studied in Ontario were revisited six to twelve months later by the observer who had not made the original visit. The differences between the original scores and the second scores, expressed as percentages of the total possible score, were all less than 12 per cent. There is no evidence that one observer consistently gave a higher score than the other, as is shown by the fact that, when the scores assigned by one observer are subtracted from the corresponding scores assigned by the other observer, the differences for the five practitioners are $+11.9$, $-11.4$, $-1.6$, $-7.7$, and $+5.4$ per cent, and the mean difference for the five practitioners is less than 1 per cent.

In an evaluation of these differences, several factors must be taken into account. First, the revisits had to be limited to one day each, whereas the original visits were of three days' duration. Secondly, the score given a particular physician on a particular day probably depends, to some extent, on the state of physical and emotional well-being of the observer on that day. If he is tired or angry or feeling unwell physically, he may be more harsh in his judgments than he might otherwise be; or, realizing the danger of this, he may lean too far in the opposite direction.

Finally, as a cause of variation in score, there is the possibility of variation in the quality of the doctor's practice from one time to another. It may be assumed that variation does occur, since it is quite inconceivable that any doctor could maintain an unvarying quality of practice. Quite apart from any improvement or deterioration that might take place over a period of months or years, it seems entirely reasonable to suppose that the quality of the doctor's work is affected, from month to month or week to week, or even from day to day or hour to hour, by such factors as his general state of health, his state of rest or of fatigue, the pressure of the practice upon him, domestic problems, financial problems, and many other factors. Two illustrations from the Survey will suffice. The revisits were made at the time when Asian influenza was epidemic in Ontario. One result of this was that a doctor, whose practice usually included difficult diagnostic problems for which he allowed ample time for a methodical investigation, was rushed off his feet by influenza cases during the revisit and had had to postpone much of his usual office work. Another doctor was running a high fever himself by the end of the day of the revisit. It was these two physicians—each of whom was visited twice under quite different circumstances—whose scores differed, between the one visit and the other, by 11.4 and 11.9 per cent; and, in each case, the score assigned under the more adverse circumstances was the lower of the two scores assigned to the particular physician.

How much of the difference between the original score and the score at the time of the revisit should be attributed to defects in the method and how much to real variation in the quality of the doctor's work cannot be determined. Certainly the preciseness of measurement that can be achieved with certain procedures in analytical chemistry cannot be expected in work of the present type. Yet, if we may anticipate our findings on quality, the differences, from one practice to another, were so gross that by comparison the imprecision that is inherent in the method may be considered negligible.

Though the major emphasis of the observations was put on quality of practice, some attention was given also to the physical characteristics of the practitioner's office, to his nursing and secretarial assistants, to matters of organization within the practice, and to his use of hospitals.

We have described two of our methods, the listing of the cases seen by the practitioner and the observation of his practice. For both of these methods, except for minor modifications, we are indebted to Peterson. Our third method was the use of a long and detailed questionnaire. Though Peterson used a questionnaire, parts of which we incorporated into our own, our questionnaire was designed with the hope that it would shed light on some of the dark spots that were apparent in earlier studies of general practice. We have discussed this in chapter 1, but we repeat that we were particularly interested in finding out whether the doctor's medical education had prepared him adequately for general practice. In the preparation of our questionnaire, we discussed the problems with so many people, mulled over so many ideas, revised so often and then so often again, that, though we must acknowledge that the sum total of our debts is great, we cannot give credit to our individual benefactors.

Since the individual questions number more than four hundred, we shall neither list them nor classify them at this stage. They will be encountered from time to time as we explore various by-ways of general practice. At that time we hope that their relevance will make them interesting, whereas at the present time a catalogue of questions would merely be wearisome. Instead, we shall describe briefly the way in which the questionnaire was used.

Before we commenced the study proper, we made a preliminary trial of our methods on a small number of doctors. Regarding the questionnaire, it was necessary to find out whether the questions, as worded, would be clear to the doctors. It was necessary, also, to decide what procedure to follow with the questionnaire and to discover how much time the doctors would require to fill it in. Though our preliminary experience resulted in many revisions and in curtailment of some parts, it was not until we were well on towards the end of our field work in Ontario that we discovered how greatly the practitioners could vary with regard to the time required to answer the questionnaire. The shortest time was about three hours, the longest about eight hours. The time required was determined by many factors, such as the doctor's ability to grasp quickly what the question meant, his quickness in organizing his thoughts, his ability to express

himself clearly, his conciseness or verbosity, his interest in the particular matter under discussion. Because, at best, it was a very long
questionnaire, we encouraged the doctor to break it into parts and
preferably to do some of it on each day of the visit. The occasional
man insisted, however, on doing it all at one sitting; and, on a few
occasions, we were just coming down the home stretch with him as our
train was coming into view.

All the advice that we had had was against mailing a questionnaire
to the doctors, as a significant proportion could be expected not to
answer even a short questionnaire. The long one we were using
obviously had to be delivered in person; but we were uncertain
whether to read the questions to the practitioner and write down his
answers ourselves or to give it to him and ask him to fill it in
during the visit and return it to us. Our early experience showed that
the former method was greatly superior. When the questionnaire was
handed over to the doctor, it might be some weeks before he filled
it in and returned it, and a number of telephone calls might have
been necessary to urge him to get it done. The other serious drawback
was that, in spite of our best efforts, the practitioner might misinterpret
certain questions or fail to understand them at all. When the observer
was writing down the doctor's answers, these difficulties could be
dealt with at once, while the subject was fresh in the doctor's mind. In
addition, the questionnaire often was the starting point of a discussion that went far beyond the questions listed and contributed much
valuable material.

A description of the qualifications of the workers who carried out
the study has been postponed to this point since it appeared that the
requirements would be seen more clearly in the light of the methods
that were to be used. Because of the long hours of observation and
the great amount of travel in all sorts of weather, it was necessary
that the observer have both good health and stamina. In addition,
he had to be able to fit into the offices of many different physicians
without unduly disturbing them or their patients. This required
some one who was neither too shy nor too aggressive; and at least
one member of the group had to be willing and able to make the
initial contact with the practitioner and to win his co-operation.

By far the most important qualification, from the point of view
of the validity of the results, was the ability to make and to record
the necessary observations. The method required a man who had a
sound knowledge of clinical medicine, on the basis of which he not
only could evaluate what he saw and heard but also would be aware

of omissions in the investigation or treatment of a patient. It would have been ideal if the observer had been highly competent in internal medicine, surgery, obstetrics, and all the other specialties. Since such a paragon was not forthcoming, it was necessary to settle for less.

Influenced by Peterson's report of a relationship between quality of practice and duration of training in internal medicine (a relationship that Peterson attributed to internal medicine's "comprehensive viewpoint and emphasis on the basic techniques of diagnosis"; see page 10 above), the Steering Committee in collaboration with the University of Toronto appointed as Director of the Survey a paediatrician, who was engaged in private practice and was a member of the staff of a large children's teaching hospital. His formal qualification was Fellowship in the Royal College of Physicians of Canada; besides his paediatric training, his background included experience in psychiatry, pathology, and research. In addition to the emphasis that the discipline of paediatrics lays on the "comprehensive viewpoint" and "the basic techniques of diagnosis," the kinship of paediatrics to (adult) internal medicine is evidenced by the fact that the Fellowship which the Royal College of Physicians of Canada grants to paediatricians is granted, not in paediatrics as such, but in internal medicine with emphasis on paediatrics.

When the author, in the early days of the study, sought a suitable associate, he recommended to the Committee and to the University the appointment of a man who, in addition to having had teaching and research experience and some training in statistics, had completed his specialist training in internal medicine. The author and his principal associate worked together through four and a half years of the six-year study. Their different backgrounds of experience, covering the age range from the newborn period to old age and including subsidiary disciplines, complemented each other in a most fortunate manner.

When the third member of the group was appointed for a limited period of time to carry out the field work in Nova Scotia, he brought with him a background of postgraduate training in public health and of general practice in the United Kingdom and the Far East. Though he had not had postgraduate training in internal medicine (either adult or paediatric), he was recommended highly by his instructors in the University of Edinburgh as having a sound knowledge of clinical medicine. Before starting on his work in Nova Scotia, he spent two months in Toronto in order to become familiar with the details of the method. During this period, he was sent out to visit a number of doctors, including some whom we had already visited. These latter visits allowed us to compare the observations made by

our new associate with those which had been made previously by
us and of which, of course, our associate was not apprised until after
he had reported his own observations. As he proved himself a keen
observer of detail, it was possible to satisfy ourselves that his knowledge of clinical medicine was, indeed, adequate for the work. We
have already described the very close supervision that was maintained
throughout the course of the study in Nova Scotia.

A question that may be in the mind of the reader and that certainly
exercised the Steering Committee is whether a study of general practice should be done by general practitioners or by physicians who are
not general practitioners. Since no intelligent person, however hard
he may try to clear his mind of preconceived ideas, can approach
such a study with a completely blank mind, it follows that a director
of such a study and his associates, whoever they may be, even before
they embark on the project, must each have his own thoughts about,
and his own attitudes towards, general practice. A general practitioner
may be optimistic or pessimistic about general practice, as we know
from our discussions with general practitioners; he may be eager to
forward the interests of general practice or he may be apathetic. A
specialist, in turn, may be sympathetic to the problems of general
practice, or he may be antagonistic, or he may be neutral. In the
final analysis, the wisdom of the choice must depend on adequate
recognition and evaluation of the qualities of the particular individual
who is chosen. In addition, the Committee had to try to select a man
who could collect the relevant data, analyse them, and resynthesize
the findings. In weighing the various requirements, the Committee
decided that a physician who was not a general practitioner was
no less likely, and was perhaps more likely, than a general practitioner
to see the problems of general practice clearly and dispassionately.
How far the Committee was correct, each reader must decide for
himself. We, finding ourselves critical of a number of the organizations
that are concerned with medical education and with the maintenance
of standards of practice, and at the same time sympathetic with each
of them, are encouraged in our hope that we have maintained a
reasonable degree of objectivity.

Having completed our description of the methods used in the actual
field work and of the qualifications of the members of our group, we
have still to deal with certain other preliminaries that were essential to
the study proper. Before we can apply our methods, we must know
to whom we are going to apply them. Who is a general practitioner?

How do we distinguish him from other physicians? When we were preparing for the Ontario study in 1956, we were so fortunate as to be allowed access to the Physicians Register, Department of National Health and Welfare. This list, which designated those physicians who were general practitioners, had been revised at the time of the Survey of Physicians in Canada, June 1954.* The fact that the list did not include those who had started to practise in the intervening two years was an advantage, since for two reasons we preferred to exclude physicians whose practices were just being established. In an incipient practice, an inordinate amount of time might be required to see the number of cases necessary for an adequate assessment of the practice; also these physicians would be answering the questionnaire without having had experience of practice.

How had the Department of National Health and Welfare decided whether a physician was a general practitioner or not? They had accepted the physician's own statement about himself. If we were not satisfied with this method, we should have to try to lay down criteria and then classify more than five thousand doctors, about many of whom we should have inadequate information on which to base a decision. This would be particularly difficult, since some physicians, though qualified in a specialty, carry on a general practice. These doctors we wished to include in our study, and they were listed as general practitioners in the Department's list. We decided that the list based on each doctor's decision about his own practice was likely to be more satisfactory than any list that we might compile. Thus we defined a general practitioner as a physician who called himself a general practitioner, with the added proviso that at least 50 per cent of his working time should be given to what he regarded as general practice. This provision was designed to exclude a certain number of practitioners who did a small amount of general practice—and for that reason called themselves general practitioners—but the major portion of whose working time was devoted to some other type of work, such as insurance work or industrial work.

The number of active general practitioners in Ontario in 1954 was given in the Survey of Physicians as 2,649 (page 23). Since an intensive study of such a number of practices was manifestly impossible, our plan was to select a random sample for study. Because of its high reputation in this field, we sought the advice of the Dominion Bureau

*Survey of Physicians in Canada, June 1954; General Series, Memorandum No. 2, 6th ed., Research Division, Department of National Health and Welfare, Ottawa, April 1955.

of Statistics about the size of the sample and the method of picking the sample. Mr. T. G. Donnelly,* who worked with us on this problem, advised a sample of 56 physicians and set forth the details of the method.

Before the sample could be selected, we had to decide whether it was to be drawn from the total body of general practitioners in Ontario or whether there were to be any exclusions. If our sole objective had been to discover the quality of the general practice that was available to the people of Ontario, we should have chosen to draw the sample from the entire body of general practitioners. We hoped, however, to investigate factors affecting the quality of practice, and we were specially interested in matters having to do with medical education. Since the data that would be obtained from certain general practitioners could not contribute to this kind of investigation, we decided to compromise by excluding certain groups of general practitioners before we chose the sample.

First of all, we deleted from the list the names of all the practitioners who were not graduates of Canadian medical schools. Since these physicians had no experience of undergraduate medical education in this country on which to base their answers to our questions and since their academic records would not be available to us and since, in observing their practices, we should not be seeing the result of Canadian medical education, it was obvious that the effective size of the sample would be reduced by the number of these physicians who were included in the sample. In view of the time-consuming and expensive nature of the work, we did not feel justified in reducing the effective size of the sample merely in order to discover the quality of the practice of these foreign graduates.

Secondly, we excluded all physicians born before 1896. Because a period of thirty years or more separated these men from their undergraduate and postgraduate medical education, a study of their practices was not likely to cast a great deal of light on educational problems. On the other hand, because the study was expected to take several years to complete, our findings were unlikely to be of much practical value to these men, who were already over sixty years of age.

Finally, we excluded the female general practitioners. This was not a case of discrimination against women. In 1954, the female physicians comprised less than 5 per cent of the total body of physicians in Canada. Our sample, then, could have been expected to contain two or three female doctors. This number is so small that useful compari-

*Assistant to Senior Research Statistician, Dominion Bureau of Statistics, Ottawa.

sons of practices of male and female physicians could not have been made. Nor would any light have been thrown on the problems of female practitioners or on the quality of their practices. Yet the difference in sex would have been a complicating factor in various ways. For example, in adding together the cases seen by the various physicians, we should have had no way of knowing whether the sex of the female general practitioner had an effect on the type (or the sex or the age) of the patients who came to her. In short, the number of female general practitioners would have been too small for anything definite to be learnt from their practices; but, at the same time, their presence in the sample would have complicated the analysis of our data.

After the exclusion of these three groups, we were left with 1,798 general practitioners, from whom the Ontario sample was to be drawn. As we wished to be certain that different age groups and communities of different sizes would be represented in the sample in proportion to their representation within the larger group of 1,798 practitioners, we stratified this larger group, i.e. we divided it into a number of smaller groups based on the age of the physician and on the population of the community in which he practised. From each of these smaller groups, a random sample of approximately 3 per cent was drawn, according to accepted principles of sampling. This gave us 56 doctors.

Our final problem was to win the practitioners' co-operation. If the group of practices studied was to be representative of the larger group from which it was chosen, it was important to keep the number of refusals to a minimum. For this reason, we chose not to hazard the success of the study on the persuasive power of a letter or a telephone call. After a brief introductory letter from Dr. W. V. Johnston, Executive Director of the College of General Practice of Canada, and a telephone call from us to arrange an appointment, one of us visited each doctor to explain what we were doing, to ask his co-operation, and to arrange a mutually convenient date for the three-day visit. Though these preliminary trips involved some thousands of miles of travel, they proved worthwhile. Without any doubt, many of the practitioners would have refused to participate—and understandably so —if they had not had the opportunity of having a look at us and of asking questions before committing themselves. These preliminary interviews served, also, to eliminate from the study five physicians who had called themselves general practitioners but who were devoting the major portion of their working time to some other type of work.

In spite of our best efforts, we lost a certain number of men from the Ontario sample of 56, in addition to the five who turned out not to be general practitioners according to our criteria. One man died shortly after the field work was begun and before his co-operation had been solicited; and another was too ill to participate. Five other doctors refused to take part in the Survey (see page 32); and one doctor, though co-operating, could not be assessed because of technical difficulties. Thus, of the 51 who were doing general practice when the sample was drawn, 44 completed the questionnaire and 43 were assessed as to the quality of their practices. A few of the doctors turned out to be practising in communities of different sizes, and one to have been born in a different year, than we had believed at the time of the sampling. In Table 1 is shown the distribution, by year of birth and by population of community, of the Ontario physicians whose practices were studied.

TABLE 1

PHYSICIANS WHO PARTICIPATED IN THE STUDY IN ONTARIO
(Distribution according to year of birth and population of community
in which practice was located)

| Population of community | Year of birth | | | | Total number of physicians | Number of communities visited |
|---|---|---|---|---|---|---|
| | 1896–1899 | 1900–1909 | 1910–1919 | 1920–1929 | | |
| Over 500,000 (Metropolitan Toronto) | 0 | 2 | 2 | 3 | 7 | 1 |
| 100,001 to 500,000 | 1 | 1 | 1 | 1 | 4 | 3 |
| 10,001 to 100,000 | 2 | 4 | 6 | 3 | 15 | 12 |
| 1,001 to 10,000 | 2 | 3 | 4 | 5 | 14 | 14 |
| 1,000 and under | 0 | 2 | 1 | 1 | 4 | 4 |
| Totals | 5 | 12 | 14 | 13 | 44 | 34 |

When we were preparing for the Nova Scotia study in 1958, our problems in connection with the sampling differed somewhat from the ones that we had encountered in Ontario. In the first place, the Department of National Health and Welfare informed us that its list had not been revised since 1954. Though we did not wish to visit practitioners who had been in practice less than two years, neither did we wish to exclude those who had been in practice more than two years but less than four. We had no alternative but to construct our own list. However, because the number of physicians in Nova Scotia was about one-tenth of the number in Ontario and because the majority of those who would be difficult to classify were concentrated in the Halifax area, where it would be easier to make inquiries about their practices, the task was not nearly as formidable as it would have been in Ontario.

The list was based on the most recent editions of the Canadian Medical Directory and the American Medical Directory. As we had done in Ontario, we excluded foreign graduates, female physicians, and physicians over sixty years of age (i.e., those of the Nova Scotia physicians who were born before 1898). The most recent graduates included in our list were those who had completed their junior interneship in 1956. Finally, Dr. M. R. Macdonald, Registrar of the Provincial Medical Board of Nova Scotia, and Dr. C. J. W. Beckwith, Executive Secretary of the Medical Society of Nova Scotia, very kindly checked the list with us and assisted us in deciding whether certain physicians were or were not general practitioners. The list, when completed, totalled 234 names.

On the size of the sample we sought the advice of Professor D. B. W. Reid,* who gave as his opinion that a sample of approximately the same number as in Ontario would be most satisfactory for our purposes. Thus, comparison of the two samples would be facilitated. For technical reasons, the exact number decided upon was 42. As we expected, in the light of our Ontario experience, that there would be some losses and as we could not predict the number of these, it was decided to start with a sample of 42 and it was agreed that, whenever a man was lost, another belonging to the same age group and practising in a community of the same size would be chosen. The distribution of the Nova Scotia physicians whose practices were studied is shown in Table 2.

TABLE 2

PHYSICIANS WHO PARTICIPATED IN THE STUDY IN NOVA SCOTIA
(Distribution according to year of birth and population of community
in which practice was located)

| Population of community | Year of birth | | | | Total number of physicians | Number of communities visited |
|---|---|---|---|---|---|---|
| | 1898–1902 | 1903–1912 | 1913–1922 | 1923–1932 | | |
| Over 100,000 (Metropolitan Halifax) | 1 | 1 | 4 | 3 | 9 | 1 |
| 10,001 to 100,000 | 1 | 3 | 3 | 1 | 8 | 4 |
| 1,001 to 10,000 | 1 | 5 | 7 | 4 | 17 | 14 |
| 1,000 and under | 1 | 1 | 4 | 2 | 8 | 8 |
| Totals | 4 | 10 | 18 | 10 | 42 | 27 |

*Department of Epidemiology and Biometrics, School of Hygiene, University of Toronto.

In order to fill our quota, it was necessary to approach 56 practitioners. Of these, 8 turned out either to have left the province or not to be engaged in general practice, and 6 refused to take part in the Survey.

In the two provinces the number of outright refusals to participate was 11. Though these men gave various reasons, it was apparent that the real reason in most cases was that the physician was uncomfortable about having anyone observe his practice. As to the quality of these practices, there was no evidence to suggest whether they were better, worse, or about the same, on the average, as those that were assessed.

Because statistics are somewhat of a mystery to those who have had no training in them and because observations made on small samples are often greeted with scepticism, it is perhaps worthwhile to discuss briefly what can be accomplished with samples such as we used in the two provinces. As Snedecor points out,* a sample, if randomly drawn, provides an "unbiased estimate" and "a confidence interval." If, for example, 33 (i.e., 75 per cent) of the 44 physicians in the Ontario *sample* answer a certain question in the affirmative and the remainder in the negative, the percentage, 75 per cent, is an unbiased estimate of the percentage of affirmative answers that would be received from the *larger body of physicians* from which the sample was drawn. It is only an estimate, however. Indeed, it is unlikely that the true percentage (i.e., the percentage in the whole population of physicians) would be exactly 75 per cent. It is possible to set limits within which it may be said with confidence that the true percentage lies. In the case of the above example, it can be stated that the true percentage lies between 60 and 87 per cent approximately, unless the sample is the very unusual one that may be expected to occur by chance five times in every hundred. The interval between the 60 per cent and the 87 per cent is the "95 per cent confidence interval" yielded by our sample of 44 physicians. The example given illustrates Snedecor's statement that "only broad confidence intervals can be based on small samples" (page 14). Broad though this interval is, in some contexts such figures are impressive evidence; and, in the final analysis, samples do not furnish proof but provide evidence, which must be weighed with whatever other evidence is available.

There is one other statistical matter about which we must say a few words before we proceed: the matter of "statistical significance." To take an example, on page 40 and in Table 5, it will be found that,

*G. W. Snedecor: Statistical Methods (4th ed.; Ames, Iowa: Iowa State College Press, 1946), p. 29.

of the Ontario doctors visited by us, those born after 1910 were, on the average, 4.5 years younger at the time of marriage than were those doctors who were born up to 1910. The difference between the mean ages of the two groups at the time of marriage is "statistically significant." The last sentence means that statistical tests have been applied and show that, with a difference as great as the one that we found in the *sample*, it is reasonable to conclude that a difference exists between the two groups (those born after 1910 and those born up to 1910) in the *whole body of general practitioners* from which the sample was drawn. For those readers who are familiar with statistical theory, probability values are added in parenthesis: ($p < 0.01$). When $p$ is less than 0.05, the difference is said to be significant; when $p$ is less than 0.01, the difference is said to be highly significant; when $p$ is greater than 0.05, the difference is not significant. These are commonly accepted critical values. Since a simple explanation of the meaning of the statement, "$p < 0.01$," is not possible, because of the complex nature of statistical theory, and since the $p$ values are not essential to the argument, it is suggested that the reader who is not on easy terms with statistics confine his attention to whether the finding reported by us is or is not (statistically) significant.

From the outset of the Survey, we have regarded ourselves as highly privileged in being permitted to observe other men's practices and have felt bound to preserve the anonymity of the physicians whom we have visited. To this end, we have taken numerous precautions, including the use of code numbers and the keeping of our records in locked cabinets. Again, in choosing the examples with which we shall illustrate various points in the following chapters, we have borne constantly in mind that there must be no possibility of the particular practitioner's being identified. In these studies, we have seen much that has delighted us and other things that have disturbed us. We hope that these latter can contribute to the progress of medical practice; but they must not bring embarrassment to the men who have trusted us in allowing us to see their practices.

# THE GENERAL PRACTITIONER

# 3 / The General Practitioner's Background

To understand the problems of general practice, it is necessary to have some knowledge of the man who carries on the practice—the general practitioner. What sort of man is he? What is his background? What induced him to choose medicine, and specifically general practice, as his career? What general education and what medical training has he had? What has been his experience of practice up to the time at which we meet him? What sort of home life does he have? What is his income? What are his interests outside his practice? What are his ethics? Most of us, hearing the word "doctor," conjure up a visual image, determined largely by our personal experience and partly by reading and hearsay. Our image is likely to be static rather than dynamic; it is likely to be as narrowly circumscribed as our own experience, with little approximation to the variation that exists. In the series of chapters that comprise this section of the book, it is our purpose to give a picture of general practitioners, not as stereotypes, but as living beings, having their strengths and weaknesses and differing from one another in many ways. This will lead up to a description of the general practitioner's work, which will be examined in the chapters of the next section. After that, in a series of chapters, we shall discuss a number of problems in the light of our findings about the general practitioner and his work.

This introductory chapter is designed to sketch in the practitioner's background. The detail of various parts of the picture will emerge in succeeding chapters.

Of the group of practitioners who were studied in each province, Ontario and Nova Scotia, approximately 80 per cent were born in the province in which they were practising when visited by the Survey; the remainder were born in other parts of Canada or in other countries. Of the last group, all had moved to Canada by the age of seven years, some much earlier. The geographic stability during the formative years of the majority of these children is apparent in the fact that 84 per cent of the Ontario group and 62 per cent of the Nova Scotia group passed the entire period of their primary and secondary education in one community. This, with few exceptions, was the community in which the boy had been born. The remaining boys had less continuity of experience, a few having spent parts of their childhood in countries whose cultures are foreign to our own, others having lived in several different communities during their school years. Those who grew up in communities of under 1,000, of from 1,000 to 10,000, of from 10,000 to 100,000, and (in Ontario) of over 100,000 form groups that are roughly equal in numbers* (Table 3).

TABLE 3

POPULATIONS OF PLACES OF ORIGIN OF ONTARIO AND
NOVA SCOTIA PHYSICIANS

| Population* of place of origin† | Ontario physicians | | Nova Scotia physicians | |
|---|---|---|---|---|
| | Number | % | Number | % |
| Over 100,000 | 13 | 29.5 | 0 | 0.0 |
| 10,001 to 100,000 | 10 | 22.7 | 15 | 35.7 |
| 1,001 to 10,000 | 9 | 20.5 | 14 | 33.3 |
| 1,000 or less | 12 | 27.3 | 13 | 31.0 |
| Total physicians | 44 | 100 | 42 | 100 |

*According to the census figures for the year nearest to the year when the physician was 10 years of age.
†The place where the physician spent most of the years between the ages of 5 and 18 years.

In each province, the boys' fathers were engaged in occupations of many and widely differing kinds, including several professions, finance, farming, various commercial enterprises, and a number of skilled trades. In Ontario, 14 per cent were physicians' sons and in Nova Scotia, 19 per cent; similarly, 9 per cent and 12 per cent had fathers in other professions and 18 and 14 per cent were farmers' sons.

After leaving high school, 59 per cent of the Ontario men went directly into a medical course† or into a course that was specifically

*We have taken, as the place of origin, the community where the physician spent most of his youth between the ages of 5 and 18 years.
†Several men entered courses that combined the requirements for degrees in both medicine and either arts or science.

designated as a premedical course. A second group, 14 per cent, went directly from high school to other university courses, including general arts, general science, and engineering. Half of these men spent only one year in the particular course, before they changed to medicine; the other half completed the requirements for the bachelor's degree. The remaining 27 per cent, after leaving high school, were engaged in a variety of activities, including farm work, service in the armed forces, and industrial work of various sorts. For these men, except one who worked at a skilled trade for nearly two decades before starting the study of medicine, the period between high school and university varied between one year and four.

Whereas all but a few of the Ontario doctors had completed Grade XIII at high school, all the Nova Scotia doctors stated that there was no Grade XIII at high school and many that there was no Grade XII so that the first year or two at college were equivalent to the Grade XIII of the Ontario doctors. For this reason, the picture of the period between the young man's leaving high school and his entry to medical school is less clear in the case of the Nova Scotia, than of the Ontario, group. The data do show, however, that, prior to entering medicine, 38 per cent of the Nova Scotia men had at least one academic degree and 48 per cent had engaged in various types of work, including military service, for periods varying in length from one to twelve years.

The physicians' medical education, undergraduate and postgraduate, will be described in the next chapter. The ages at which the physicians completed their postgraduate work cover a wide span of years (Table 4). Half of those in each province were at least 27 years of age by this

TABLE 4

AGES OF ONTARIO AND NOVA SCOTIA PHYSICIANS AT
COMPLETION OF POSTGRADUATE WORK

(This table does not take into account the fact that several physicians, after some time in practice, returned to a teaching centre for further training.)

| Age of physician | Ontario physicians | | Nova Scotia physicians | |
|---|---|---|---|---|
| | Number | % | Number | % |
| Under 24 | 1 | 2.3 | 2 | 4.8 |
| 24–26 | 13 | 29.5 | 16 | 38.1 |
| 27–29 | 20 | 45.5 | 13 | 31.0 |
| 30–32 | 8 | 18.2 | 8 | 19.0 |
| 33–35 | 1 | 2.3 | 2 | 4.8 |
| 36–38 | 0 | 0.0 | 1 | 2.4 |
| Over 38 | 1 | 2.3 | 0 | 0.0 |
| Total physicians | 44 | 100 | 42 | 100 |

time.* Those men who entered the medical course after military service or whose postgraduate training was delayed by such service were somewhat older when they completed their postgraduate training.

All but one of the Ontario physicians, and all but three of those in Nova Scotia, married. Of those in each province who were born not later than 1910, more than half were at least 30 years of age before they married, whereas, of those in each province who were born after 1910, more than half were married before the age of 27 years (Table 5). The difference between the mean ages of the two groups at the

TABLE 5

Ages of Ontario and Nova Scotia Physicians at Time of Marriage

| | Number of Ontario physicians born: | | Number of Nova Scotia physicians born: | |
|---|---|---|---|---|
| Age at marriage | 1896–1910 | 1911–1926 | 1898–1910 | 1911–1931 |
| Under 20 | 0 | 0 | 0 | 1 |
| 21–23 | 1 | 4 | 1 | 3 |
| 24–26 | 2 | 10 | 1 | 10 |
| 27–29 | 5 | 8 | 3 | 9 |
| 30–32 | 3 | 4 | 2 | 3 |
| 33–35 | 4 | 0 | 3 | 1 |
| 36–38 | 0 | 0 | 1 | 0 |
| 39–41 | 2 | 0 | 1 | 0 |
| Total physicians | 17 | 26 | 12 | 27 |
| Mean age at marriage | 30.6 | 26.1 | 30.8 | 26.5 |

time of marriage is statistically significant, both in the case of the Ontario physicians and in the case of the Nova Scotia physicians ($p < 0.01$).† Similarly, the doctors born after 1910 married earlier in their careers than those who were born up to 1910 (Table 6). Of the latter, only 18 per cent in Ontario and 17 per cent in Nova Scotia were married by one year after graduation, whereas more than half in each province had been out of medical school three years or more before they were married. On the other hand, of the doctors who were born after 1910, 65 per cent in Ontario and 70 per cent in Nova Scotia were married by the time they had been graduated one year. On the average, the Ontario physicians in the younger group had been out of medical school 1 year, those in the older group 4.3 years when they were married. In Nova Scotia, on the average, the older group had

*This statement is true even if we exclude those whose studies were interrupted by service in the armed forces.

†The meaning of this statement is explained on pages 32–33.

TABLE 6

NUMBER OF YEARS BETWEEN GRADUATION FROM MEDICAL SCHOOL
AND MARRIAGE OF ONTARIO AND NOVA SCOTIA PHYSICIANS

| Number of years* between graduation† and marriage | Number of Ontario physicians born: | | Number of Nova Scotia physicians born: | |
|---|---|---|---|---|
| | 1896–1910 | 1911–1926 | 1898–1910 | 1911–1931 |
| − (more than 3) | 1 | 0 | 0 | 2 |
| −3 | 0 | 3 | 1 | 1 |
| −2 | 0 | 0 | 0 | 4 |
| −1 | 1 | 2 | 0 | 4 |
| 0 | 1 | 6 | 1 | 3 |
| 1 | 0 | 6 | 0 | 5 |
| 2 | 3 | 5 | 1 | 3 |
| 3 | 4 | 0 | 1 | 3 |
| 4 | 0 | 0 | 1 | 1 |
| 5 | 2 | 3 | 1 | 1 |
| 6 to 10 | 2 | 1 | 5 | 0 |
| More than 10 | 3 | 0 | 1 | 0 |
| Total physicians | 17 | 26 | 12 | 27 |

*A minus sign indicates that marriage preceded graduation.
†In order that all the physicians may be comparable, those who did not receive their degrees until after their junior interneship are regarded as having graduated a year earlier than this. This is explained on page 42.

been out of medical school 5.4 years, and the younger group were still about a month short of their graduation, at the time of marriage.

Of the married doctors in Ontario, approximately 12 per cent had no children or one child, 70 per cent had two or three children, and 19 per cent had four, five, or even more children. The corresponding figures for Nova Scotia were 8 per cent, 56 per cent, and 36 per cent.

When the 86 physicians were visited in the course of the Survey, they had been in practice for periods that ranged from less than 5 to more than 35 years.

Such is the background of the general practitioners in the two samples. These men were drawn from communities of all sizes, where their fathers were engaged in many different occupations. In the majority of cases, the boy grew up in one community. Some went directly from high school to a medical, or a clearly designated premedical, course; others had a variety of experiences, academic, military, and other, before they undertook the study of medicine. Though some men were younger, half of the total group in each province were at least 27 years of age, some considerably older, by the time they had completed their postgraduate training and were ready to establish themselves in the private practice of their profession.

4  /  The General Practitioner's
          Education


The preparation for the practice of medicine, after a student leaves high school, may be said to consist of formal university courses in the various medical subjects, preceded by courses in the basic sciences and by some education in the liberal arts and followed by practical experience gained during a period of service on the house staff of a hospital. Some medical schools in Canada grant the medical degree prior to the interneship (i.e., at the completion of the formal university courses), whereas other schools withhold the degree until the student has completed one year of interneship. Because the undergraduate interneship of these latter schools is the equivalent, except in name, of the postgraduate interneship served by the graduates of the former group of schools and because the first year of interneship, whatever it may be called, is more akin to any succeeding postgraduate hospital training than to the formal university courses, we have chosen, arbitrarily, to regard as *post*graduate training *all* house-staff appointments that followed the completion of the formal university courses. Only in this way is it possible to compare the postgraduate training of physicians who are graduates of different medical schools.

Examining the data collected by the Survey, we found that the portion of the student's education that had to do with the liberal arts varied according to the organization of the particular medical school he had attended. Some schools required that a student should have completed his work in the liberal arts and in the basic sciences (physics, chemistry, and biology) before he might be admitted to medical school. Other medical faculties, admitting students straight from high school, devoted either the first year of the medical course or two "premedical years" to this preliminary phase of a student's education. It is not possible, nor would it likely be profitable, to describe in detail the education of the various physicians in the liberal arts. The diversity is illustrated by the fact that some men were graduates of general arts courses, while others, in the entire period of their university education, had only a single non-scientific subject, English, and that for only one year. Though the number of liberal arts subjects studied by a particular man varied, among the Ontario practitioners, from none to eight, 70 per cent of these doctors took either two or three of these subjects. It is interesting to note that only three subjects appeared frequently among those listed by the Ontario doctors, namely, English (the only subject studied by more than 50 per cent of the doctors), history of science and civilization, and French. The study of other liberal arts subjects was uncommon, no one of the subjects being listed by even one-quarter of the doctors.

In the case of the Ontario practitioners, between 5 and 13 years elapsed from the time of the student's first experience of university work to his completion of his undergraduate medical training. For two-thirds of the men, this period was either 5 or 6 years. Of the remaining one-third, some were held up by serious academic difficulties, others had completed the several years of university work required for an arts or science degree before they entered medicine, while a few were delayed by illness, military service, or indecision whether to continue with the study of medicine.

Because of the difference, already referred to (page 39), between the high school education of the Ontario doctors and that of the Nova Scotia doctors, it is not possible to give a comparable statement either of the education of the Nova Scotia physicians in the liberal arts subjects or of the number of years that elapsed between the beginning of their university work and the completion of the undergraduate medical course.

In Table 7 is shown the incidence of academic difficulties that occurred during the medical course and during the premedical part of the training when the latter was given under the auspices of the medical faculty; not included are any difficulties that the men may have had in a general arts or science course. Academic records were available for 41 of the 44 Ontario practitioners and for 39 of the 42 in Nova Scotia. Fifty-six per cent in Ontario and 44 per cent in Nova Scotia passed each year without being required to write any supplemental examinations; 32 per cent and 46 per cent in Ontario and in Nova Scotia, respectively did not have to repeat any year but did have

TABLE 7

ACADEMIC DIFFICULTIES OF ONTARIO AND NOVA SCOTIA PHYSICIANS
IN MEDICAL COURSES*

| Number of failed years | Number of years with supplemental examinations | Number of Ontario physicians | | Number of Nova Scotia physicians | |
|---|---|---|---|---|---|
| None | None | | 23 | | 17 |
| | One | 9 | | 9 | |
| | Two | 3 | 13 | 7 | 18 |
| | Three | 1 | | 1 | |
| | Four | 0 | | 1 | |
| One | None | 1 | | 1 | |
| | One | 2 | | 0 | |
| | Two | 0 | | 1 | |
| | Three | 0 | 5 | 2 | 4 |
| | Four | 0 | | 0 | |
| | Five | 1 | | 0 | |
| Three | | | 1 | | 0 |
| Records incomplete or not available | | | 3 | | 3 |
| Total number of physicians | | | 44 | | 42 |

*See page 43 for comment on inclusion of premedical courses.

supplemental examinations in one or more years; and 12 per cent and 10 per cent in the two provinces, respectively, were required to repeat one or more years. The differences between the Ontario group and the Nova Scotia group are not statistically significant.

Over 90 per cent of the men in each province took their entire medical course in one university. The few who transferred did so either because of academic difficulties or because the medical school in which they started offered only the first half of the course. Of the 44 Ontario physicians whom we visited, 25 graduated from the University of Toronto, 7 from the University of Western Ontario, 6 from Queen's University, and the remaining 6 from several other universities; of the 42 physicians in Nova Scotia, all but 3 graduated from Dalhousie University.

After completing the university portion of their medical education, the physicians, both in Ontario and in Nova Scotia, had postgraduate training experiences that show a remarkable variation in duration, in content, and probably in quality. Before describing these, however, we must define the two classes to which, arbitrarily, we have assigned all the hospitals in which the physicians took their postgraduate training. These are teaching hospitals and non-teaching hospitals.

Teaching hospitals are defined as those hospitals in which medical students (i.e., undergraduates) are continually receiving instruction in general medicine, surgery, obstetrics, or paediatrics. Those hospitals whose activities are narrowly limited within the major fields (e.g., infectious diseases hospitals) are not counted as teaching hospitals, except when the physician was sent to such a hospital for a short period in order to round out the rotation of a major teaching hospital.

Of the Ontario group of general practitioners, 2 had no post-graduate hospital training. Both went directly from medical school into general practice, one man joining an established practitioner as his assistant, the other working for a year as assistant to a group of doctors. In Nova Scotia, one physician went into practice on his own without any postgraduate hospital training.

Of those Ontario physicians who had some postgraduate training, 50 per cent had it entirely in teaching hospitals, 31 per cent entirely in non-teaching hospitals, and the remaining 19 per cent in both types of hospital. The corresponding figures in Nova Scotia were 20 per cent, 17 per cent, and 63 per cent. Most of these physicians had a rotating interne-ship,* which usually lasted for 12 months, though, for some men during war-time, it was only 8 or 9 months, and a few others extended this experience to 18 or even 24 months. A few Ontario physicians interned in hospitals that did not have organized services. The rotating internships of the Ontario doctors were, with few exceptions, taken entirely in one hospital, whereas many of the Nova Scotia doctors served a few months in each of several hospitals. In later chapters, we shall consider the type of training that is required as preparation for general practice and the relationship between postgraduate training and quality of practice. We might mention here, however, a combination of experiences that one physician had, which struck us as a singularly inappropriate preparation for general practice. After graduation, he had three years of experience divided between mental defectives and tuberculous patients and six weeks on an obstetrical service; but, of postgraduate training in general medicine, general surgery, or general paediatrics, he had none.

Sixty-three per cent of the Ontario practitioners who interned, but only 34 per cent of those in Nova Scotia, took additional training beyond their rotating internship. The difference between the two groups is statistically significant ($p < 0.05$).† The additional training of the

---

*An internship during which the physician works on a number of different services in succession (medicine, surgery, paediatrics, etc.), the period spent on each service ranging from a few weeks to a few months.

†This is explained on pages 32–33.

Ontario men ranged in length from 3 to 36 months and of the Nova Scotia men from 6 to 48 months, with a median length of approximately 12 months and 13 months in the two provinces respectively. Most of the men who took additional training proceeded to it directly from their rotating interneship, though in a few instances a period of military service or of practice intervened. The extra training after the rotating interneship was in one or more specific subjects. These included internal medicine, general surgery, obstetrics, paediatrics, anaesthesia, otolaryngology, psychiatry, diagnostic radiology, and urology. In each of the two provinces, those whose extra training beyond the rotating interneship was in one subject only and those who took training in more than one subject were about equal in number.

In Table 8 are shown both the numbers of physicians, in the Ontario group and in the Nova Scotia group, who had postgraduate training in various clinical subjects and the median duration of the training in each of these. The most noteworthy points in this table are that there was no experience in paediatrics and that there was no experience

TABLE 8

DURATION OF POSTGRADUATE TRAINING IN VARIOUS CLINICAL
SUBJECTS OF 38* ONTARIO PHYSICIANS AND OF 39* NOVA SCOTIA PHYSICIANS

| | Ontario physicians | | | Nova Scotia physicians | | |
|---|---|---|---|---|---|---|
| | Number who had no time on the service | Those who had some time on the service | | Number who had no time on the service | Those who had some time on the service | |
| Clinical subject | | Number | Median duration (months)† | | Number | Median duration (months)† |
| Medicine | 1 | 37 | 3.0 | 1 | 38 | 3.0 |
| Paediatrics | 22 | 16 | 2.0 | 13 | 26 | 1.5 |
| Surgery | 2 | 36 | 4.0 | 0 | 39 | 3.3 |
| Obstetrics and gynaecology | 1 | 37 | 2.5 | 2 | 37 | 2.0 |
| Emergency and admitting | 14 | 24 | 1.0 | 25 | 14 | 1.0 |
| Anaesthesia | 14 | 24 | 1.0 | 36 | 3 | 1.0 |
| Ophthalmology | 32 | 6 | 0.5 | 27 | 12 | 0.5 |
| Otolaryngology | 24 | 14 | 0.5 | 25 | 14 | 0.5 |
| Psychiatry | 36 | 2 | 2.0 | 31 | 8 | 1.5 |

*Six Ontario physicians are excluded from this table, 2 because they had no postgraduate training, 2 because they took their training in hospitals that did not have organized services, and 2 because they could not remember the amount of time spent on the various services. Three Nova Scotia physicians are excluded, 1 because he had no postgraduate training, and 2 because they could not remember the amount of time spent on the various services.

†These figures are for total postgraduate training, i.e. training in both teaching and non-teaching hospitals.

TABLE 9

DISTRIBUTION OF ONTARIO AND NOVA SCOTIA PHYSICIANS ACCORDING
TO DURATION OF POSTGRADUATE TRAINING IN THE MAJOR CLINICAL SUBJECTS

| Duration of postgraduate training | Ontario physicians | | | | Nova Scotia physicians | | | |
|---|---|---|---|---|---|---|---|---|
| | Medicine | Paediatrics | Surgery | Obstetrics | Medicine | Paediatrics | Surgery | Obstetrics |
| Nil | 1 | 22 | 2 | 1 | 1 | 13 | 0 | 2 |
| Up to 1 month | 1 | 6 | 0 | 4 | 2 | 9 | 1 | 5 |
| Over 1 and up to 2 months | 4 | 6 | 6 | 13 | 11 | 13 | 6 | 19 |
| Over 2 and up to 3 months | 13 | 2 | 9 | 12 | 10 | 2 | 12 | 8 |
| Over 3 and up to 4 months | 7 | 1 | 10 | 2 | 9 | 0 | 7 | 1 |
| Over 4 and up to 6 months | 2 | 1 | 3 | 1 | 2 | 2 | 4 | 2 |
| Over 6 and up to 12 months | 4 | 0 | 4 | 4 | 3 | 0 | 4 | 2 |
| Over 12 and up to 24 months | 4 | 0 | 3 | 1 | 1 | 0 | 2 | 0 |
| Over 24 months | 2 | 0 | 1 | 0 | 0 | 0 | 3 | 0 |
| Total number of physicians* | 38 | 38 | 38 | 38 | 39 | 39 | 39 | 39 |

*The omission of 6 Ontario and 3 Nova Scotia physicians is explained in a footnote to Table 8.

in an emergency department in the postgraduate training of considerable numbers of the men visited in each province. Table 9 gives the distribution of the physicians according to the duration of their postgraduate training in the four major clinical subjects, medicine, paediatrics, surgery, and obstetrics.

Total duration of the postgraduate training is shown in Table 10

TABLE 10

TOTAL DURATION OF POSTGRADUATE TRAINING OF ONTARIO
AND NOVA SCOTIA PHYSICIANS

| Duration of postgraduate training | Ontario physicians | | Nova Scotia physicians | |
|---|---|---|---|---|
| | Number | % | Number | % |
| Nil | 2 | 4.5 | 1 | 2.4 |
| 6 months | 0 | 0.0 | 1 | 2.4 |
| Over 6 and up to 12 months | 14 | 31.8 | 26 | 61.9 |
| Over 12 and up to 18 months | 8 | 18.2 | 2 | 4.8 |
| Over 18 and up to 24 months | 10 | 22.7 | 4 | 9.5 |
| Over 24 and up to 36 months | 7 | 15.9 | 5 | 11.9 |
| Over 36 and up to 48 months | 3 | 6.8 | 0 | 0.0 |
| Over 48 months | 0 | 0.0 | 3 | 7.1 |
| Total physicians | 44 | 100 | 42 | 100 |

where it may be seen that a small percentage of the men in each province had no postgraduate training, that 32 per cent in Ontario and 64 per cent in Nova Scotia had 12 months or less, that 41 per cent in Ontario and 14 per cent in Nova Scotia had more than 1 year and up to 2 years, and that 23 per cent and 19 per cent in the two provinces, respectively, had postgraduate training exceeding 2 years in duration and extending even to 5 years. The percentage of Ontario physicians whose postgraduate training was more than 12 months in length was significantly greater than the corresponding percentage of Nova Scotia physicians ($p < 0.01$).

Of postgraduate training in *teaching* hospitals, 34 per cent of the Ontario men had none, 34 per cent had between 9 and 12 months, 18 per cent had more than 1 year and up to 2 years, and 14 per cent had over 2 years and up to 4 years. In Nova Scotia, approximately 19 per cent of the practitioners had no postgraduate training in teaching hospitals, another 19 per cent had 3 months or less, 10 per cent 6 months, 36 per cent between 8 and 12 months, 10 per cent over 1 year and up to 2 years, and 7 per cent over 2 years and up to 52 months. The two groups did not differ significantly in the percentage with more than 12 months of postgraduate training in teaching hospitals.

A description of the details of the individual practitioner's postgraduate experience would serve no useful purpose. We would emphasize, however, the lack of uniformity of this period of training in length, in content, and probably also in quality. The physicians themselves made many comments, both descriptive and critical, about their undergraduate and postgraduate education. Though these comments contributed greatly to the picture that we obtained of the training period, we shall defer them to later chapters, where, in a discussion of problems of medical education, they will have greater relevance.

At the time of the Survey's visit, four of the Ontario physicians, though continuing to do general practice, had been granted the specialist certificate of the Royal College of Physicians and Surgeons of Canada, one in internal medicine, one in surgery, one in obstetrics and gynaecology, and one in anaesthesia. In Nova Scotia, two of the physicians held the Royal College's certificate in surgery.

5 / The General Practitioner's Career
*Vicissitudes of*
*Planning and Practice*


After university work lasting at least 5 years, and in some cases more than 10 years, and after postgraduate training varying in length from 0 to 48 or even 60 months and, in some cases, either interrupted or followed by military service, the physicians of the Survey began private practice. Their ages, at this time, ranged from 23 to 41 years, in Ontario, and from 23 to 38 years, in Nova Scotia, with a mean, in each province, of approximately 28 years. The present chapter will cover the period of practice prior to the Survey; in subsequent chapters, we shall describe the organization of the doctor's practice as it appeared when we visited him. Because it is easy to assume, however, as we see the general practitioner at a particular point in time, that he always wished to be a general practitioner, that the various parts of his training were chosen with this end in view, and that he followed a straight road to his goal, we shall first go back to the time when he entered medical school and examine the vicissitudes of his career even while it was in the planning stage.

Each of the doctors was asked, "When you entered medical school, what type of practice did you intend to do after graduating?" Of the 44 Ontario physicians, 45 per cent intended to do general practice, 20 per cent had one or another of the specialties in mind—obstetrics, internal medicine, otolaryngology, psychiatry, or surgery (the last being mentioned as frequently as all the others combined)—and 32 per cent said that they were not sure or that they intended to "wait and see." The one remaining doctor entered medicine with the intention of going into research. Of the 42 Nova Scotia physicians, on the other hand, 79 per cent entered medical school with the intention of being general practitioners, 14 per cent with the intention of practising a specialty—internal medicine, paediatrics, surgery, ophthalmology and otolaryngology, or psychiatry—5 per cent without any definite plans, and the one remaining man with the hope of becoming a teacher of medicine. Those who planned to be general practitioners gave a number of reasons. The sole reason of some was said to have been the influence of a general practitioner, who was either the family doctor or a member of the young man's family. A few doctors did not give any reason; and the remainder mentioned, either singly or in various combinations, that they liked to know people well, that they liked the variety of the work, that they could not afford the training required for a specialty, that they were not interested in any of the specialties or thought that a specialty would be too confining, that general practice appeared the most satisfying career, that general practice was the accepted thing, or that they liked small towns. Two of them mentioned admiration for the general practitioner but without reference to any particular practitioner.

Of the men who had surgery in mind when they entered medical school, two had relations who did surgery, another had a "hero complex" (i.e., admired a surgeon with whom he had associated closely), still another referred to the glamour of the movie portrayals of surgeons and said that "everyone at that time thought of being a surgeon," and one man's parents, neither of whom was a doctor, suggested that he be a "top surgeon." One man thought of obstetrics and gynaecology, because they constituted a "clear-cut" type of practice. The one man who contemplated a research career said that this interest arose from intellectual curiosity. The reason given by one of the two men who named internal medicine, that internal medicine represented the real field of medicine, that surgery was only a technique, and that the only good surgeon was the internist who did surgery, strikes one as too sophisticated to be the thinking of a boy just entering medical school.

Of the men who entered medical school with the intention of doing general practice, 60 per cent in Ontario and 70 per cent in Nova Scotia never gave more than a passing thought to any other type of medical career. The remainder either seriously considered, or actually embarked upon, specialty training. Some of them changed their minds in favour of specialties while they were still in medical school, some while they were interning, and the rest after some time in practice. Three reasons were given for choosing the specialty, some men giving more than one reason. One man mentioned that the specialist was better paid than the general practitioner, and several that the specialist's life was not as hard as the general practitioner's. In most cases, however, interest in the specialty was stated as a reason for the choice. One man attributed his enthusiasm to the stimulating teaching of one clinical professor of internal medicine, another to the influence of an obstetrician who was described as a "dynamic lecturer," whereas yet another man had become interested while he was studying on his own to repair defects in his knowledge of a particular subject. In several cases, the specialty training that was contemplated was not undertaken, either because it was financially impossible or because it did not seem worth the time and money that would be required. Those who did undertake training in a specialty (25 per cent of those in Ontario, and 6 per cent of those in Nova Scotia, who on entering medical school intended to do general practice) returned to general practice for one or more of several reasons, some of them after completing the training in their specialty. One doctor was unable for financial reasons to complete the training, another was unable owing to illness in his family. Two others, after qualifying in their specialties, found them not sufficiently remunerative. One man mentioned the impersonal nature of the specialist's life, and another the monotony of his particular specialty. In several cases, attractive openings at least partially determined the man's decision to enter general practice.

Of the 16 men (14 in Ontario, 2 in Nova Scotia) who did not know, when they began the medical course, what type of medical career they wished, almost half made a choice while they were still in medical school, almost half while they were interning, and a few while they were in the armed services. General practice was the initial decision of about half of these men. The reasons given for this choice were lack of money, a desire to get settled down, and the length of specialty training; these men occasionally mentioned also a liking for people and lack of any wish to be a specialist. The remainder of those who entered medicine without knowing what type of medical career they wished gave serious thought to at least one, and some of them to two, of surgery, obstetrics, internal medicine, and paediatrics. The reason usually given for the choice of a specialty was interest in that phase of medicine, though one man initially decided upon internal medicine because he believed, erroneously, that he was not skilful with his hands, whereas another chose surgery partly out of interest and partly because "surgery is easier than medicine" and because surgery made possible more definite action than did medicine at that time. The most commonly mentioned reasons for abandoning plans for training in a specialty were inability to finance further training, the inordinate length of the training, and (even in cases in which the training was financially possible) a wish to settle down and to start living "a reasonable life." One man was unable to get a training appointment, and another, while waiting for a promised appointment, became so fond of the area in which he was temporarily practising that he decided to relinquish his opportunity for training and stay where he was. The doctor who thought himself not skilful with his hands, finding during his internship that he was wrong in this and that he enjoyed obstetrics, surgery, and anaesthesia, gave up the idea of being an internist and entered general practice.

Finally, there were 10 practitioners in Ontario and 7 in Nova Scotia who had begun the study of medicine with the intention of practising a specialty or of having a career in research or teaching. These plans were abandoned at various stages, by some men during the years in medical school, by some during their internship, by some on leaving the armed forces, by some after two or three years of what had been considered temporary general practice, and by one man after a prolonged period of training in a specialty. The commonest reason, given by more than half of these doctors, for the change of plans from a specialty to general practice was financial necessity. Other reasons were unwillingness to leave a wife "to a lonely existence" throughout the period of hospital training, a desire to earn a living and raise a family, a growing interest in general practice, a waning interest in a specialty, and a feeling of responsibility towards a community that had no other physician.

The effect of finances on postgraduate training will be discussed more fully in chapter 13; but the description of the vicissitudes of the physicians' planning for their careers would be incomplete without a brief statement of the part played by financial factors. Financial difficulties were said by approximately one-quarter of the practitioners in each province to have been the determining factor, and were said by almost as many to have been a contributing factor, in their decision to bring their training to an end and enter general practice. Some of these men were prevented, by their financial problems, from taking further training in preparation for general practice; others were diverted to general practice from the specialist career that they would have preferred (see pages 185–186).

In an attempt to determine the relative importance of the influence of various groups upon the young man's decision to enter general practice, the interrogator asked each doctor, "Who do you think exercised the greatest influence on your decision to go into general practice?" It was explained that the name was not required but merely an indication whether it was a friend, a relative, a physician, a teacher in medical school, etc. Fifty-seven per cent of the physicians, both in Ontario and in Nova Scotia, replied that no one had influenced their decisions. Thirty-nine per cent in Ontario and 33 per cent in Nova Scotia named physicians, including the doctor's own father, other relatives who were physicians, medical school teachers, and doctors who were neither relatives nor teachers. One man had been influenced most by his father, who was not a physician, and one thought that he had been influenced most by a movie portrayal of a general practitioner.

Turning now to the practice experience of the physicians, we find that, of the 44 in Ontario, only 10* had practised in communities other than those in which they were established when visited by the Survey. These included 2 men who had previously practised in other provinces, one of whom had given up his original practice in order to take several years of postgraduate training and, on completing this, settled in Ontario, and the other of whom moved because of dissatisfaction with the poor quality of medicine being practised by his partner. Only 8 physicians (18 per cent of the Ontario sample) had practised in more than one Ontario community. Two of these men moved to very small places, in order to get away from the turmoil and the rapid pace of the larger cities. An additional reason given by one of these men was that in Toronto he had so little access to hospital facilities that he had a heavy load of house calls. One doctor left a large city because the area in which he lived was "down at the heels"; he later made two more moves, from one small village because of "the dead winters" and from another because there were "too many old people."

The moves made by 5 of the doctors who had practised in more than one Ontario community were necessitated by lack of enough practice to produce a reasonable living. Some of these men had to move several times before they found communities in which they were able to establish satisfactory practices. On the average, these 5 practitioners had had 2½ years of practice before they settled in the

*This number excludes 1 doctor who spent his first year of practice in another town as a salaried assistant. This appointment was understood to be only temporary.

communities in which they were located at the time of the Survey. The average duration of these practices, since the last move, was approximately 22 years. The eventual success of these physicians, after their early discouragements, is, at least in part, a reflection of the general prosperity of Ontario since the depression years.

Of the doctors visited in Nova Scotia, one had practised in another province but had given up his practice to take additional training, after which he settled in Nova Scotia; 17* others (40 per cent of the Nova Scotia sample) had practised in more than one Nova Scotia community. As in Ontario, a few of these moves had been dictated by financial necessity; the remainder were said to have been made for a variety of reasons. Some men had moved to larger centres in order to get away from the monotony, the primitive living conditions, the poor facilities for education, or the isolation, of the small communities in which they were living. Others had moved away from large communities in order to be more on their own. One man had been forced to move in order to escape from a load of work that had become unendurable.

Moves within a community were not common, such moves having been made by only 18 per cent of the Ontario doctors and by only 10 per cent of the Nova Scotia doctors. Most frequently, according to the Ontario men, the purpose of these moves was to have more satisfactory office space or living accommodation. A desire for a larger income prompted some of the moves, a few of which involved disagreements with a partner or employer and disruption of existing practice arrangements. In Nova Scotia, almost all of the moves within a community were made by men who had been serving as salaried assistants of other physicians but wished to practise on their own.

The physicians' reasons for choosing the communities in which they were practising when visited by the Survey fell into two groups: professional opportunities and preferences regarding their living arrangements. Some doctors returned to practise with their fathers or with other relatives who were physicians. One mentioned that his father's reputation gave him a good start. A number of men were offered partnerships or assistantships. Some communities were short of doctors. In one case, a doctor's house was for sale and would be suitable for office accommodation. One man's choice was determined by the opportunity to join a clinic, with better hours and a higher income than

---

*Not included are 3 physicians who practised for short periods, either as assistant or as locum tenens, in what were clearly recognized as temporary positions.

he had had on his own. Another, who was interested in surgery, chose a particular town, at least in part, because of the high incidence of injuries occurring in the district's major industry. Two others, also interested in surgery, settled where they did because the local hospitals did not demand specialist qualifications of those undertaking surgery. Some men said that there had been an "opening" in the town in which they had settled, but did not elaborate on this. A wish to return to their home towns played a major part in determining the location of practice of approximately one-third of the doctors both in Ontario and in Nova Scotia. Other, less frequently mentioned, reasons were that they liked a small town, that the community was new and growing, that it was near a large city or that it was away from "well-established regions," and that this was "a good place to live."

Each physician was asked whether he would settle where he was, if he had the choice to make again. In Ontario, only 1 physician, practising in Toronto, answered in the negative and explained that he would settle further out in the suburbs in order to get away from the dirt, the noise, and the traffic of the older part of the city. Of the remaining 43, who were satisfied, 2 added qualifying comments to their answers. One pointed out that, though practice in one's home town was made easier by the detailed knowledge that one had of the background of patients, it was difficult to charge many patients whom one had known from boyhood. The other commented that he missed the library facilities and the cultural opportunities of a large city and remarked on the great number of "uninteresting people" in his medium-sized city. In Nova Scotia, 8 practitioners replied that they would not choose the same community again. One would have liked a larger city; another would have liked to avoid the Nova Scotia winters. The remaining 6 (14 per cent of the Nova Scotia group) were all located in mining towns. They complained of the contract system of practice that was in operation, which they said imposed too heavy a work load, remunerated them inadequately, and was abused by some of the patients. Though these men had been in their present communities for 14 years on the average, they seemed to be there as prisoners of circumstance rather than by choice.

In spite of the dissatisfaction expressed by this group of Nova Scotia practitioners, we were impressed, throughout the course of the field work in both provinces, by the feeling of permanency that we had about most of the practices. Analysis of the numerical data has shown this impression to be well founded. Even the 8 doctors who had practised in more than one community in Ontario, whose average number of years of practice was approximately 21,* had been in their present communities for a little over 14 years on the average. Similarly, the 18 Nova Scotia physicians who had practised in more than one community, with an average of approximately 18 years of practice behind them, had spent almost 14 of those years in their present communities. On the other hand, the careers of a small proportion of the general practitioners may undergo major changes even after some years of practice, as was shown by the facts that one practitioner, of more than ten years' standing, planned within a year or two to give up general practice for a specialty and that another, after nearly ten years of practice, intended to abandon his medical career completely in favour of some type of business enterprise. The average duration of practice in Ontario of the entire group of 44 physicians was 15 years, of which almost 14 had been spent in the community in which the physician was visited by the Survey. The figures for the 42 Nova Scotia doctors were almost the same, approximately 14 years of practice, on the average, of which almost 13 had been in the physician's present community.

*In computing the number of years of practice in Ontario or in Nova Scotia, we have taken the total number of years from the time when the doctor established practice in the particular province, even though, in some cases, illness, further postgraduate training, or military service later interrupted practice.

# 6 / Arrangements for Practice
## *Within the Office*

In this chapter and the two succeeding ones, we shall consider the physician's arrangements for carrying on his practice. These are included in the section on the General Practitioner, because we believe that something of the man is reflected in them.

Among doctors differing so much from one another in background and in educational experience, it is not surprising to find also great variation in their arrangements. The extent of the variation we shall illustrate by picturing two offices.

Dr. A's office suite comprised waiting room, consulting room, examining room, utility room, and lavatory. The waiting room was large and attractive, with excellent furnishings and a variety of recent magazines neatly displayed. Near the door leading to the consulting room, in a location easily accessible to the doctor, were his secretary's desk and filing cabinets. The doctor's consulting room was spacious, attractively finished with wall panelling and built-in bookcases, and comfortably and tastefully furnished. The examining room, which was bright and neat, contained an examining table of excellent quality and a cabinet for instruments and supplies. In the utility room were refrigerator, autoclave, centrifuge, microscope, and laboratory reagents. Counters on either side of the sink provided adequate space for laboratory work. Large cupboards were stocked with supplies, so arranged that they could easily be found. The lavatory was clean; it contained a toilet but no facilities for patients to wash and dry their hands.

Dr. B's office suite consisted of waiting room, consulting room, and examining room, which were situated one behind the other. The waiting room was shabby and dusty and contained large piles of old magazines and numerous cheap pictures. The consulting room was cramped, poorly lighted, dingy, dirty, and untidy, with masses of books, papers, and drug samples piled on desk, tables, examining couch, and bookcases. Before the examining couch could be used, the things heaped on it had to be moved; it was used seldom. The examining room was large but poorly lighted. Its walls, cracked and peeling, were partially covered with ancient, luridly coloured diagrams depicting the abdominal and pelvic organs. On a table beside the sink was a hot-water sterilizer. The remaining space, here and on the other side of the sink, was loaded with bottles, most of them covered with dust. Piles of rubbish, medical and non-medical, cluttered the room.

Neither of these pictures is a composite or an exaggeration. Each was the office of a practising physician; and most, if not all, of the good and bad features of these two offices were encountered in many other offices.

Although most physicians' offices differed from one another in at least some respects, there were enough similarities to enable us to give a general picture of the practitioner's office facilities. Naturally, the size of the premises varied with the number of physicians using them. Sixty-six per cent of the Ontario doctors were practising by themselves; 20 per cent were practising in association with another doctor, either an employer, an employee, or a partner; and the remaining 14 per cent were members of groups of three or more. The corresponding percentages for Nova Scotia were approximately 67 per cent, 10 per cent, and 24 per cent. Only 18 per cent of the Ontario doctors and 31 per cent of the Nova Scotia doctors, all except one of whom were located in communities with populations of less than 100,000, had their offices in their own homes. The communities in which it was commonest for the doctors to have their offices in their homes were those with populations of 1,000 or less. The percentages of physicians in different age groups who practised from their homes did not differ significantly in either Ontario or Nova Scotia.

Every doctor had some area that served as a waiting room, though its adequacy and comfort varied from one office to another. Of the 29 men who were engaged in solo practice in Ontario, a few had a combined consulting-and-examining room, but the majority had separate consulting and examining rooms. In Nova Scotia, on the other hand, less than a quarter of the 28 solo practitioners had separate consulting and examining rooms. In actual practice, however, some physicians saw the majority of their patients in their consulting room

only and used their examining room for such special purposes as prenatal examinations, well-baby care, and injections or other therapeutic
procedures, whereas other men used the two rooms almost inter-
changeably. In those offices, in each province, in which two doctors
were practising together, it was uncommon for each doctor to have more
than one room. Usually, in these offices, each doctor had a consulting-
and-examining room; and, in a few offices, the two doctors staggered
their hours so that each of them was able to use the same space. In
most of the offices, of the men in solo practice and of those in groups
of two, there were one or two other rooms that served as dispensary,
store room, utility room, laboratory, secretary's room, treatment room,
or various combinations of these. All except 10 of the solo practitioners,
5 in each province, and all but 1 of the men in groups of two had
lavatory facilities. Of these and of the provision for laboratory work,
more will be said presently.

The larger groups, to which 6 of the Ontario and 10 of the Nova
Scotia physicians belonged, had more extensive premises, one group
occupying most of a three-storey building. In several cases, the building had been constructed specially to provide accommodation for
the group. Each doctor would have one or two, or possibly even three,
rooms in which to see his patients. In addition to a common waiting
room, the group would share other facilities, which differed from one
practice to another. Among the facilities available to one or more
of these groups were a laboratory with a full-time trained technician,
a small operating room (for tonsillectomies and minor surgical procedures) with a recovery room, a room in which electrocardiograms and
basal metabolic rates were done, rooms for radiology, rooms for eye,
ear, nose, and throat examinations, rooms for secretarial workers and
office managers, store rooms, and cloak rooms. All but one of these
groups had lavatory facilities.

The facilities that the doctors had provided for themselves for
doing laboratory work varied, both in Ontario and in Nova Scotia,
from being almost non-existent to being more than ample. A few
examples will illustrate the variation. In one office, the laboratory
space was a cupboard having neither a window nor a source of artificial light. In another, the space intended for laboratory work had
long since been usurped by empty bottles, samples, and other miscellaneous objects, until the working space available had been narrowed,
literally, to the rim of the sink. Another doctor's only laboratory equipment was indicator-type paper strips, which were kept in his desk
drawer and brought out when he wished to test urine for protein or
sugar. In only one office, was there no sign either of space or of any

sort of equipment for laboratory work. Some men preferred to do haemoglobin determinations at their desk, but did the chemical urinalysis at a sink, perhaps in another room. Sometimes the laboratory facilities were in a hall or a lavatory; frequently they were in a room that was used also as a dispensary, a treatment room, or a store room. Though only an occasional office devoted a whole room to laboratory work, in a number of instances ample counter space was set aside for this purpose, with glassware and reagents neatly arranged and convenient to a sink and with a microscope in good working order and provided with a suitable source of light.

Whereas we observed the physician's use of laboratory procedures in his handling of patients and took it into account in assessing the quality of practice, we did not determine in any detail what equipment was available in the physician's office; but the presence or absence of a few items was noted. These are listed in Table 11. Approximately 70 per cent of the Ontario, and 50 per cent of the Nova Scotia, doctors had adequate facilities for refrigerating such products as required refrigeration. Most of these had a refrigerator in their office or made use of the refrigerator in their living quarters if these were close to

TABLE 11

MAJOR LABORATORY EQUIPMENT OR FACILITIES IN ONTARIO AND NOVA SCOTIA PHYSICIANS' OFFICES

| | Ontario | | | Nova Scotia | | |
|---|---|---|---|---|---|---|
| | Number of physicians | | | Number of physicians | | |
| Item | With | With-out | Un-known | With | With-out | Un-known |
| Refrigeration facilities | 30 | 12 | 2 | 19 | 20 | 3 |
| Equipment for sterilization by boiling | 42 | 2* | — | 38 | 4† | — |
| Autoclave | 8 | 36 | — | 9 | 33 | — |
| Microscope | 35 | 8 | 1 | 26 | 16 | — |
| Centrifuge | 6 | 37 | 1 | 4 | 38 | — |
| ECG machine | 4 | 40 | — | 5 | 37 | — |
| BMR machine | 5 | 39 | — | 2 | 40 | — |
| X-ray equipment | | | | | | |
| None | | 34 | | | 38§ | |
| Fluoroscopy only | | 4‡ | | | 0 | |
| Fluoroscopy and films | | 6‡ | | | 4‖ | |

*These 2 physicians had autoclaves.

†Three of these physicians had autoclaves.

‡Included in each of these counts is 1 physician whose equipment, though located in a hospital separate from his office, was owned and operated by him.

§One of these physicians did own equipment for taking films, but it was located in a hospital and was not operated by the doctor.

‖One of these physicians had ceased using the equipment.

the office; a few arranged with a nearby pharmacist to store their supplies in his refrigerator.

The most commonly used method of sterilizing instruments in the office was boiling, usually in a commercial hot-water sterilizer, occasionally in a saucepan. Over 90 per cent of the offices in each province had facilities for this method, though one doctor was using a "sterilizer" that he said would not bring the water to a boil. About 20 per cent of the doctors in each province had autoclaves.

Eighty per cent of the Ontario offices had microscopes; 18 per cent had none. One of the doctors who had no microscope was questioned about the importance of this instrument in general practice and replied that it was needed only to do hanging-drop preparations in suspected cases of trichomonas infection. Of the doctors who did have microscopes, two made comments that were of interest in that they made clear that one cannot assess a practice merely on the basis of the facilities available. It is the use that is made of them that counts. One man said that his microscope was "not working." He did not know what was wrong with it and apparently had no intention of having it repaired. It later turned out that the microscope *was* working. Another doctor said that he used his microscope seldom—only when he suspected cystitis—and could probably do without it. In one other office, the microscope was in such poor condition as to be virtually useless. In effect, then, one-quarter of the Ontario practitioners lacked facilities for microscopic work in their offices; and several, though possessing microscopes, gave evidence of using them seldom, if ever. It is likely, however, that some of them either did microscopic examinations, or had them done, at their hospitals. Of the Nova Scotia doctors, 62 per cent had microscopes, and 38 per cent did not. More will be said on the subject of clinical microscopy in the chapter that deals with quality of practice.

Four other pieces of equipment, namely, centrifuges, machines for making electrocardiograms, equipment for determining basal metabolic rates, and X-ray equipment, were encountered in only a small proportion of the offices in either Ontario or Nova Scotia.

Since by far the greatest part of the laboratory work done by the doctor himself in his office consisted of haemoglobin determinations and examinations of urine for sugar and protein, a few words will be said about the methods used. Of the 68 physicians whose method of doing haemoglobin determinations is known with certainty, 17 in Ontario and 10 in Nova Scotia used the Sahli type of haemoglobinometer, 9 in Ontario and 20 in Nova Scotia used an improved type of visual colorimeter, 1 in each province had a photo-electric colorimeter, and 5 in each province were satisfied with the inaccurate Tallqvist method.

The test for glucose in the urine by Benedict's reagent and the heat-and-acetic-acid method of testing for protein were rarely seen. Glucose was frequently tested for by means of a commercially prepared tablet to which prescribed amounts of water and of urine were added. The methods commonly used to test for protein were the sulphosalicylic acid method in Ontario and Roberts' test in Nova Scotia. In some offices, all of these tests had been supplanted by the more recently invented indicator-type paper strips. Tests for blood, acetone, bilirubin, and urobilinogen in the urine were seldom done in the physicians' offices. Indeed, some of the offices did not possess the materials necessary for these tests.

Thirty-nine per cent of the Ontario physicians dispensed drugs, though a few of these indicated that their dispensing was on a minor scale; of the Nova Scotia physicians, 21 per cent dispensed. Some had a whole room for their dispensary, whereas in other offices the same room served as dispensary, laboratory, and perhaps general storage room. Some of the dispensaries were extremely well organized, every item in its place and easy to find; in others the lack of organization was tantamount almost to chaos.

In order to make an estimate of the adequacy of the offices from the point of view of the patients' comfort, both physical and psychological, the observer rated each office as good, fair, or poor on each of 13 items. These, with the ratings, are shown in Table 12.

Every one of the offices was judged to be conveniently located. For all but 3, the parking facilities were at least fair. The necessity for patients to park a considerable distance from 3 of the offices reflects present-day traffic congestion with its inevitable parking restrictions. Stairs were rated as good when there was not more than half a flight or when there was an elevator in operation in the building. A full flight of stairs was called fair. More than one flight or a single flight that was unusually long (as in some old, high-ceilinged buildings) or steep or dangerous was designated as poor. The stairs were poor in 5 per cent of the Ontario, and in 33 per cent of the Nova Scotia, practices. It is unlikely that either the stairs or the parking facilities could have been improved, except by a move to another office, which in some communities might not have been available. These disadvantages are mentioned, however, as part of the total picture and as points that are worthy of consideration by a doctor at the time of choosing the location of his office.

TABLE 12

ASSESSMENT OF ONTARIO AND NOVA SCOTIA PHYSICIANS' OFFICES

| Item | Ontario Number of offices assessed as: | | | Nova Scotia Number of offices assessed as: | | |
|---|---|---|---|---|---|---|
| | Good | Fair | Poor | Good | Fair | Poor |
| Convenience of location | 44 | 0 | 0 | 42 | 0 | 0 |
| Parking | 27 | 15 | 2 | 38 | 3 | 1 |
| Stairs | 32 | 10 | 2 | 23 | 5 | 14 |
| Daylight | 26 | 10 | 8 | 29 | 7 | 6 |
| Artificial light | 38 | 5 | 1 | 30 | 10 | 2 |
| Ventilation | 41 | 3 | 0 | 40 | 1 | 1 |
| Heating | 39* | 4 | 1 | 38* | 2 | 2 |
| Furnishings | 35 | 5 | 4 | 18 | 14 | 10 |
| Cleanliness | 40 | 2 | 2 | 29 | 4 | 9 |
| General attractiveness | 28 | 12 | 4 | 11 | 20 | 11 |
| Lavatory facilities | 18 | 16 | 10 | 4 | 13 | 25 |
| Privacy | 37 | 5 | 2 | 36 | 1 | 5 |
| Chaperoning of female patients† | 6 | 2 | 35 | 8 | 0 | 33 |
| Total number of physicians | 44 | | | 42 | | |

*Included in these numbers are some physicians who were visited during those parts of the year when the heating system was not having much demand made on it or was not in use at all.

†In each province, one physician could not be assessed on this item.

In contrast with these two inconveniences on the way to the office, the remaining items of Table 12 refer to the interior of the suite, and all, except possibly daylight, reflect the doctor's ability to organize an office. Ventilation, heating, and privacy were considered to be good in more than 80 per cent of the offices in each province. Of the offices that were rated as poor in the matter of heating, one was cold, especially in the examining room, on all three days of the observer's visit. Though several patients noticed this, the practitioner himself seemed oblivious of the cold and made no use of the auxiliary heater that stood by. In another office, a stove in the consulting room kept the temperature unbearably high, while the waiting room was chilly. Some offices were cold at times but not continuously. The occasional office boasted an air-conditioner, which added immeasurably to the comfort of the rooms on a hot summer day.

Privacy was considered to be good when conversation between the doctor and his patient could not be overheard in the waiting room or in other rooms to which patients might have access. Some doctors, who were concerned about this matter, had taken such precautions as having the door between their consulting room and their waiting room covered with plywood or sound-proofing board or even having two doors between the rooms. In the 15 per cent of offices that were rated as less than good in this respect, conversations between doctor and patient could be overheard, sometimes with great ease, through thin or poorly fitted doors. Two partners, who almost always left open the doors that led from their consulting rooms into an intervening room, appeared quite unheedful of the fact that their conversations with patients were clearly audible to other patients.

Daylight was good in about two-thirds of the offices in each province. In some cases, the doctor could have effected an improvement by rearranging the furniture to take advantage of the light or by raising the Venetian blind during the hours of daylight. In other offices, however, little or no improvement seemed possible. Artificial light, though poor in only the occasional office, was judged to be only fair in 11 per cent of the Ontario, and 24 per cent of the Nova Scotia, offices.

Cleanliness was rated as good in 91 per cent of the Ontario, and 69 per cent of the Nova Scotia, offices. Some offices were untidy and unclean in a few areas; others were dirty throughout. Ninety-one per cent of the Ontario, and 76 per cent of the Nova Scotia, premises were at least fairly well, and some of them very well, furnished. The remainder were poorly furnished, some of them containing only a few pieces of old, battered furniture.

General attractiveness was judged to be good in 64 per cent of the Ontario, and 26 per cent of the Nova Scotia, office suites. Many of these were most attractive indeed, reflecting thought for the patient's comfort in such matters as lighting, agreeable colours, one or two well-chosen pictures, ash trays conveniently located, and in the waiting room a supply of recent magazines. In some offices, the cleanliness and the good quality of lighting and furniture were obscured by the overpowering impression of shabbiness and dinginess created by the drab, dull paint or wall paper from bygone decades.

It may be objected that, in assessing the office suites, we have made subjective judgments. This is true, since no objective means of measuring the various items are available. In the matter of general attractiveness, it is particularly true that our ratings are based on subjective impressions. Nevertheless, we are not quibbling about minor points. This is clear from the following description of an office that we considered poor from the point of view of general attractiveness.

The waiting room, which had no window and a single electric bulb on the ceiling, was both cramped and dirty. It contained half a dozen side chairs, no table, and a magazine rack stuffed with old issues of various magazines. The consulting room was attractively painted, but this tended to escape notice because of the poor furniture, the cot that was used as an examining couch but that, after a few patients had rumpled its two sheets, looked like an unmade bed, and mountains of papers piled higgledy-piggledy on the desk and the bookcase. Behind the desk, in one corner of the room, was a large pile of trash, which had been aimed at the waste basket but had missed it. The same disorder prevailed in the other rooms, with bottles, packages, pamphlets, dressings, empty cartons, and instruments, all hopelessly mixed up. The floors needed cleaning, the other horizontal surfaces were too well covered to permit of any cleaning. Offices such as the last (or Dr. B's, described above), which were in marked contrast with the attractive offices of some physicians, suggested that these men gave little or no thought to the comfort of their patients or to their own dignity as practitioners of medicine.

Two matters had been given less thought than they deserved by a sizable number of doctors: lavatory facilities and chaperoning of female patients. The latter was assessed on the conduct of the vaginal examination. Of 84 doctors whom it was possible to assess on this, only 14 routinely had another woman present, either a nurse, a secretary, or the physician's wife. Two were sometimes chaperoned, sometimes not. The remaining 68 did their vaginal examinations without having a chaperone present. One of these doctors stated that prior to coming to his present town he had always had a chaperone but that he quickly discovered that here the women did not wish another woman present. Another man stated that he did have a chaperone if he had any reason to be suspicious of a patient. Quite apart from the fact that many women would probably be more comfortable if they had another woman present, we were impressed with the risk incurred by many doctors from the legal point of view.

In judging lavatory facilities, we took into account whether they were accessible to the patient, whether they gave the patient a reasonable degree of privacy, whether toilet paper was available, whether there were facilities for washing and drying the hands, and whether the room was clean and had enough light to enable the patient to see. Judged by these criteria, 41 per cent of the Ontario, and 10 per cent of the Nova Scotia, offices had good lavatory facilities. In Ontario 36 per cent and in Nova Scotia 31 per cent were considered only fair for one or more of several reasons. To reach many of these washrooms, it was necessary to pass through the doctor's consulting room, examining room, or both, which would be enough to discourage many patients from using the washroom unless their need were urgent. Some lavatories lacked a wash basin or towels or both. In some cases, the washroom was an unusual distance away; in other cases, the patient had to negotiate a flight of stairs in order to reach the room; and some washrooms were crowded and untidy.

Twenty-three per cent of the Ontario, and 59 per cent of the Nova Scotia, offices were rated as poor in the matter of lavatory facilities. In about a third of these, there were no facilities at all. Others did not have their own washrooms but adjoined the doctor's living quarters. Since it was apparent, however, in each of these cases that the domestic bathroom was not equipped for use by patients and since patients would be even more hesitant about asking to use it, such facilities can only be considered unsatisfactory. In a number of cases, the lavatory facilities combined so many of the undesirable features mentioned in the preceding paragraph that the over-all picture was poor in the extreme. It was not uncommon to find that the washroom was dirty and smelly and had neither soap, towels, hot water, nor, sometimes, even toilet paper. This picture is applicable mainly to those washrooms that were shared by several tenants in a building.

Having dealt with the premises, we pass on now to the non-medical personnel employed by the physicians. Of the 29 Ontario physicians who were engaged in solo practice, 19 had assistance (16 of these physicians had 1 secretary, 1 had 1 nurse, 1 had 1 secretary and 1 nurse, and 1 had 2 nurses); of the 28 solo practitioners in Nova Scotia, 13 had assistance (6 of these physicians had 1 secretary, 2 had 2 secretaries, and 5 had 1 nurse). The difference between the two provinces is not statistically significant. The other 25 solo practitioners had no secretarial or nursing assistance, except such sporadic help as some of their wives were able to give. Most of these physicians were not, as one might think, men who were just establishing themselves. In Ontario, they averaged more than eighteen years of practice, and none of them had been in practice less than nine years; in Nova Scotia, they had been in practice more than fifteen years on the average, and all but 2 had been in practice eight years or more. Most of them did not give any indication why they had never had any assistance; but a few men thought that they could not afford to pay a secretary. They did not seem to have considered that to be without help was probably more costly since, after years of training in medicine, they were using their own time to do many things that did not make use of that training and that someone with experience in typing, filing, and other office procedures could probably have done much more efficiently. The occasional man was afraid that his wife would object to his having a secretary.

Of the 15 Ontario, and 14 Nova Scotia, physicians who were practising in association with one or more other physicians, all but 2, both in Nova Scotia, had assistance in their offices. Most of them employed 1, 2, or 3 persons, though a few of the larger groups had even more employees. In some offices, where the hours were very long, there were 2 or 3 secretaries with staggered hours, perhaps overlapping during the busiest part of the day. Some groups made use of 2 secretaries concurrently but assigned them different duties, one woman, for example, acting as receptionist and answering the telephone, the other handling the records. In the occasional larger group practice, there might be a laboratory technician, an X-ray technician, or a telephone switchboard operator. Table 13 summarizes the assistance available in the 86 offices.

TABLE 13

DISTRIBUTION OF ONTARIO AND NOVA SCOTIA PHYSICIANS ACCORDING
TO THE NUMBER OF NON-MEDICAL ASSISTANTS IN THEIR OFFICES

| Assistants in physician's office | | | Number of physicians | | | |
|---|---|---|---|---|---|---|
| Total number | Number of secretaries | Number of nurses | Ontario | | Nova Scotia | |
| None | None | None | 10 | 10* | 17 | 17† |
| One | One | None | 19 ⎫ | 20 | 8 ⎫ | 15 |
| | None | One | 1 ⎭ | | 7 ⎭ | |
| Two | Two | None | 4 ⎫ | | 2 ⎫ | |
| | One | One | 4‡ ⎬ | 9 | 2 ⎬ | 4 |
| | None | Two | 1 ⎭ | | 0 ⎭ | |
| Three | Three | None | 1 ⎫ | | 0 ⎫ | |
| | One | Two | 1 ⎬ | 2 | 0 ⎬ | 1 |
| | None | Three | 0 ⎭ | | 1 ⎭ | |
| Four or more | § | § | 3 | 3 | 5 | 5 |
| Total number of physicians | | | 44 | | 42 | |

*Some of these physicians were assisted by their wives, regularly in one office, sporadically in others.

†One of these physicians had no assistance at the time of the Survey's visit but said that he usually employed a part-time secretary. Two of these physicians were assisted by their wives; but, in 1 of these offices, the assistance was very occasional.

‡One of these offices employed 2 nurses, as well as a secretary, during the few months of each year that were particularly busy.

§The workers in these offices included receptionists, secretaries, clerical workers, nurses, technicians, business managers, and switchboard operators.

The major duties most frequently assigned to the secretary were answering the telephone, making appointments for patients in the doctor's own office, arranging for X-rays, consultations, and admissions to hospital, looking out records and filing them again after the patients' visits, ushering patients into the doctor's consulting room, keeping financial records and accepting payments, typing letters, accounts, and, in a few offices, clinical records, and filling out forms for insurance companies and prepaid medical plans. Some doctors had taught their secretaries to do haemoglobin determinations and to test the urine for sugar and protein, and an occasional one to do red blood cell and white blood cell counts and to make blood smears. Rarely, we encountered a secretary who gave injections, both intra-muscular and subcutaneous. In a few offices, the secretary chaperoned examinations of female patients. Occasionally, the ordering of supplies and the dispensing of drugs were done by the secretary under the doctor's supervision.

Nurses were used partly for duties that drew upon their nursing training but also for some of the duties listed in the preceding paragraph, such as answering the telephone, making appointments, keeping accounts, looking out records, and conducting and chaperoning patients. Their professional ability was utilized in giving injections, sterilizing supplies, doing laboratory tests, applying dressings, and setting up for, and assisting at, minor surgical procedures.

In answer to the question, "Are good nursing and secretarial assistants fairly easy to get?" 48 per cent of the Ontario, and 43 per cent of the Nova Scotia, physicians replied in the negative; 32 per cent of the Ontario, and 57 per cent of the Nova Scotia, physicians replied in the affirmative; and the remainder could not answer, most of them because they had never looked for such assistants. A number of men, who were well satisfied with their own workers, emphasized that it was difficult to find a *capable* woman to do this type of work. Occasional mention was made of the higher salaries that industry could afford to pay. The hours also were thought to be of importance, one doctor stating that many women were not willing to work in the evening, another saying that it was easy to obtain part-time workers, especially for the afternoon. There was no clear evidence, in Ontario, that good office assistance was easier to obtain in a community of one size than in a community of another. In Nova Scotia, however, 88 per cent of the physicians in communities of over 10,000, but only 36 per cent of those in communities of less than 10,000, said that assistance was fairly easy to obtain ($p < 0.01$).*

Though the practitioners were not questioned in detail about their nurses and secretaries, such comments as they made were noted. A remark that we heard frequently, as did Peterson and his associates

*This is explained on pages 32–33.

while studying the general practitioners in North Carolina,* was that a secretary was preferable to a nurse. The doctors said they needed a woman who could answer the telephone, make appointments, and keep financial records, and stressed the last particularly. An occasional man had taught his secretary to do simple laboratory work and even to give injections. The few men who expressed a preference for a nurse rather than a secretary found it helpful to have a woman who could interpret patients' stories over the telephone, sort out patients in the office, do dressings and injections, and run an autoclave. Among qualities listed as necessary in an office worker, whether nurse or secretary, were honesty, intelligence, and ability to meet patients.

Though we did not make specific inquiry, about one-third of the Ontario doctors mentioned that they made use of the services of men with accounting experience. Several physicians retained chartered accountants, one made use of a retired bank manager, and others did not specify the qualifications of their "accountants." The three principal functions of these men were to prepare income tax returns and advise on matters connected with income tax, to check the doctor's books, monthly or even, in the occasional office, semi-monthly, and to fill out insurance forms and the cards of Physicians' Services Incorporated and supervise the sending out of monthly accounts to patients. In one office, in addition to the semi-monthly checking of the books, there was a quarterly audit. One practitioner had a modern accounting system installed by, and supervised by, a firm of accountants and declared himself thoroughly pleased.

From our consideration of the office premises and the personnel employed by the physicians, we turn now to what might be called the mechanics of carrying on the work of the office. Under this heading we shall include arrangements for answering the telephone, appointments, and the keeping of records, and we shall describe briefly, with examples, systems that struck us as unusually efficient or inefficient.

Forty-one per cent of the Ontario, and 31 per cent of the Nova Scotia, doctors had a telephone-answering service of one sort or another. There was no relationship, in either province, between the age of the physician and whether he made use of such a service. On the other hand, 62 per cent of the Ontario, and 59 per cent of the Nova Scotia, doctors in places of over 10,000, but only 11 per cent of the Ontario, and 12 per cent of the Nova Scotia, men in places of 10,000

*O. L. Peterson *et al.*: Journal of Medical Education, *31*, No. 12, Part 2: 1–165, 1956; see his page 109.

or less, used such a service. The difference is statistically significant for each province ($p < 0.01$). While this difference probably results partly from the greater availability of answering services in larger cities, this is not the whole explanation, since in several cities we observed that one physician did, while another did not, have an answering service. That the attitude of the individual physician was important in determining whether he availed himself of a service that existed in his community is shown by the fact that several doctors commented that an answering service was not necessary, whereas an approximately equal number asserted that it was essential. It was interesting to see that some doctors, living in communities where commercial answering services were not available, had provided themselves with efficient services which they would likely not have had if they had not believed in the need for such a service. For example, one Nova Scotia physician, in solo practice, provided twenty-four-hour coverage of his telephone by arranging with a widow to take, and relay to him, all calls occurring outside his office hours. In another community in Nova Scotia in which there was no established answering service, a group of doctors practising together paid a family to take their telephone calls. One large group in Ontario had its own switchboard with girls working eight-hour shifts around the clock. In some cities the doctor's telephone was connected to a commercial answering service, in others to the Nurses' Registry or to the Academy of Medicine. Whatever calls were urgent the service would pass on to the doctor at once; the remainder would be listed and kept until the doctor called the service at periodic intervals.

With such arrangements as these, it was possible for the physician to see his office patients without continual interruptions and to have some moments of relaxation, especially during his meals. In the larger cities, some of the practitioners with answering services had their home telephones listed under their wives' names. It is believed by many doctors that, in a *small* community, it is not possible for the doctor to protect himself from the constant ringing of the telephone. Indeed, some men told us that, in order to have a break from the endless series of calls, they had to leave town and go somewhere—fishing or visiting in another town—where they could not be located. Peterson was told the same thing in North Carolina (see his page 120). This method of escaping from the many non-urgent or even trivial calls carries with it the risk of being absent in a real emergency. Because of the belief that there was no other way of achieving some degree of privacy, we observed with great interest a doctor, in a community of less than 2,500, whose home telephone number was not listed and all of whose calls were taken by the hospital switchboard. There was no evidence that he neglected his patients, and he appeared to be respected in the community. By asserting himself, however, he had made plain that he and his family, like other people, had a right to a certain amount of privacy.

By and large, the physicians who made use of answering services seemed satisfied with them, though they pointed out that sometimes a call was missed and that occasionally the service was not as courteous to a patient as the doctor could have wished. One man illustrated how useful he found the service by stating that, during the first month, the service took 486 calls for him.

The doctors who stated that an answering service was not necessary said that there was always, or almost always, someone at home to answer the telephone. Some men had the office telephone and the house telephone connected, so that at times when they were out or when they did not wish to be disturbed in the office they could have their wives take the calls. Some of the practitioners who did not have a regular answering service did make use of either the Nurses' Registry or their hospital switchboard, while they were on vacation or while they were taking a regular half-day in the middle of the week, to take their calls or to relay them to whatever doctor was covering the practice.

Next we shall consider appointments. To see patients by appointment was the policy of 59 per cent of the Ontario, but of only 24 per cent of the Nova Scotia, physicians ($p < 0.01$). This policy was not rigidly adhered to, since these doctors saw urgent cases, of course, without appointment and would see an occasional patient whose need was not urgent and who had not made an appointment, if he was willing to wait until the scheduled patients had been seen. Thirty-four per cent of the Ontario men, and 74 per cent of those in Nova Scotia, gave no appointments, and the remaining few doctors had a policy of making a limited number of appointments for special purposes, such as insurance examinations, but of seeing most of their patients without appointments.

The percentages of younger doctors and older doctors who saw patients by appointment did not differ significantly in Ontario. In Nova Scotia, 37 per cent of the doctors up to 45 years of age, but none of those over 45 years of age, had appointment systems. The difference is significant ($p < 0.05$). Seventy-seven per cent of the Ontario practitioners in places of over 10,000, but only 33 per cent of those in places of 10,000 or less, had appointment systems. The difference between the two groups is significant ($p < 0.01$). The corresponding figures for Nova Scotia are 41 per cent and 12 per cent. Though the trend is in the same direction in Nova Scotia, the difference between places of more than 10,000 and places of 10,000 or less does not reach the level of statistical significance.

Every practitioner who did not see his patients by appointment was asked the reason for this. The most impressive reason, given by three doctors in small isolated communities in Ontario, was that many of their patients did not have telephones. Two of these men said that an appointment system had been tried, either by them or by a colleague in the same community, and had failed. The most frequent reason for not giving appointments, both in Ontario and in Nova Scotia, was that patients were not used to an appointment system and liked to be able to come in at any time. Some of the men who gave this reason recognized that this could result in patients' having to wait, but said that patients did not mind waiting and usually did not have to wait long. That the latter statement is perhaps not quite accurate is suggested by a story told us by a doctor who attached some importance to seeing patients by appointment. He reported that he had a patient who regularly came twenty miles for prenatal visits because the dotcor to whom she had previously gone had no system and kept patients waiting most of the afternoon. By coincidence, a doctor whom we had visited in this lady's town was one of those who had told us that patients did not mind waiting.

The feelings of one patient about being kept waiting were expressed in a letter to the Editor of the *Ontario Medical Review*, from which we quote the following excerpts:

I guess I've been in doctors' offices across Canada about ten times in the past ten years. I cannot recall when I did not have to wait at least one-half an hour for my appointment. During my last two visits to two different doctors I had to wait over an hour each time. . . .

At all these visits I have wondered why doctors never apologize for keeping me waiting. Don't any of them have any consideration for their patients' feelings? Some patients have to take time off from work for which they do not get paid in order to see their doctors. Don't the doctors realize this? What about mothers with one or more young children in tow? How would doctors feel if I kept them in my office for an hour or two for an appointment which they had made weeks before? They would certainly expect an explanation.*

Another physician, who stated that patients sometimes did have to wait a long time to see him, maintained that they seemed to wait

*J. W. Patterson: Ontario Medical Review, 27: 1157, 1960.

just as long for doctors who had an appointment system. His reason for not having one was that he had no secretary to answer the telephone and give appointments. Somewhat incongruous was his later statement that he had no need for a telephone-answering service "because somebody is always here." Some doctors who made use of an answering service told us that they left a duplicate appointment book with the service and checked the appointment book in their office against the duplicate book at intervals during the day.

In several offices, apathy or lack of organizing ability seemed to stand in the way of an appointment system. We heard such statements as, "I thought of doing it the odd time but never got around to it," "Our time is so indefinite," and "It is too hard to apply—having no appointments saves phoning and arranging—most people don't want it anyway." Peterson, commenting on the lack of an appointment system in some of the North Carolina practices, thought that the failure of some men to systematize their practices in this way "was due at least in part to the physician's own reluctance to discipline himself to this degree" (see his page 126).

On the other hand, concern for his patients prevented one Ontario doctor from having appointments, since he was afraid that he would "get booked up," so that patients would not be able to see him on the same day on which they called. Since it may be that other men have the same fear of an appointment system and since it is true that some specialists with appointment systems are "booked up" even weeks ahead, we might linger a moment to consider the implications of this doctor's statement. The first implication, that patients should be seen on the very day on which they call, need not detain us long. This depends on the urgency of the situation. A patient who has just developed a coronary thrombosis or meningitis must be seen with dispatch; a patient who has had a skin condition for the past six months and decides today that he would like his doctor to do something about it cannot justifiably feel aggrieved if he has to wait a day or two for an appointment.

Since the doctor who sees patients by appointment can, if he has time for an additional patient, tell a patient who calls and asks to be seen today to come in later this afternoon, the fear expressed by the doctor that he would "get booked up" so that patients would not be able to see him the same day suggests that a doctor can see more patients without an appointment system than he can see by appointment in the same amount of time. This was explicitly stated to be the case by one doctor and was implied by several others in Nova Scotia, who said that an appointment system was not practical because of the numbers of patients seen by them. From this one must conclude either that the amount of time allotted to each patient under the appointment system is too great (and this should be possible to correct without too much difficulty) or that doctors working without appointments are seeing some patients too briefly, the length of time given to each patient being determined perhaps by the number of patients to be seen on the particular day. Without any doubt, this is what happens in the outpatient departments of certain teaching hospitals when the staff is too small to cope with the number of patients.

In Nova Scotia, a number of doctors gave two other reasons for not having appointment systems, that patients had to come great distances from the farms and that it was not possible to have an appointment system for those who were employed in the mines either because it could not be co-ordinated with the miners' shifts or because the miners, being covered by a prepaid medical plan, thought that they should be seen whenever they wished to be seen. Since the latter statement has important implications for the future of medical care we shall comment upon it in chapter 26.

In describing the practitioners' office premises, we mentioned that 39 per cent of the Ontario, and 21 per cent of the Nova Scotia, doctors dispensed drugs. Only 19 per cent of the Ontario practitioners in places of over 10,000, but 67 per cent of those in places of 10,000 or less, did their own dispensing. The difference between the two groups is significant ($p < 0.01$). The corresponding figures in Nova Scotia, 6 per cent and 32 per cent, show that the trend is in the same direction, but the difference between places of more than 10,000 and places of 10,000 or less does not reach the level of statistical significance. Between the various age groups, there was no significant difference in either province in the matter of dispensing.

The doctors' attitudes towards dispensing varied from active enjoyment on the part of one man to dislike on the part of several others. Most of the Ontario men gave several reasons for having a dispensary. The most frequent was that, in the particular practice, to dispense was customary. One doctor stated that the tradition of a physician's practising and dispensing in his present premises extended back for 75 years. It was pointed out by some men that the dispensing of drugs by the doctor was a great convenience for the patient, especially if he needed the drugs at an hour when the drugstore was closed or if he lived, as patients out in the country did, at a distance from the drugstore. In 2 practices, the dispensing of drugs was not merely a convenience, but a necessity, since there was not a drugstore within

25 miles of either place. Each of these doctors found dispensing a nuisance, of which he would have been glad to be rid. One of them, whose dispensary was very well organized, explained that his inventory was worth about $1,700 and that taking stock, which had to be done several times a year, required his working right through the night.

Several doctors stated that dispensing maintained the contact between them and their patient, since the patient had to return to the doctor's office when he wished a refill. Other men, including one who would have liked to be rid of dispensing, said that patients were not willing to pay for the doctor's time and advice unless they received something tangible. Indeed, one doctor, who seemed to think that his patients expected it, dispensed something to everyone. Some men dispensed in order to save their patients from the pharmacists' prices, which they regarded as much too high. Reasons that were each mentioned only once were that the local pharmacist would not co-operate with the doctor in stocking what was needed, that dispensing was financially "worthwhile" for the doctor himself, and that the particular doctor found dispensing easier than prescription-writing, since he was "not too well up on this."

In contrast with their Ontario colleagues, the Nova Scotia physicians who had dispensaries each gave a single reason for this. Three-quarters of these men said that the nearest drugstore was many miles away. The remainder said that the check-off contract under which they cared for most of their patients required that they dispense drugs.

The keeping of clinical records, like so many other things, varied greatly from one practice to another. The *adequacy* of these will be discussed in the chapter on quality of practice. Here, we shall limit ourselves to describing the *methods* used by the various physicians. Of the Ontario practitioners, 20 per cent kept no clinical records at all and 7 per cent kept no records except for their obstetrical, and occasionally their paediatric, cases. The corresponding figures for Nova Scotia were 38 per cent and 14 per cent respectively. Of the physicians who kept records, well over half in each province recorded the data on cards, which varied in size from 3 by 5 inches to 8½ by 11 but were most frequently 5 by 8. The remainder kept their records on sheets of paper, 8½ inches by 11, which were filed in folders. A few doctors had had forms printed to their own specifications. These were used for the initial history and examination, and subsequent visits were recorded on plain sheets of paper. Occasionally, also, there were special forms for paediatric patients or for obstetrical patients.

Though the practitioners were not asked why they had chosen their particular method of keeping records, it appeared that cards of medium size were popular because of the greater ease with which they could be handled and stored. There is one serious disadvantage, however, to the use of cards: the difficulty of filing with them the numerous reports and letters that pertain to the particular case. Indeed, one doctor said that for this reason he was thinking of changing over from cards to paper and folders. Other expedients were to file the cards, either from the start or as soon as there were any extra papers, in folders or in envelopes. Still other doctors filed the cards in one place—in a drawer, in a Kardex holder, or on a wheel—and filed the reports and letters separately.

In dealing with members of one family, some physicians kept a separate folder or envelope for each member of the family, some had separate cards or sheets of paper for each individual but a single folder or envelope for the family, whereas some kept their notes about several members of the family on a single card or sheet of paper. This last method appeared unsatisfactory, since only with difficulty could the course of a particular member of the family be followed through the maze of entries.

Only the occasional doctor dictated his notes to be typed later by his secretary. For men who are too busy to write up detailed notes or who dislike writing, a dictating machine would appear to be a worth-while piece of equipment. One doctor, who made a habit of doing thorough physical examinations but was too busy to write out his findings, was able, by dictation, to keep excellent records containing not only the positive findings but significant negative findings. He dictated his notes immediately after seeing a patient, because, as he explained, he did not have a good enough memory to defer the dictation. This doctor used his machine also to instruct his nurse to make notes of things that should be attended to some days, or even weeks, later.

In discussing telephone-answering, appointments, the keeping of records, and the use of dictation, we have dealt with a few important items among the many that determine whether the conduct of the practice is efficient or not. We should mention also that it was surprising how few men delegated to their helpers such easy duties as the weighing of patients and the taking of temperatures. To illustrate how varied are the factors that must be considered in attempting to assess this aspect of a practice, we shall describe a few practices as we saw them in operation.

Dr. X was carrying on a solo practice, without either nursing or secretarial assistance, in a large city. At the beginning of a patient's visit, he might spend between five and ten minutes questioning the patient about what medicines he had been taking. While doing this, he would search through his record, sometimes reading parts of it aloud to himself. If he could not find a note of the medication, he would have to telephone the drugstore to find out what he had previously prescribed for the patient. At the end of one patient's visit, he spent ten minutes searching though a disorganized drawer of drug samples for an empty bottle in which he might give the patient a small portion of a sample. Having found a satisfactory bottle, he took several more minutes to wash it out, scrape off the label, dry it, and pour just the right amount of the sample into it.

His records were written on cards, but these were not kept in folders or envelopes. After he had followed a patient for some time, he might have used half a dozen cards, all of which were filed separately. In addition, he did not use markers to indicate the alphabetical divisions in his filing drawers. He stated that he now had so many cards filed under each letter that it was difficult to find a record quickly unless the patient's name began with X, Y, or Z. The observer repeatedly saw him take five minutes or more to find a patient's complete record. He did not seem to give any consideration to changing his filing system.

His records of charges made and of fees paid were as incomplete as his record of drugs prescribed. He expressed concern about whether he had given patients credit for payments that they had made and said that it was difficult for him to make up his statements to his patients at the end of the month. He did all his secretarial work himself, because he was trying to keep his overhead as low as possible.

When he stopped at a service station, where he obviously was known, he did not charge the cost of the gasoline but paid for it in cash. On his return to the office, after lunch, he got out his books and entered the amount that he had paid.

This doctor, who was a man of middle age, made no secret of the fact that he did not enjoy his practice. Perhaps better organization would not have increased his fondness for practice; but, if he had delegated to a secretary, to a pharmacist, and to the accounting department of an oil company those functions which they would have carried out much more efficiently than he, at least his burden would have been lightened.

Dr. Y's office appeared to function efficiently except in the keeping of financial records. At the end of each day, the doctor spent about an hour going through the records of all patients seen that day and writing out a list of the patients, of cash received, and of charges to be billed. This list could equally well have been compiled by his secretary; the doctor need only have decided upon the charge to be made. Lists of patients and fees were sent to a firm in another city, where the accounting was done. The patients' bills were sent out by the doctor's own secretary. When asked how the system worked, the doctor said that he did not understand it himself, that he was a "babe in the woods."

In two other offices, different physical arrangements could have saved the doctors many unnecessary steps. Dr. M's consulting room and examining room were at opposite ends of his suite. Though each room had a desk, the doctor used only the desk in the consulting room. This room, however, had no examining table. In order, then, to examine a patient in the reclining position, the doctor, after taking the patient's history at the desk in the consulting room, had to make his way to the examining table in the examining room, a distance of about forty feet. Because the doctor did not use his two rooms for alternate patients, it was necessary, also, for him to wait while patients undressed and dressed. Dr. N, on the other hand, had both his desk and an examining couch in his consulting room, in which he saw the majority of his patients. However, he kept his otoscope and his tongue depressors in his laboratory or in his examining room, which was used relatively seldom. To obtain these articles each time they were needed and to return them afterwards involved much unnecessary walking back and forth.

Dr. O's office suite had the unusual and highly fatiguing feature of being divided between two floors. Each patient was greeted by the doctor on the first floor, taken down to the basement for examination, and afterwards escorted back to the first floor.

Dr. Q, who worked more than 80 hours a week, drove more than 10 miles each way to tell a patient that it was time for him to come to the hospital to have further X-rays of a fracture. This doctor also visited at home a patient with an affection of the shoulder, which, though painful, was not so severe as to keep him in bed or as to preclude an office visit. In each of these cases, time that the physician desperately needed for his patients he used to drive unnecessary miles.

Of the many examples that we could cite of smoothly running offices, we have chosen two. Dr. C practised with a partner in a large city. They employed two nurses and a typist. One of the nurses answered the telephone, made appointments, and conducted patients from the waiting room to the rooms used by the doctor. The other nurse chaperoned female patients, laid out sterile trays for the doctor, and did whatever cleaning up was necessary between successive patients. The doctor alternated between his consulting room and his examining room. As soon as he had finished dictating his notes about the patient whom he had just seen, he proceeded to the other room where the nurse had another patient ready for him. The nurse had laid out the patient's record and, if it had seemed likely to her that an extensive examination would be necessary, she had had the patient undress before the doctor came in. The typist was employed on a part-time basis to type the case records that the doctor had dictated and to look after correspondence. When no one was in the office, the telephone was answered by an answering service.

Dr. D, on the other hand, was in practice by himself in a small town. His nurse answered the telephone and made appointments. When a telephone call had to be passed on to the doctor himself, she signalled by a buzzer. An intercommunication system made it possible for him to give her instructions without leaving his desk. At the beginning of the office hours, she set the patients' records on his desk, and she sent the patients into the consulting room as the doctor was ready for them. The arrangements made by Dr. D illustrates that an office can function efficiently without the advantages, which Dr. C had, of an answering service and of a partner to share the overhead.

Before we leave the doctors' offices, a few general comments and recommendations will be made. The office suites of many of the practitioners were of good quality on the average, though, in some of them, there were opportunities for improvements. A number of premises, on the other hand, could be regarded only as extremely unsatisfactory throughout. In two matters that concern patients' comfort—chaperoning and lavatory facilities—there was room for improvement in a substantial proportion of the offices. Other matters called for attention less often. Peterson, also noting great variation among the offices that he visited, considered almost a third of them "unacceptable for the use to which they were put" (see his page 105).

Though the Survey was planned to study quality of practice rather than the efficiency with which a practice was conducted—and, indeed, a detailed examination of each doctor's office arrangements would have been a large study by itself—nevertheless it was impossible to see so much of practice without being impressed with the efficiency of some practices and the inefficiency of others. In particular, it was surprising to find that 23 per cent of the Ontario practitioners and 40 per cent of those in Nova Scotia, almost all long-established, had no regular assistance in their offices and that it was the policy of 41 per cent of the Ontario, and 76 per cent of the Nova Scotia, doctors to see most, if not all, of their patients without appointments. The doctor's need for assistance in his office increases as the external pressures increase. These latter include the necessity for correspondence with consultants, hospitals, social agencies, and government agencies, the demand of government for accurate financial records for income tax purposes, and the demands of insurance companies and prepaid medical plans for reports on patients covered by these plans, to name only some of the many pressures that were virtually unknown to the doctor of fifty years ago.

We must mention especially two modern conditions that, in combination, have a particularly disturbing, if not disrupting, effect on practice. These are the ubiquity of the telephone and the average person's greater concern about his health today than at any time in the past. Whether the latter stems more from the public's awareness of medical advances or from a shift in interest from the life hereafter to the present life, as the present life attains a degree of security unknown in earlier ages, is immaterial. The fact remains that doctors are called today about myriads of details which no one, a generation or two ago, would have thought an adequate reason for a consultation.

The adverse effect of the telephone is twofold. People who would consider their question unimportant if they had to walk even one block to ask it are able, by means of the telephone, to bridge the distance effortlessly at any hour. Some members of the public are thoughtful in their use of the telephone, others thoughtless. So great is the public's concern with things medical that even otherwise thoughtful, responsible persons may at times abuse the telephone. Secondly, the telephone has a psychological effect that completes its tyranny. Very few persons would dream of not answering the telephone. This is well illustrated by the observation, recently made to us by a prominent member of the legal profession, that a colleague who would resent being interrupted by a knock at the door would raise no protest at the same degree of interruption by telephone. A doctor, any one of whose calls *may* be urgent, is even less able to deny the telephone. Yet repeated interruptions of a consultation are distracting to a doctor, whose attention should be concentrated on his patient, and may be keenly resented by the patient, who suspects that the doctor has only half a mind for him. Since it is as unlikely that thoughtless use of the telephone will decrease as it is that the telephone itself will disappear, a doctor's telephone will continue to ring endlessly. This must be accepted as a condition of modern medical practice. For this reason, if for no other, it is essential that a doctor have assistance in his office and perhaps also make more use than at present of telephone-answering services.

Turning now to the matter of appointments, we can see very little justification for doctors' continuing to operate their practices without appointments, except in a few isolated communities where telephone service is poor. To the doctor who says that he is "always here and available," it is perhaps fair to put the question, "Are you really available when a patient has to sit and wait several hours in a crowded waiting room?" Except in urgent cases or with patients who have come long distances, there would appear to be little reason why patients whose conditions could not be handled fully in the allotted time should not be requested to come back in a day or two when the necessary time would be set aside. In this way, a doctor would not be faced with the alternative either of giving insufficient time and thought to the present case or of keeping his other patients waiting unduly long.

We have dwelt at some length on the efficiency of the conduct of the practices, because we think that, in this area, doctors have lagged behind the rest of the community. Since there are likely those who will decry efficiency as cold and inconsistent with humanity, we would point out that for a doctor to save himself unnecessary steps or to save himself interruptions from a continually ringing telephone does not make him less human but does allow him to have *more* time to deal with his patient.

# 7 / Arrangements for Practice
## Outside the Office

The previous chapter limited itself, with minor exceptions, to the physician's own office. In the present chapter, we shall consider those arrangements that entail relationships with professional individuals or groups outside the physician's office: with other general practitioners, consultants, laboratories, the provincial department of health, and the local medical officer of health. One organization, the hospital, because of its special importance to the physician, we shall treat in a separate chapter.

Owing to the nature of the physician's work, some of his arrangements are determined by the physical distance between him and his nearest colleague. In particular, his ability to arrange time off, whether for recreation or for study, depends on the availability of a standby. So unpredictable are emergencies, including obstetrical deliveries, that the practitioner who has no colleague within a reasonable distance can hardly absent himself for a few hours, let alone the time necessary for a vacation or for attendance at a medical convention or a postgraduate course. On the other hand, the practitioner with a colleague close at hand is able, in theory at any rate, not only to arrange for time off duty, but also to call on his colleague for assistance with procedures that he cannot carry out single-handed and for a second opinion in difficult cases.

To determine to what extent physical isolation was a problem, we asked each doctor how far away his nearest colleague was located. Forty-one of the 44 Ontario doctors and 38 of the 42 Nova Scotia doctors were not more than one mile from their medical neighbours.

Those who were more widely separated from their colleagues constituted approximately 7 per cent and 10 per cent of the Ontario and
the Nova Scotia practitioners, respectively, the most isolated doctor
being 30 miles from his nearest colleague. When 95 per cent confidence
limits are set,* the upper limit, for the percentage of general practitioners who are more than one mile from the nearest colleague, is 19
per cent for the Ontario group and 24 per cent for the Nova Scotia
group. Thus we can feel reasonably confident that not more than one-
fifth of the Ontario general practitioners, and not more than one-
quarter of the Nova Scotia general practitioners, from whom the
samples were drawn are more than a mile from another physician,
and the fractions may well be much smaller than these.

When the practitioners are considered from the point of view of
the relationship that exists between each of them and the other
general practitioners in the area, they appear to fall into three groups.
Those practising as members of groups of two or more (details of
which are shown in Table 14) made up 34 per cent of the Ontario,

TABLE 14

DISTRIBUTION OF ONTARIO AND NOVA SCOTIA PHYSICIANS
BY SIZE OF GROUP

| Type of practice | Ontario physicians | | Nova Scotia physicians | |
|---|---|---|---|---|
| | Number | % | Number | % |
| Solo—no arrangements with other doctors during time off | 9 | 20.5 | 4 | 9.5 |
| Solo—arrangements with other doctors to cover practice | 20 | 45.5 | 24 | 57.1 |
| Group of two | 9 | 20.5 | 4 | 9.5 |
| Group of three, four, or five | 5 | 11.4 | 6 | 14.3 |
| Group of six or more | 1 | 2.3 | 4 | 9.5 |
| Total physicians | 44 | 100 | 42 | 100 |

and 33 per cent of the Nova Scotia, physicians. Those who were
engaged in solo practice but made arrangements with other doctors
to cover their practices whenever they were not available constituted
45 per cent and 57 per cent of the Ontario and the Nova Scotia
practitioners, respectively. The remaining doctors, 20 per cent in
Ontario and 10 per cent in Nova Scotia, were in solo practice but did
not have such arrangements with other doctors. It is interesting to
note than men belonging to groups of two or more made up a

*For an explanation of this term, see page 32.

comparable proportion (27 per cent) of the practitioners studied by Peterson in North Carolina.°

Each of the doctors was asked to state the advantages and the disadvantages of his type of practice. Of the 13 men who were practising entirely on their own, 6 did not name any advantage of this type of practice. Of the other 7, one man said that he could make more money alone than in a partnership; another was able to meet the demands of certain personal and domestic circumstances in a way that might not have been possible had he had to consider the interests of a partner or of a group; and the remainder felt that it was an advantage to be "independent" or to be one's "own boss." An additional reason given by one doctor was that working alone helped him by increasing his self-confidence.

Of the disadvantages of solo practice, the one mentioned by most of the doctors was that one was always on call, that there was no time off. Another disadvantage, named by several men, was the lack of another doctor to talk to. They amplified this by saying that they would have liked to have a colleague to share the worry of difficult cases; and one wished that he had a colleague to stimulate his interest in medicine. One practitioner who was 30 miles from his nearest medical neighbour mentioned the inconvenience of making arrangements when he needed this doctor to assist him with operative procedures. Only two doctors found solo practice without any disadvantages. The attitude of one of these men is best given in his own words: "None [i.e., disadvantages] as far as I'm concerned. I don't mind being on call twenty-four hours a day. I don't mind working four evenings a week. What else would I do? I'm not socially inclined and I haven't any particular hobbies."

When the 20 Ontario physicians who were in solo practice but who arranged with other men to take their calls during their time off duty were questioned as to the advantages of *their* type of practice, more than three-quarters of them mentioned one or both of two advantages that are probably really different facets of the same attitude. These were their wish to be their "own boss" and their fear of personal friction, or of differences arising out of management of patients, or of legal or financial entanglements, if they had to work closely with someone else. These fears were expressed in such statements as, "I've never seen a partnership yet that worked" and "I just don't trust clinics." One younger man, however, though stating

°O. L. Peterson *et al.*: Journal of Medical Education, *31*, No. 12, Part 2: 1–165, 1956; see his page 100.

his wish to be independent, gave as his opinion that solo practice was "out of date."

Several other advantages of this type of practice were named, but only once or twice each. Two men derived satisfaction from the knowledge that they were personally responsible for the practice. One doctor pointed out the closeness of the relationship possible between doctor and patient; another said that patients wanted their "own doctor" and were not happy when the calls were taken by another man, as would occur in a group practice. One physician was pleased that, except at vacation time, there was no need, as there would be in a group practice, to arrange work schedules with others, but that during his vacations colleagues designated by him covered his practice efficiently. Only one doctor mentioned the possibility of making arrangements to be off duty at times other than his vacation. Financially, this type of practice was considered superior to group practice by two doctors, one of whom, however, would gladly have accepted the lower income that he thought would be likely with a group, in order to have better working hours.

Of the 24 Nova Scotia physicians who were in solo practice but who made arrangements with colleagues to take their calls during time off, about two-thirds said, as did their counterparts in Ontario, that the advantage of this type of practice was that they were independent or were their "own boss." Unlike the men in Ontario, however, the Nova Scotians did not make any mention of fear of friction or of legal entanglements if they were to engage in group practice. Two of those who liked to be independent added that it was an advantage to have the responsibility of practice all to themselves. Another doctor, who thought that he could accomplish more by being on his own and retaining his initiative, said, "Competition is the driving force to work, even in medical practice." Only two doctors mentioned as an advantage that it was possible to arrange to be off duty; these carried on solo practices but each shared an office suite and secretarial services with a colleague. These men both said, too, that this type of arrangement reduced their expenses. About one-quarter of the Nova Scotia doctors who were in solo practice but arranged for their practices to be covered did not name any advantage of this type of practice.

Of the disadvantages of this type of practice, one was mentioned by 60 per cent of the Ontario doctors and by 75 per cent of those in Nova Scotia: the long hours on call. The doctors felt that they were tied twenty-four hours a day, seven days a week, except when they signed out to another doctor, and this they hesitated to do with any frequency. It was pointed out by some of them that being on call, i.e. knowing that the telephone might ring at any time, was as much of a strain as actually working and that this uncertainty interfered with reading and studying, was hard on family life, and made social activities difficult, especilly such activities as golf or bridge which called for definite commitments. Even more difficult was arranging to be away long enough to attend postgraduate courses. The coup de grâce of continuous, unrelieved hours, days, and weeks on call was thought by one doctor to be the obstetrical delivery, which, coming after a long day at the office, was "killing."

Other disadvantges that were mentioned by one or another doctor were inability of the doctor to be available at all times (since he might already be tied up by a case or might be ill himself), periodic inability to handle the volume of practice, difficulty at times in finding another doctor to cover his calls, financial loss if he took time off, the high cost of providing the necessary facilities and services to carry on practice by himself, and the fact that no colleague was closely enough associated with him to share his worries in difficult cases and to keep a critical eye on the quality of his work.

Finally, of the 44 doctors who practised alone but arranged at times for other doctors to cover their practices for them, 5 in Ontario and 4 in Nova Scotia said that there was no disadvantage to this type of practice. One of these men delegated almost all of his night work to a younger man who had his own independent practice; one had no strong objection to evening office hours or to night calls, except "silly ones"; and one appeared rather to welcome the long hours, since, as he said, he never read and had no interest in television but liked to be with people and to be "on the go."

When we compare the two groups of physicians that have been described so far, those who practised entirely on their own and those who practised by themselves but arranged at times to have other men cover their practices for them, the two groups show a remarkable similarity. The principal advantage mentioned by each group was the independence of the individual physician. The principal disadvantage, given by more than half of each group, was that the doctor was tied almost continuously to his practice, that it was next to impossible to arrange free time for study, non-medical interests, and family. Thus, although initially these appeared to be two distinct groups, the distinction turns out to be less than might have been expected, in that those who had reciprocal arrangements with colleagues had not developed this system to anything like full advantage (see also pages 111–112).

The surprising thing is that, though so many doctors complained about the long hours and the lack of free time and though more than 90 per cent of those in each province were within a mile of a colleague, there was little evidence that they were attempting to improve the conditions of practice. Certainly, of those practitioners who had their own individual offices (i.e., who were not members of groups), it was only the occasional one, in either province, who had an arrangement, or indicated that he ever had had an arrangement, with one or two other men whereby they covered one another's practices on a *regular* rotational system. Since we did not specifically ask each doctor why he did not work out a more satisfactory system with his colleagues, our clues are few. One man who was on his own said that he hesitated to ask his "competitors" to take his calls. It may be mere coincidence that he spoke of "competitors" instead of colleagues, or his choice of the word may have indicated a distrust that was the counterpart of the lack of concern expressed by another doctor, a member of a group, when he said that an advantage of belonging to a group was that one's practice was covered in one's absence and yet was handed back on one's return. Another possible reason for not arranging to have another doctor take one's calls might be lack of confidence in the other's professional ability, though none of the doctors visited made such a suggestion. Other possible explanations are lack of originality and adherence to tradition.

Having considered those physicians who were practising entirely on their own and those who were in solo practice but made arrangements with other doctors to cover their practices at times, we turn now to the third group, the 15 Ontario physicians and the 14 Nova Scotia physicians who were practising in association with one or more other physicians. Two advantages of this type of practice were each claimed by more than half of the group in each province. First, it was possible to schedule working hours and time off. Thus the schedule could make provision for evenings, nights, week-ends, and holidays. Several men stressed both their own and their patients' peace of mind at knowing that the practice was covered at all times. As a result of this, the doctors felt that they could take longer holidays and attend postgraduate courses more frequently. The other advantage frequently mentioned was the fact that another opinion was always available to the doctor without the inconvenience, delay, and expense involved in a formal referral by a solo practitioner. The amount of moral support, however, that could be derived from an associate depended on his status in relation to one's own. In usual circumstances, neither a salaried assistant nor a very much junior partner could share responsibility to any significant degree.

Just as some of the men in solo practice would have liked to have someone to talk to, so several of the men belonging to groups said that they enjoyed the stimulation and the companionship. One man said that it was "not so lonely," another that "on my own, I often dreaded going to the office; now I look forward to it." One source of stimulation was said to be the fact that the individual doctor was able to see a greater number of interesting and unusual cases, since he saw such cases from his colleagues' practices as well as from his own. Other advantages of group practice were occasionally mentioned: that emergencies could be covered more quickly; that assistance was always available for those procedures that a doctor could not expeditiously carry out single-handed; that each man in the group, while carrying on a general practice, could concentrate on a field in which he was particularly interested; and that, if one were sick, one's patients would still receive satisfactory medical care. Against the possibility of being overwhelmed during peak periods, one doctor had made quite unusual provision, which would not have been possible had he been working alone. He and another doctor located several hundred miles away, each of whom had an associate in his office, had an agreement to go to each other's assistance in times of need or to send the associate.

On the economic side, group practice was considered to have a number of advantages. Since costs were shared, it was thought possible for a doctor to have better facilities than he could provide on his own and to have a higher income. (The reader is reminded that several of the solo practitioners thought that *their* type of practice produced a higher income.) Absence from work did not result in financial loss, and expenses of postgraduate courses, it was said, were paid by the group instead of by the individual. Other advantages were said to be that there was no "throat-cutting" during one's time off, that one had a guaranteed income from the beginning of the association with an established group, and that there was security for old age in that the younger members of the group sustained the older men's incomes. One doctor introduced a somewhat ghoulish note when he said that partnership gave an introduction to many more patients in the event of the partner's death.

Two of the advantages listed above call for comment. The fact that the group, rather than the individual doctor, pays the expenses of postgraduate courses is probably a psychological, rather than a real, advantage of group practice as contrasted with solo practice, since, if each member's expenses for courses are roughly the same, each is really paying his own expenses whether he pays from his own pocket or from the group's profits before distribution. In the matter of absence from work, however, whether because of illness, postgraduate study, or vacation, the member of a group has a real advantage over the solo practitioner, since the other members of the group, by taking over his work, are, in effect, protecting him against financial loss during his absence. This type of mutual insurance is particularly effective in allaying his apprehension lest his own income might suddenly be cut off by illness.

One practitioner who employed a salaried assistant stated, as an advantage of this type of practice, that the assistant "screened" the majority of the patients and took care of the "routine things," so that he himself was left with more time to deal with more difficult cases. We found it surprising that no mention was made of this by any other physician. Of this, we shall have more to say in chapter 26.

We turn now to the reported disadvantages of practising with one or more other doctors. Five of the 15 Ontario men and 4 of the 14 in Nova Scotia said that there was no disadvantage. Many of the others mentioned the problem of disagreements between the members of the group. Matters over which differences might arise were said to include organization of the practice, medical standards, and honesty. The apportionment of the work tended to be difficult, since one man was likely to feel that he was doing more than his share. What has been described above as the security that group practice offers the older doctor was regarded quite differently by a younger man, who said that his elderly partner intended to do less and less so that the younger man felt that in the near future he would be "carrying" the older man as far as both work and income were concerned. Peterson (see his page 117) reports that some of the physicians in North Carolina who started practice in association with an older doctor stated that "they had to do all the work and the older doctor took all the money," whereas established physicians "often complained that younger partners wanted larger salaries but did not want to do the work necessary to earn them." One of our doctors pointed out that the junior partner had to be willing to be subservient. This man was one who had stated, as an advantage of group practice, that a regular schedule could be arranged but who, as the junior man—he was not yet fifty—found this advantage largely negated by the fact that he was required to do almost all the night work. The subservience of another

man who was a junior partner was apparent in the fact that, though
he wished to have an appointment system, he had not yet been able
to institute it because his senior partner had never had one. As some
of the men made clear, to practise in association with others required
some sacrifice of personal independence. The advice given by one
man who seemed satisfied with his arrangements was, "Everything
should be down in black and white." To this might be added the
sound observation of one older man that the doctors' wives must not
interfere.

Several doctors thought that they would have made more money
on their own than they were making as members of groups. It was
suggested occasionally that group practice tended to reduce the
individual doctor's initiative and competitiveness. A disadvantage of
a group from a patient's point of view was said to be that the patient
who does not like his doctor cannot without embarrassment switch
to another member of the same group. Finally, a disadvantage that
was mentioned by only one of the men who had salaried assistants and
by none who had junior partners was responsibility of the older man
for the younger man's mistakes.

From the general practitioner's working relationships with other
general practitioners, we turn our attention now to the consultants to
whom he referred difficult cases. Other aspects of the relationship
between general practitioner and specialist will be discussed in later
chapters. Here we limit ourselves to ascertaining whether facilities
for consultation were available in the referring physician's own community or whether he had to refer a patient to a physician in another
community when he needed a consultant's services in one or another
branch of medicine. In order to collect the data, we asked each of the
general practitioners in what communities were located the consultants
to whom he usually referred patients. The consultants named by the
practitioners have been divided into those located in the same community as the referring doctor and those located elsewhere.

The divisions of medicine about which the practitioners were
questioned as to referrals were internal medicine, surgery, obstetrics,
paediatrics, ophthalmology, otolaryngology, and diagnostic radiology.
In communities of 10,000 or less, both in Ontario and in Nova Scotia,
the vast majority of referrals were made to physicians located elsewhere, i.e. in larger cities, except in the case of diagnostic radiology,
of which we shall say more presently. In communities of between
10,000 and 33,000, almost all the paediatric referrals were made to

physicians located in larger cities; almost all the referrals in ophthalmology, otolaryngology, and diagnostic radiology were made within
the referring physician's own community; and internal medicine and
surgery occupied an intermediate position, some referrals being made
within the community and some being made to physicians located
elsewhere. Obstetrical problems in Ontario communities of this size
were referred within the community and out of the community by
equal numbers of doctors, whereas, in Nova Scotia, 6 physicians out
of 7 referred their obstetrical problems within their own communities;
but the difference between the two provinces is not statistically significant. In cities of between 33,000 and 100,000, all of which were
located in Ontario, referrals to doctors in other communities became
less common in relation to referrals made within the referring physician's own city. In cities of over 100,000, there were said to be few
referrals out of town, presumably only in those cases that demanded
the facilities of a large medical centre.

It is interesting to note that some Ontario cities, with populations
of between 10,000 and 33,000, which could not perhaps have provided
enough work to support a full-time ophthalmologist or otolaryngologist, were served on a part-time basis by consultants in these fields,
who visited the cities at certain specified times each week. No mention of such arrangements was made by the Nova Scotia doctors. In
both provinces, however, some smaller communities were served
by radiologists from larger cities, who visited once or twice a week
to interpret films and to carry out examinations requiring their
special skill. Almost all the physicians in cities of 10,000 or more, and
more than half of those in communities of between 3,300 and 10,000,
had a radiologist available, at least on a part-time basis, in their own
community. A radiologist's services were not available in any of the
Ontario communities visited that had populations of 3,300 or less,
but were available on a part-time basis in certain of the Nova Scotia
communities of this size. The difference between the two provinces
was not statistically significant.

In the previous chapter, the laboratory facilities of the physician's
own office were described; but all of the laboratory work in pathology
and serology, most of the work in bacteriology, and a good many
of the haematological and chemical tests demand more specialized
training and more elaborate equipment than are possessed by any
but the most exceptional practising physicians. Each of the physicians
was asked where he had these types of laboratory work done. Forty
of the 44 Ontario physicians made use both of the laboratories of the

Department of Health of the Province of Ontario and of the laboratories in their local hospitals, and 3 relied entirely on the Provincial Department of Health. One practitioner had no laboratory work done, beyond the few simple tests that he performed in his own office, as he thought that there was "no need" for it. One other doctor, who made use of the facilities of the Provincial Department for chemical and serological work, never required any bacteriological or pathological tests. Of the 41 Nova Scotia doctors who answered the question, 7 depended entirely on the laboratories in their hospitals, 4 used only the facilities of the Department of Health of Nova Scotia or of Dalhousie University, and the remaining 30 had their laboratory work done both in the laboratories of their hospitals and in the laboratories of the Department of Health or of the University.

When they were questioned further about the use that they made of the services of the Provincial Department of Health, 98 per cent of the Ontario practitioners said that they used them frequently. All except the occasional doctor made use of the laboratory service, about one-fifth mentioned that they obtained immunizing agents from the Department, and several men stated that they used such services as the provision of free insulin for indigent patients, the advice and the free penicillin that may be obtained for the treatment of syphilitic patients, the booklets that are available for distribution to patients, and the facilities of the chest clinics. Fifteen of the doctors did not indicate whether they were satisfied or dissatisfied with the Department's services. The comments of the remainder ranged from "satisfactory" and "no complaints" through "good" (the comment of half of the doctors) to "excellent" and "invaluable." In particular, there was appreciation of the rapidity with which the results of important tests, such as cultures of blood and of spinal fluid, were reported.

In Nova Scotia, the services of the Provincial Department of Health were said by 81 per cent of the physicians to be used frequently, by the remainder seldom. Almost all of those who made frequent use of the Department obtained their immunizing agents from it and made use of it for help of one sort or another in the management of cases, or suspected cases, of tuberculosis. Many doctors said, also, that they used the Department's laboratory service. Occasionally physicians said that they turned to the Department for advice about infectious diseases other than tuberculosis, for literature on health education, and to obtain penicillin for syphilitics. About one-quarter of the doctors did not comment on the Department; most of the remainder expressed satisfaction with what was being done. A few men showed some resentment at the Department's tendency to interest itself in matters that these doctors thought should be left to the private practitioner. One doctor, half in earnest, half in jest, said, "If the preventive medicine men keep on, they will eliminate all the work of the G.P. The only thing they can't prevent is obstetric work."

Since matters of public health at the local level are in the hands of a medical officer of health for the community, it was deemed appropriate to inquire about the relationship between him and the general practitioners. The two questions asked were, "How often do you make use of the local medical officer of health? Never? Seldom? Or frequently?" and "What use do you make of him?"

These questions were not applicable to 9 of the doctors in each of the two provinces, because either they were the local medical officers of health themselves or else they did the work for partners who were the actual incumbents. Of the remainder, 9 per cent in Ontario and 41 per cent in Nova Scotia said that they "never" used the medical officer of health, 74 per cent in Ontario and 47 per cent in Nova Scotia that they used him "seldom," and 17 per cent in Ontario and 12 per cent in Nova Scotia "frequently." Almost half of the doctors in each province had no contact with him, except the reporting to him of certain communicable diseases, as is required by law. (In passing, we might remark that several of these practitioners stated that their reporting of these cases was "occasional" or "often neglected.") Each of the remaining practitioners named one or more ways in which the medical officer of health was of use to him, although many of them availed themselves of his services "seldom." The most frequently mentioned help given by him in Ontario was making arrangements for transportation and admission of patients to mental hospitals and to hospitals for tuberculosis or other infectious diseases. He was also helpful in arranging visits to mental health clinics, chest clinics, and well-baby clinics. Advice was said to have been sought from him on a variety of subjects, including contagious diseases, isolation and quarantine, immunization, and contaminated wells. Finally, his help was requested in epidemics and outbreaks of food poisoning. In Nova Scotia, only rarely did a practitioner mention any use that he made of the local medical officer of health except the obtaining of advice about the handling of cases of tuberculosis or other infectious diseases.

Sixteen physicians in Ontario did not express any opinion on the ability of their medical officers of health. Four were most unenthusiastic, complaining that these men had no interest in medicine, were deficient in their medical knowledge, had queer personality problems, or never attended meetings—in short, that they hardly seemed to belong to the medical community. The remaining 15 practitioners described their local medical officers of health as good.

In Nova Scotia, 18 doctors made no comments on their local medical officers of health, 3 regarded them as satisfactory, and 3 were neutral in their remarks. Three, including a former local medical officer of health, felt that the position was superfluous, that problems having to do with water supply and sewage disposal could be handled much better by the provincial department's sanitary inspector than by a local doctor. The remaining 6 doctors regarded their medical officers of health as unsatisfactory. Such remarks were made as "the local MOH knows no more about public health problems than I do," "he's a politician, who never sees or recognizes situations in which the MOH is required," and, in several cases, "he's an old retired G.P." who was described as "hitting the bottle" or as not being "on the ball."

We shall conclude this chapter with a discussion of one oft-forgotten activity that deserves mention because it consumes much of some general practitioners' time, namely, the driving of their automobiles on calls. Each of the men was asked to state approximately his annual milage in connection with his practice. In Ontario, the answers varied between 1,000 and 30,000 miles; in Nova Scotia, between 4,000 and 40,000 miles. A few doctors were located in regions where the roads were so few that driving was automatically limited. At the other end of the scale were doctors whose visits to their hospitals, quite apart from any house calls that they might make, called for forty to fifty miles of driving daily. The Ontario physicians had a mean milage, exclusive of driving done for pleasure or other personal reasons, of approximately 11,400 miles; the mean for the Nova Scotia physicians was approximately 16,500 miles. The considerably greater mean milage of the Nova Scotia physicians may be accounted for by the fact that, whereas the Ontario physicians reported a total of 661 home visits made during a period of 290 days, the men in Nova Scotia reported 1,102 home visits made during a period of 253 days. (See Table 58, on pages 242–243.)

In Table 15 are shown the milages of the physicians in communities of different sizes in Ontario and in Nova Scotia. We would point out that the mean milage of the Ontario physicians in communities of between 10,000 and 100,000 was very much lower, and the mean milage of the Nova Scotia physicians in communities of 1,000 or less

TABLE 15
DISTRIBUTION OF PHYSICIANS ACCORDING TO ANNUAL
PRACTICE MILAGE AND POPULATION OF COMMUNITY

| Population of community | Thousands of miles of driving | | | | | | Mean practice milage (thousands) |
|---|---|---|---|---|---|---|---|
| | 0–5.0 | 5.1–10.0 | 10.1–15.0 | 15.1–20.0 | 20.1–30.0 | 30.1–40.0 | |
| A. *Ontario* | | | | | | | |
| Over 500,000 | 0 | 1 | 5 | 1 | 0 | 0 | 12.9 |
| 100,001 to 500,000 | 0 | 1 | 2 | 1 | 0 | 0 | 12.8 |
| 10,001 to 100,000 | 1 | 13 | 1 | 0 | 0 | 0 | 7.9 |
| 1,001 to 10,000 | 3 | 2 | 5 | 3 | 1 | 0 | 12.7 |
| 1,000 and under | 0 | 0 | 2 | 2 | 0 | 0 | 16.3 |
| Totals | 4 | 17 | 15 | 7 | 1 | 0 | 11.4 |
| B. *Nova Scotia* | | | | | | | |
| 100,001 to 500,000 | 0 | 0 | 7 | 0 | 1 | 0 | 13.5 |
| 10,001 to 100,000 | 0 | 3 | 3 | 2 | 0 | 0 | 12.3 |
| 1,001 to 10,000 | 2 | 4 | 5 | 3 | 2 | 1 | 15.3 |
| 1,000 and under | 0 | 0 | 2 | 1 | 2 | 3 | 26.0 |
| Totals | 2 | 7 | 17 | 6 | 5 | 4 | 16.5 |

very much higher, than the mean milages of their confrères in communities of other sizes. Whether these differences can be ascribed to differences in the number of home visits made by the physicians, we are unable to say with the data available to us.

Miles, in themselves, have little meaning. If it is assumed, however, that, in cities of 10,000 or more, a physician is unable to average more than 25 miles an hour, and that, in communities of less than 10,000, he is unable, even with the greater amount of rural driving, to average more than 40 miles an hour, and if 8 hours is taken as today's usual working-day, then the average general practitioner in cities of over 100,000 in Ontario spends roughly 64 entire working-days each year just driving his car. His colleagues in Ontario communities of between 10,000 and 100,000, of between 1,000 and 10,000, and of 1,000 or less spend approximately 40 days, 40 days, and 51 days, respectively, in this activity. The corresponding figures for Nova Scotia are approximately 67 days, 61 days, 48 days, and 81 days. These estimates are probably conservative, since it is unlikely, when starts, stops, and the traffic congestion especially of the larger cities are taken into account, that the average speeds suggested above can be achieved.

In considering the efficiency with which the available medical manpower is used, we cannot but wonder whether there is not great and unnecessary waste here. No one in his senses would dream of employing a physician to drive a taxi or a bus, because this would be wasting years of training. Yet this, in effect, is exactly what is being done when a doctor is asked to make *unnecessary* house calls. By "unnecessary" we mean those calls that are made to a patient's house for other than medical reasons. What are these reasons? Usually they can be reduced to the fact that it is more convenient for a patient to have his doctor come to him or her than to make the arrangements at home and for transportation that a visit to the physician's office may necessitate. Examples have already been given (see page 78). Another physician, in a large city, was requested to visit a home five or six miles distant for the sole purpose of giving an injection of tetanus toxoid to a child who had a very minor injury and could just as well have been brought to the physician's office. Since the family owned a car and since the father was home when the physician arrived, the major portion of the time taken up by that case was spent by the physician functioning, not as a physician, but as an errand boy.

Lest our position be misunderstood, we wish to make quite clear that we believe that those patients who for *medical* reasons cannot come to the physician's office should certainly be visited at home. We think, however, that many house calls are not medically necessary. In so far as they are not, they represent an inefficient and extravagant use of physicians' time.

# 8 / Arrangements for Practice
## *Time*

In describing the arrangements made by the physicians within their own offices and in their dealings with individuals and groups beyond their offices, we have here and there touched upon their use of time. We shall now examine in some detail the ways in which the general practitioners we observed organized their time.

In this, as in so many other things, there were both similarities and differences. Most of the doctors we visited made rounds on their hospitalized patients during the morning. At this time they checked on their patient's condition, received the results of laboratory tests, and saw whatever X-ray films had been taken since the previous visit. Whatever anaesthesia and elective surgery they did were usually done in the morning; but many of the doctors did little or none of either. Most of the men made a practice of dropping in to the doctors' room for a cup of coffee sometime in the course of the morning. These contacts, partly professional, partly social, with their colleagues seemed to serve the purpose of counteracting, at least to some extent, the solo pracitioners' loneliness, of which mention was made in the preceding chapter. A small number of doctors, however, spent such a disproportionate amount of time in the doctors' room each day that it could be regarded only as a waste.

If part of the morning remained after the visit to the hospital or hospitals, this might be used by the doctor to make house calls, to see a few patients in the office, or to open his mail and attend to paper work of one sort or another.

The picture that we have given of the "average" morning is subject to many variations. Sometimes a meeting, either of the entire medical staff of the hospital or of a committee on which the doctor served, might take an hour out of a morning. The occasional practitioner who was on the staff of a teaching hospital associated with a medical school might serve, part of one or two mornings a week, in one or another of the hospital's clinics. A few doctors, who had hospital privileges but who seemed to make little effort to maintain contact with their hospitals, did not make any hospital visits in the course of our stays with them. Their mornings might be spent on house calls, office visits, or on pursuits that had nothing to do with medicine, as in the case of one doctor whose professional work rarely began before two o'clock in the afternoon.

The mid-day meal varied greatly. Some men took as much as an hour and a half or two hours at lunch time, so that they were able to relax during their meal, and then read the paper, watch television, or perhaps play with their children. In other homes, the observer had barely finished answering his hostess's hurried inquiries about the Survey before the practitioner's "Come on, doctor; let's be on our way" forced him to cram a whole sandwich into his mouth and wash it down at one gulp with a cup of boiling coffee. The usual lunch time, however, was about an hour—time to get home, wash, and eat comfortably, but no time for anything else.

It was virtually universal practice to have office hours during the afternoons of the week-days,\* except Wednesday or Thursday afternoon, on one or other of which some doctors were off duty. Usually the office hours began about two o'clock. In some offices, they might end around five o'clock or half past, whereupon the doctor might make a house call or two or might go straight home. Other men might not complete their afternoon office work until seven or half past or even, occasionally, as late as eight o'clock.

The evening meal, like the noon one, might be relaxed or might be rushed. It was likely to be the latter if a busy evening lay ahead. Sixty-eight per cent of the Ontario, and 93 per cent of the Nova Scotia, physicians had office hours at least one evening between Monday and Friday. The difference between the two provinces is significant ($p < 0.01$).† Even more striking, however, is the difference between the two Canadian provinces and North Carolina, where only 7 per cent of Peterson's practitioners "maintained formal office hours during

---

\*Throughout this chapter the words, "week-days" and "week-nights," are to be understood to mean the five days, Monday to Friday inclusive.
†This is explained on pages 32–33.

TABLE 16

FREQUENCY OF EVENING OFFICE HOURS OF ONTARIO AND NOVA SCOTIA PHYSICIANS

| Number of evenings on which physician had office hours (Monday to Friday) | Ontario physicians | | Nova Scotia physicians | |
|---|---|---|---|---|
| | Number | % | Number | % |
| None | 13 | 29.5 | 2 | 4.8 |
| One per week | 3 | 6.8 | 1 | 2.4 |
| Three in two weeks | 1 | 2.3 | 1 | 2.4 |
| Two per week | 9 | 20.5 | 9 | 21.4 |
| Three per week | 4 | 9.1 | 9 | 21.4 |
| Four per week | 9 | 20.5 | 8 | 19.0 |
| Nine in two weeks | 1 | 2.3 | 0 | 0.0 |
| Five per week | 3 | 6.8 | 11 | 26.2 |
| No set times | 1 | 2.3 | — | — |
| Unknown | — | — | 1 | 2.4 |
| Total | 44 | 100 | 42 | 100 |

the evening."* As is shown in Table 16, the three commonest patterns in Ontario were no evening office hours (in 30 per cent of the practices), office hours on 2 evenings a week (in 20 per cent), and on 4 evenings a week (in 20 per cent), whereas, in Nova Scotia, the great majority of the practitioners were divided fairly evenly into those with office hours on 5 evenings a week (26 per cent), 4 evenings (19 per cent), 3 evenings (21 per cent), and 2 evenings (21 per cent). Since some physicians had had their evening meal and were ready to start their evening office hours by half past six or seven o'clock, whereas others were only completing their afternoon office work by that time, we have arbitrarily defined evening office hours as those occurring after the evening meal. These hours usually began abou seven or eight o'clock. In some offices, the work was completed by nine o'clock or even earlier; in others, the doctor was still seeing patients at half past ten or eleven.

On Saturday, some physicians tried to complete their routine work by the middle of the day and to deal later only with urgent cases, but other physicians had office hours during the afternoon and some also during the evening. Twenty-three per cent of the Ontario practitioners and 33 per cent of those in Nova Scotia had both afternoon and evening office hours on Saturday. Roughly 40 per cent in each province had afternoon, but not evening, hours. Thirty-six per cent in Ontario and 21 per cent in Nova Scotia had no Saturday office hours after mid-day. The two provinces did not differ significantly with respect either to the percentage of physicians who had Saturday

*O. L. Peterson *et al.*: Journal of Medical Education, *31*, No. 12, Part 2: 1–165, 1956; see his page 124.

TABLE 17

DISTRIBUTION OF PHYSICIANS ACCORDING TO FREQUENCY OF
EVENING OFFICE HOURS, MONDAY TO FRIDAY, AND ARRANGEMENTS
FOR SATURDAY AFTERNOON AND EVENING OFFICE HOURS

| Number of evenings on which physicians had office hours (Monday to Friday) | Arrangements for office hours on Saturday afternoon and evening | | | | Total number of physicians |
|---|---|---|---|---|---|
| | No office hours | Office hours in afternoon only | Office hours in evening only | Office hours both afternoon and evening | |
| A. *Ontario* | | | | | |
| None | 6 | 6* | 0 | 1 | 13 |
| One to two per week | 6 | 5 | 0 | 2 | 13 |
| Three to four per week | 4 | 6 | 0 | 3 | 13 |
| Five per week | 0 | 0 | 0 | 4† | 4 |
| Total number of physicians | 16 | 17 | 0 | 10 | 43‡ |
| B. *Nova Scotia* | | | | | |
| None | 1 | 1 | 0 | 0 | 2 |
| One to two per week | 5 | 4 | 0 | 2 | 11 |
| Three to four per week | 2 | 9§ | 1 | 5 | 17 |
| Five per week | 1 | 3 | 0 | 7 | 11 |
| Total number of physicians | 9 | 17 | 1 | 14 | 41‖ |

*One of these physicians had Saturday afternoon office hours only every other week.
†Included is 1 physician who had evening office hours on 9 evenings in 2 weeks.
‡One other physician is excluded because he had no set time for office hours.
§One of these physicians had Saturday afternoon office hours only every other week; another had Saturday afternoon office hours only one Saturday in four.
‖The office hours of the one remaining physician are not known.

afternoon office hours or to the percentage who had office hours on Saturday evening. Peterson (see his page 125) found that 72 per cent of the doctors studied by his group had office hours after noon on Saturday.

Table 17, in which is given the distribution of the doctors according to their evening office hours on week-days and their arrangements for Saturday afternoon and Saturday evening office hours, shows clearly the great diversity that existed. At one extreme was a group of men who had no office hours on any evening or on Saturday afternoon; at the other was a group who had office hours six evenings a week as well as Saturday afternoon.

Before we close the description of evening office hours and Saturday office hours after mid-day, we must make one further point, namely, that the fact that a physician did not have office hours at these times did not necessarily mean that he was not working. Some, it is true, did little or no work on Saturday afternoon or in the evenings. Others, after their office hours were over, had still hours of work before them. One practitioner in a large city had no office hours on Saturday afternoon or on any evening. On the five week-nights, however, he made house calls from eight o'clock until ten, and on Saturday afternoon till four o'clock. Another practitioner in a large city had no evening office hours but spent three hours on each of four evenings a week to make house calls and answer telephone inquiries; and, though his office hours on alternate Saturdays were over by three o'clock, he still had seven hours of house calls before him. Many other physicians gave similar accounts of their evenings and their Saturdays.

Sunday also varied greatly from one practice to another. The only work done by some doctors was looking after the very occasional emergency and obstetrical deliveries. A few were so busy on Sunday that this day was almost indistinguishable from the other days. One young doctor, for example, on two out of every three Sundays, made hospital rounds and house calls from ten o'clock until noon, house calls from one to two in the afternoon, had office hours from two until five, and made more house calls from seven o'clock until ten in the evening. On the third Sunday, his Sunday "off," he made about half a dozen house calls. Another physician, over forty-five years of age, worked from nine in the morning until eleven at night on his Sunday "on," and from nine in the morning until six in the evening on his Sunday "off." Eighteen per cent of the Ontario practitioners and 5 per cent of those in Nova Scotia said that they did no Sunday work, whereas 30 per cent of the Ontario, and 43 per cent of the Nova Scotia, physicians did more than 3 hours—in some cases, considerably

TABLE 18

DISTRIBUTION OF ONTARIO AND NOVA SCOTIA PHYSICIANS
ACCORDING TO NUMBER OF HOURS OF WORK ON SUNDAY

| Number of hours of work on Sunday* | Ontario physicians | | Nova Scotia physicians | |
|---|---|---|---|---|
| | Number | % | Number | % |
| None | 8 | 18.2 | 2 | 4.8 |
| One-half | 1 | 2.3 | 1 | 2.4 |
| One | 10 | 22.7 | 6 | 14.3 |
| Over one and up to three | 12 | 27.3 | 15 | 35.7 |
| Over three and up to five | 9 | 20.5 | 9 | 21.4 |
| Over five and up to ten | 4 | 9.1 | 6 | 14.3 |
| Over ten | 0 | 0.0 | 3 | 7.1 |
| Total | 44 | 100 | 42 | 100 |

*If the number of hours of work varied from one Sunday to another for a particular physician, the number shown is the mean for that physician.

more (Table 18). The average figure for Sunday work was about 2½ hours in Ontario and about 3¾ hours in Nova Scotia.

We have said nothing of those calls (including time-consuming obstetrical deliveries) that occur in the middle of the night, because the shortness of our visit precluded our estimating the frequency of night calls. Otherwise, we have endeavoured to present a picture of the hours of work of a "typical"* general practice throughout the week and also to give some idea of the many variations that may be encountered. In Table 19 are shown the working hours for each day

TABLE 19

NUMBER OF HOURS OF WORK OF ONTARIO AND NOVA SCOTIA PHYSICIANS FOR EACH DAY OF THE WEEK

| | Ontario physicians | | Nova Scotia physicians | |
|---|---|---|---|---|
| | Number of hours of work | | Number of hours of work | |
| Day | Range | Mean | Range | Mean |
| Monday | 5–16 | 9.3 | 6.5–15 | 10.2 |
| Tuesday | 2.5–16 | 9.1 | 6–14 | 10.2 |
| Wednesday | 2–13 | 6.5 | 0–14 | 8.1 |
| Thursday | 1–16 | 9.2 | 3–15 | 10.0 |
| Friday | 4.5–16 | 8.9 | 3–13 | 9.9 |
| Saturday | 2–16 | 7.0 | 2.8–14 | 8.1 |
| Sunday | 0–10 | 2.5 | 0–14 | 3.7 |
| Total | 23–103 | 52.5 | 40.5–89 | 60.2 |

of the week in each of the two provinces. In Ontario, the number of hours of work per week varied from 23 to 103, with a mean of 52.5; in Nova Scotia, the range was from 40.5 to 89 hours, with a mean of 60.2 hours. The means differ significantly ($p < 0.05$). The distribution of the physicians according to the number of hours of work per week is given in Table 20. Nine per cent of the Ontario men, but none in Nova Scotia, had a work week of 35 hours or less; 73 per cent of the Ontario, and 81 per cent of the Nova Scotia, physicians were working more than 45 hours a week; and 18 per cent and 36 per cent in the two provinces, respectively, were working more than 65 hours a week.

The arrangements of physicians of different ages, of physicians in communities of different sizes, and of physicians who were and who were not members of groups were compared, with respect to evening office hours, Saturday office hours, and number of hours of work per week. No significant differences were found between different

*The problem of describing the "typical" practice is discussed on page 258.

TABLE 20

<small>DISTRIBUTION OF ONTARIO AND NOVA SCOTIA PHYSICIANS ACCORDING TO NUMBER OF HOURS OF WORK PER WEEK</small>

| Number of hours of work per week | Ontario physicians | | Nova Scotia physicians | |
|---|---|---|---|---|
| | Number | % | Number | % |
| 16–25 | 1 | 2.3 | 0 | 0.0 |
| 26–35 | 3 | 6.8 | 0 | 0.0 |
| 36–45 | 8 | 18.2 | 8 | 19.0 |
| 46–55 | 16 | 36.4 | 9 | 21.4 |
| 56–65 | 8 | 18.2 | 10 | 23.8 |
| 66–75 | 6 | 13.6 | 11 | 26.2 |
| 76–85 | 1 | 2.3 | 2 | 4.8 |
| 86–95 | 0 | 0.0 | 2 | 4.8 |
| 96–105 | 1 | 2.3 | 0 | 0.0 |
| Total | 44 | 100 | 42 | 100 |

age groups, either in Ontario or in Nova Scotia, with regard to Saturday afternoon or Saturday evening office hours or number of hours of work per week. Nor was there any striking difference between the different age groups in evening office hours between Monday and Friday, with the one exception that, in Ontario, the few physicians who had office hours on every one of these five evenings were all over forty-five years of age.

Between those physicians who were practising entirely on their own, those who were in solo practice but had arrangements with colleagues to cover their practices at times, and those who were members of groups, there were no significant differences in Nova Scotia with respect to frequency of evening office hours between Monday and Friday, Saturday afternoon office hours, Saturday evening office hours, or total number of hours of work per week. In Ontario, on the other hand, there were differences with respect to total number of hours per week and to Saturday afternoon and Saturday evening office hours, but not with respect to frequency of evening office hours between Monday and Friday. In the matter of total number of hours of work per week, those Ontario physicians who were practising in association with one other physician worked longer hours (68.2 hours per week on the average) than either those who were entirely on their own (44.6 hours per week on the average) or those who were in solo practice but arranged for their calls to be taken in their absence (50.8 hours of work per week of the average). Again, of the Ontario men who belonged to groups or who were in solo practice but had arrangements with other doctors to cover their calls at times, 49 per cent had

Saturday afternoon office hours, whereas 100 per cent of the men who were entirely on their own had office hours on Saturday afternoon ($p < 0.01$). Finally, in Ontario, those who practised entirely on their own differed significantly from those who were either members of groups or at least had arrangements for their calls to be taken for them, in that 67 per cent of the completely solo practitioners, but only 11 per cent of the remainder, had office hours on Saturday evening ($p < 0.01$). The corresponding figures for Nova Scotia, namely 50 per cent and 35 per cent, do not differ significantly. Indeed, among the physicians who either belonged to groups or had arrangements for their practices to be covered, the percentage (11 per cent) in Ontario who had Saturday evening office hours was significantly smaller than the corresponding percentage (35 per cent) in Nova Scotia ($p < 0.05$).

Between physicians practising in communities of different sizes, differences were found both in Ontario and in Nova Scotia. In each province, the percentage (88 per cent in Ontario, 92 per cent in Nova Scotia) of the men in communities of under 10,000 who had Saturday afternoon office hours was significantly greater than the percentage (46 per cent in Ontario, 50 per cent in Nova Scotia) with Saturday afternoon office hours in communities of over 10,000 ($p < 0.05$ for Ontario; $p < 0.01$ for Nova Scotia). Saturday evening office hours in Ontario were encountered in 8 per cent of the practices in places of over 10,000, but in 47 per cent of the practices in places of under 10,000 ($p < 0.05$). The corresponding figures for Nova Scotia, 19 per cent and 48 per cent, do not differ significantly. The number of evenings between Monday and Friday on which office hours were held appeared to be more closely related to size of community in Nova Scotia than in Ontario. In Nova Scotia, 31 per cent of the practitioners in communities of over 10,000, but 92 per cent of those in communities of under 10,000, had office hours on three or more of the five evenings ($p < 0.001$). The corresponding figures for Ontario, 35 per cent and 47 per cent, do not differ significantly. Rather, the physicians in Nova Scotia communities of under 10,000 differed significantly from their counterparts in Ontario in the percentage having office hours on three or more of the five evenings ($p < 0.01$). In neither province was there a significant relationship between size of community and total number of hours of work per week.

It must be pointed out that the figures used in our account of working hours were obtained from the practitioners' descriptions of each of the days of the week. The men were *not* asked to estimate how many hours they worked. They *were* asked to describe, in chronological order, what they did each day from the time they left the house in the morning until their work was over in the evening. The calculation of the number of hours of work was made by us. In arriving at the figures, we included whatever time was given to paper work and to attendance at medical meetings. We included also whatever time was taken up with salaried medical work, such as insurance, industrial, or public health work, and with voluntary unpaid medical work, such as work in public clinics of teaching hospitals. Since these activities were all part of the professional work of general practitioners, it seemed appropriate to include the time devoted to them when we were computing the practitioners' working hours. For the same reason, time set aside for regular medical reading would have been included, but no practitioner mentioned this activity in giving the details of his week. On the other hand, in calculating the hours of work, we excluded the mealtimes. We excluded also the estimates, which were made by some men, of the number of hours per week they spent on night calls, including obstetrical deliveries, *after* they had finished the evening's office work and round of house calls.

It may be asked how reliable our figures for number of hours of work are. In a few cases, the hours described by the practitioner differed from those observed during the visit. In the majority of cases, however, there was a close correspondence; and particularly was this so at both extremes of the range. We think that, over all, the figures presented give a reasonably reliable picture of the doctors' working hours and that, so far as they are in error, they are more likely an under-estimate than an exaggeration.

Though we have described the hours of work, it would be erroneous to conclude that the remaining hours constitute time off. Many of the practitioners are on call much or all of the time during which they are not actually working. This is a fact of importance, since it means that they are not free to go to a movie, to go for an afternoon's drive, or even to become involved in activities around the house from which they cannot quickly disengage themselves. In a word, as certain men pointed out to us, they are not able to relax.

Since the medical profession could well be accused of arrogance if it were to claim that the relaxation and recreation that it prescribes for others were unnecessary for its own members, it is fitting that we find out how much time off duty the various practitioners had arranged. Each of the practitioners was asked how often he had an evening off, between Monday and Friday, how often he had half of one of these days off, how often he had a week-end off, and the duration of his vacation or vacations during the course of the year. Several doctors took four- or five-day "week-ends" at intervals of a month or two. Most, however, began their week-ends either at mid-day or in the evening of Saturday; and, as the remarks in Tables 23 and 24 indicate, some of the "week-ends" were Sunday only or any successive twenty-four hours occurring on Saturday and Sunday.

Before reporting our findings about time off duty, we must say briefly what we mean by the term, "off duty." Because the doctor who is on call is severely restricted in his activities even if he is not actually working, our aim was to find out how much time the physicians had in which they could expect to give their attention to personal interests—or, for that matter, to study—*without interruption.* We wished to know how often they were *completely* off duty, i.e. how often they were not responsible for taking *any* calls except those that might occur in such very unusual circumstances as, for example, a community catastrophe. As it became apparent, however, when we were dealing with the Ontario data, that some of the practitioners had not fully understood what we meant and had included, as time off, during which they were on call for obstetrical cases and perhaps

TABLE 21

FREQUENCY OF EVENINGS OFF DUTY OF ONTARIO AND NOVA SCOTIA PHYSICIANS

| Frequency of evenings off duty (Monday to Friday) | Ontario physicians | | Nova Scotia physicians | | | |
|---|---|---|---|---|---|---|
| | | | Number | | Total physicians | |
| | Number | % | Completely off duty | Off duty except for obstetrical calls | Number | % |
| None | 14* | 31.8 | — | — | 31 | 73.8 |
| Very seldom or almost never | 5 | 11.4 | — | — | 0 | 0.0 |
| One every two months | 2 | 4.5 | — | — | 0 | 0.0 |
| One every month | 5 | 11.4 | — | — | 0 | 0.0 |
| Two to three per month | 4 | 9.1 | 1 | 0 | 1 | 2.4 |
| One to two per week | 6† | 13.6 | 3 | 4 | 7 | 16.7 |
| Five to six every two weeks | 3 | 6.8 | 0 | 3 | 3 | 7.1 |
| Four per week | 3† | 6.8 | — | — | 0 | 0.0 |
| No answer | 2 | 4.5 | — | — | — | — |
| Total | 44 | 100 | — | — | 42 | 100 |

*Not included in these 14 are 2 physicians who took obstetrical calls on their evenings off.
†One physician in each of these groups took obstetrical calls on his evenings off.

even for other cases, the figures that we shall present indicate more frequent time off duty than was actually the case for the Ontario physicians. In Nova Scotia, we attempted to obtain more accurate information by dividing the evenings, week-ends, etc., into those on which the doctors were completely off duty (i.e., were accepting no calls), those on which they were taking only obstetrical calls, and those on which they were on duty for any calls that might come.

On the basis of evenings off duty between Monday and Friday, the practitioners in each province can be divided into those who had evenings off less often than once a week or even not at all (68 per cent of the Ontario physicians and 76 per cent of those in Nova Scotia) and those (27 per cent in Ontario, 24 per cent in Nova Scotia) who were off duty one or more evenings per week between Monday and Friday. The two provinces did not differ significantly in the percentages of those who were off one or more evenings per week. Whether, as Table 21 suggests, more physicians did take *occasional* evenings off in Ontario than in Nova Scotia or whether the Nova Scotia physicians did not consider it worthwhile to mention evenings taken less frequently than once a week, we have no way of knowing. It is noteworthy that only 10 per cent of the Nova Scotia physicians had any evenings, between Monday and Friday, on which they were *completely* free of calls.

TABLE 22

FREQUENCY OF HALF-DAYS OFF DUTY OF ONTARIO AND NOVA SCOTIA PHYSICIANS

| Frequency of half-days off duty (Monday to Friday) | Ontario physicians | | Nova Scotia physicians | | | |
|---|---|---|---|---|---|---|
| | | | Number | | Total physicians | |
| | Number | % | Completely off duty | Off duty except for obstetrical calls | Number | % |
| None | 17 | 38.6 | — | — | 29 | 69.0 |
| Very rarely, seldom, or almost never | 5 | 11.4 | 1 | 0 | 1 | 2.4 |
| One to five per year | 3 | 6.8 | 1 | 1 | 2 | 4.8 |
| Six to twelve per year | 2 | 4.5 | 0 | 0 | 0 | 0.0 |
| Over one and up to three per month | 2 | 4.5 | 0 | 1 | 1 | 2.4 |
| One or more* per week | 14† | 31.8 | 3 | 6* | 9 | 21.4 |
| Not answered | 1 | 2.3 | — | — | — | — |
| Total | 44 | 100 | — | — | 42 | 100 |

*One of these physicians had 1 whole day off in the middle of each week.
†Three of these physicians had 1 afternoon off per week except for obstetrical calls; another took 1 afternoon per week in the summer only.

In the matter of half-days off between Monday and Friday, we found that 66 per cent of the Ontario doctors and 79 per cent of those in Nova Scotia either had no half-days off or else had them less frequently than once a week, in some cases very infrequently, whereas 32 per cent in Ontario and 21 per cent in Nova Scotia had a half-day off each week (Table 22). The difference between the provinces is not significant. It does appear, however, that, among the doctors who did not have a half-day off as often as once a week, a considerably greater proportion of the Ontario, than of the Nova Scotia, men did have half-days off now and then, though, as in the case of evenings off, the difference may not be real but may be due to a different interpretation of the question in the two provinces.

The frequency of week-ends off duty and the details regarding the duration of the week-ends are shown in Tables 23 and 24. In brief,

TABLE 23

FREQUENCY OF WEEK-ENDS OFF DUTY OF ONTARIO PHYSICIANS

| Frequency of week-ends off duty | Physicians | | Details of time "off duty" |
| --- | --- | --- | --- |
| | Number | % | |
| None | 9 | 20.4 | 1: every second Sun. evening<br>1: one Sat. evening per month |
| Very seldom or almost never | 3 | 6.8 | 1: every Sun. evening |
| Two to six per year | 14 | 31.8 | 1: 4 days every 2 months.<br>1: from Thurs. evening to Mon. morning once in 2 months<br>1: Sat. evening and Sun., every ninth week |
| One every two or three weeks | 9 | 20.4 | 1: Sat. evening and Sun.<br>1: Sat. evening and Sun. off, except for obstetrical calls<br>1: Sat. afternoon and evening and Sun. off<br>1: Sun. off, except for obstetrics<br>2 others took obstetrical calls<br>1: off every third week-end; 8 every second week-end |
| Most week-ends | 7 | 15.9 | 1: three out of four week-ends off from the end of Sat. afternoon<br>2: every Sat. afternoon and four out of five Sundays off<br>1: every week-end off from noon on Sat.<br>1: every Sun. off (except for obstetrics)<br>1: 24 hours off every week-end<br>1: "most" week-ends off, except for hospital rounds |
| Five days per month (May to October) | 1 | 2.3 | |
| Not answered | 1 | 2.3 | |
| Total | 44 | 100 | |

TABLE 24
FREQUENCY OF WEEK-ENDS OFF DUTY OF NOVA SCOTIA PHYSICIANS

| Frequency of week-ends off duty | Physicians | | Details of time "off duty" |
|---|---|---|---|
| | Number | % | |
| None | 16 | 38.1 | |
| One to two per year | 1 | 2.4 | Sunday 2–10 p.m. (except for obstetrical calls) |
| Two to six per year | 6 | 14.3 | 3: completely from 2 p.m. Sat. until midnight Sun. |
| | | | 2: completely from 4 p.m. Sat. until Sun. evening |
| | | | 1: all day Sunday except for obstetrical calls |
| Eight to twelve per year | 6 | 14.3 | 2: completely from 2 p.m. Sat. until late Sun. evening |
| | | | 1: completely from 8 a.m. on Sun. until midnight |
| | | | 1: completely, sometimes from 2 p.m. on Sat., sometimes from 9 a.m. Sun. until midnight Sun. |
| | | | 1: except for obstetrical calls, sometimes from 2 p.m. Sat., sometimes from 10 a.m. Sun., to midnight Sun. |
| | | | 1: sometimes completely, sometimes except for obstetrical calls, from 5 p.m. Sat. until 9 a.m. Mon. |
| One every two or three weeks | 5 | 11.9 | 2: except for obstetrical calls, from 2 p.m. on Sat. until midnight Sun. |
| | | | 1: completely on Sun., 10 a.m. to 7 p.m. |
| | | | 1: from 4 p.m. Sat. until 8.30 a.m. Mon., except for obstetrical calls and 1 hour of rounds at noon on Sunday |
| | | | 1: from 2 p.m. Sat. to midnight Sun., except for obstetrical calls and 1 hour of rounds at noon on Sunday |
| | | | 2: every third week-end; 3: every second week-end |
| Most week-ends | 8 | 19.0 | 2: completely from 2 p.m. Sat. until midnight Sun., three week-ends out of four |
| | | | 1: completely from 9.30 p.m. Sat. until 10 a.m. Mon., three week-ends out of four. |
| | | | 1: except for obstetrical calls, from 2 p.m. Sat. to midnight Sun., three week-ends out of four |
| | | | 1: completely from midnight Sat. to midnight Sun., two week-ends out of three |
| | | | 1: except for obstetrical calls, from 4 p.m. Sat. to midnight Sun., two week-ends out of three |
| | | | 1: except for obstetrical calls, from 2 p.m. Sat. until midnight Sun., one week-end out of three and all Sun. one week-end out of three |
| | | | 1: except for obstetrical calls, the whole of every Sun. |
| Total | 42 | 100 | |

20 per cent of the Ontario doctors and 38 per cent of those in Nova Scotia had no week-ends off; 39 per cent of the Ontario, and 31 per cent of the Nova Scotia, men had some week-ends off, but not more than 1 per month and, in most cases, fewer than this; 20 per cent in Ontario and 12 per cent in Nova Scotia were off every second or third week-end; and 16 per cent and 19 per cent in Ontario and Nova Scotia, respectively, had most of the week-ends off. The differences between the two provinces are not statistically significant.

Vacations varied in duration from none, in the case of a few doctors in each province, to several months each year in the case of one older physician who practised in a remote part of Ontario. Twenty-five per cent of the Ontario doctors took vacations not exceeding 2 weeks in length, 50 per cent took more than 2 weeks and up to 1 month, and 20 per cent were away more than 1 month out of the year. The corresponding figures for Nova Scotia were 38 per cent, 45 per cent, and 10 per cent (Table 25). The differences between the provinces are not significant.

TABLE 25

ANNUAL VACATIONS TAKEN BY ONTARIO AND NOVA SCOTIA PHYSICIANS

| | Ontario physicians | | Nova Scotia physicians | |
|---|---|---|---|---|
| Duration of vacation(s) | Number | % | Number | % |
| No vacation | 2 | 4.5 | 3 | 7.1 |
| One week or less | 4 | 9.1 | 3 | 7.1 |
| Over one week and up to two weeks | 7 | 15.9 | 13 | 31.0 |
| Over two weeks and up to three weeks | 9 | 20.5 | 9 | 21.4 |
| Over three weeks and up to one month | 13* | 29.5 | 10 | 23.8 |
| Over one month and up to six weeks | 7 | 15.9 | 4 | 9.5 |
| Over six weeks | 2 | 4.5 | 0 | 0.0 |
| Total | 44 | 100 | 42 | 100 |

*One of these physicians said, "One month at least."

As with hours of work, so in the matter of time off duty we compared physicians of different ages, physicians in communities of different sizes, and physicians who were working alone and those working in groups. In Ontario, no significant differences were found in the matter of evenings off duty between Monday and Friday, half-days off, week-ends off, or vacations. In Nova Scotia, physicians in different age groups did not differ significantly with respect to these items; nor did physicians in communities of different sizes show appreciable differences with regard to half-days off, week-ends off, or duration of vacation. In the matter of evenings off, however, there was a significant difference, in that 88 per cent of the physicians in communities of less than 10,000, but only 53 per cent of those in communities of more than 10,000, had no evenings off between Monday and Friday ($p < 0.05$). As we have stated above, no such difference was found in Ontario. Comparison of Ontario and Nova Scotia showed that, in places of 10,000 or more, there was no significant difference between the percentages who had no evenings off between Monday and Friday, whereas, in communities of less than 10,000, there was a significant difference between the percentage (50 per cent) of Ontario physicians and the percentage (88 per cent) of Nova Scotia physicians who had none of these evenings off ($p < 0.05$).

Finally, when the Nova Scotia physicians practising entirely alone, those practising alone but having arrangements with colleagues to cover their practices in their absences, and those who were members of groups were compared, certain differences were found with respect to frequency of week-ends off and duration of vacations. The physicians practising entirely on their own differed both from those who were in solo practice but had covering arrangements with colleagues and from those who were in groups, in that 100 per cent of those in completely solo practice but only 33 per cent of the solo practitioners with covering arrangements and 29 per cent of those in groups had no week-ends off ($p < 0.05$). Again, the Nova Scotia physicians in group practice differed from those in solo practice with covering arrangements and from those in entirely solo practice in that, of the men in group practice, 86 per cent had vacations of over 2 weeks whereas only 46 per cent of those in solo practice with covering arrangements and none of those who were completely on their own had more than two weeks ($p < 0.05$ and $p < 0.01$). Those in entirely solo practice, those in solo practice with covering arrangements, and those in group practice did not differ significantly with respect either to half-days off or to frequency of evenings off between Monday and Friday.

More interesting and important, perhaps, than the differences that we *found* are the differences that might have been expected but were *not* found to exist, especially between the physicians who were in solo practice and those who were members of groups. When we compared the percentages of solo practitioners and of those in groups who had at least one evening off *each week* between Monday and Friday there was no significant difference in either province. Even of those who were practising in groups, more than 50 per cent in each province had an evening off duty, between Monday and Friday, *less* often than once a week, and some of them rarely or never. Finding this, one may wonder whether the physicians who are practising in groups are really taking advantage of the benefits that are possible with this type of practice. Similarly, of the solo practitioners who had arrangements with other physicians to cover their calls during time off, 55 per cent in Ontario and 79 per cent in Nova Scotia rarely or never had one of the week-evenings off, and another 20 per cent and 2 per cent in Ontario and Nova Scotia, respectively, had one of these evenings off less often than once a week. The members of this group also, it appears, might benefit from extending their arrangements with their colleagues. In the matter of week-ends, 55 per cent of the solo practitioners in Ontario who had covering arrangements and 47 per cent of those men who were in groups had week-ends off less often than once a month. The corresponding figures for Nova Scotia are 71 per cent and 36 per cent, respectively. Again, in Ontario, 65 per cent of those in solo practice with covering arrangements and 60 per cent of those in groups had a half-day off during the week less often than once a week. In Nova Scotia, the corresponding figures were 79 per cent and 71 per cent, respectively. Finally, in Ontario, one-quarter of those in solo practice with covering arrangements and one-quarter of those in group practice had two weeks or less of vacation per year. In Nova Scotia, though the great majority in group practice had more than two weeks of vacation, more than half of those who were in solo practice with covering arrangements had two weeks or less of vacation. Each of these findings suggests that, in spite of the comments that were made by the physicians about their dislike of the long hours and the advantage of group practice in this respect, less is being done to solve this problem than might be expected.

We have dealt with the various practitioners' time off duty, and it now remains only for us to say a few words about the arrangements made to cover their practices during their absences. All of the men who were practising as members of groups had their practices covered by the other members of the groups. All the physicians whom we have described as being in solo practice but as arranging with other doctors to cover for them made definite arrangements of one sort or another before going away. Some of these men said that on week-ends and on half-days there was a doctor on call for the community, according to a definite schedule. Other men before short periods off duty, and all of them before going on longer vacations, arranged with one or two colleagues to look after their patients in their absence. One doctor stated that he did not take on any obstetrical patients who were likely to deliver during the time of his vacation, whereas another left his obstetrical patients to be looked after by a certificated obstetrician. A locum tenens was mentioned by only 1 Ontario practitioner, who was shortly going to try this expedient for the first time, and by 4 practitioners in Nova Scotia.

There were 9 Ontario physicians who were in solo practice and did not have arrangements with other doctors to cover their practices during time off duty. Two of these men were more than twenty-five miles distant from their nearest colleagues. One of these two, before going away, would write to his obstetrical patients and suggest whom they might call if they should need care in his absence. Other patients urgently in need of care would have to depend on whatever physician was closest. One of the 9 doctors "usually" arranged for his practice to be covered during annual vacation but would sometimes go away for shorter periods, including week-ends, and leave it to his patients to find another doctor if they needed one. No provision was made by the remaining 6 doctors, except that 2 of them sometimes arranged for obstetrical patients to be under another doctor's care and a third doctor said that he would come back from his vacation if one of his patients went into labour.

Six of the doctors who failed to make definite arrangements with other doctors were practising less than a mile from their nearest colleagues. Yet we must point out that the fact that another doctor is practising near by is not a guarantee that the patient's interests are safeguarded, since in a large city he may not know whom to call and in a small place he may find that the only other doctor in the town is also absent. Indeed, one doctor told us that he and the other doctor in town had formerly checked with each other before they went away, but that in recent years they had stopped doing so, and that he knew that occasionally they had both been away at the same time.

In Nova Scotia, there were 4 practitioners who said that they did not have arrangements with other local doctors to cover their calls during their absences. Two of these men engaged a locum tenens during their vacations. One doctor went out of town a short distance but came in each day to see seriously ill patients and could be reached by telephone between these daily visits. In effect, he did not take a vacation. The fourth of this group said that, if he went away, his practice would not be covered, but that he had had no vacations during the preceding fourteen years.

This chapter has brought to light certain problems. We have just indicated that, in 20 per cent of the Ontario practices, the arrangements made by the doctors for periods when they will be away are less than ideal, since it depends upon chance whether adequate care will be available in an emergency. Probably an even greater problem, however, is presented by the length of working hours and the paucity of time off duty in many practices. This statement is applicable both to Ontario and to Nova Scotia, though perhaps somewhat more to the latter in that a number of our findings suggest that the Nova Scotia doctors, and especially those in places of under 10,000, are working longer hours and having less time off duty than their counterparts in Ontario. From what we have reported, it seems reasonable to conclude that a great deal could be done by many of the practitioners to improve their working hours. To the problem of time we shall return later (pages 465 ff.), when its importance will be more apparent in the light of other findings.

# 9  /  The General Practitioner and the Hospital

Though by far the greater part of a general practitioner's work can be done, and is done, in his office and in his patients' homes, certain types of case, if they are to be managed competently and safely, require the facilities of a hospital. Briefly, these are the more serious medical (i.e., non-surgical) cases, obstetrical deliveries and complications, and all but the most minor surgical cases. In addition, a hospital serves another, and an important, purpose: it brings physicians, many of whom would otherwise be practising in almost complete isolation, into touch with their local colleagues and, through them, with the rest of the medical world. Though this purpose is served in part by medical meetings, either of a hospital staff or of a local medical society, it is probable that the informal and frequent contacts of the doctors' room exert a stronger and more consistent influence.

Because a physician who lacks hospital facilities is seriously hampered in his management of certain cases, we asked each of the physicians to what hospitals he had access for the care of his patients and what limits, if any, the hospitals set to the work that he might undertake. Every one of the physicians, both in Ontario and in Nova Scotia, had privileges in at least 1 hospital, and more than half of them in 2 or more hospitals (Table 26). Some of the physicians said that they were on the "active" staffs of their hospitals, others that they were on the "courtesy," "visiting," or "associate" staffs. Some men were on the "active" staff of one hospital and the "courtesy" staff of another. These terms had different meanings in different hospitals. The active staff of one hospital, for example, included doctors who lived and practised outside the community in which the hospital was located,

TABLE 26

| Number of hospitals in which physician had privileges | Ontario physicians | | Nova Scotia physicians | |
|---|---|---|---|---|
| | Number | % | Number | % |
| None | 0 | 0.0 | 0 | 0.0 |
| One | 19 | 43.2 | 19 | 45.2 |
| Two | 20† | 45.4 | 12 | 28.6 |
| Three | 4 | 9.1 | 1 | 2.4 |
| Four | 1‡ | 2.3 | 10 | 23.8 |
| Total | 44 | 100 | 42 | 100 |

*In most hospitals, the doctor was appointed as an "active," "associate," or "courtesy" member of the staff; a few men said that no appointment was necessary in their hospitals.
†One of the 2 hospitals was a "private hospital" in the cases of 2 of the physicians.
‡One of the 4 hospitals was a "private hospital."

whereas a hospital in another community made its facilities available to out-of-town doctors as members of the courtesy staff, who had no hospital responsibilities and no vote regarding hospital business.

Since these designations of staff members are so varied in their meanings, we shall not take further time with them. The point of importance is not the name, but what the member of the staff is permitted to do. Of the 44 Ontario practitioners, 18 stated that there were no restrictions upon their work in any of their hospitals, though 3 of these indicated that restrictive regulations were being drawn up but had not yet come into effect. One man was unrestricted in 3 hospitals, but in 1 hospital he was not permitted to do major surgery. Three others were not interested in doing surgery. One of these 3 had never inquired whether his hospitals would grant him surgical privileges, and the other 2 did not make clear whether they would have been limited by their hospitals if they had not limited themselves. Similarly, of the 42 Nova Scotia physicians, 19 stated that they were subject to no restrictions in their hospitals and 2 that they were restricted in one hospital but not in another. In short, then, 50 per cent of the doctors in each province either had full privileges in at least 1 hospital or else regarded whatever restrictions there may have been as too unimportant to report to us.

Of the other 43 doctors, 21 in Ontario and 20 in Nova Scotia were restricted in their surgery, 8 in Ontario and 10 in Nova Scotia in anaesthesia, 7 in Ontario and 12 in Nova Scotia in obstetrics, and 1 in each of paediatrics and psychiatry in Ontario. The regulation regarding psychiatry forbade the use of electroshock therapy. The sole paediatric restriction, if it can be called that, was a requirement of one hospital that unusually sick babies, including prematures, must be referred to a paediatrician. The 7 Ontario physicians who stated that their obstetrical work was subject to hospital restrictions were allowed to manage normal cases themselves but were required to refer for consultation all cases in which there were complications. In Nova Scotia, 4 doctors gave, as the sole obstetrical restriction, that they were not permitted to perform Caesarean sections; 8 said that they were required to have a consultation whenever they encountered various complications. Among the complications listed by one or another doctor were toxaemia of pregnancy, antepartum haemorrhage, breech presentations, Rh incompatibility, and situations in which a Caesarean section was being considered for the first time for the particular patient. One other doctor, who was subject to no restrictions in his local hospital, was permitted to deliver patients in a Halifax hospital, but only if he arranged for a Halifax doctor to be on call in case he ran into difficulties.

Of the 8 doctors in Ontario who were subject to restrictions in anaesthesia, 3 were limited to local anaesthetics. Two others were "limited" but did not define the limitation; but 1 of them, who had had no training in anaesthesia during his interneship, said that he gave no anaesthetics as he believed that other men could do this better than he. One practitioner was limited to minor work in anaesthesia, 1 was allowed to use an open mask but was not permitted to use the gas machine, and the eighth member of this group did what he described as "intermediate" anaesthesia. In Nova Scotia, 7 doctors said that they were not permitted to do any general anaesthesia, 1 that he was not allowed to give anaesthetics in "major" surgical cases, and 2 that their use of general anaesthetic agents was restricted to obstetrical cases only. One other doctor thought that his hospital would have restricted him in anaesthesia, but he had never been sufficiently interested in this type of work to make inquiry.

Restrictions were most frequently encountered in the field of surgery. Of the 21 Ontario practitioners whose surgical privileges were limited, 2 men, both in the city of Toronto, stated that they were not allowed to do surgery, 2 had minor privileges only, and 6 were not allowed to do major surgery. One doctor said that the "minor surgery" that he was allowed to do was out-patient department surgery only and did not include excision of tonsils and adenoids; another, who was not allowed to do "major surgery," said that the operations forbidden to him included uterine curettage. Apart from these two comments, the terms "major" and "minor" surgery were not elaborated upon by these doctors.

Another group of 9 Ontario doctors stated that the major surgery that their hospitals permitted them to do was limited. Three did not define the limits, but 1 of these said that he did no surgery because other men could do it better than he. Four were allowed to remove tonsils and adenoids and to perform uterine curettage. Three of these 4 added that they might manage "simple" fractures and 1 that he was not permitted to perform appendectomies or Caesarean sections. Each of the remaining 2 of the 9 said that, to do major surgery, he must have a more senior surgeon present at the operation. One of these 2 said that he was allowed, with a more senior surgeon assisting, to repair hernias and remove appendices, but that actually he limited himself to excision of tonsils and adenoids, uterine curettage, circumcisions, and the handling of lacerations.

Of the 21 Ontario practitioners who were restricted in the surgery that they might undertake, the remaining 2 said that they were allowed to do "intermediate" surgery. One man did not define this term; the other was permitted to repair hernias and to do appendectomies, but was not allowed to remove gallbladders or perform Caesarean sections.

In Nova Scotia, 11 doctors said that they were limited to minor surgery. Most of these men specified that this included, not only such procedures as the suturing of skin wounds and the removal of superficial cysts, but also the removal of tonsils and adenoids and the management of simple fractures. The remaining 9, of the 20 who were limited in surgery, were subject to a variety of restrictions on their major surgery. Thus, 2 were permitted to do major surgery only in an emergency. Two others were permitted to do "no major surgery." Both, however, did Caesarean sections and removed appendices, and one removed gallbladders, which he said, in answer to a question, was not "major surgery" in the eyes of the Credentials Committee of his hospital. Three other physicians said that, when they did certain operations, they were required to have a senior man available. This senior man might or might not have to be a certificated specialist in surgery; he might have to be scrubbed up or he might merely have to be within the hospital; and the operations for which he was required to stand by might include appendectomies or might include only those operations that were considered to be more difficult than removal of the gallbladder. Yet another 2 doctors were permitted to do any operation, except those involving the chest or the central nervous system, with the provision, in the case of one doctor, that a senior surgeon should be in the hospital. Finally, the sole limitation imposed upon 1 doctor was that he should have a consultation before performing a hysterectomy on any woman under forty-five years of age.

The limitations imposed by the hospitals have been described in detail because, in the past few years, repeated expressions of dissatisfaction in this regard on the part of the general practitioners have been voiced publicly or have appeared in print. In November, 1957, the *Bulletin* of the College of General Practice of Canada reprinted from the *Bulletin* of the Toronto Academy of Medicine an article entitled, "Bill of Rights for the General Practitioner."* The author, Dr. Struan Robertson, begins with the statement, "I believe it is time that we, in General Practice, sought recognition of certain fundamental rights." In the course of discussing a number of these rights, he says:

Another fundamental right is that of being enabled to perform any service or procedure in hospital of which he has proven himself capable.

Another is the right of the General Practitioner for equal opportunity with the specialist to admit his patients to hospital. . . .

Another is the right of the General Practitioner to admit his patients to hospitals in the district even though it is not the hospital on which staff he happens to be. . . .

Six months later, in May, 1958, in the *Bulletin* of the College of General Practice of Canada, under the caption, "Hospital Integration of G.P. is Major Convention Subject,"† it was reported that "At the College annual meeting and at the Board of Representative session immediately preceding the convention, the College heard committee chairmen report: 1. Need for greater integration of general practitioners into their community hospitals in many parts of Canada. . . ." The retiring president of the College was quoted as saying, "The College has achieved some success in the matter of hospital integration. In large general hospitals in some cities of Canada today general practitioners are beginning to play an active and rightful role." Further on, the report says, "With reference to hospital privileges for general practitioners which was an important subject of discussion during the three-day College convention Dr. Young [Dr. Morley A. R. Young, President of the Canadian Medical Association] said 'every medical practitioner should have hospital privileges. In the West this need is not as great as in other parts of the country. Whenever hospital privileges are denied, someone has caused a step to be taken which lowers the standard of practice.' "

*S. Robertson: College of General Practice (Medicine) of Canada, Bulletin, 4: 2, 32, 1957.

†College of General Practice (Medicine) of Canada, Bulletin, 4: 4, 19, 1958.

In November, 1958, the College of General Practice returned to this topic in its *Bulletin*. Under the heading, "College Information— The G.P. in Accredited Hospitals,"* it is stated:

The Board of Representatives of the College of General Practice last spring forwarded the following resolution to the Canadian Medical Association:

"RESOLVED THAT the representatives of the Canadian Medical Association on the Joint Commission on Accreditation of Hospitals be instructed to stimulate action by that body leading to the warning of provisional accreditation, or removal of accrediation of hospitals which exclude or arbitrarily restrict hospital privileges of general practitioners as a class regardless of their individual professional competence, after appeal by the local medical society concerned; and

"BE IT FURTHER RESOLVED THAT the Canadian Medical Association use its full influence to discourage any arbitrary restrictions by hospitals against general practitioners as a group or as individuals."

In January, 1959, in an article entitled "The General Practitioner in the Hospital,"† Dr. Lorraine Trempe, Editor of the French Section of the *Bulletin* of the College of General Practice of Canada, states:

The time has come to put an end to class consciousness in the profession. The "dignus es intrare" must not be reserved for a small proportion of doctors and be subject to arbitrary choice, but competence alone should be the determining factor. . . .

It is painful to notice that it is not the hospital administration which is opposed, at the out-set, to the entrance of the general practitioner but rather his own colleague, the hospital doctor, whose attitude is prompted, in most cases, by personal rather than scientific interests.

This exclusion, an insult to our universities which train doctors; to our provincial college which gives them the right to practice; to the hospitals themselves which afford them their clinical teaching, is inadmissible on a professional level. And Dr. Gobeil suggests [Dr. Trempe is referring to an earlier article of Dr. L. J. Gobeil], and rightly so, that one should consider as an action derogatory to professional honour that of preventing a colleague from exercising his profession, of belittling a colleague not only on the professional but also on the scientific level, at the bedside of patients and often in the presence of medical students.

How can one explain logically the attitude of these hospital doctors, chiefs of services, of intern or resident doctors, whose abilities they have appreciated to the point of allowing them to examine their patients, complete their charts, collaborate in their scientific research, collect documentation and even occasionally share their service responsibilities? Then overnight when these same interns or resident doctors have become practitioners, they have become in the minds of these same hospital doctors merely inept competitors. . . .

*College of General Practice (Medicine) of Canada, Bulletin, 5: 2, 17, 1958.
†College of General Practice (Medicine) of Canada, Bulletin 5: 3, 25, 1959.

Our College of General Practice (Medicine) of Canada . . . cannot but share the views of one of its members whose own experience is expressed with such foresight and conviction."

A few pages further on in the same issue of the College's *Bulletin* under the heading, "General Practitioners in Hospitals by Dr. Merrell Carleton, Past Chairman, Committee on Hospitals,"* is an article which contains the following statements:

Summarizing the findings of the hospital committee at the conclusion of their survey, Dr. Merrell Carleton gives a province by province picture of the general practitioner's position in relation to his local hospital. All hospitals in Canada of seventy-five beds or more were surveyed.
. . . Only five of thirteen hospitals in Nova Scotia completed their questionnaires. None of these were in larger centres. The Canadian Medical Association were told at their annual meeting that general practitioners have lost most of their privileges in the Halifax area. . . .
In Ontario 53 out of 77 hospitals replied to the College study. "In the large cities and teaching centres, general practitioners' hospital privileges have been drastically curtailed. However, a large number of departments of general practice have been organized" Dr. Carleton reported.

We have quoted in full what was said about Ontario and Nova Scotia, the two provinces studied by the Survey of General Practice. We may summarize what Dr. Carleton said of the other provinces. He found that the general practitioners had full privileges in all hospitals of Newfoundland and of Prince Edward Island and that in New Brunswick they had "a reasonable amount of privileges although surgery is restricted in some degree." One statement about Quebec indicated that there was no problem except in the larger city hospitals, whereas another statement, attributed to a member of the provincial legislature, was that 75 per cent of Quebec hospitals were "closed." Dr. Carleton stated that there were "full privileges in all Manitoba hospitals" and in Alberta and Saskatchewan hospitals except the teaching hospitals. In British Columbia there were full privileges "except in one or two city hospitals." One may suspect, though it is not stated, that these also were teaching hospitals.

Again, in the *Fourth Annual Report* of the College of General Practice, dated June 1, 1959, the Executive Director writes:

The position of the general practitioner in some city general hospitals continues to give the College much concern. Though more and more large hospitals are integrating the general physicians into their medical staff organization, there still remain too many hospitals where they are denied participation in staff organizations. The College is now able to demonstrate

*College of General Practice (Medicine) of Canada, Bulletin, 5: 3, 29, 1959.

and prove that full integration of the general practitioner is highly desirable to all concerned.*

We quote also from a speech made in the Ontario Legislature, on March 19, 1958, by Dr. J. A. McCue, the Member for Lanark.† Speaking on "the position of the general practitioner or family doctor in the present day scheme of medical affairs as it exists in this province," Dr. McCue, who was not, so far as we know, a member of the College of General Practice, says:

. . . there is a condition existing in this province today which I believe is unjust and completely intolerable. This is the fact that there are many hospitals in existence today which will not allow a family doctor to become a member of their staff nor to treat any patient of theirs within the hospital. In the type of hospital of which I speak he cannot have the services of his own doctor. He is stopped at the front door—no matter how much the patient may want him as the doctor he has confidence in. . . .

But there are in this province today people who want their own doctor and cannot have him because he is not on the staff of the hospital and they have to be turned over to a stranger. . . .

That in certain areas a man who has spent possibly at least 8 years of his life in training to become a doctor should be put in the position that all he is allowed to do is to practice in his office and make house calls is a condition which makes him a second class medical citizen that is at once demoralizing and degrading and devastating in a medical sense. This is a condition which I contend lowers the standard of medicine in the overall picture in this province. . . .

Here we are, Mr. Speaker, at a time when this province is expanding faster than it ever was in its history, talking about a shortage of doctors, and yet there is a certain amount of medical talent in certain areas in this province which is denied its proper release and the public are therefore suffering from a lack of this treatment, which these doctors are willing and ready to give if they are given a chance. . . .

I have no axe to grind . . . but I am here to speak and I think it is about time that somebody got up on their feet and spoke on behalf of these men who I think are getting choked off in their medical efforts. . . .

. . . I would like to see legislation introduced which would require every hospital board at present not doing so, to take the family doctor onto their staffs. In other words, *let the doctors into the hospitals*‡ wherever they now cannot do so—why should there be any medical caste system anywhere? Why should there be any discrimination in a democracy such as ours?"

Whether general practitioners *should* have hospital privileges is a question the consideration of which we defer to later chapters (see pages 462 and 514–515). At present we are intent upon discovering how

*College of General Practice (Medicine) of Canada, *Fourth Annual Report*, 1959, p. 11.
†Legislature of Ontario, Debates, Official Report, 1958, pp. 1026–9.
‡The italics are used in the official report of the speech.

many *do* have unrestricted hospital privileges and how extensive are the restrictions laid upon the remainder. That these questions of fact need to be asked is amply demonstrated by the quotations given in the last few pages. Dr. McCue's speech in particular is couched in emotion-laden phrases calculated to impress upon the hearer that in Ontario a bad state of affairs exists in "many hospitals," although he does not bring forward any evidence in support of what he says. Dr. Trempe, also, by his choice of expressions, makes an emotional appeal but again does not adduce any evidence in support of his contention.* Thus, though neither Dr. McCue nor Dr. Trempe supports his allegations with a single concrete example, their words cannot be ignored because of the response that such words tend to elicit from uncritical hearers or readers, both within the profession and among the laity. The other writers whom we have quoted are more moderate in their choice of words, but they too speak with a conviction that the problem is one of considerable magnitude.

Earlier in this chapter, we have reported the hospital connections of the Ontario and Nova Scotia physicians and the limits set to their work by some of the hospitals. Let us now re-examine these data against the background of the published expressions of dissatisfaction that we have cited. First of all, there was no general practitioner visited by us either in Ontario or in Nova Scotia who did not have privileges in at least one hospital,† though a few men did not go near their hospital during the Survey's visit and made it plain in their conversation that they made little use of their hospital connection. Next we found that more than 50 per cent of the practitioners in each province had privileges in two or more hospitals. In the matter of restrictions, our finding was that 50 per cent of the doctors in each of the two provinces were, for all practical purposes, unrestricted by their hospitals, while the other 50 per cent were subject to restrictions in one or more of the clinical fields.

We do not presume to state categorically whether the restrictions are reasonable or unreasonable, but we put forward a few facts for the reader's consideration. The sole restriction that was mentioned in

---

*It is conceivable that Dr. Trempe intended his remarks to apply only to the province of Quebec, with which the Survey of General Practice has had no experience, though no such geographical limit is set in either the French or the English version of his statement.

†Similarly, the College of General Practice of Canada has recently reported that replies to a questionnaire sent to its members and answered by 46 per cent of them show that only "1.4 per cent of those answering . . . are not members of hospital staffs." Canadian Medical Association Journal, *84:* 1156, 1961.

psychiatry prevented the use of electroshock therapy; this is a technical procedure that a doctor not specializing in psychiatric practice would rarely, if ever, have occasion to use. The doctor who was restricted in this way did not evince any dissatisfaction. The only restriction of which we were told in paediatrics was that unusually sick babies, including prematures, must be referred. To care for the "unusually sick" would seem to be the prime function of the specialist. The inclusion of prematures among those to be referred must be viewed in the light of such a statement (typical of many that could be cited) as that of Waldo E. Nelson, Professor of Pediatrics at Temple University School of Medicine, that "Prematurity is the most important problem of the neonatal period. During the first month of life infants born prematurely account for almost half of the total number of deaths."*

Of the 8 Ontario physicians who were restricted by their hospitals in their giving of anaesthetics, 4 had had no experience with this during their internships, 2 had had 1 month on an anaesthetic service, 1 had had 3 months during which his time was divided between anaesthesia and the demands of two other services, and 1 man could not recall the duration of his anaesthetic training. Among this entire group only one man had had his training in anaesthesia, of 1 month's duration, in a *teaching* hospital. Of the 10 Nova Scotia practitioners who were limited by their hospitals in the field of anaesthesia, only 1 had had any experience with this during his period of postgraduate training. He had had 1 month in a non-teaching hospital.

Seven Ontario doctors stated that, in obstetrics, they were permitted to handle normal cases but were required to ask for consultation in all cases that developed complications. Two men could not recall the duration of their training in obstetrics during their internships, though in one case it was more than 4 months. The remaining 5 men had spent from 1 to 3 months on an obstetrical service as internes. Four had had their internships in non-teaching hospitals, 3 in teaching hospitals. Of the 12 Nova Scotia physicians who were restricted in their handling of various obstetrical complications, 1 had had 12 months of obstetrical training, of which 9 months were spent in a teaching hospital; 2 had had no obstetrical experience during their internships; and the remaining 9 had had from 1 to 3 months on an obstetrical service. Of these 9, 6 had gained their postgraduate obstetrical experience entirely in non-teaching hospitals.

*Waldo E. Nelson: Textbook of Pediatrics (7th ed.; Philadelphia, W. B. Saunders Company, 1959), p. 4.

Though it is self-evident that only cases that develop, or may develop, complications require a specialist's services, it is not for us, who are not specially trained in obstetrics, to say which of such cases should be referred. That the complications of pregnancy are formidable, however, unless due precautions are taken is illustrated by a recent report, in the *Nova Scotia Medical Bulletin*, of several cases of still birth and neonatal death.* These cases, which had been studied intensively, had been abstracted from a report of the Maternal and Child Welfare Committee of the Medical Society of Nova Scotia. The point of particular importance in this report is that the dangers of toxaemia, of prematurity, and of maternal anaemia apparently either were not recognized by the physicians or were not taken seriously enough. The importance of recognizing and treating the complications of pregnancy is further emphasized by the statement made by Nicholson J. Eastman, Professor of Obstetrics at Johns Hopkins University, about a single group of complications, the toxaemias. He says, "The toxemias of pregnancy . . . account for some 1,000 maternal fatalities in the United States each year . . . and it can be estimated conservatively that at least 30,000 still births and neonatal deaths each year in this country are the result of toxemia of pregnancy. . . . This huge toll of maternal and infant lives . . . is in large measure preventable."† Though the figures for Canada are different and not necessarily proportional to those given for the United States, it is clear that the complications of pregnancy are to be taken seriously. In the light of these facts, the demand of certain hospitals that patients with complications be referred does not seem to be unreasonable.

Still to be considered are the restrictions upon the practitioners' surgical work. At this point, however, in order that the reader may have a clear impression of the value of the training that a doctor receives as an interne and may be able to assess the limitations imposed upon a general practitioner in the light of the training that the practitioner has had, we must digress briefly to explain what an interne does. When a patient is admitted to the hospital, an interne takes his history and does a physical examination. Both of these he is required to record, together with his tentative diagnosis or the various diagnostic possibilities, his suggestions for further investigation, and his proposed plan of treatment. This ideal is approached closely in most,

*B. S. Morton and P. M. Sigsworth: Nova Scotia Medical Bulletin, 39: 405, 1960.
†Nicholson J. Eastman: Williams Obstetrics (11th ed.; New York: Appleton-Century-Crofts, 1956), p. 687.

if not all, teaching hospitals and in some non-teaching hospitals. In other non-teaching hospitals, however, case records are scanty or non-existent, except for a few laboratory reports.

From this point on, the rôle of an interne varies from one hospital to another and from one branch of medicine to another. The ultimate responsibility for a patient rests with the attending physician, whether the patient is one of his own private patients or is on a public ward of which the attending physician is in charge. The amount of responsibility that devolves upon any particular interne depends upon many things, including the ability of the interne, the structure of the house-staff hierarchy* in his hospital, the particular branch of medicine, and the philosophy of the individual attending physician. Most attending physicians, as would be expected, delegate less responsibility for those patients who have retained their services privately than for the public ward patients, though this is not to imply by any means that they are heedless of the welfare of the latter group. Many practising physicians delegate little or no responsibility for their private patients. In medical cases, as opposed to surgical or obstetrical cases, an interne can learn by making up his own mind what he *would* do, even if he is not permitted to proceed without the authorization of the attending physician. The value of this type of experience is limited, however, since it is one thing to say what one *would* do, when one will not have to face any of the unhappy consequences that may ensue, but quite a different thing to have to decide between one and another course of action and, whichever one chooses, accept responsibility for the results.† In other words, only *by* assuming responsibility, preferably in increasing amounts, does one *learn* to assume responsibility. Thus the value of training received in a hospital where there are few or no public ward patients is definitely limited, even in medicine (including paediatrics). In surgery and obstetrics, the limitation is much more severe. A private patient who has retained a physician to deliver her baby or to perform an operation has every right to expect that the work will be done by the doctor selected, not by someone less experienced. Though an interne may deliver the occasional private

*For example, a junior interne who has no one placed between him and his attending staff physician is in a different position, both as to the amount of responsibility that he is allowed to assume and as to the degree of intimacy between him and the attending physician, from a junior interne who has, between him and his attending physician, a senior interne, an assistant-resident, and a resident.

†See also, on page 356, Janeway's opinion of the limited effectiveness of teaching that has "a make-believe element to it."

obstetrical patient when the attending physician does not arrive in time, similar opportunities do not occur in surgery. Since most of the non-teaching hospitals have few or no public ward patients, the opportunity for learning the techniques, as opposed to the theory, of obstetrics and of surgery is slight.

In teaching hospitals, where public ward patients predominate,* the situation is quite different. In the handling of medical cases, an interne, though under the watchful eye of more senior members of the house staff and of the attending physician, is allowed much more, and constantly increasing, responsibility. In obstetrics, he delivers the public ward patients himself, at first under direct supervision, then more on his own. On a busy obstetrical service of a large teaching hospital, an interne will have carried out enough deliveries in a few months to be able to feel confident of his ability to handle normal cases. Such short experience, however, will not enable him either to acquire the techniques or, more important, to develop the judgment, that are necessary for the handling of obstetrical complications.

On the surgical service of a teaching hospital, many of the operations, including the very difficult ones, are performed by the house staff. Of necessity, this is a type of training that extends over several years. In the final phase of this training, a young surgeon is assuming as much responsibility as he will in his own practice, except that nominally the final responsibility rests with a member of the attending staff. A surgeon-in-training, however, does not have such a measure of responsibility during the earlier years when he is acquiring technique and developing his critical faculties. Indeed, during the first year of interning, which in this country is usually a rotation through a number of the hospital services, an interne's few months on the surgical service are occupied mainly with taking histories, examining patients, doing laboratory work, and carrying out various routine procedures on the wards. He may be permitted or expected to be present in the operating room, but seldom, in a teaching hospital, will he be the first assistant at an operation, and not very frequently even the second assistant. He may possibly be allowed, under very close supervision, to remove one appendix during his period of service on the surgical wards.

The description that we have just given of the work done by an interne and the responsibility assumed by him has been given at this

---

*This is becoming less true today with the increase in prepaid medical care plans. The decrease in the number of public patients poses serious problems for medical education in the future. Consideration of this, however, is beyond the scope of our study and would have no bearing on our present discussion.

particular point in order that the reader may have it fresh in his mind as he considers the limits set by some of the hospitals to the surgical work of our practitioners. Almost half of the practitioners that we visited in each of the two provinces were restricted in the surgery that they were permitted to do. The great variation in the restrictions has already been described in some detail.* The duration of the postgraduate surgical training of these 21 Ontario, and 20 Nova Scotia, physicians is shown in Table 27.† It will be observed that, of the 21

TABLE 27

DURATION OF POSTGRADUATE SURGICAL TRAINING OF THE 21 ONTARIO, AND THE 20 NOVA SCOTIA, PHYSICIANS WHOSE SURGICAL WORK WAS RESTRICTED BY THEIR HOSPITALS

| Duration of postgraduate surgical training (total)* | Number of physicians | | Duration of surgical training (teaching hospital only) | Number of physicians | |
|---|---|---|---|---|---|
| | Ontario | Nova Scotia | | Ontario | Nova Scotia |
| None | 1 | 1 | None | 8 | 9 |
| One month | 0 | 0 | One month | 0 | 1 |
| Two months | 3 | 5 | Two months | 3 | 3 |
| Three months | 6 | 4 | Three months | 3 | 2 |
| Four months | 6 | 3 | Four months | 3 | 2 |
| Five months | 1 | 1 | Five months | 1 | 0 |
| Six months | 1 | 2 | Six months | 0 | 1 |
| Eleven months | 0 | 1 | Eleven months | 0 | 1 |
| Fifteen months | 1 | 0 | Fifteen months | 1 | 0 |
| Sixteen months | 0 | 1 | Sixteen months | 0 | 1 |
| Several years | 1 | 0 | Several years | 1 | 0 |
| Not known | 1 | 2† | Not known | 1 | 0 |

*Total includes time spent in teaching hospitals *and* non-teaching hospitals.
†The total duration of surgical training of 1 of these men is known to be less than a year and of the other to be less than 18 months and probably less than a year.

Ontario doctors, 18 had had 6 months or less of experience as internes on surgical wards. In fact, 15 had had between 2 and 4 months, and 1 had had no time, on a surgical service. In *teaching* hospitals, 8 of these 18 had had no surgical interning. Similarly, in Nova Scotia, 16 of the 20 physicians whose surgery was restricted had spent 6 months or less on surgical wards as internes; and 7 of these 16, as well as 2 other doctors whose *total* time on surgical wards is unknown, had spent no

*See pages 117–119.
†The median duration of the postgraduate surgical training (both the total training and the part taken in teaching hospitals) of those doctors whose surgical work was not restricted by their hospitals did not differ at all in Ontario, and did not differ appreciably in Nova Scotia, from the corresponding median for the doctors whose surgical work was restricted. Some of the non-restricted doctors, however, though not restricted by their hospitals since their hospitals did not yet have any restrictive regulations, nevertheless limited their own work.

time on surgical wards in *teaching* hospitals. None of the 18 Ontario men had gone on, in surgical training, beyond the rotating interneship as described in the preceding paragraph, though some had taken more advanced training in *non*-surgical fields. This statement applies equally to the surgical training of the 16 Nova Scotia physicians who had had 6 months or less of surgical training. In other words, the surgical training of these 18 Ontario, and 16 Nova Scotia, practitioners had not proceeded beyond the elementary level.

Of the remaining doctors shown in Table 27, the one in Ontario whose surgical training was of unknown duration *is* known not to have taken training beyond the level of the rotating interneship. This is true, also, of 1 of the 2 Nova Scotia doctors who were unable to state accurately the duration of their surgical training. The man in Ontario who had had 15 months of surgical training in a teaching hospital, i.e. a year of surgical experience after the rotating interneship, was permitted to do appendectomies and to repair hernias, but not to remove gallbladders. This doctor, whose surgical training had proceeded beyond the elementary stage but not as far as the advanced stage, was limited to "intermediate" surgery. The same apparently was true of the Nova Scotia doctor with 11 months of surgical training, who, though not permitted to do "major" surgery, was permitted to do appendectomies and Caesarean sections. The Nova Scotia doctor who had had 16 months of surgical training in a teaching hospital was not allowed to do major surgery except in an emergency. It is interesting to note that this man, whose surgical training had been exceeded in length by that of only 3 out of the entire sample of 42 Nova Scotia doctors and who had had more surgical training than any of the other Nova Scotia doctors who were restricted in their surgical work, was Chief of Staff of his hospital and was himself the author of the limitations that were imposed. Commenting on the fact that he did not do appendectomies, except in an emergency, he said, "Why should I hazard a patient, when there is a surgeon up the road?" Finally, the Ontario doctor who had had "several years" of surgical training in teaching hospitals was not permitted to do surgery. Apparently, the restriction was imposed because he did not hold a specialist's certificate in surgery, as was required by his hospital, which was a teaching hospital.

In the last case, and in the case of 1 of the Nova Scotia physicians who could not remember how much surgical training he had had, we are not in possession of enough information to express an opinion about the reasonableness of the restriction. In the cases of the other men who were restricted, if it be urged that their formal training does not reflect their surgical ability, i.e. that they have acquired experience and have matured their judgment during their years in private practice, one can reply only that this may be so or that it may not be so and that there is no way of evaluating such experience. Viewed against the background of interneship training, which, in the absence of formal specialist qualifications, is the only criterion available, the surgical restrictions upon all the physicians, except possibly the two whom we have mentioned at the beginning of this paragraph, do not seem unreasonable, if the welfare of the patient is assumed to be of first importance.

There is a group whose comments on hospital restrictions we have not yet heard—the doctors themselves whom we visited. What had they to say? They said surprisingly little, especially in contrast with what has been said publicly by others. Only 6 of the 44 Ontario practitioners commented on this matter. One, who was not restricted in his hospital work, said that there were no limitations in his hospital, that each new member of the staff, after the first six months, had full privileges, and that each physician "must know his own limitations." Another man, whose hospital did not yet have any restrictions but was likely to institute them, thought that hospital authorities should not have the power to limit a man's work, that it was up to each doctor to decide for himself what he was capable of doing.

One man who had surgical privileges in two hospitals but not in a third hospital said that hospitals should not be closed to general practitioners. Another man, who had limited hospital privileges, said that regulations were probably needed, although they were aggravating to an experienced doctor. Still another physician, a member of the College of General Practice, on the staff of a teaching hospital, and subject to restrictions laid down by the hospital, said:

I have no complaints myself. I got on the staff of this hospital in the old days. Now, it's almost impossible for a non-specialist to do so. However, if a young general practitioner can't get on the staff, he's got to face facts. If he wants a hospital appointment, he's got to move to a smaller place, or get a certificate [i.e., qualify for a specialist's certificate], or both. It's only natural that the hospitals should pick men with more training. A young man should get a certificate in something before going into general practice. Then he will be able to specialize later, if this becomes desirable. . . . I'm against excess planning and spoon-feeding. Each man has to work for what he gets. If he wants to be a big shot with extra prestige, he's got to figure out what to do and do it without moaning.

Much less satisfied was a doctor who was on the visiting staff of another teaching hospital. He was not permitted to do major surgery because he was not certificated. He said that, if he did not call for a consultation at the slightest hint of difficulty with an obstetrical case, the nursing staff supervisor would report to the "head office." His medical cases, he was allowed to treat himself, theoretically: in actual practice, beds were so few, he said, that it was necessary to refer these patients also to members of the active staff of the hospital in order to get them into the hospital. He said that he had once been bitter about the situation in his hospital, but was now reconciled to it.

When we embarked upon the Survey in Ontario, we were not fully aware how strong were the feelings of some doctors on the subject of hospital privileges for general practitioners. As the strength of feeling was brought home to us by some of the statements that we have already quoted deploring the exclusion of general practitioners from hospitals or the restriction of their privileges, we decided, in carrying out the Nova Scotia study, to ask certain specific questions. The first of these was, "Do the hospital facilities to which you have access meet your needs?" Sixty-two per cent of the Nova Scotia doctors answered unreservedly in the affirmative, 33 per cent in the negative; of the 2 remaining doctors, one qualified his affirmative answer with "except for a shortage of beds," and the other was satisfied with the facilities in one hospital but dissatisfied with those in another. Those who were dissatisfied were asked to explain in what way the facilities did not meet their needs. The complaints included such things as lack of technicians and nurses, shortage of space, inadequate laboratory facilities, and even unsatisfactory plumbing. Nineteen per cent of the entire sample of Nova Scotia doctors complained either of a shortage of beds or of a shortage of beds for private patients. The percentages of physicians in various age groups who made this complaint did not differ significantly. On the other hand, these men constituted 56 per cent of the doctors who were visited in Halifax (with which is included Dartmouth) but only 9 per cent of those who were visited in other communities. The difference is significant ($p < 0.05$).* It is to be noted, however, that no doctor, in answering the question, made any mention of being dissatisfied with the restrictions upon what he might do.

The next question was, "Are you satisfied with the limitations placed upon you by your hospitals?" Forty-five per cent of the physicians were subject to no restrictions, 45 per cent were limited but were satisfied with the limitations, and the remaining 10 per cent were dissatisfied with the limitations set by their hospitals. Three of the 4 men who

*This is explained on pages 32–33.

were dissatisfied were speaking of teaching hospitals. One of them, who had had 2 months of surgical training in a teaching hospital, objected to surgical restrictions and specifically to the fact that he was not allowed to remove tonsils. Another, who had had 3 months of surgical training and 2 months of obstetrical training in a non-teaching hospital, was protesting not being allowed to do tonsillectomies and being required to have consultations for certain obstetrical and gynaecological conditions. It developed that the latter restriction had its origin in the religious affiliation of the particular hospital. The third doctor of this group said that the limitations barred his access to further training experience under specialists—a complaint the meaning of which was not clear to our interrogator. Finally, one practitioner in a smaller community, who had had 2 months of surgical training in a non-teaching hospital and who was permitted to perform any operation, except those involving the chest or the central nervous system, provided that a certificated surgeon was present in the hospital, objected to this proviso.

The last of this series of questions was, "Are you excluded from any hospital to which you think you should have access?" Forty-one of the 42 doctors replied in the negative. The one doctor who said that he was excluded was referring to the fact that, when a close friend was being operated on in a community many miles distant from where his own practice was located, he was not permitted to assist at the operation.

The problem of hospital restrictions is further illuminated by the stories told by two Ontario doctors. One of these, practising in a community of less than 10,000, said that a small group of doctors in that community were continually complaining of the limitations on major surgery. Only men who were certificated in surgery were allowed full surgical privileges. The doctor telling of this, who was not certificated but had had a good deal of experience in surgery, agreed with this policy, but he said that other men, who were clumsy surgeons, were resentful of the surgeons who held certificates in surgery, though in the informant's opinion these latter were the only men in town who were competent to do such operations as the removal of stomach or gallbladder. It is significant that the disgruntled group, men who were considered incompetent surgeons, thought that the College of General Practice should see that the general practitioner was not restricted in any way. Of the dissatisfaction of these men, whom we chanced to meet, our own observations left us in no doubt; the remainder of the story, since it could not be verified by direct observation of the surgical work being done, must be accepted with that certain caution which is always appropriate to such second-hand evidence.

The other story is not subject to such a reservation, since the doctor being visited by us was recounting his own experience (see also page 306). He said that, some years earlier, assisted by a certificated surgeon, he had been repairing a hernia. In the course of the operation, he lost his bearings. Not only did he ask his "assistant" to take over, but he explained the situation afterwards to the patient and arranged for the certificated man to receive the surgeon's fee while he received the assistant's fee; and, more important and significant, from that time on, he turned over *all* major surgery to men who were certificated in surgery. This man's internship in a non-teaching hospital had included 4 months on a surgical service; and the operation was one that repeatedly we have heard included among those that general practitioners should be allowed to perform.

To sum up, a minority of the doctors in each of the two provinces commented on the matter of hospital restrictions, and only about 10 per cent in each province made comments that showed any antipathy to the hospitals' policies in this regard.

After examining all the evidence available to us from the Survey, we find it impossible to conclude that the charges that general practitioners are excluded from use of the hospitals have any basis in fact, so far as either Ontario or Nova Scotia is concerned, except, perhaps, in the teaching hospitals.[*] It is true that some hospitals have set limits to the work that may be undertaken by members of their staffs. These limits, however, when examined in relation to the duration of the practitioner's training in the particular field of medicine, seem not unreasonable,[†] but rather, as some practitioners themselves asserted, they appear to be in the public interest. Indeed, in each province, the practitioners who expressed dissatisfaction with the restrictions in their own hospitals formed but a small percentage of the total group. It is interesting to note that Peterson says[‡] of North Carolina, "there appears to be little basis for any complaint on the part of North Carolina general practitioners that they have been crowded out of

[*]In this connection, we note that of 967 members of the College of General Practice of Canada who answered a recent questionnaire (46 per cent of those to whom the questionnaire was sent), 241 are on the staffs of university teaching hospitals. D. I. Rice: Canadian Medical Association Journal, *84*: 1156, 1961.

[†]See page 491 for J. T. Wearn's comments on the inadequacy of a single year of a rotating internship as preparation for "practice involving advanced problems in internal medicine or major surgery."

[‡]O. L. Peterson *et al.*: Journal of Medical Education, *31*, No. 12, Part 2: 97, 1956.

hospitals by specialists. Some physicians were not allowed the full range of hospital practice which they may have desired, but in no instance did a physician state that he had been unable to obtain any hospital staff appointment."

We find ourselves in sympathy with the doctor who complained that he had to refer even his medical cases in order to have them admitted to hospital. We do not think, however, that this is a matter of discrimination against the general practitioner and in favour of the specialist, since we have repeatedly heard the same complaint from specialists in internal medicine, men who are on the "active" staffs of teaching hospitals and are devoting many hours each week, without pay, to teaching or to the care of public patients, namely, that private beds are so scarce that it is only rarely that they can get a bed for one of their private patients (see also page 373).

We do not propose to discuss further whether general practitioners should or should not have the privilege of treating their patients in *teaching* hospitals, because we do not feel competent to do so. This is a matter of great complexity and of vital importance to medical education and so to the country as a whole. This whole problem needs, in our view, a thorough re-examination, either by the general practitioners and the specialists working in concert, or, if either group should refuse that, then by an independent commission, probably one having both lay and professional representation.

We now leave the controversial matter of hospital privileges and go on to consider the relationships between the physicians and those responsible for the administration of the hospitals. Each of the doctors was asked, "Are you satisfied with the relationship that exists between the administration of your hospital(s) and the professional staff?" Eight-six per cent of the Ontario doctors and 79 per cent of those in Nova Scotia replied in the affirmative, 9 per cent in Ontario and 14 per cent in Nova Scotia in the negative, and the remaining 5 per cent in Ontario and 7 per cent in Nova Scotia expressed satisfaction with one hospital but dissatisfaction with another. Of the 6 Ontario physicians who were dissatisfied, 3 were using hospitals located in communities with populations of between 1,000 and 10,000, 1 was on the staff of a hospital in a place of between 10,000 and 100,000, and 2 were complaining of Toronto hospitals. None of these six hospitals was a teaching hospital. Of the 9 Nova Scotia practitioners, 1 was complaining of a hospital in a community of less than 1,000, 3 of hospitals in communities of between 1,000 and 10,000, 2 of hospitals in communities of between 10,000 and 100,000, and 3 of hospitals in Halifax, including teaching hospitals.

Each of the 15 physicians was asked in what way he was dissatisfied. The core of every one of the complaints in Ontario was that there was too much lay control. One physician said that the laymen had complete control, that the only medical representative on the hospital board was the president of the medical staff, usually an older man who would not "push things" with the board. Another physician, speaking of a large city hospital, called it "a very unhappy place," though he considered another large hospital "excellent." Another physician, in a community of between 1,000 and 10,000, complained that the hospital board and the administration tried to dictate medical policy. In another community of a similar size, the complaint was made that there is "a gap between the administration and the medical staff. The board asks for recommendations and then very often turns them down. The board has too much to say in minor matters. It interferes in matters that should be settled by the nursing and medical staff." Another practitioner, in a city of between 10,000 and 100,000, said that the administration did not ask the advice of the medical staff "as they should," and that, when advice was given, it was not taken. This doctor informed us that the superintendent, apparently at least in part because he was not a physician, was considered by the doctors to be "the board's man." He added, however, that the medical men probably could not "do the job, since they cannot agree on policy."

In Nova Scotia, a few of the complaints referred to the fact that the administrator was inadequately prepared to cope with his or her responsibilities; but the majority were concerned with the fact that laymen, either the administrator or the hospital board, went their own way with little regard for the professional staff. Matters about which the doctors' wishes either were not ascertained or were ignored included such things as admitting procedures and operating hours. One doctor, who told us most emphatically that he was not satisfied with the relationship existing between the professional staff and the administration of one of the hospitals used by him, said that there were poor relations between the board and the doctors owing to "personality differences" with certain trade union members of the board.

After the physicians had answered the more general question about the relationship existing between the hospital administration and the medical staff and had explained the reason for any dissatisfaction that they had expressed, they were asked the more specific question, "In your hospital(s), does the division of administrative control strike an optimal balance between laymen and medical men? or have the medical men too much control? or have the laymen too much control?" Approximately three-quarters of the physicians in each province said that there was an optimal balance in their hospitals; the remainder in each province thought that the laymen had too much control, with the exception of 1 Nova Scotia doctor who said that the medical men had too much control.

In discussing the relationships between the practitioners and those hospitals in which they had privileges, we have had occasion to refer to the teaching hospitals, since some of the physicians were on the staffs of these hospitals. Other doctors, who have no direct connection with the teaching hospitals, do have another, more indirect, relationship, in that, now and then, they refer difficult cases to these hospitals for investigation or treatment. From time to time one hears complaints levelled at these hospitals, and it seemed desirable to find out whether they had a substantial basis. Each doctor was therefore asked, "With regard to the *teaching hospitals to which you refer patients*, are you satisfied with the relationship that exists between you and these hospitals?" This question was not applicable to 6 Ontario doctors who were themselves on the staffs of teaching hospitals. Five others did not refer patients to teaching hospitals. Another was satisfied with one teaching hospital and dissatisfied with another. Of the remaining 32 Ontario physicians, 4 were dissatisfied, 28 satisfied. Yet, of this latter group, about one-quarter were critical of one or another of the teaching hospitals with which they had had experience.

Some of the complaints referred to specific teaching hospitals, others did not. One doctor, for example, said, "I work the case up and then I'm right out of it. I lose the patient. It's hard to make a living." Another, who also complained that the patient was lost to him, said that he was treated as an outsider and that, to rectify this, "it would require an atom bomb." Several practitioners complained that the teaching hospitals to which they referred patients did not send them reports on their patients, even when a letter accompanied a patient on his admission to hospital. Some asserted that certain large teaching hospitals were "frosty" or "frigid" and that the occasional member of their attending staffs or even the hospital superintendents had been downright rude to them. Others, to avoid being treated in this way and to ensure that they would receive a report on their patients, stressed that they referred patients to particular doctors in the teaching hospitals.

In Nova Scotia, 9 of the doctors were on the staffs of teaching hospitals. Of the remainder, 26 were satisfied, and 7 dissatisfied, with the relationship existing between them and the teaching hospitals to which they referred patients. The causes of dissatisfaction were said to be that the teaching hospitals were too slow in sending out reports to the referring doctor, that outside doctors were "looked down upon," and that the teaching hospitals tended to disregard the investigative work that the referring doctor had already done on a case. One doctor commented, "The gap is so wide that I can't see any solution until the Haligonians realize that there is such a place as Cape Breton." On the other hand, another practitioner, who said that he was satisfied with the teaching hospitals, added, "Actually they go out of their way to give you a bed."

So far we have discussed the hospitals as institutions that are useful to the practitioner in the conduct of his practice. Another aspect of the relationship between the physician and those hospitals in which he has privileges is the responsibilities of the physician to the hospital itself as distinct from his responsibility for the care of his own private patients while they are in hospital. Each of the doctors was asked what hospital responsibilities he had. Thirty-four per cent of those in Ontario and 31 per cent of those in Nova Scotia had no responsibilities at the time of the Survey's visit; 66 per cent in Ontario and 69 per cent in Nova Scotia had one or more responsibilities. These are shown in detail in Table 28. Briefly, they fall into four groups: medical care, instruction, a variety of offices, and membership on one or more of a number of boards and committees. Whether the doctors remembered to mention all their responsibilities we have no way of knowing.

Nothing more need be said about the offices and committees, since the type of responsibility involved is obvious. What we were told of the staff ward work, the outpatient department work, and the emergency call rotations will be described briefly.

One doctor, located in a city of between 100,000 and 500,000, looked after ward patients on the obstetrical and gynaecological service of his hospital, for one month each year. Another in a city of between 10,000 and 100,000 cared for public ward surgical cases in rotation with the other doctors at his hospital. Two physicians were responsible, for two months each year, for the care of the patients on the medical wards of their hospitals. One of these doctors was located in a community of less than 10,000; the other was on the staff of a non-teaching hospital in Toronto, where he shared his responsibility with a second general practitioner.

The outpatient department work was all done either in the general

TABLE 28

HOSPITAL RESPONSIBILITIES OF THE 30 ONTARIO, AND THE
29 NOVA SCOTIA, PHYSICIANS WHO HAD SUCH RESPONSIBILITIES*

|  | Responsibilities | Number of physicians | |
|  |  | Ontario | Nova Scotia |
|---|---|---|---|
| Medical care | Emergency call | 8 | 5 |
|  | Staff ward work | 4 | 0 |
|  | Outpatient department | 6 | 2 |
|  | Examination and care of nurses | 3 | 2 |
| Instruction | Lectures to nurses | 5 | 3 |
|  | Instruction of internes | 1 | 0 |
| Offices | Hospital superintendent | 1 | 0 |
|  | Chief of staff | 2 | 5 |
|  | Vice-president of medical staff | 2 | 0 |
|  | Chief of advisory committee to hospital board | 0 | 1 |
|  | Chief of a clinical section | 5† | 2‡ |
|  | Secretary of the medical staff | 3 | 0 |
|  | Secretary of the medical advisory board | 2 | 0 |
|  | In charge of the laboratory | 0 | 1 |
| Boards and committees | Board of governors | 3 | 6 |
|  | Medical advisory board§ | 2 | 0 |
|  | Building committee | 2 | 0 |
|  | Credentials committee | 3 | 4 |
|  | Executive committee | 0 | 1 |
|  | Interne committee | 0 | 2 |
|  | Laboratory committee | 0 | 2 |
|  | Liaison committee of nurses and hospital board | 0 | 1 |
|  | Library committee | 0 | 1 |
|  | Negotiations committee | 0 | 1 |
|  | Nurses' education committee | 0 | 1 |
|  | Obstetrics committee | 1 | 0 |
|  | Pharmacy committee | 1 | 2 |
|  | Purchasing committee (for new hospital) | 1 | 0 |
|  | Records committee | 3 | 5 |
|  | Records, library, and programs committee | 1 | 0 |
|  | Staff committee | 0 | 1 |
|  | Standards committee | 0 | 11 |
|  | Tissue committee | 2 | 6 |
| Miscellaneous‖ |  | 0 | 2 |

*The term "hospital responsibility" is explained in the text.
†Two were chief of anaesthesia, and one each of medicine, obstetrics, and general practice.
‡One was chief of medicine, the other of surgery.
§Exclusive of those who were secretaries of these boards.
‖One of these physicians screened all admissions for length of stay in the hospital and reported on this to the hospital board. The other physician, though having no official position in his hospital, determined the hospital's policies in the final analysis.

medical part of the outpatient department or in special subdivisions of internal medicine. The amount of time given to this type of service varied. One physician gave one morning each week during two months each year, whereas another gave two mornings per week throughout the year, one morning to each of two hospitals. Others fell in between, perhaps working in the outpatient department one morning, or the better part of it, per week. The hospitals in which the 8 physicians were doing outpatient department work were all located in cities of over 100,000. It should be made clear that the outpatient department work and the work on the public wards were service for which none of the practitioners received any financial remuneration.

Eight doctors in Ontario and 5 in Nova Scotia took turns with their colleagues at being on call for emergencies, including particularly automobile accidents. This type of arrangement was mentioned by doctors in communities of all sizes, except in places of less than 1,000, in most of which, presumably, no such rotation system was possible. The arrangements varied from one hospital to another. One physician, for example, was on call throughout every thirteenth week, another physician for the whole of every tenth week, whereas still another had this responsibility every third day. This was a free service, in the sense that the physicians kept themselves in readiness during the specified times and recived no compensation for being available. On the other hand, whatever emergency patients they *were* called to treat, they would charge as they would their own private patients.

The age groups did not differ appreciably in the percentages of their members who had hospital responsibilities. Nor was there any significant relationship between size of community and whether the practitioner had hospital responsibilities.

Because the College of General Practice has been desirous that departments of general practice should be established in the teaching hospitals, we questioned the practitioners about this, in order to find out what need they thought would be met by these departments and what part they would play in the functioning of the hospitals. Each practitioner was asked, "Do you think that there should be departments of general practice in teaching hospitals?" and, regardless of the answer, "Why?" Sixty-eight per cent of the Ontario physicians thought that there should be departments of general practice in teaching hospitals, 27 per cent said that there should not be, and the rest gave indefinite answers. Affirmative answers were given by approximately the same percentages, 73 per cent and 67 per cent respectively, of those who were located in cities that contained teaching hospitals and of those who were located elsewhere. In Nova Scotia, 88 per cent of the practitioners said that there should be departments of general practice in teaching hospitals, and 12 per cent that there should not be.

The two points that were repeatedly mentioned were that the physicians who were members of departments of general practice in teaching hospitals should teach and that they should give the medical students and internes a "true picture" of general practice. Many suggestions were made regarding the part that should be played by the general practitioner in teaching. It was said that he should "assist in all phases of teaching and demonstrations, including lectures on the mechanics of general practice," that he should give a course of lectures on "office and house call matters," that he should teach on an obstetrical ward and on a medical ward, that he should lecture on "routines, ethics, hospital duties, and status." Many of those who said that he should teach did not elaborate; and very few named any topic of a *medical* nature (as opposed to economics, ethics, organization, etc.) that should be taught by general practitioners.

Many of the physicians said that the general practitioners in a teaching hospital should give the medical student a true picture of general practice. These men thought that, in this way, the student would have a greater respect for general practice and would be encouraged to choose this as his career. It was felt by some men that students got mistaken ideas from the specialists. One doctor's words sum up this attitude, "G.P.'s are just as important as specialists . . . they should be *teaching students* . . . so many boys end up as specialists because that's all they ever hear."

Three other points that were mentioned when the practitioners were asked why they thought there should be departments of general practice in teaching hospitals were that the general practitioner would do outpatient department work, that he would take part in the care of ward patients, and that he would be able to treat his own patients in hospital. A number of men thought that the general practitioners should run the outpatient department or that they should be in charge of its medical clinic and perhaps serve in rotation in the other clinics. Several thought that departments of general practice in the teaching hospitals would increase the prestige of the general practitioner. Other ways in which these departments would be useful were each named by one or two men and included instruction of nurses, arranging preceptorships for medical students or preferably internes, keeping the general practitioner in contact with other doctors and interested in hospital medicine, and relieving the specialist staff of a great deal of work that was "at the general practitioner level." Of those men who thought that there should be departments of general practice in teaching hospitals, only the occasional one specified that the general practitioner should take no part in teaching and that he should have nothing to do with the care of patients on the public wards.

We have said that 27 per cent of the Ontario doctors and 12 per cent of those in Nova Scotia thought that there should not be departments of general practice in teaching hospitals. A few gave no reason for their negative answer. The remainder said that they could not see the need for such departments. One man, himself on the staff of a teaching hospital, said that a general practice ward would be "silly— a duplication of effort," that the general practitioner was not able to teach, that he had no special knowledge to offer students, that teaching should be done by specialists only, and that in his hospital it was difficult to get the general practitioners to take on responsibility, that many of them wanted beds but were unwilling to do extra work in the outpatient department. Several physicians, who felt that specialists were the logical men to teach students, pointed out that general practitioners, though usually knowing enough to do good practice, did not have the specialized knowledge of minutiae that was necessary for teaching.

One practitioner, in a moderate-sized city, said that general practitioners should not be separated from other doctors, as they would be by the creation of a department of general practice. He thought that the general practitioner should be called a "physician" and be skilled in basic diagnosis like the internist. He suggested that training equivalent to the training for certification in internal medicine would be ideal, though he doubted that it would be economically possible for many men.

A few men who did not favour departments of general practice in teaching hospitals did specify that the general practitioners should do some teaching and that they should be allowed to treat their patients in these hospitals.

From the last few pages two things are plain. The majority of the practitioners, but not all of them, were in favour of departments of general practice in teaching hospitals. There was no uniformity of opinion, however, about the purpose that would be served by these departments. It is true that some men had given little thought to the matter and said little in reply to our questions; but those who apparently had thought about this expressed quite divergent opinions. This is in keeping with what we have said above about the complexity of the problems of the teaching hospitals.

# 10 / The General Practitioner and the Medical Profession

The general practitioner, whom so far we have seen carrying on his practice by himself or with a few associates, is a part of the general society in which he lives and of that more limited society which is the medical profession. In these days, when the interrelationships between groups and between individuals are ever increasing in complexity, it would be puerile to imagine that an individual physician could go his own way, completely unaffected by the beliefs and the strivings of his fellow-physicians and of his fellow-citizens. Even though he takes no part in the affairs of his profession beyond the limits of his own practice, he will still be affected by the policies that are formulated by his colleagues, and he in turn will have an influence on those policies if only because the silence of disapproval and the silence of lethargy cannot be distinguished by the policy-makers and either may be mistaken for assent.

To examine in any detail the relationship between the general practitioner and his fellow-members of the medical profession would be a large study in itself—one to which someone might profitably turn his attention in the future. In the present study, however, because of the number of aspects of practice being examined and because of the demanding nature of the actual assessment of quality of practice, it was necessary to set severe limits to our examination of the relationship between the general practitioner and the medical profession. Of the many aspects that might have been considered, we chose to confine our attention mainly to the Canadian Medical Association (the body that speaks for the doctors), the College of General Practice of Canada (which is interested primarily in quality of practice), and the specialists as a group.

First, we turn to the professional societies in which the general practitioners held membership. Each man was asked to list these. Over 90 per cent in each of the two provinces belonged to the provincial medical society and to the Canadian Medical Association; 64 per cent in Ontario and 88 per cent in Nova Scotia belonged to one or more local societies; and 32 per cent and 40 per cent, in the two provinces respectively, were members of the College of General Practice of Canada. The occasional physician belonged to special societies

TABLE 29

MEMBERSHIP OF ONTARIO AND NOVA SCOTIA PHYSICIANS IN
PROFESSIONAL SOCIETIES

| Society | Ontario physicians | | Nova Scotia physicians | |
|---|---|---|---|---|
| | Number | % | Number | % |
| Canadian Medical Association* and Ontario Medical Association or Medical Society of Nova Scotia | 42 | 95.5 | 39 | 92.9 |
| Local medical societies† | 28‡ | 63.6 | 37§ | 88.1 |
| College of General Practice of Canada | 14 | 31.8 | 17 | 40.5 |
| Canadian Public Health Association | 2 | 4.6 | 2 | 4.8 |
| Canadian Anaesthetists' Society | 3 | 6.8 | 0 | 0.0 |
| Alpha Omega Alpha | 1 | 2.3 | 0 | 0.0 |
| American Association of Railway Surgeons | 0 | 0.0 | 1 | 2.4 |
| American Industrial Physicians' Association | 0 | 0.0 | 1 | 2.4 |
| American Society of Anesthesiologists, Incorporated | 1 | 2.3 | 0 | 0.0 |
| Association des médecins de langue française du Canada | 1 | 2.3 | 0 | 0.0 |
| Association of Life Insurance Medical Directors of America | 1 | 2.3 | 0 | 0.0 |
| Defence Medical Association | 1 | 2.3 | 0 | 0.0 |
| Halifax Medico-Legal Society | 0 | 0.0 | 1 | 2.4 |
| International Association of Anesthesiologists, Incorporated | 1 | 2.3 | 0 | 0.0 |
| Life Insurance Medical Officers Association of Canada | 1 | 2.3 | 0 | 0.0 |
| Maimonides Society | 1 | 2.3 | 0 | 0.0 |
| New England Psychiatric Society | 0 | 0.0 | 1 | 2.4 |
| University of Toronto Medical Alumni Association | 1 | 2.3 | 0 | 0.0 |

*These are listed together because the provincial society is a division of the national society and it is not possible to belong to one without belonging to the other.
†These include county medical societies and academies of medicine which exist in the larger cities.
‡Seven physicians belonged to 2 local societies; the remaining 21 belonged to 1.
§Two physicians belonged to 2 local societies; the remaining 35 belonged to 1 society.

interested in such matters as anaesthesia, public health, or life insurance or to one or another of a miscellany of societies that are listed in Table 29. The number* of societies varied from 0 to 6 in the case of the Ontario physicians and from 0 to 4 in the case of those in Nova Scotia. The greatest percentage, however, in each province belonged to 2 societies (Table 30). Physicians of different ages did not differ significantly, in either province, in the number of societies to which they belonged.

TABLE 30

NUMBER OF PROFESSIONAL SOCIETIES TO WHICH
ONTARIO AND NOVA SCOTIA PHYSICIANS BELONGED

| Number of societies | Ontario physicians | | Nova Scotia physicians | |
|---|---|---|---|---|
| | Number | % | Number | % |
| None | 1 | 2.3 | 1 | 2.4 |
| One | 10 | 22.7 | 4 | 9.5 |
| Two | 16 | 36.4 | 19 | 45.2 |
| Three | 9 | 20.5 | 13 | 31.0 |
| Four | 6 | 13.6 | 5 | 11.9 |
| Five | 0 | 0.0 | 0 | 0.0 |
| Six | 2 | 4.5 | 0 | 0.0 |
| Total | 44 | 100 | 42 | 100 |

Each physician was asked why he did, or did not, belong to the Canadian Medical Association. Among the reasons given by the few physicians who did not belong were that the fee was too high, that the physician had neglected to renew his membership, that the Association's conventions were held in inconvenient places, and that the physician was dissatisfied with those administering the affairs of the provincial society. Of the 81 practitioners who were members of the Canadian Medical Association, about 70 per cent gave as their reason, or as one of their reasons, that the Association represented the medical men collectively, that "medical organization is of paramount importance," and that they belonged in order to support the negotiating body of organized medicine. The next most common reason for belonging, mentioned by less than a fifth of the doctors, was to receive the Association's *Journal*. Other reasons, each of which was given by one or a few men, included to obtain the Blue Cross coverage that was available through the Ontario Medical Association, to keep in

*The Canadian Medical Association and the provincial medical society have been counted as one, since it is not possible to belong to one without belonging to the other.

touch with what was going on in the profession, to meet physicians who were doing various types of medical work, and to support the body that was helping to provide life insurance and health insurance for doctors.

The reasons reported in the preceding paragraph were given singly or in various combinations by 71 per cent of the Ontario members and by 92 per cent of those visited in Nova Scotia. The remaining 29 per cent in Ontario, and 8 per cent in Nova Scotia, said that they belonged to the Canadian Medical Association because "it's a good thing to belong to," "because it's the thing to do," "because it's a parent body—no real reason," "because it's automatic—belonging to the O.M.A." or out of "loyalty" or "duty." None of these reasons was explained further.

Every one of the practitioners, whether a member of the Canadian Medical Association or not, was asked, "*In general*, are you satisfied with the way in which the C.M.A. is handling the affairs of the profession?" In Ontario 77 per cent and in Nova Scotia 74 per cent replied that they were satisfied, 16 per cent and 21 per cent in the two provinces, respectively, said that they were not satisfied, and the remainder were unable to answer. There was no significant relationship, in either province, between the answers given and either the size of the physician's community or the age of the physician.

Those who had given negative answers were asked, "In what way are you not satisfied?" and "What action would you like the C.M.A. to take?" One physician complained that surgeons were overpaid and that general practitioners were "just chore boys"; he wished for a change in the fee schedule. Another thought that the Association should press for action on the "unfair income tax." He pointed out that doctors' hours of work were long but yet they were penalized for extra work. Other complaints were that the Ontario Medical Association was "not running" Physicians' Services Incorporated "properly," that the Canadian Medical Association was "not doing enough," and that it was "not doing enough for the fee." Several men who complained that the Association was not doing enough, when questioned further, stated that they did not read the Association's reports and did not really know what was being done. One extraordinary complaint was, "Why are they interested in W.H.O. and that junk? Why should an ordinary joker like a G.P. in a small town contribute to giving rice to Chinese kids?" A number of the Nova Scotia physicians maintained that there was little or no contact between the Canadian Medical Association and the mass of its members. Suggestions as to what the

Association should do included improving the *Journal* and arranging for the standardization of insurance forms, both those used in examinations for insurance and those used in prepaid care plans, in order that the expenditure of time and the confusion connected with paper work might be reduced. Those who complained of lack of contact between the Association and its members thought that the Association should take steps to make its policies known and to give leadership to its members, even to the extent of having the officers of the Association visit the various local societies at frequent intervals.

The final two questions having to do with the Canadian Medical Association were, "*In particular*, are you satisfied with the way in which the C.M.A. is handling the issue of private medical care versus some form of governmental control?" and "What action do you think the C.M.A. should take in this regard, or what policy should it adopt?" The former question was answered in the affirmative by 68 per cent of the Ontario physicians and by 74 per cent of those in Nova Scotia, and in the negative by 7 per cent and 19 per cent in the two provinces respectively. The remaining doctors said that they did not know enough about what the Association was doing to give any answer. There was no discernible relationship between the physicians' answers and either their ages or the populations of the communities in which they were practising.

The question about what action the Canadian Medical Association should take or what policy it should adopt was answered by 41 per cent of the Ontario physicians. Of the remainder, who had no suggestions, one man said that this was "better left to the people in medical politics," whereas another, who said that he knew little of the matter, was "afraid some C.M.A. jokers are going to hand it over to the government." The percentage of physicians in different age groups who had suggestions to make did not differ significantly. In Nova Scotia, the question was answered by 86 per cent of the physicians.

Because this issue, which seemed important when the Survey was planned, has increased greatly in prominence in the past year or two and has already been the central issue, and given rise to acrimonious debate, in one provincial election,\* the views expressed by our two random samples of physicians should be of interest. To avoid the possibility of giving undue weight to one or another suggestion, we

\*Indeed, since this book went to the printer, the issue of governmental control of medical care has been the main plank in the platform of one political party in the federal election of June 18, 1962, and has precipitated a doctors' "strike" in Saskatchewan.

shall not summarize them but shall report what each of the 18 Ontario, and 36 Nova Scotia, physicians said. We remind the reader that the statements of the Ontario physicians were made between July, 1956, and October, 1957, and the statements of the Nova Scotia physicians between December, 1958, and February, 1960.

ONTARIO

*Physicians 46 to 61 years of age*

NUMBER 1. The patient should pay something, no matter what plan comes in, except that the poor and the old should be subsidized. Governments don't realize the terrific expense of state medicine, but it is a vote-getter.

NUMBER 2. There is little to do. Just wait and see. Maybe state medicine is inevitable.

NUMBER 3. The C.M.A. should fight it [i.e., governmental control].

NUMBER 4. Strive to prevent nationalization of medicine.

NUMBER 5. The doctors have made too much fuss about it in the past. Better to wait for definite move by government and then make suggestions. Regarding the Ontario government hospitalization scheme, they should get after the government and remind them that they promised that the doctors would have some say in the scheme.

*Physicians 36 to 45 years of age*

NUMBER 6. Stick to the P.S.I. idea—voluntary, prepaid, medically controlled, fee-for-service.

NUMBER 7. The starting of P.S.I. was good. Also it is good to have public relations men.

NUMBER 8. The present policy is correct. Some socialization is inevitable. Should try to preserve the doctor-patient relationship.

NUMBER 9. Definitely opposed to a per capita scheme as in England.

NUMBER 10. We have to do what the majority of the people want. If our present practice is so undesirable that people do not want it, that's our own fault. We must discipline ourselves and control our fees.

NUMBER 11. The C.M.A. has not been handling it well but they have been becoming more realistic recently. The C.M.A. should be unalterably opposed to state control of physicians' services—by more public education.

*Physicians 31 to 35 years of age*

NUMBER 12. Look after the pensioners better before taking on more people, i.e. pay the doctors more adequately for what they *are* doing. Doctors to run the scheme. Government to look after only the finances but the Ontario Medical Association to pay the doctors on a fee-for-service basis.

NUMBER 13. Fee-for-service is very important. A government scheme is O.K. if this is a proviso.

NUMBER 14. There should be a health insurance scheme run by government with the doctors having an adequate say. *Adequate* fee for service is important, not per capita payment. Such a scheme would remove worry over the patient's finances from the doctor's mind.

NUMBER 15. There should be a firm policy of co-operation with schemes such as P.S.I. People not co-operating are harming themselves and the profession. This also should be stressed to the undergraduates.

NUMBER 16. I'm against government control.

NUMBER 17. It is obscure what the C.M.A. has done. They should come out with a clear-cut policy and present it to the government and should also make the policy clear to the profession. It should have specific recommendations. Also, present-day bargaining between management and labour includes costs of medical care. Whichever side loses in each of these disputes and has to pay the costs of medical care finds it to its advantage to have the government take over the burden of these costs. Thus in the struggle between labour and management, the medical profession must inevitably be squeezed between the two unless it allies itself with one or other. A clear picture of the medical situation should be presented to the labour leaders.

NUMBER 18. Good public relations are important.

### NOVA SCOTIA
*Physicians 46 to 60 years of age*
NUMBER 1. The C.M.A. should be prepared to acquiesce in whatever the Canadian Government should decide in this regard, and should be fully prepared to give an outline of the profession's position.

NUMBER 2. The C.M.A. should rigorously oppose state medicine.

NUMBER 3. Maintain the present policy of the C.M.A.

NUMBER 4. The C.M.A. accepts the principle of a national health service, but the details of the doctors' participation in this scheme and their status and conditions of service are what the C.M.A. must make policy decisions on. The fear is that the state will make medicine its slave.

NUMBER 5. Leadership in organizing and directing the medical profession nationally (and, when requested, provincially). For example, the C.M.A. should work with the new agencies.

NUMBER 6. Should adopt policy which will protect the interests and dignity of the medical profession, to see that we have a voice in the conduct of hospitals, medical schools, and therapy of patients.

NUMBER 7. The C.M.A. should bring to the government's attention the need for adequate care of the indigent. A fee-for-service plan is best. A scheme embodying this on a federal basis is needed.

NUMBER 8. The C.M.A. should present to the government a workable prepaid plan designed by the medical profession, in which the government cannot find flaws.

NUMBER 9. They should be adamant and *united* in opposing governmental control.

NUMBER 10. The C.M.A. should support private and plan care until the national health service comes.

NUMBER 11. Keep on with the present policy.

*Physicians 36 to 45 years of age*
NUMBER 12. They should insist on private control of medicine and oppose governmental control.

NUMBER 13. It should take a constructive attitude. A national health service is for the betterment of the public. The C.M.A. should associate themselves with the formulation of policies for such a service in order that the profession may have an adequate say in the administration of the health services.

NUMBER 14. The C.M.A. should have a unified opposition which will oppose any plan not acceptable to the C.M.A.

NUMBER 15. A policy must be made which will preserve medical unity. The form of the scheme should be left to the doctors to formulate and not to the politicians or the lay public.

NUMBER 16. Medicine should not be in the least socialized. The C.M.A. should oppose any trend in this direction.

NUMBER 17. Changes are inevitable. The medical men should lead the way to changes.

NUMBER 18. We are living in a socialistic age, where the politicians use the gimmick of "something for nothing." Therefore, some sort of insurance scheme will be demanded by the public. This scheme should be worked out by professional men representing the medical profession so that the doctors will have some say in the scheme's operation.

NUMBER 19. Plans like Maritime Medical Care should be promoted. Doctors should keep good public relations with the public. They should make it clear to the public that the medical profession is not responsible for high drug costs which play a major role in current medical costs.

NUMBER 20. Any national health service should allow the present mode of payment and choice of doctor.

NUMBER 21. Stipulate that private initiative and fraternity between doctors should be encouraged.

NUMBER 22. They should make the best deal they can with the Government: as long as doctors are independent they shouldn't be against a national health set-up.

NUMBER 23. The C.M.A. should put out more data on these issues, *available* to the G.P.; the profession is not adequately informed. The C.M.A. should approach all doctors on their views on this issue. Representatives of all groups should put their views forward. Halifax, for instance, doesn't have the same view in this matter as this area.

NUMBER 24. I'm a firm believer in free enterprise. This principle should be a keystone in all negotiations. I feel free enterprise should apply to all the professions.

NUMBER 25. A government-controlled scheme is O.K. if medical men are allowed to run it.

NUMBER 26. There is a tendency to wait and see—the C.M.A. is not pushing ahead fast enough. They are not pushing the government sufficiently. They may wait too long and see too little.

NUMBER 27. The C.M.A. should oppose regimentation of the profession and any tendency to government control.

NUMBER 28. The C.M.A. should work in co-operation with the government because *in time* a national health service is inevitable. The C.M.A. must stress the necessity, however, to maintain good medicine within such a service and should do this by educating both the doctor and public to their responsibilities. Remuneration must be adequate and should combine salary with fee for service. Any complaints in a health service against the doctor must be substantiated.

*Physicians 28 to 35 years of age*
NUMBER 29. The C.M.A. should be organizing a policy which the doctors know about.

NUMBER 30. They should have no socialized medicine but should have some federal or inter-provincial medical plan.

NUMBER 31. Have a medical economics committee evaluating a program of medical care coverage completely satisfactory to the C.M.A. and patients. The government's scheme (which is eventually going to come) should be met with constructive criticisms. The C.M.A. is a union and should have some say in what format any new medical care scheme may take.

NUMBER 32. Maintain the present policy.

NUMBER 33. The C.M.A. should take a more definite stand, so that they won't end up with laymen organizing their profession and setting standards for the doctors to meet.

NUMBER 34. Should take strong stand against Government control.

NUMBER 35. They should take a firm stand on private medicine until it has been proven that other care schemes are superior.

NUMBER 36. Satisfied with the majority policy at present shown by the C.M.A. The C.M.A. should not be as militant as the A.M.A.—too militant an approach leads to poor public relations.

In our discussions with the physicians about the issue of governmental control of medical care, the points that struck us most forcibly were that some physicians seemed to have given little constructive thought to this—indeed, in Ontario, only 41 per cent of the men had any comments to make—and that among those who did comment there was no unanimity. It appeared, moreover, that to the vast majority of these men the Canadian Medical Association was an impersonal, infinitely remote body with which the average physician neither had, nor expected to have, any contact. There seemed to be a great need for more direct communication between the practising physician and those who serve the Association full time.

We turn now from the Canadian Medical Association to the College of General Practice of Canada, the organization whose thought and efforts brought the Survey of General Practice into being. The College had its formal inauguration on June 17, 1954, under the auspices of the Canadian Medical Association. The objectives the founders had in mind were clearly stated on that occasion by Dr. Murray Stalker, in his Presidential Address:

. . . The formation of this College . . . marks the fulfilment of an unsatisfied need in our profession. . . . It is our hope that this new College of General Practice will help and stimulate the family doctor to retain his position in this changing world, to the advantage of both the profession and the public. . . . Our efforts will not be political. It will be our main function to develop efficient family doctors, to accredit them and to maintain standards. . . . Our broad objective is educational. This educational approach is undergraduate, immediate postgraduate and through the life of the practitioner.*

The first Newsletter sent out by the College, and quoted in the *Canadian Medical Association Journal*, stated:

THE COLLEGE OF GENERAL PRACTICE OF CANADA is a collective effort by general practitioners to aid themselves in operating good general practices. ... It is not a medical-political organization. It is not simply a protest movement. It is planned to be a sort of academic headquarters with emphasis on training and education. It is a serious attempt to do some of those things for the shock troops of the profession that the Royal College of Physicians and Surgeons has done for the specialist.†

Of the practitioners visited by the Survey, 32 per cent in Ontario and 40 per cent in Nova Scotia stated that they were members of the College of General Practice. When the physicians were grouped by age, the groups did not differ significantly, either in Ontario or in Nova Scotia, in the percentages who were members of the College. Nor was there any significant difference in this respect between groups based on size of community.

Each physician was asked why he was, or was not, a member of the College. Three reasons were commonly given by the members. First, they were interested in the extension of postgraduate education for general practitioners; and some stated that they would be encouraged and stimulated themselves to keep up their studying. Secondly, there was felt to be a need to organize the general practitioners, and some men were quite specific in saying that this was to counterbalance the specialties. Thirdly, though this perhaps was just another aspect of the preceding reason, some men were supporting the College in order to improve the status of general practitioners. One man said that he had the feeling that the general practitioner was being "pushed around," especially in the big cities. Another said, "I like the idea of giving the G.P. a boost back up where he belongs." A few men gave vague reasons for joining the College, such as that it was "the thing to do," that it was a "darned good idea," or that they believed in its aims, without further elaboration.

Of the doctors who were not members of the College, almost one-third in Ontario and two-fifths in Nova Scotia had not "got around to considering it very seriously." Another one-third of the non-members in Ontario, and a smaller fraction in Nova Scotia, either were unaware

*M. Stalker: Canadian Medical Association Journal, 71: 174, 1954.
†W. V. Johnston: Canadian Medical Association Journal, 71: 398, 1954.

of the College's existence or else had only the slightest knowledge of it. One man, for example, when asked whether he was a member, said, "I don't think I belong," and another thought that the member of the Survey team who was visiting him was from the Section of General Practice of the Ontario Medical Association. A few of those who were not members of the College had not been in practice long enough to qualify for membership. The remainder gave various reasons for not belonging. One physician said, "There is too much division already between specialists and general practitioners. I feel that the College of General Practice was organized as a reaction against specialists." Several men said that the College's fee was too high, and one that he thought that he would be refused membership because he did not belong to the Canadian Medical Association. Lack of time was the reason given by a number of those in each province who were not members, some of whom specified that they did not have time to do the amount of postgraduate study demanded by the College. Finally, a few men said that they could see no advantage in belonging to the College.

Two other questions were asked about the College of General Practice: "Do you think that the College is accomplishing anything of value for the general practitioners of Canada?" and "What is it accomplishing and what should it be accomplishing?" The former question was given an affirmative answer by 59 per cent of the Ontario, and 62 per cent of the Nova Scotia, doctors, and a negative answer by 7 per cent and 5 per cent respectively. The remaining 34 per cent in Ontario and 33 per cent in Nova Scotia said that they did not know or that it was still too early to say. Of the doctors who said that they did not think that the College was accomplishing anything of value, only one added any explanatory comments. He had been unfavourably impressed by the College's public relations campaign and thought that "The College should avoid public relations work. It depends on the individual G.P." Regarding the raising of standards, he said: "The standards of the College may keep young fellows up to date as they get older. You can't reform the old boys now."

Forty-one per cent of the Ontario physicians and 50 per cent of those in Nova Scotia stated a number of ways in which they felt that the College was already accomplishing something of value. It was pointed out that the College was bringing the general practitioners together, "instead of," as one man said, "being rugged individualists, which does not accomplish anything." Results of this organization were said to be that a general practitioner had a sense of belonging to something (i.e., to the local chapter of the College in his own community); that the individual general practitioner was brought to realize that his problems were not unique but that other general practitioners had the same problems;* and that, in the College, the general practitioners had, to quote one Nova Scotia practitioner, "a spokesman against the rampaging specialists."

Another accomplishment of the College, mentioned repeatedly both in Ontario and in Nova Scotia, was that it was increasing the prestige of general practitioners. The importance attached to this was apparent in the remark of one young doctor that the general practitioner was "no longer sneered at." It was felt that the College was making the public aware of the value of the general practitioner. His *self*-esteem, also, was thought to have been increased.

More concretely, the College was given credit for encouraging general practitioners to keep up postgraduate study and for organizing postgraduate courses, both of which it was thought would bring about improvement in the quality of practice. The College was said to be interesting young men in general practice as a career and to be fostering recognition of the general practitioners by hospitals.† A few doctors commended the College for instituting the Survey of General Practice. One commented, "Such a survey is long overdue."

Approximately 60 per cent of the Ontario, and 50 per cent of the Nova Scotia, practitioners stated what they thought the College should do. Their suggestions were concerned with four matters: preparation for general practice, postgraduate education, the general practitioners' working conditions, and the status of the general practitioners. Apropos of preparation for general practice, it was felt that the College of General Practice should try to bring about improvements in those parts of the undergraduate teaching that had to do with general practice and in the interneship as a preparation for general practice. It was suggested, also, that the College should try to increase medical students' interest in general practice and should arrange preceptorships‡ for undergraduates and for recent graduates in order that they

*We have already mentioned on pages 84 and 88 the loneliness of some of the men in practice by themselves.

†The general practitioner's relationship to the hospital has been discussed at length in chapter 9.

‡A preceptorship is an arrangement whereby a student or recent graduate spends some time with a general practitioner, who acts as a preceptor, or instructor. The purpose of the preceptorship is to afford a student or young doctor an opportunity of learning about some of those aspects of practice that he does not see in his hospital training. For further discussion of the preceptorship, see pages 403–406. It should be noted that, at the request of medical students, the College of General Practice has arranged preceptorships for some of them.

might have enough knowledge of general practice to decide whether they wished that as a career.

The means by which it was suggested that the College might improve postgraduate education included arranging courses, seminars, and clinics, advising about courses, arranging financial assistance for physicians taking such courses, helping the practitioner to obtain a locum tenens to look after his practice in his absence, making recommendations about reading material, and seeing that regular postgraduate work was done by the physician. These measures, it was hoped, would raise the standard of practice.

Two recommendations having to do with the general practitioners' working conditions were made by a number of practitioners in each province: that the College should maintain their claim to the right to make use of the hospitals and should "stick up for the rights" of the general practitioners if "state medicine" came. One doctor urged that the College should promote the organization of group practice. Another said that the College should take steps to improve the general practitioners' "bad hours," to increase their remuneration, which he regarded as only one-third to one-half of what it should be, and to reduce the number of early deaths of general practitioners. Yet another wished to see the College give guidance on matters of ethics; and he specifically deprecated the tendency of some of his colleagues to "fuss about patient-stealing."

Finally, one group of suggestions had to do with the status of the general practitioner. A number of men, both in Ontario and in Nova Scotia, thought that the College could increase the practitioners' prestige with the public and with the specialists. Some men had in mind public relations work. This was not universally favoured, however, as is shown by the adverse comment reported above* and by the opinion expressed by another doctor that he did not think that the College should do public relations work, that the best method of improving public relations was to improve the standard of general practice, not to "publish blurbs for the public." A few men said that there was a need to engender mutual respect between general practitioners and specialists. Divergent opinions were expressed about the need to improve the position of general practitioners in teaching hospitals. On the one hand, it was urged that they should have an important part in teaching; on the other hand, doubt was expressed whether they would have anything definite to teach and it was pointed out that "it's rather difficult to teach an attitude."

*See page 153.

One of the most interesting and thought-provoking comments was made by a young doctor who said that he would like to see it possible for a general practitioner to improve his status when he was in practice. He said that the fact that one could not "move up" killed initiative. He did not advocate removing hospital restrictions but felt that there should be some way whereby a general practitioner could qualify further, i.e. be allowed to take increasing amounts of responsibility. We shall return to this in chapter 26.

Since the entire body of physicians who are engaged in clinical practice may conveniently be divided into general practitioners and specialists, it is appropriate that the relationship between these two large groups should be examined. Because we had from time to time heard remarks (see, for example, some of the quotations given in the preceding chapter) that suggested that the *status* of general practitioners might possibly be a problem,* we asked a question that we hoped would enable us to ascertain the general practitioner's attitude towards the specialists and would give him an opportunity to express his feelings about the specialists. The question, put to each general practitioner, was, "Do you think that general practitioners have as much prestige as they merit in the eyes of their specialist colleagues?" In each province, the doctors were divided fairly evenly in their opinions, affirmative answers being given by 48 per cent in Ontario and 43 per cent in Nova Scotia and negative answers by the remainder. There was no significant difference, between the various age groups or between physicians from communities of different sizes in either province, in the percentages giving affirmative or negative answers.

Those who said that general practitioners did not have as much prestige as they merited with the specialists were then asked, "Why

*That the status of the general practitioner *is* a problem is confirmed in a recent issue of the Canadian Medical Association Journal (84: 1155, 1961). In a section devoted to the College of General Practice, under the title "Should There be a Fellowship for General Practitioners?" is an article that begins as follows:

"One of the most contentious problems within the medical profession today stems from the certification distinction that is made between specialist and general practitioner.

"The current emphasis on 'specialist thinking' in our medical schools has brought about a common misconception that the general practitioner is a doctor who didn't have the brains, ability or money to become a specialist.

"It has been suggested that one answer to the problem is to establish standards whereby the G.P. may become a specialist in general practice and be so designated, and to develop a career structure for general physicians comparable to that for specialists."

not?" and "What measures would you suggest to correct this situation?" All except one of the Ontario physicians suggested one or more reasons for this lack of prestige. The explanations offered may be grouped under four headings: the comparative abilities of general practitioners and of specialists as physicians, the power of these groups to influence policy, lack of adequate understanding between the groups, and the influence of the teaching centres. By far the most frequent reference was made to the first of these, i.e. to the comparative abilities of general practitioners and specialists. Thirty-nine per cent of those in Ontario who were dissatisfied with the prestige that general practitioners had in the eyes of specialists (20 per cent of the entire sample) attributed the lack of prestige to the fact that the specialists' work was of superior quality. This opinion was expressed in various ways. Thus a few physicians said that it was difficult for a general practitioner to keep up with modern medicine or that specialists knew more about specific subjects and that a general practitioner was not expert in *any* one thing, but the majority referred more directly to the failure of some general practitioners to "work up" cases adequately before referring them, to the fact that some practitioners continued on with cases too long before referring them, and to "poor performance" by certain general practitioners. One physician, who thought that general practitioners did have as much prestige as they merited with specialists, commented to us, "Let's face it. A lot of G.P.'s do pretty poor work. The superintendent of —— Hospital showed me some charts when we had an argument about this. I had to back down and admit that some men were ignorant." The reason for quoting these words has not been to shed light on the quality of general practice, since such evidence, being second-hand with regard to quality of practice, is of little value for that purpose. These words are first-hand evidence, however, of the *concern* that is felt by some general practitioners in Ontario about the quality of the work that is being done by general practitioners and about the deleterious effect of this on the standing of the general practitioners in the sight of the specialists.

In addition to the physicians who suggested that the superior quality of the specialists' work was a reason for the general practitioners' lack of prestige with them, another 18 per cent of the Ontario sample said that the specialists *thought* that they knew more than the general practitioners. Some men felt that it was "just human nature" for a specialist to feel superior, especially in view of the greater length of his training. One physician said that the specialists thought the general practitioners too lazy or too stupid to specialize and added, "Maybe they're right."

Another reason for the general practitioners' lack of prestige with the specialists, a reason given by a number of Ontario physicians including some who referred to the superior work of the specialists, was said to be the greater weight of the specialists in determining policy. It was felt by some men that in the hospitals, and especially in the teaching hospitals, there was a tendency for the positions of authority to be filled by specialists. There was also the belief that the specialists were more highly organized than the general practitioners.

Some doctors referred to lack of understanding between the specialists and the general practitioners and to the influence of the teaching centres as reasons for the diminished prestige of the general practitioners in the eyes of the specialists. It was stated that some specialists, having never been in general practice, were not aware of the problems of the general practitioners and that they based their judgment of a general practitioner's work on his most unsatisfactory results, i.e. on the cases that he had to refer, and never had the opportunity to see the cases that he handled successfully. One physician pointed out that the general practitioners fraternized with general practitioners and the specialists with specialists and that in this way a caste system was created unintentionally. The universities were thought to have an effect on the prestige of the general practitioner in that there was a lack of general practitioners in the teaching hospitals and in that "snobbishness is ingrained in specialists during their university courses."

Of the 24 Nova Scotia physicians who had said that general practitioners did not have as much prestige as they merited with the specialists, all but 1 suggested a reason for this. Only 1 said that he considered that the specialist's work was superior to the general practitioner's, whereas 18 said that the specialist *thought* he knew more than the general practitioner. Comparing the 23 Ontario, and the 24 Nova Scotia, physicians who said that the general practitioner did not have the prestige that he merited with the specialist, we found that a significantly greater proportion of the Ontario, than of the Nova Scotia, doctors said that the specialist's work was superior ($p < 0.01$),[*] whereas a significantly greater proportion of the Nova Scotia, than of the Ontario, physicians said that the specialist *thought* that he knew more ($p < 0.02$). A few Nova Scotia physicians referred to the lack of understanding between the two groups and attributed

[*]This is explained on pages 32–33.

this to the specialists' lack of knowledge of general practice. Only 1 doctor in Nova Scotia ascribed the general practitioners' lack of prestige to the specialists' carrying greater weight in determining policy.

Of the Ontario doctors who thought that general practitioners were not held in high enough regard by the specialists, one-third were unable to suggest any remedy for this. Another one-third said that the standard of general practice must be raised. Specific recommendations by means of which this might be achieved were few, but included improving postgraduate education for general practitioners and teaching general practitioners to realize their own limitations and to refer patients to consultants. In order that specialists might be made aware of the problems of general practice, one man thought that, if specialists and general practitioners co-operated in the care of patients on the wards and in the outpatient department, the specialists would become acquainted with the *average* work of the general practitioners instead of knowing only the poor results of their most difficult cases, whereas another doctor said that the medical schools and the junior interneship should stress training for general practice. Other suggestions, each made by one doctor, were that a general practitioner should be paid more,* that his prestige would be increased if he had a better name than "G.P." ("general physician" was suggested but it was not made clear what good such a change of name would do), that the general practitioners should organize (this was suggested by a doctor who, prior to our visit, was not aware of the existence of the College of General Practice), and that the general practitioner should take a more active part in medical meetings in order to demonstrate that "he does know something."

In Nova Scotia, one-quarter of those who said that the general practitioners had not the prestige that they deserved with the specialists were unable to suggest any remedy. A few men said that the specialists' outlook should be broadened; and, to this end, they would make it compulsory for them to spend between two and five years in general practice before specializing. A few others thought that the standard of general practice should be raised. The remaining doctors gave voice to a multitude of suggestions, among which were that the fees of specialists and general practitioners should be brought close together, that their work and their fees should be more sharply differentiated than at present, that certification should be abolished as a specialty qualifi-

---

*For a discussion of the fees of general practitioners and specialists, see pages 205–210.

cation and only the Fellowship of the Royal College of Physicians and Surgeons of Canada be recognized, that general practice itself should be a specialty, that the work of general practitioners should be "expanded," and that general practitioners should do some teaching of medical students.

The practitioners were asked another, more direct, question about the relationship existing between them and the specialists: "Do you think that the specialist treats the general practitioner, by and large, with the courtesy and consideration which are his due?" Every one of the 44 Ontario doctors, but only 32 of the 42 Nova Scotia doctors, replied in the affirmative ($p < 0.01$). Some of the men added comments, the most frequent of which, made by almost one-quarter of the Ontario doctors and by a few of those in Nova Scotia, was to the effect that the specialist *had* to be courteous because his "bread and butter" depended on the general practitioners' referrals. A few men expressed annoyance at what they regarded as attempts by consultants to "steal" their patients. There were complaints, for example, about dermatologists and ophthalmologists who kept patients coming to them instead of sending them back to the referring general practitioner. One general practitioner was greatly displeased with a gynaecologist who had made a follow-up examination of a patient six months after operation without asking the general practitioner's permission. One young physician made quite apparent his hostility towards specialists. He said that no specialist had held office for some time in the medical organizations in his area and stated emphatically that there would not be a specialist in office there again. He himself refused to look after people who, routinely, had either an obstetrician or a paediatrician for those parts of their medical care. He referred to "educating" patients who came from other communities regarding the fact that, if he was going to look after them at all, he was going to do their obstetrics and their paediatrics. Another general practitioner, who gave a good many anaesthetics for other doctors, was so concerned about doing the "correct" thing that, though he thought that he should examine patients before giving them an anaesthetic, he did not examine the adults because he feared that the referring doctor might misinterpret his action as an attempt to "steal" the patient.

Comments such as those just cited point up in a sad way the pettiness and distrust that exist in the relationships between some general practitioners and some specialists. If a genuinely better relationship could be established, it would be to the advantage both of patients and of the profession. The suggestion made by a number of the general practitioners themselves that the standard of general practice should be raised will be discussed later when the quality of practice has been examined. The examples given in the preceding paragraph, however, raise other questions which are appropriately discussed here.

First it may be asked whether it is only the specialists who do not understand the general practitioners' problems or whether the general practitioners also fail to understand the specialists' problems. We do not know the details of the dermatological and ophthalmological cases referred to, but a number of questions come to our mind. Did the referring general practitioner, at the time of making the referral, have clearly in mind what he wished the consultant specialist to do? Did he wish the consultant merely to examine the patient and diagnose the condition but to leave the treatment to him, the general practitioner, to carry out? Or did he wish the consultant also to institute treatment but to leave the follow-up care to him? Or did he wish the specialist to follow the case until the condition was either cured or unlikely to benefit further by the specialist's attention? If the referring physician was clear in his own mind about what he wished of the consultant, did he communicate his wishes effectively to the consultant? If he did not, did the consultant attempt to find out from the referring physician what he wished?

There is also the matter of a consultant's responsibility to the patient. If the referring doctor merely wishes the case to be diagnosed and then sent back to him for treatment but the consultant honestly feels that the patient will do better under his own care, whose interests must the consultant consider first, the referring doctor's or the patient's? Was the gynaecologist, who examined the patient six months after operation, obligated to ask the permission of the doctor who had originally referred the patient to him? This probably did not occur to him. Suppose he had asked the general practitioner's permission and had been refused (unlikely, but not impossible), what then would his responsibility have been—to examine or not to examine? Or, to refer again to the physician who gave anaesthetics, was his responsibility to avoid incurring the illwill of the referring doctor or was it to carry out the examination that was demanded by his own opinion of what constituted good medical practice?

We have asked some questions that were brought to mind by general practitioners' complaints about specialists and by one general practitioner's uncertainty about his responsibility when he was himself functioning as a specialist. No answers can be given, because the details of the particular cases are not known to us. It seems to us, however, that the occurrence of such problems might be prevented, if the student or the young doctor were led, early in his career, to consider carefully the issues involved. Perhaps the medical schools and the College of General Practice of Canada could devote some thought to how students could be brought to a clearer understanding of these problems.

Another question that needs attention here concerns the claim of a doctor on his patient. We were greatly disturbed by the attitude manifested by certain doctors that their patients *belonged* to them and had no right to go to another doctor without their permission. Such an attitude was exemplified by the doctor who made clear to his patients, according to his own statement, that, unless he was permitted to give routine obstetrical and paediatric care, he would not have anything to do with them at all. Perhaps such an attitude is a carry-over from the days when practices were bought and sold more commonly than they are today and when such a transaction involved not only house and equipment but also, and more significantly, the goodwill of patients. Or perhaps, as in human families older brothers sometimes do not take kindly to younger brothers with whom they must compete, so general practice resents the specialties, much junior in age, which have sprung up to threaten its long-established sense of security. However accurate or inaccurate these speculations may be, today it is generally accepted that a doctor may start a practice wherever he wishes; and it is regarded by organized medicine as fundamental that a patient have freedom of choice of doctor. Under these circumstances, each individual doctor must recognize and accept that his patients do *not* belong to him, that they come to him of their own free choice, and that they must be free to leave him if they so choose. The development of such an attitude, it seems to us, is the responsibility of each doctor and should be fostered during the doctor's training years.

# 11 / The General Practitioner and the Pharmaceutical Industry

In the last quarter of a century, new drugs have followed one another onto the market with a bewildering rapidity unmatched in the history of medicine. One problem that this has presented to the physician—the decision about what drugs to use in his own practice—we shall consider in chapter 24. Here, our concern is with the physicians' reactions to the advertising methods used by the manufacturers, who, understandably, are eager to sell their products.

Besides advertisements in medical journals, two other, more direct, approaches are made to physicians. Daily, the postman brings a flood of advertising material of all shapes and sizes—letters extolling one or another product, magnificent brochures, and boxes containing samples of drugs; and at regular intervals, the practitioner is visited by the companies' local representatives, sometimes by several of these "detail men" in a single afternoon, who take from five to fifteen or twenty minutes to describe their companies' products and usually leave more samples.

How much of a physician's day, on the average, is taken up with detail men and advertisements, we do not know. We do know that all the printed material that arrives in many offices could not be read critically in less than several hours, but much of it is not read at all. Some finds its way, along with samples, straight into the waste paper basket; some, tossed unlooked-at into a drawer or a cupboard, must rest there for weeks or months before rejoining the flow of waste material to the garbage pit; some grows into mountains that threaten to force the physicians from their very desks; and some items, especially certain samples, they find useful.

To discover the general practitioners' attitudes towards these advertising efforts of the pharmaceutical industry, we asked the physicians several questions about detail men, advertisements, and drug samples. The first question was whether or not the physician saw detail men. In each of the two provinces, all replied that they did, though a few specified that they would see some detail men but refused to see others. They were then asked whether they were glad to see the detail men, whether they were neutral, or whether they were antagonistic. Fifty-five percent of the Ontario physicians and 48 per cent of those in Nova Scotia said that they were glad to see detail men—though 16 per cent of the Ontario doctors added such qualifying comments as, "but not too many" or "as long as they don't stay too long"—; 27 per cent in Ontario and 48 per cent in Nova Scotia were neutral; and 14 per cent and 5 per cent in the two provinces, respectively, were antagonistic. One of those who was basically antagonistic to the idea of detail men said that he hated to turn away a man who was trying to earn a living.

Regarding the advertisements sent to them by pharmaceutical companies, the practitioners were asked whether they were pleased to receive them, were neutral, or were antagonistic. Only 9 per cent of the Ontario group and 24 per cent of the Nova Scotia group declared themselves pleased to receive the advertisements, 36 per cent in Ontario and 40 per cent in Nova Scotia were neutral, and 55 per cent and 38 per cent in Ontario and Nova Scotia, respectively, were antagonistic. A few of the doctors added comments, to the effect that heavy advertising increased the cost of drugs, that many of the advertisements were thrown out without being opened, and, in the words of one man, "their only value is increased tonnage for the Scouts' paper drive."

In answer to the question whether they were pleased to receive drug samples or whether they found them a nuisance, 55 per cent of the Ontario physicians said that they were pleased to receive them, 43 per cent that they were a nuisance, and one man took a neutral position. Similarly, in Nova Scotia, 60 per cent were pleased and 40 per cent regarded samples as a nuisance.

The final question having to do with the pharmaceutical industry was whether the physician made use of more than half the samples that he received or whether he used about half and threw out about half or whether he threw out more than half. In Ontario, approximately 61 per cent replied that they threw out more than half of the samples, 18 per cent that they used about half and threw out about half, and 20 per cent that they used more than half. The corresponding figures for Nova Scotia were 26 per cent, 17 per cent, and 57 per cent. A significantly greater percentage of the Nova Scotia, than of the Ontario, physicians used more than half of the samples, and a significantly greater percentage of those in Ontario than of those in Nova Scotia used less than half.

# 12 / The General Practitioner and the Community

As a member of a community, a general practitioner functions not only in his special capacity as a physician, but also in the more general capacity of a citizen. Inasmuch as a community is a social and political body, active citizenhood implies an interest in contemporary political and social problems. To examine general practitioners in these terms would be an immense study, far exceeding the resources of the Survey of General Practice. Therefore we shall do no more than touch upon a few aspects of a physician's relationship to his community.

Though it is convenient, for descriptive purposes, to talk of a general practitioner now as a physician and now as a citizen, as though these were separate, the fact is, of course, that he is one individual. At different times, however, different parts of his personality are somewhat more prominent. Thus when he is treating a patient in his office, his concern is with the needs of that particular patient rather than with the problems of contemporary society. On the other hand, as a member of the local school board, for example, he is faced with community problems, which do not, except perhaps rarely, call upon his special knowledge for their solution. Between these two extremes, is an area in which a privately practising physician functions as a physician, but does so in order to meet the needs of his community rather than because his services are sought by a particular patient. To these activities we shall first direct our attention.

We have already catalogued the various hospital responsibilities undertaken by the physicians whom we visited (pages 137–139, Table 28). Twenty per cent of those in Ontario donated their services for the care of indigent patients on the wards or in the outpatient departments of their hospitals. These physicians, though forming roughly the same percentage of the different age groups, constituted 64 per cent of the practitioners in the cities of over 100,000 but only 6 per cent of those in communities of less than 100,000. The difference, which is significant ($p < 0.01$),[*] reflects the fact that hospitals with public wards and outpatient departments are located mainly in the large cities. This type of responsibility was mentioned by only an occasional doctor in Nova Scotia. Many doctors, in both provinces, assumed other hospital responsibilities, especially service on various boards and committees. Furthermore, some physicians who did not have hospital responsibilities at the time of the Survey's visit had made significant contributions in the past. One physician, for example, had arranged to have a radiologist visit the hospital once a week; another had organized a "walking blood bank," i.e. had arranged for about two hundred young adults to have their blood typed and to be listed and available to give blood quickly.

If we have seemed in the preceding paragraph to be repeating what we said in discussing the relationships of the general practitioners to their hospitals, the repetition is deliberate. Our reason is that these services performed by the physicians constitute a part of the relationship between them and their communities. In looking after indigent patients and in doing committee work for hospitals that have no salaried physicians to perform these functions, the physicians practising in the community are meeting needs of the community. These services, given without remuneration, are seldom, if ever, mentioned by those elements in the community that in recent years have been outspoken in denouncing physicians as thinking more of their own financial interests than of service to the public.

Some physicians gave service to the public in other ways, which had no connection with their hospitals. These included volunteering to look after the high school rugby team, to assist with the immunization of school children, and to examine children each year for day camp. One physician, who stated that he had been an alcoholic some years before, devoted his efforts to helping alcoholics, whose problems he felt he understood better than most people in the community. Probably many doctors have some patients whom they continue to see in spite of their failure to pay for the services rendered. One physician, afraid that he might be prejudiced against patients who were not paying him, instructed his secretary to send out accounts to these patients but not to tell him which patients paid and which did not. Sixty-six

[*]This is explained on pages 32–33.

per cent of the Ontario physicians and 79 per cent of those in Nova Scotia named one or more types of voluntary medical service that they were giving at the time of our visit. We know, also, that some who were not giving any such service at that time had served on committees in recent years.

In order to explore further the practitioners' relationships with the society of which they were a part, the interrogator asked each of them to list the civic, fraternal, and religious organizations to which he belonged and to enumerate any offices, local, provincial, or federal, which he was holding or had held in the past. Among the organizations to which they belonged, 59 per cent of the Ontario, and 55 per cent of the Nova Scotia, doctors included the church. Of the Ontario doctors who mentioned the church, about one-third stated that they were "not active" or that they "hardly ever" attended; about one-quarter served in such capacities as elder, warden, delegate to the synod, sidesman, trustee, or member of the board of stewards or other boards or committees; and the remainder did not give any indication of the extent of their participation in church affairs. Of the Nova Scotia doctors who stated that they were members of the church, about one-sixth said that they were elders and the remainder did not elaborate upon their relationships with the church. The remaining physicians, 41 per cent of the Ontario group and 45 per cent of the Nova Scotia, either made no reference to the church or, occasionally, were so vague as to be unintelligible. Since the doctors were asked about "religious organizations," but not specifically about their relationship to the church, it is not possible to say whether failure to mention the church indicates lack of interest in it or whether these men, taking for granted that everyone would belong to a church, did not think to mention it. All, then, that can be said with certainty is that at least 16 per cent of the Ontario, and 10 per cent of the Nova Scotia, physicians were actively involved in church affairs and that at least another 43 per cent in Ontario and 45 per cent in Nova Scotia were, nominally at any rate, members of the church. Neither in Ontario nor in Nova Scotia did the various age groups differ significantly either in the percentages of physicians who mentioned the church or in the percentages of those who made clear that they took an *active* part in church affairs.

The organizations, other than the church, to which the practitioners belonged are listed in Table 31. In Ontario, 46 per cent of the practitioners who were visited in cities of over 10,000 did not belong to any civic, fraternal, or religious organization other than the church, whereas only 11 per cent in places of less than 10,000 did not belong

TABLE 31

NON-PROFESSIONAL ORGANIZATIONS, OTHER THAN THE CHURCH, TO
WHICH THE ONTARIO AND NOVA SCOTIA PHYSICIANS BELONGED OR
WITH WHICH THEY WERE ASSOCIATED

| | Number of physicians | |
| Name of organization | Ontario | Nova Scotia |
|---|---|---|
| Masonic Order | 8 | 12 |
| Board of Trade or Chamber of Commerce | 6 | 4 |
| Rotary Club | 6 | 3 |
| Knights of Columbus | 1 | 6 |
| Lions International | 5 | 1 |
| Kinsmen Club | 3 | 1 |
| St. John Ambulance | 3 | 1 |
| Young Men's Christian Association | 1 | 3 |
| Canadian Legion | 1 | 2 |
| Board of governors of hospital | 1* | 1* |
| Gyro Club | 0 | 2 |
| Kiwanis Club | 1 | 1 |
| United Appeal (collectors) | 2 | 0 |
| Victorian Order of Nurses | 2 | 0 |
| Others | † | ‡ |

*Each of these physicians specified that he was a member of the board, not as a physician, but as a citizen.
†Each of the following was named once: AKO (a fraternal order promoting sports for older boys), Alcoholics Anonymous, Children's Aid Society, Red Cross, school for retarded children, Sons of England, town planning board, Tuberculosis Association (of county).
‡Each of the following was named once: B'nai B'rith, Canadian Arthritis and Rheumatism Society, Canadian Order of Foresters, community betterment association, Holy Name Society, John Howard Society, Knights of Pythias, Nova Scotia Opera Association, Odd Fellows, recreation fund of parish (chairman), Young Men's Hebrew Association.

to one or more of these organizations ($p < 0.05$). In Nova Scotia, the corresponding percentages, 24 per cent and 12 per cent, did not differ significantly. Between the different age groups, there were no significant differences in this respect in either province.

None of the Ontario physicians reported having been elected to public office at the provincial or the federal level. Six had served their municipalities, 1 as a member of the board of health, 4 as members of school boards, and the remaining doctor both as a member of the school board and as a municipal councillor. In Nova Scotia, 1 practitioner had been a Member of the Legislative Assembly and 13 of the 42 had served at the local level, 7 as members of school boards, 4 in connection with civil defence, 3 as municipal councillors, 2 as members of local boards of health, and 1 as coroner and justice of the peace. Some of the periods of service ran into a number of years.

The next subject to engage our attention is what the practitioners themselves thought of doctors'* participation in community activities. The first question asked about this was, "Do you think that doctors generally take as active an interest as they should in non-medical community affairs?" In Ontario, 55 per cent replied in the affirmative, 45 per cent in the negative; in Nova Scotia, 40 per cent in the affirmative, 60 per cent in the negative. The difference between the two provinces is not statistically significant. One-quarter of the Ontario, and almost one-half of the Nova Scotia, practitioners added that doctors were "too busy" or had "not enough time." Other comments, made by an occasional doctor, were that in a large city a physician had "too many other interests," that participation in community activities depended on a doctor's personality (as well as on availability of time), and that doctors were "too narrow-minded," "too selfish," or "too lazy" to participate. An occasional doctor in Nova Scotia said that doctors were afraid that they might jeopardize their patients' good opinion of them if they took on an appointment, or engaged in an activity, of which their patients did not approve.

Next, the physicians were asked, "Do you think that the doctor's education prepares him adequately to take an active part in the non-medical activities of the community?" In Ontario, 61 per cent replied affirmatively, 39 per cent negatively; in Nova Scotia, 43 per cent affirmatively, 57 per cent negatively. Some of those who gave affirmative answers amplified these with comments. These included such statements as that the physician received "a good, broad education, better than most," that he was "ten times better prepared than the average person" to participate in community affairs, and that he was adequately prepared but that teachers and lawyers were better prepared. Suggestions were made by a few men and included training in public speaking, "more humanities," and "orientation in social principles" in the final year of the medical course.

Of those who said that a doctor's education did *not* prepare him adequately to take an active part in the non-medical activities of the community, some were unable to suggest any improvements. One man said, "This is postgraduate education which he acquires after settling in a community," another that, as a doctor was too busy for community affairs, educating him to play a part in community affairs would

---

*It should be pointed out that the questions that were asked referred to "doctors" rather than specifically to "general practitioners." In their answers, none of the physicians made any distinction between general practitioners and specialists.

be a waste of time. Other men recommended courses in "civics," "the humanities," "the cultural arts," "law," "political science," and "business matters." Instruction in public speaking was advocated by a few, including one man who asserted that too few doctors could speak at all well in public. One young doctor said that the premedical training should be on a "broader base—more in keeping with modern living," while an older man, who said that "there was nothing in our education" to prepare a doctor to participate in community affairs, suggested that "if it were stressed in college, there would be more interest taken later." Yet another thought that a premedical education emphasizing the liberal arts subjects might prepare a doctor adequately for participation in community affairs, but maintained that the present premedical education was not adequate for this purpose.

Finally, coming to the picture that the general practitioner had of his own standing in the community, we asked, "How appreciative are patients generally of what doctors do for them? Very? Fairly? Slightly? Or not at all appreciative?" In Ontario, 66 per cent thought that patients were very appreciative, 27 per cent fairly appreciative, and 5 per cent fell between these two answers. The one remaining physician regarded them as only slightly appreciative. In Nova Scotia, 40 per cent considered patients very appreciative, 55 per cent fairly appreciative, and 5 per cent slightly appreciative. The percentage of physicians in Ontario who regarded patients as very appreciative was significantly higher than the percentage in Nova Scotia ($p < 0.05$).

The physicians were then asked, "Do you think that general practitioners today have as much prestige as they merit in the eyes of the community?" Those who gave negative answers were asked, "Why not?" and "How might this situation be corrected?" In Ontario, 70 per cent answered the first question in the affirmative, 27 per cent in the negative, and one physician was not certain. In Nova Scotia, 48 per cent gave affirmative answers, 50 per cent negative answers, and one physician's answer was indefinite. The difference between the answers received in Ontario and those in Nova Scotia is significant ($p < 0.05$). In neither province, however, did the different age groups or the groups based on different community sizes differ significantly in their replies to this question.

In Ontario, most of those who thought that general practitioners did not have as much prestige as they merited in the eyes of the community either attributed this to the rise of specialization* or at

*See also pages 156–162, where the relationship between general practitioners and specialists was discussed.

least regarded the two as related phenomena. Their answers varied from terse utterances such as "the public is specialist-conscious" and "the specialists have caused this" to longer statements that attempted to explain the public's enthusiasm for specialists. One young practitioner said that more and more people refused to accept a serious or incurable ailment or a prolonged illness unless they had been seen by a specialist. Another man referred to the glamour associated with the specialties, particularly surgery. Yet another compared the specialist, who is seldom seen by the patient and who may be located at a great distance, with the general practitioner, whose prestige he thought was lessened by the patient's closer acquaintance with him. Nine per cent of the Ontario practitioners laid at the general practitioner's own feet either all or part of the blame for his diminished prestige in the eyes of the community. They said that some general practitioners had "not kept up enough," that some were money-minded, careless, or did unnecessary operations, and that there were too many "crocks" in general practice.* Other reasons for a specialist's being consulted were said to be the fact that people were better able now to afford a specialist's services and the fact that they trusted a specialist's formal qualifications as a guarantee of adequate training, but could not differentiate between a good general practitioner and a poor one. An occasional man ascribed the decrease in the prestige of doctors to the "propaganda" of such groups as the Christian Scientists, the faith healers, and the chiropractors, or mentioned that, whereas the news media seldom paid attention to the unpaid accounts and the long hours of doctors, they were quick to publicize, with adverse comment, a patient's inability to obtain a doctor.

In Nova Scotia, only one-third of those who said that a general practitioner did not have as much prestige as he merited in the eyes of the community ascribed this state of affairs to a predilection, on the part of the public, for specialists. Frequent mention was made of the fact that medical matters were so much discussed in newspapers and lay journals that the public either knew, or thought that it knew, much more about medicine than was the case a generation ago. As a result, it was said, physicians were held in lower esteem. One practitioner said, "General public education has destroyed the myth of the G.P."; another said, "The physician's cloak has been removed by knowledge." It was said, also, by a few doctors, that the social level of workmen

*The 4 physicians who made these comments were in addition to the 9 (20 per cent of the sample), mentioned on page 157, who said that the work of the specialist was superior to that of the general practitioner.

had risen and that they tended to push the white-collar workers, including the physicians, down to their own level or below it. One doctor felt that labour unions had had a good deal to do with bringing about a "disparaging attitude" towards doctors. Other causes to which a few doctors attributed the general practitioners' lack of prestige included diminution of the loyalty that patients felt towards their doctors in former years, the public's lack of awareness of doctors' problems, a desire on the part of some doctors to make too much money, a tendency of doctors to undervalue their own work, failure on the part of medical men to participate actively in community affairs, and the tendency of patients who are covered by prepaid plans to look upon a doctor as a civil servant and to expect him to jump at their bidding.

About half of the men in each province who were dissatisfied with the general practitioners' prestige in the community thought that the remedy was "public relations" or "education of the public." They suggested that the importance of the family doctor be stressed in advertisements in newspapers and magazines, that the public be advised to see a general practitioner first and to leave to him the calling in of a specialist, and that the public be told more of what doctors do. Several physicians said that a practitioner's prestige depended mainly on his doing "a good job" and advocated raising the standard of practice and of membership on hospital staffs.* One man even recommended that a general practitioner should have to pass written, and perhaps oral, examinations every three years.† Economic changes that an occasional physician visualized as likely to increase the general practitioners' prestige included raising the fees, since it was thought that the public tended to value a man by his fees and his earnings, and approximating the fee schedules of the general practitioners and the specialists. Several men did not have any suggestions to make.

A few of the Ontario doctors who thought that the general practitioner did have enough prestige in the community added comments. One said that the situation had improved greatly during the previous five years, another that general practitioners often had more prestige than they deserved, and another that it was up to each man to deserve prestige on the basis of his own performance in practice. One young man, who was satisfied with the situation in his own small community but whose colleagues in large cities reported that the general practitioners' prestige was low, thought that the answer lay in insisting that all specialists confine their work to referred cases.

*This subject will be discussed on pages 514–515.
†For comment on this recommendation, see page 492.

The final question asked each of the physicians was, "How do you think the public rates the specialist? Does it underrate him, overrate him, or rate him correctly?" In Ontario, 70 per cent replied that the specialists were overrated and 30 per cent that they were correctly rated. The corresponding figures for Nova Scotia were 67 per cent and 29 per cent. Two Nova Scotia doctors considered that the specialists were underrated, one of whom added, "The public doesn't realize the time and money that go into making a specialist."

This exceedingly cursory examination of the general practitioners' relationships to the communities in which they lived and practised shows that the majority, quite apart from their private practices, were serving their communities, in various ways, as physicians. Their non-professional contacts with the community were through membership in various non-medical organizations, which was almost the rule in Nova Scotia and in the smaller places in Ontario, but was less common in the larger cities in Ontario. Active participation in politics was quite uncommon. Almost half of the Ontario, and more than half of the Nova Scotia, practitioners thought that doctors took a less active part in non-medical community affairs than they should and—perhaps of more importance—that their education did not prepare them adequately for active participation.

# 13 / Financial Aspects of the
General Practitioner's Career

In the course of his career, a medical man is confronted by a series of financial problems. The first of these, which must be faced either by him or by his parents, is the cost of his medical education. We asked the practitioners of the Survey certain questions in order to gain some idea of the magnitude of this problem in their own experience. In order that the reader may be able to view our findings from the proper perspective, however, he must first know how much a medical education costs. Since the cost of this, as of almost everything else, has increased tremendously over the years, it would be ideal if it could be stated for various times during the past forty years; but this is not possible. In fact, to our surprise, we have not been able to find any satisfactory statement of the cost of medical education *to the student*.

James S. Thompson, Assistant Dean of the Faculty of Medicine of the University of Alberta and Secretary of the Association of Canadian Medical Colleges, has made an estimate, which he states "may have an error of 15 to 20%," that in Canada "the total cost of four years of medical education (not including pre-medical work) for each graduating medical student is at least $12,000 and of this the student himself, in his fees, pays only 20%."* In addition to having omitted the cost of the premedical years (two years following senior matriculation), Thompson has been concerned with the cost to the *medical school* rather than with how much the *student* has invested in his education

*J. S. Thompson: Canadian Medical Association Journal, 82; 728, 1960.

between the time of leaving high school and the time of graduating from medical school. Similarly, the most recent figures available for the twelve Canadian medical schools (the figures given in the Fifty-Ninth Annual Report on Medical Education in the United States and Canada by the Council on Medical Education and Hospitals of the American Medical Association), while showing the total fee for the four-year medical course as ranging between $2,003 and $3,000 with a mean of $2,253,* give a picture of only part, and a minor part, of the student's investment.

Dealing with the year 1952–1953, Counts and Stalnaker, of the Association of American Medical Colleges, added together the fees, the cost of books and equipment, and the living expenses reported by 6,251 medical students in the United States and concluded that "The average medical student to-day spends some $9,200 for his four years in medical school."† Whiting, Powers, and Darley, of the Association of American Medical Colleges, who sent out a questionnaire in April and May of 1959 to each of the 6,827 final-year students in the seventy-eight medical schools in the United States, say, on the basis of replies received from 4,899 students, "The average direct cost to the student of a medical school is about $1,000 a year, or $4,000 for 4 years of medical education leading to the M.D. degree."‡ The items that they have included in the term, "direct cost," are "tuition, fees, books, and instruments." Again, apart from the fact that the cost of the premedical years is omitted from the estimates both of Counts and Stalnaker and of Whiting and his associates, neither of these approaches is satisfactory for our purposes. Doubtless the student or his parent is greatly interested in knowing how much he will have to pay out during the years in medical school. In calculating the cost of a medical education, however, one cannot fairly include living expenses, since these would have to be met even if the young man did not study medicine.§ On the other hand, it is necessary to include, as part of a student's financial invest-

*W. S. Wiggins *et al.*: Journal of the American Medical Association, *171*: 1507, 1959. The figures are calculated from Table 2, pp. 1516–17.

†S. Counts and J. M. Stalnaker: Journal of Medical Education, 29: 2, 23, 1954.

‡J. F. Whiting *et al.*: Journal of Medical Education, *36*: 748, 1961.

§Some of the young men, of course, taking a job but living in their parents' homes, would be able to live less expensively than if they went to medical school and had to live away from home. We do not know, however, what percentage of those going to medical school must move away from home. Nor do we know how long those going straight into jobs from high school would continue to live under the parental roof. For these reasons, in calculating the cost of medical education, we prefer to omit living expenses. This omission will cause the estimated cost to err on the low side, if at all.

ment, what he might reasonably expect to earn (less income tax) had he gone from high school into a job.

Data gathered from more than one thousand medical students in Canada show that, in the summer of 1956, the median monthly salary of those who had summer jobs was $234.* It seems reasonable to assume that these same individuals, if they had elected to take a full-time job rather than to study medicine, would have been able to earn at the same rate or, being in permanent jobs, at a higher rate.† At a rate of $234 per month, the man's yearly salary would be $2,808. If he remained single, his income tax, at the 1960 rate, would be $277. His yearly income, after income tax, would be $2,531. On the other hand, a medical student, if he worked for four months in the summer—and he is not likely to work as long as this—would earn $936, on which he would pay no income tax. The difference between the earnings of the medical student and the non-student would amount to $1,595 per year, or, over a period of six years, $9,570.

At the University of Toronto, the fees for the two premedical years and for the four medical years, for the academic year 1961–1962, total $3,770. (The fees for women students for the entire six-year period total $126 less.) When to this amount are added (as listed in the Calendar of the Faculty of Medicine) $140 for microscope, $160 for other instruments, and $400 for books, the total expenditure (other than living expenses, which are not a legitimate item to include) becomes $4,470 for the six years. When the figure of $9,570 in lost earnings during those six years is added, our estimate of a medical student's total investment, from completion of senior matriculation to graduation from medical school, is a little in excess of $14,000. Of necessity, this is a rough estimate. Since we think, however, that we have overestimated the medical student's summer earnings and have underestimated what he would have earned had he gone from school to a steady job, with the likelihood of promotions during the years, and since we have not included in our calculations interest on the difference between the earnings of the medical student and the non-

*Canada, Dominion Bureau of Statistics, *University Student Expenditure and Income in Canada, 1956–57* (Ottawa, 1959), pp. 26–27.

†Sixteen per cent of those who had summer jobs had medical internships, which pay poorly even at the graduate level (see page 180); 7 per cent were "lab and research technicians"; 8 per cent "student assistant, research worker and trainer"; less than 1 per cent X-ray technicians; 11 per cent "R.O.T.P., armed forces personnel"; and the remainder were in forty-five other types of job that appeared to have no relationship either to medicine or to the fact that the incumbent was at university. Canada, Dominion Bureau of Statistics, *University Student Expenditure and Income in Canada, 1956–57*, pp. 87–88.

student, we regard our estimate of $14,000 as very conservative. What the corresponding figures would be for the physicians visited by the Survey, all of whom graduated between the early 1920's and the mid 1950's, we cannot say. It seems reasonable, however, to assume that they would be of similar magnitude in relation to the cost of goods and services at the time.

Each practitioner in the Survey was asked: "How difficult was it for you to finance your medical school education? Very difficult? Fairly difficult? Not very difficult? Or not at all difficult?"* In Ontario, 11 per cent replied "very difficult," 32 per cent "fairly difficult," 27 per cent "not very difficult," and 30 per cent "not at all difficult." The corresponding figures for Nova Scotia were approximately 10 per cent, 29 per cent, 29 per cent, and 33 per cent, respectively. The financing of this part of their education was either very difficult or fairly difficult for 18 per cent of the Ontario men up to thirty-five years of age, for 53 per cent of those between thirty-six and forty-five, and for 50 per cent of those over the age of forty-five; in Nova Scotia, 50 per cent, 32 per cent, and 40 per cent, respectively, of the men in the youngest, the middle, and the oldest of the three age groups found it either very difficult or fairly difficult to finance the undergraduate part of their medical education. In neither province are the differences between the age groups statistically significant. Whiting and his associates, on the basis of replies received from 4,899 medical students in the United States, have recently said, "the 1959 graduating students were divided approximately 50–50 between those who felt that medical school had been very rough financially (48 per cent) and those who felt that finances were of little or no concern to them in medical school (48 per cent)."†

Postgraduate education will be considered in two parts, the first year of internship and further training. We make this division because the first year is necessary for general practice and was taken by all but a few of the doctors whom we visited, whereas further training, though obligatory for a doctor who wishes to become a qualified specialist, is entirely optional for a general practitioner. In estimating the cost of

*This question and a few others were taken, either in their original form or with modifications to suit the needs of our study, from a questionnaire that was used by Robert K. Merton and his associates and that has since been published in *The Student-Physician: Introductory Studies in the Sociology of Medical Education*, edited by Robert K. Merton *et al.* (Published for the Commonwealth Fund by Harvard University Press, 1957). We wish to acknowledge the kindness of Professor Merton's group in giving us a copy of their questionnaire when we were planning our study.

†J. F. Whiting *et al.*: Journal of Medical Education, *36*: 759, 1961.

the first year of postgraduate work, we have no university fees to take into account.* The cost of this year to a young doctor is, therefore, the difference between what he is paid as an interne and what he would likely have earned had he not been an interne.

So necessary today is the first year of interneship that, in estimating how much a man might have earned in some other way, we cannot take into consideration his medical training, since, without a year of interneship, he would have little opportunity to profit financially from his undergraduate medical training. This is not to suggest that the six years of premedical and medical education are not of value, nor is it to imply, as some hospital personnel have tended to maintain,† that the work done by an interne, during his first year of interneship, is almost without value to the hospital. In the labour market, however, the man who has the medical course behind him but who has not interned is unlikely to be able to turn his training to account. For this reason, in considering what he might have earned in some other way than by interning, we regard him as having a high school education and six years of experience in a job.

If a medical student can average $234 a month in summer earnings (see page 177), then it seems highly unlikely that a man with the same intellectual ability, employed full-time for six years, would be earning less than $300 per month, i.e. $3,600 per year. If it is assumed either that he is not married or that he is married but that his wife is earning too much for him to claim married status for income tax purposes,‡ his income tax, at the 1960 rate, would be $430; and his earnings, after deduction of income tax, would be $3,170.

Turning now to what an interne is paid in the first year of interneship, we found that the salaries vary greatly from one hospital to another and from one part of the country to another. In Tables 32 and

*This is not true of at least one Canadian medical school, which requires its students, during their interneship year, to pay the university a fee of approximately $375. As this is not generally the case, however, we have chosen to ignore it for the purpose of calculating the cost of the year of interneship.

†This problem is discussed at greater length in chapter 23. See also pages 187–188.

‡In view of our findings, reported in chapter 3, about the time of marriage of the younger doctors, it seems more reasonable to assume that the majority are either not married or just married at this time. In the case of a man who has been out of high school and in a job for over six years, this assumption is less likely, since he may well have been married long enough to have children, in which case he will be able to claim exemptions for his children and likely also for his wife. To give him the status of a single man, however, is to err on the side of underestimating, rather than overestimating, the cost of the year of interneship to the medical man.

TABLE 32

Mean Monthly Salaries* of Junior (first year) Interneships in Approved† Hospitals with University Affiliations and in Approved† Hospitals without University Affiliations, by Provinces, in 1956

| Province | University affiliation | | No university affiliation | |
|---|---|---|---|---|
| | Number of interneships | Mean monthly salary $ | Number of interneships | Mean monthly salary $ |
| British Columbia | 74 | 112.03 | 38 | 94.74 |
| Alberta | 77 | 100.00 | 28 | 100.00 |
| Saskatchewan | 61‡ | 98.36 | 0 | — |
| Manitoba | 30§ | 48.33 | 11 | 50.00 |
| Ontario | 233 | 64.27 | 151 | 118.87 |
| Quebec (English) 89 | 161 | 31.18 / 24.69 | 0 / 8 | — / 50.00 |
| (French) 72 | | 16.67 | 8 | 50.00 |
| New Brunswick | 20 | 24.00 | 0 | — |
| Nova Scotia | 30 | 15.00 | 0 | — |
| Newfoundland | 16 | 169.00 | 0 | — |
| Total (English) 630 | 702 | 71.15 / 65.56 | 228 / 236 | 109.21 / 107.20 |
| (French) 72 | | 16.67 | 8 | 50.00 |

*These have been calculated from the data given in the Canadian Medical Association Journal, **75**: 534, 1956.

†General hospitals in Canada approved by the Canadian Medical Association for junior interne training.

‡Twelve of these had also a "bonus" of unstated amount.

§Twenty-eight other internships were available but the salaries were not stated.

33 are shown the mean monthly salaries, in 1956 and 1961 respectively, for internes in approved* hospitals with and without university affiliations, in the ten provinces. For hospitals with university affiliations, the figures for 1961 show a spread from approximately $71 per month (the mean salary paid to junior internes in such hospitals in Quebec) to $300 per month (the mean salary paid to junior internes in such hospitals in Newfoundland). The mean for the whole country is $121 per month in those hospitals having university affiliations. The mean is higher, if hospitals without university affiliations are included; but, as will become clear in a later chapter (see page 442), an internship in a hospital lacking university affiliation is, in many cases, of such

*I.e. approved by the Canadian Medical Association for junior interne training.

TABLE 33

MEAN MONTHLY SALARIES* OF JUNIOR (FIRST YEAR) INTERNESHIPS IN APPROVED† HOSPITALS WITH UNIVERSITY AFFILIATIONS AND IN APPROVED† HOSPITALS WITHOUT UNIVERSITY AFFILIATIONS, BY PROVINCES, IN 1961

| Province | University affiliation | | No university affiliation | |
|---|---|---|---|---|
| | Number of interneships | Mean monthly salary $ | Number of interneships | Mean monthly salary $ |
| British Columbia | 74 | 170.30 | 32‡ | 187.50 |
| Alberta | 68§ | 142.79 | 28§ | 100.00 |
| Saskatchewan | 35 | 184.43 | 32 | 181.25 |
| Manitoba | 64 | 118.44 | 8 | 150.00 |
| Ontario | 247‖ | 153.64 | 214# | 185.15 |
| Quebec (English) | 112** | 70.00 | 22 | 150.00 |
| (French) | 235 | 71.30 | 0 | |
| | 347 | 70.88 | 22†† | |
| New Brunswick | 22 | 127.27 | 0 | — |
| Nova Scotia | 39 | 94.23 | 0 | — |
| Newfoundland | 15‡‡ | 300.00 | 0 | — |
| Total (English) | 676 | 137.74 | 336 | 174.77 |
| (French) | 235 | 71.30 | | |
| | 911 | 120.60 | | |

*These have been calculated from the data given in the Canadian Medical Association Journal, **85**: 853–854, 1961.
†General hospitals in Canada approved by the Canadian Medical Association for junior interne training.
‡Sixteen of these have also a living-out allowance of unstated amount.
§Eight of each of these groups have also a living-out allowance of unstated amount.
‖Eighty-nine of these have also a living-out allowance of unstated amount.
#Fifty-six of these have also a living-out allowance of unstated amount.
**One hundred and three of these have also a living-out allowance of unstated amount.
††Sixteen of these have also a living-out allowance of unstated amount.
‡‡All of these have also a living-out allowance of unstated amount.

inferior quality that it can hardly be considered seriously as an educational experience. As the mean salary of a junior interne in Canada in 1961, then, we can take $121 per month, i.e. $1,452 per year.

In addition, the room and board provided by the hospitals must be taken into account. It is very difficult to find any satisfactory figure for the value of room and board, because the amounts spent on these in any community vary enormously from one individual to another, according to the income of the individual. The most satisfactory figure that we have been able to find is that given by the University of Toronto for 1961–1962 (in the Calendar of the Faculty of Medicine) as the likely minimum cost of room and board for a medical student. This amount, $20 per week, we consider reasonable for our purposes because the standard of room and board of a university student and of an interne, if unmarried, are probably fairly similar. At this rate, the value of room and board for a year is $1,040. When this is added to the direct salary of $1,452, the unmarried interne's total earnings become $2,492. After the deduction of income tax, $224 at the 1960 rate, the amount remaining is $2,268.

The difference between the earnings (after deduction of income tax) of an interne and of a man who has not gone through medical school is the cost to the interne of his first year of internship. This, the difference between $2,268 and $3,170, amounts to $902. This is a *conservative* estimate, because the man who has been employed for six years is probably earning more than we have suggested. Moreover, this is an estimate of the cost to an *unmarried* interne, to whom the room in the hospital residence has real value. For the *married* interne—and more than half of the recent graduates visited by the Survey were married before they had completed a year of internship—though the board is of value, the room is of no value, financially, because he has to provide shelter for his wife and is therefore not being saved an expenditure by having a room in the hospital.

In calculating the cost of the first year of interneship, we have used the figures for 1961 salaries. Comparison of Tables 32 and 33 shows that salaries have been increased considerably in the past five years. Figures are not available for salaries in earlier years, i.e. for the years when the physicians whom we visited were interning; but it is safe to say that most of the internships in good hospitals (i.e., good from the educational point of view) provided little or even, literally, no remuneration except room, board, uniforms, and laundry.

The cost of further training, *after* the junior interneship, must be approached in a different way. Let us imagine that the physician has so many years left to him before either death or disability supervenes to bring his practice to a close. Since the number of years varies from one physician to another and cannot be predicted for any individual physician, let us say that it is $N$ years. Let us imagine, also, that his entry into practice is preceded by $T$ years of further training—in some cases, of course, $T$ will be zero—and that his practice will go through three stages: a stage of growth, a stage of maturity (during which his earnings will be at their peak and will be relatively stable), and a stage of decline.* If the duration of the stage of growth is $G$ years and the duration of the stage of decline is $D$ years, the stage of maturity of the practice will have a duration of $[N - (T + G + D)]$ years.

The value of $G$ (growth stage) will vary from one practice to another. The determining factor, however, will be the need of the community for the doctor, i.e. whether the fledgling practice faces little or no competition, moderate competition, or severe competition. Except in the case of the physician whose training is so long that he becomes a qualified specialist doing work of a type that precludes competition from general practitioners, it is unlikely that the value of $G$ will be affected by the duration of postgraduate training. To put it another way, the community that is badly in need of a doctor will quickly provide plenty of work for the doctor who settles there, whether he has had one, two, or three years of postgraduate training; but, in the community where competition is keen, the doctor, after one year or after three years of postgraduate training, will have a slow start.

The value of $D$ (stage of decline), also, can be assumed to be unrelated to the duration of postgraduate training, since there is no reason to believe otherwise.

If, as has been assumed, the values of $N$ (total number of years), $G$ (growth), and $D$ (decline) are fixed for a particular physician in a particular practice situation, then the value of $[N - (T + G + D)]$, i.e. the duration of the stage of maturity of the practice, will be dependent on the value of $T$ (training after the junior interneship). In other words, when the training time, $T$, is lengthened, the total time available for private practice is shortened by exactly the same number of years. Even more important, it is not the growth stage of the practice that is shortened by extra training: it is the practice's stage of maturity that is shortened. The cost of the extra year or years of training must be calculated accordingly.

Since we shall discuss the incomes of general practitioners at some length later in this chapter, it is enough to say now that the median net income (i.e., income after deduction of professional expenses but before the deduction of income tax) of the 78 physicians who told us their incomes, was $13,000. Income tax on this for a married man, if no allowance is made for children, amounts to $2,610, at the 1960 rate. When this is deducted from $13,000, the physician is left with $10,390. This figure represents the lost earnings from private practice for each

*If death occurs prematurely, it may preclude the third stage; but that is irrelevant to the argument.

year of postgraduate training after the junior interneship. From this, however, must be deducted the interne's earnings during these years.

Unfortunately, we have not been able to find any published figures for salaries paid to members of Canadian house staffs *after* the first year of interneship. We are informed, however, that the salary schedule of one of the foremost teaching hospitals in Ontario, for the year 1960–1961, is $2,000 for the first year after the junior interneship, $2,400 for the next year, and $2,900 for each succeeding year. These figures represent the physician's complete earnings, since he is required to pay for whatever meals he eats in the hospital and since the room provided by the hospital is of no value to him financially, unless he is one of the few who are still unmarried at this time. On the assumption that these men can claim their wives as dependents but have no children as yet, the income tax, at 1960 rates, comes to $0, $56, and $126 respectively, for the first, second, and subsequent years after the junior interneship. Thus, the earnings, after income tax, for these three years are $2,000, $2,344, and $2,774 respectively.

Subtracting these figures from the $10,390 (the median earnings of the general practitioners after deduction of income tax) gives finally an estimate of the cost, to the physician, of his postgraduate training. The first year after the junior interneship costs him $8,390, the second year costs him $8,046, and each subsequent year $7,616.

These figures are only an estimate. Since they are based on the salary schedule of only one teaching hospital, it may well be that the *mean* salaries for the more senior members of house staffs in Canadian teaching hospitals are higher than those we have quoted. Yet, even if the salaries were double those that we have quoted, the costs of the three years of training subsequent to the junior interneship would range between $6,700 for the first of these years and $5,250 for the third and subsequent years.

These estimates refer to the present time. We are no more able to estimate the costs of postgraduate training taken ten, twenty, or thirty years ago than we were to determine the costs of undergraduate medical education at those times. In spite of this, however, the data that we obtained about the financial difficulties experienced by the general practitioners in connection with their postgraduate training are worthy of consideration.

The first question that each of the physicians was asked about the financial aspects of his postgraduate training was analogous to the one asked about medical school: "How difficult was it for you to finance your postgraduate training? Very difficult? Fairly difficult? Not very difficult? Or not at all difficult?" In Ontario, 9 per cent said that it was very difficult, 11 per cent fairly difficult, 32 per cent not very difficult, and 48 per cent not at all difficult. The corresponding figures for Nova Scotia were 17 per cent, 26 per cent, 21 per cent, and 36 per cent. In neither province did the various age groups differ significantly in their answers. A significantly larger percentage, however, of the entire Nova Scotia, than of the entire Ontario, sample said that they had found it either very difficult or fairly difficult to finance their postgraduate training ($p < 0.05$).[*]

The doctors were next asked, "Did your financial situation play a significant part in the termination of your postgraduate training?" Those who gave an affirmative answer were asked, "Were financial difficulties the determining factor or only a contributing factor in the termination of your training?" Twenty-five per cent of the entire Ontario group and 24 per cent of the Nova Scotia group stated that financial difficulties were the determining factor, and another 23 per cent in Ontario and 21 per cent in Nova Scotia that they were a contributing factor. The three age groups—up to thirty-five, thirty-six to forty-five, and over forty-five years—did not differ significantly in their answers in either province.

Finally, those who said that financial difficulties had played a part in the termination of their training were asked, "If it had not been for your financial difficulties, would you have chosen a specialty as your career instead of general practice?" Thirty-six per cent of the practitioners who were visited in Ontario and 19 per cent of those in Nova Scotia answered that they would have chosen a specialty. (Of the 16 Ontario physicians, 3 would have chosen internal medicine, 6 surgery, 4 obstetrics, 1 dermatology, and each of the other 2 was undecided between two specialties; of the 8 Nova Scotia physicians, 3 would have chosen internal medicine, 2 surgery, 1 paediatrics, 1 paediatrics or obstetrics, and 1 pathology.) The difference between the provinces is not significant; and, within each province, the different age groups did not differ significantly. Of the 24 doctors who would have made this choice, 15 (9 in Ontario and 6 in Nova Scotia) said that their financial situation had been the determining factor that prevented them from taking specialty training; for the remainder (7 in Ontario and 2 in Nova Scotia) it was a contributing factor. Five other men in Ontario and 11 in Nova Scotia would have taken further training had it not been for their financial situation, but with the intention of doing general practice. To recapitulate, 48 per cent of the entire Ontario

[*]This is explained on pages 32–33.

group and 45 per cent of the entire Nova Scotia group said that financial difficulties were at least a contributing factor, if not the determining factor, that had prevented them from taking further training; and 36 per cent in Ontario and 19 per cent in Nova Scotia would have chosen a specialty in preference to general practice. The fact that almost half of the physicians in each of our two samples wished to take further training but were financially unable to do so is startling evidence of the need for further consideration of the economics of postgraduate training by all those organizations—and particularly the teaching hospitals—that have any connection with this phase of a physician's education.

In order to ascertain what the general practitioners themselves thought internes' services were worth, we asked each of them, "Considering the question only *from the point of view of the value of the services rendered by the graduate doctor* on the house staff of the average teaching hospital, what do you think would be a fair salary in the first year after graduation and in the second year after graduation?" Most of the physicians named a figure for the total worth of an interne's services and indicated how much should be withheld for room, board, and laundry. Of the remaining few, who could not suggest a value for room, board, and laundry, some named a salary exclusive of these benefits, whereas others set a figure that included them. The figures are shown in Table 34. There was a striking similarity between the answers given by the Ontario practitioners and those given by the Nova Scotia practitioners. This is most apparent in the median figures. Quite as striking, however, as the similarity between the provinces was the very wide range covered by the answers of the physicians within each of the provinces. Thus, in each province, the greatest value assigned to the services of a first-year interne and of a second-year interne was several times the least value assigned.

The same wide divergence of opinion was apparent in the comments that some of the doctors made about internes' salaries. One doctor, for example, who considered the current salaries inadequate, said that the present system was "archaic" and that it should be put on a businesslike basis. Another said, "Internes should be part of the paid staff— just like the office personnel. It is an antiquated system—just terrible. It is the English apprenticeship system." One Nova Scotia doctor said that an interne gave good service and that his salary should be in keeping at least with that of a labourer, who, in a large industry near by, was able to make $2.50 an hour. Some men, who were not averse, in principle, to adequate salaries for internes, justified the existing

TABLE 34

OPINIONS OF PHYSICIANS ABOUT SALARIES THAT WOULD REFLECT
FAIRLY THE VALUE OF THE SERVICES RENDERED BY INTERNES IN
TEACHING HOSPITALS IN THE FIRST YEAR AND IN THE SECOND
YEAR AFTER GRADUATION

| | Physician's opinion about | | | | | |
| | Salary | | | | | |
| Year of interneship | Exclusive of room, board, and laundry | | Inclusive of room, board, and laundry | | Value of room, board, and laundry | |
| | Range | Median | Range | Median | Range | Median |
| A. *Ontario* | | | | | | |
| First year | $480–5,200 | $1,200 | $1,200–5,800 | $2,100 | $300–1,200 | $660 |
| Second year | $660–7,800 | $2,400 | $1,320–8,400 | $3,120 | | |
| Number of physicians | 41* | | 41† | | 38 | |
| B. *Nova Scotia* | | | | | | |
| First year | $300–5,000 | $1,200 | $900–6,000 | $2,000 | $480–1,700 | $850 |
| Second year | $1,200–6,200 | $2,500 | $2,000–7,200 | $3,550 | | |
| Number of physicians | 42 | | 42 | | 42 | |

*The 3 physicians who did not answer named salaries, *including* room, board, and laundry, of $1,800, $1,800, and $2,400 for the first year, and of $2,400, $2,400, and $3,600 for the second year.

†The 3 physicians who did not answer named salaries, *excluding* room, board, and laundry, of $480, $1,200, and $2,400 for the first year and of $660, $1,800, and $3,600 for the second year.

salaries on the basis that the hospitals could not afford to pay adequately. One older man, however, dismissed this argument with the remark that the money should be found for internes' salaries, "just as it is found for the janitor and the scullery maids. Why should the young doctor subsidize the hospital?" One doctor, who said that there should be adequate salaries, added, "It doesn't have to be much, especially if the wife is working." His figure for a first-year interne was $600 in cash plus room, board, and laundry, which he valued at $600. Occasionally, reference was made to an interne's need to keep his self-respect and to be "free of charity." A few men who suggested salaries that were higher than those usually paid said, "Surely an interne is worth at least as much as a graduate nurse or a floor-sweeper." Others, however, did not agree. One of these said, "A junior interne does no work for the hospital that couldn't be done by a technician." Another laid stress on the value of the training to an interne and said that an interne, for that reason, should not be paid nearly as much as an orderly. He favoured low-interest loans, instead of salaries, because the former acted as a stimulus to work hard to pay off the debt. He had never had financial difficulties. One older doctor, who had had to cope with the problem of trying to obtain internes for his hospital, a non-teaching hospital, and who thought, wishfully perhaps, that an oversupply of internes would develop in a few years, said, "Then we won't have so much trouble getting them." Other reasons that were given for paying internes low salaries were that "I was never paid as an interne" and that it was "not good psychologically for junior internes to receive too much." The latter comment was made by a doctor who set the figure at $500 in cash plus room and board, which he would value at $1,000. The one conclusion that one can draw from these remarks is that there is no unanimity among the practitioners about the value of an interne to a hospital or about the salary that he should be paid. This lack of agreement, or of anything approaching it, is additional evidence suggesting the need for further study of the economics of postgraduate training. About this we shall have more to say in chapter 23.

Having discussed at length the costs, to the physician, of his medical education, we turn now to an examination of his earnings when at last he comes to be engaged in carrying on a general practice. We must distinguish here between income earned by the physician *as a physician* (i.e., by virtue of his professional knowledge and skill) and income from investments, business enterprises, or other sources, since this second type of income has nothing to do with the fact that the man is a physician. The published statistics dealing with the incomes of Canadian doctors show the amounts derived from more than a dozen sources.* Only two of these, however, appear to be admissible as sources of income to the man *as a physician*. These two are called "professional income" and "wages and salaries." "Professional income is broadly defined as income received from the independent practice of a profession for profit. Where a professionally qualified person is employed on an annual salary basis by a company, government or institution, the remuneration is classified under . . . 'Wages and Salaries'. . . . Professional income is shown net. . . ."†

*Canada, Department of National Revenue, *Taxation Statistics, 1961* (Ottawa, 1961), p. 41.
†*Ibid.*, p. 24.

The most recent figures available are those for 1959. These show that 13,281 "medical doctors and surgeons" (12,878 whose returns were taxable and 403 whose returns were non-taxable) had "professional income" of $187,942,000 and "wages and salaries" amounting to $5,384,000.° These two items total $193,326,000. The mean income per doctor, then, from these two sources, works out to $14,557.† These figures are based on the incomes of physicians generally, without regard for the types of practice in which they are engaged. There are no published figures, so far as we are aware, that deal with the earnings of general practitioners only.

Each of the physicians visited by us was asked what his professional income was for the year prior to the one in which our field work was begun in that province, i.e. for the year 1955 in Ontario and for the year 1957 in Nova Scotia. Because we regarded this question as one of the most delicate in our entire questionnaire, we were satisfied with an approximate statement (to the nearest thousand dollars). For the same reason and also because verification of the figure by examination of the doctor's accounts would have been impossible in the existing circumstances, we did not ask for any proof of the amount stated. The very occasional doctor gave the impression that he was naming a figure that was lower than the real one in order to avoid any entanglement with the income tax authorities. In Ontario, the remainder, i.e. the overwhelming majority, showed no reluctance to answer the question; and many of them voluntarily drew out their income tax returns in order to give us the exact figures. One of the Ontario doctors, whose practice was being reorganized at the time, was unable to give any reliable figure. Four others told us their incomes for 1956, instead of 1955. There was no reason to believe that the 1955 figures would have been higher; and in some cases, because of illness or other circumstances, it was likely that the 1956 figure was substantially higher but more typical. In Nova Scotia, 6 physicians declined to state their incomes, and 1 physician had been in practice for only six months during the year 1957. The remaining practitioners were most co-operative in answering the question. What follows is based, then, on the figures given us by 39 Ontario doctors for 1955, by 4 Ontario doctors for 1956, and by 35 Nova Scotia doctors for 1957.

The physicians' net professional incomes (i.e., after deduction of the

°*Ibid.*, p. 41. The amounts of money are shown to the nearest thousand dollars.
†In connection with this figure, it should be noted that doctors working principally on a salary basis, among whom are included members of hospital house staffs and physicians engaged in practice as the salaried assistants of other physicians, are classified, not as doctors, but as "employees." *Ibid.*, p. 27.

TABLE 35

NET PROFESSIONAL INCOMES OF ONTARIO AND NOVA SCOTIA
PHYSICIANS DURING ONE CALENDAR YEAR*

| Income | Ontario physicians | | Nova Scotia physicians | |
|---|---|---|---|---|
| | Number | % | Number | % |
| $ 5,000 or less | 5 | 11.4 | 1 | 2.4 |
| 5,001 to 10,000 | 10 | 22.7 | 13 | 31.0 |
| 10,001 to 15,000 | 11 | 25.0 | 13 | 31.0 |
| 15,001 to 20,000 | 10 | 22.7 | 6 | 14.3 |
| 20,001 to 25,000 | 4 | 9.1 | 2 | 4.8 |
| 25,001 to 30,000 | 1 | 2.3 | 0 | 0.0 |
| ×××　 | — | — | — | — |
| Over 50,000 | 2 | 4.5 | 0 | 0.0 |
| Not known | 1† | 2.3 | 7‡ | 16.7 |
| Total | 44 | 100 | 42 | 100 |

*The year, 1955, in the case of the Ontario physicians, except 4 who stated their 1956 incomes; the year, 1957, in the case of the Nova Scotia physicians.
†This practice was undergoing a reorganization.
‡One physician had been in practice for only 6 months in 1957; 4 physicians declined to state either their gross or their net income. Two physicians who gave their gross incomes as between $15,000 and $15,500 declined to state their net incomes.

cost of carrying on the practice but before the deduction of income tax) are shown in Table 35. The median income for the Ontario group was $13,500 and for the Nova Scotia group $13,000.* Lest the reader assume that the men earning $5,000 or less were just establishing themselves in practice, we must state that only one of them had been in practice less than 5 years and that the mean duration of practice for this group was more than 15 years. In Tables 36 and 37 are shown the median net professional incomes of physicians in three age groups and in communities of various populations, both in Ontario and in Nova Scotia.

In chapter 8, we discussed in detail the doctors' hours of work.† To refresh the reader's memory, the number of hours worked per week ranged from 23 to 103 in Ontario, with a mean of 52.5 hours, and ranged from 40.5 to 89 in Nova Scotia, with a mean of 60.2 hours. Because of this extreme variation, the figures that we have given for the physicians' incomes have little meaning, as they stand. It was necessary to attempt to arrive at an estimate of their earnings per hour

*Because the incomes of the two Ontario doctors in the highest range carry a disproportionate weight in the calculation of the mean, the median is used as giving a fairer picture of the earnings of the "average" general practitioner.
†The method used to estimate the number of hours worked by an individual physician is described on pages 104–105.

TABLE 36

MEDIAN NET PROFESSIONAL INCOMES OF ONTARIO AND NOVA SCOTIA
PHYSICIANS OF VARIOUS AGES*

|  | Ontario | | Nova Scotia | |
|---|---|---|---|---|
| Age of physician | Number of physicians | Median annual net income | Number of physicians | Median annual net income |
| Up to 35 | 11 | $10,000 | 7‡ | $ 8,400 |
| 36–45 | 14† | 15,500 | 19 | 15,000 |
| 46–60‖ | 18 | 13,553 | 9§ | 11,800 |
| Total | 43 | 13,500 | 35 | 13,000 |

*Income for the year, 1955, in the case of the Ontario physicians, except 4 who stated their 1956 incomes; income for the year, 1957, in the case of the Nova Scotia physicians.
†One other physician did not know his income.
‡One other physician had been in practice for only 6 months in 1957.
§Six other physicians declined to state their incomes.
‖One physician was 61 by the time of the Survey's visit.

TABLE 37

MEDIAN NET PROFESSIONAL INCOMES OF ONTARIO AND NOVA SCOTIA
PHYSICIANS IN COMMUNITIES OF VARIOUS POPULATIONS*

|  | Ontario | | Nova Scotia | |
|---|---|---|---|---|
| Population of community | Number of physicians | Median annual net income | Number of physicians | Median annual net income |
| Over 500,000 | 7 | $10,000 | — | — |
| 100,001 to 500,000 | 4 | 13,750 | 7‡ | $13,000 |
| 10,001 to 100,000 | 14† | 18,000 | 6‡ | 12,400 |
| 1,001 to 10,000 | 14 | 11,103 | 15§ | 14,000 |
| 1,000 and under | 4 | 8,875 | 7‖ | 9,000 |
| Total | 43 | 13,500 | 35 | 13,000 |

*Income for the year, 1955, in the case of the Ontario physicians, except 4 who stated their 1956 incomes; income for the year, 1957, in the case of the Nova Scotia physicians.
†One other physician did not know his income.
‡Two other physicians in each of these groups declined to state their incomes.
§One other physician declined to state his income; and one other had been in practice for only 6 months.
‖One other physician declined to state his income.

of work. Subtracting the number of weeks of vacation—which, we remind the reader, varied from 0 to more than 6 per year—from the total year, we arrived at the number of weeks worked. This number multiplied by the number of hours of work per week gave us an estimate of the number of hours of work per year. In Ontario, this varied from less than 1,200 to more than 5,000, with a median of 2,302 hours of work per year; in Nova Scotia, the range was from a little under 2,000 to a little over 4,600, with a median of 2,908 hours of work per year (Table 38).

TABLE 38

DISTRIBUTION OF ONTARIO AND NOVA SCOTIA PHYSICIANS
ACCORDING TO ESTIMATED NUMBER OF HOURS OF WORK PER YEAR

| Number of hours of work per year | Ontario physicians | | Nova Scotia physicians | |
|---|---|---|---|---|
| | Number | % | Number | % |
| 1,500 or under | 1 | 2.3 | 0 | 0.0 |
| 1,501 to 2,000 | 8 | 18.2 | 2 | 4.8 |
| 2,001 to 2,500 | 17 | 38.6 | 10 | 23.8 |
| 2,501 to 3,000 | 11 | 25.0 | 11 | 26.2 |
| 3,001 to 3,500 | 4 | 9.1 | 11 | 26.2 |
| 3,501 to 4,000 | 2 | 4.5 | 4 | 9.5 |
| 4,001 to 4,500 | 0 | 0.0 | 3 | 7.1 |
| 4,501 to 5,000 | 0 | 0.0 | 1 | 2.4 |
| Over 5,000 | 1 | 2.3 | 0 | 0.0 |
| Total | 44 | 100 | 42 | 100 |

The estimated net earnings per hour of professional work are shown in Table 39. They ranged from \$1.51 to \$29.07 in Ontario and from \$0.58 to \$9.01 in Nova Scotia. The median earnings were \$5.18 in Ontario and \$4.34 in Nova Scotia. In Tables 40 and 41 are shown the estimated median earnings per hour of practitioners in various age

TABLE 39

NET PROFESSIONAL INCOMES* PER HOUR OF WORK OF ONTARIO
AND NOVA SCOTIA PHYSICIANS

| Income | Ontario physicians | | Nova Scotia physicians | |
|---|---|---|---|---|
| | Number | % | Number | % |
| \$1.00 or less | 0 | 0.0 | 1 | 2.4 |
| 1.01 to 3.00 | 8 | 18.2 | 6 | 14.3 |
| 3.01 to 5.00 | 10 | 22.7 | 18 | 42.9 |
| 5.01 to 7.00 | 11 | 25.0 | 7 | 16.7 |
| 7.01 to 9.00 | 9 | 20.4 | 2 | 4.8 |
| Over 9.00 | 5 | 11.4 | 1 | 2.4 |
| Not known | 1† | 2.3 | 7‡ | 16.7 |
| Total | 44 | 100 | 42 | 100 |

*Estimated from the incomes reported by 39 Ontario physicians for the year, 1955, by 4 Ontario physicians for the year, 1956, and by 35 Nova Scotia physicians for the year, 1957.

†This practice was undergoing a reorganization.

‡One physician had been in practice for only 6 months during the year, 1957; the other 6 declined to state their incomes.

TABLE 40

MEDIAN NET PROFESSIONAL INCOMES* PER HOUR OF WORK
OF ONTARIO AND NOVA SCOTIA PHYSICIANS OF VARIOUS AGES

| | Ontario | | Nova Scotia | |
|---|---|---|---|---|
| Age of physician | Number of physicians | Median hourly net income | Number of physicians | Median hourly net income |
| Up to 35 | 11 | $4.41 | 7‡ | $2.85 |
| 36–45 | 14† | 6.14 | 19 | 4.56 |
| 46–60 | 18 | 6.46 | 9§ | 4.58 |
| Total | 43 | 5.18 | 35 | 4.34 |

*Estimated from the incomes reported by 39 Ontario physicians for the year, 1955, by 4 Ontario physicians for the year, 1956, and by 35 Nova Scotia physicians for the year, 1957.
†One other physician did not know his income.
‡One other physician had been in practice for only 6 months in 1957.
§Six other physicians declined to state their incomes.

TABLE 41

MEDIAN NET PROFESSIONAL INCOMES* PER HOUR OF WORK OF ONTARIO
AND NOVA SCOTIA PHYSICIANS IN COMMUNITIES OF VARIOUS POPULATIONS

| | Ontario | | Nova Scotia | |
|---|---|---|---|---|
| Population of community | Number of physicians | Median hourly net income | Number of physicians | Median hourly net income |
| Over 500,000 | 7 | $3.42 | — | — |
| 100,001 to 500,000 | 4 | 5.67 | 7‡ | $4.21 |
| 10,001 to 100,000 | 14† | 8.43 | 6‡ | 4.79 |
| 1,001 to 10,000 | 14 | 4.66 | 15§ | 4.48 |
| 1,000 and under | 4 | 4.51 | 7‖ | 3.29 |
| Total | 43 | 5.18 | 35 | 4.34 |

*Estimated from the incomes reported by 39 Ontario physicians for the year, 1955, by 4 Ontario physicians for the year, 1956, and by 35 Nova Scotia physicians for the year, 1957.
†One other physician did not know his income.
‡Two other physicians in each of these groups declined to state their incomes.
§One other physician declined to state his income; and one other had been in practice for only 6 months during 1957.
‖One other physician declined to state his income.

groups and of practitioners in communities of various sizes in each of the two provinces.

The hourly earnings of the physicians who included surgery in their work and of those who did not do surgery were compared. In Ontario, the median hourly earnings of the group doing surgery were $7.17, of the group not doing surgery $4.87. Although those men in the Ontario sample whose practices included surgery were earning substantially more per hour than the rest of the general practitioners, the difference is not statistically significant. In Nova Scotia, the estimated median earnings of those doing surgery were $4.57, and of those not doing surgery $4.05, per hour of work.

In Table 42 are shown the median hourly earnings of physicians in solo practice, with and without secretarial or nursing assistance, physicians practising in association with one other physician, and physicians belonging to groups of more than two. (These types of practice arrangement have been discussed on pages 83–90.)

TABLE 42

MEDIAN NET PROFESSIONAL INCOMES* PER HOUR OF WORK OF ONTARIO AND NOVA SCOTIA PHYSICIANS WITH VARIOUS TYPES OF PRACTICE ARRANGEMENT

| | Ontario | | Nova Scotia | |
|---|---|---|---|---|
| Type of practice | Number of physicians | Median net income per hour | Number of physicians | Median net income per hour |
| Solo† | | | | |
| without nursing or secretarial assistance | 9 | $4.19 | 11§ | $3.24 |
| with nursing or secretarial assistance | 19 | 5.17 | 12‖ | 4.57 |
| Group of two# | 8‡ | 6.09 | 4 | 4.99 |
| Group of more than two —with assistance | 6 | 8.17 | 8** | 4.29 |

*Estimated from the incomes reported by 39 Ontario physicians for the year, 1955, by 4 Ontario physicians for the year, 1956, and by 35 Nova Scotia physicians for the year, 1957.
†One Ontario physician is omitted, whose wife functioned as his secretary.
‡One other physician did not know his income.
§One other physician had been in practice only 6 months in 1957 and was unable to state his income. Three other physicians declined to state their incomes.
‖One other physician declined to state his income.
#All of these physicians had assistance except 1 in Nova Scotia, whose hourly income was slightly above the Nova Scotia median.
**Two other physicians declined to state their incomes.

When physicians with appointment systems were compared with those who operated their practices without appointments,* we found that the median hourly earnings of the two groups did not differ appreciably. In Ontario, the median was $5.18 for those with appointment systems and $4.95 for those without; in Nova Scotia, the medians were $4.37 and $4.34 respectively.

We remind the reader that our figures are estimates only. The

*A few of these men made a limited number of appointments for special purposes. The subject of the appointment system has been discussed on pages 71–74.

figures for net *annual* professional income we think are reliable approximations. To come appreciably nearer to the true figures, one would have to carry out a detailed audit of the doctors' accounts. Our estimates of the number of hours of work done by the various practitioners may be more erroneous; but we think it more likely that we have underestimated than overestimated the number of hours (see pages 104–105). If this is so, then it is more likely that our estimates of *hourly* earnings are too high than that they are too low. In short, the figures that we have given for hourly earnings of general practitioners, though they are estimates only, are, we think, close enough to the truth to merit attention, especially in view of the lack of any other figures.

The next matter to consider is the *way* in which the practising physician is remunerated. Whereas, in times past, a physician submitted his account to his patient and was paid by him, today many accounts are settled by commercial insurance companies, by insurance companies set up by the medical profession itself, or by government agencies. As we said in an earlier chapter (page 15), each of the practitioners visited by us was asked to keep a list of the patients seen by him during a period of seven days. For each patient, the doctor was asked to state, among other things, how he was likely to be paid, whether privately (i.e., by the patient directly) or through one of the agencies just mentioned or not at all. In the last of the three groups were to be included both those patients whom the doctor was treating free of charge and those who he knew from previous experience were unlikely to pay his account. Not all the doctors kept complete records, especially of the hospital visits (this is discussed more fully on page 237 and page 241). Records of non-hospital visits were kept by 43 Ontario physicians for a total of 290 days and by 42 Nova Scotia physicians for a total of 253 days; hospital visits were recorded by 41 Ontario, and 42 Nova Scotia, physicians for a total of 275 days and 253 days, respectively. The physicians' expectations regarding payment are shown in Table 43. It is to be noted that in Nova Scotia the percentage of office visits for which payment was not expected was more than one and one-half times the percentage in Ontario ($p < 0.01$) and that the percentage of home visits for which payment was not expected in Nova Scotia was almost double the percentage in Ontario ($p < 0.01$). The latter observation is the more striking in view of the fact that 661 home visits were reported in Ontario during a total of 290 days and that 1,102 were reported in Nova Scotia during 253 days.

TABLE 43

NUMBERS OF OFFICE VISITS, OF HOME VISITS, AND OF HOSPITAL
VISITS* REPORTED BY THE PHYSICIANS

(Grouped according to whether the physician was likely to be paid privately
or through a third party, i.e. a prepayment plan or an agency, or not at all)

### A. *Ontario*

| Payment | Office visits (43 physicians) | | Home visits‡ (43 physicians) | | Hospital visits (41 physicians) | |
|---|---|---|---|---|---|---|
| | Number | %† | Number | %† | Number | %† |
| Private | 1768 | 51.3 | 332 | 55.6 | 368 | 35.2 |
| Third party | 1582 | 45.9 | 241 | 40.4 | 539 | 51.5 |
| Not expected | 99 | 2.9 | 24 | 4.0 | 139 | 13.3 |
| Not recorded | 199 | — | 64 | — | 78 | — |
| Total | 3648 | | 661 | | 1124 | |

### B. *Nova Scotia*

| Payment | Office visits (42 physicians) | | Home visits§ (42 physicians) | | Hospital visits (42 physicians) | |
|---|---|---|---|---|---|---|
| | Number | %† | Number | %† | Number | %† |
| Private | 1369 | 55.7 | 551 | 51.1 | 702 | 44.9 |
| Third party | 979 | 39.8 | 444 | 41.2 | 665 | 42.5 |
| Not expected | 110 | 4.5 | 83 | 7.7 | 196 | 12.5 |
| Not recorded | 23 | — | 24 | — | 28 | — |
| Total | 2481 | | 1102 | | 1591 | |

*In Ontario, non-hospital visits were reported for a total of 290 days, hospital visits for a total of 275 days; in Nova Scotia, both non-hospital and hospital visits were reported for a total of 253 days.

†The percentages shown are percentages of those visits for which the likely method of payment was reported.

‡Included are 12 visits made in places other than home, office, or hospital.

§Included are 52 visits made in places other than home, office, or hospital.

In order to find out the attitudes of the practitioners towards the various methods of payment other than direct payment by the patient himself, we listed the methods and asked each doctor, "How well satisfied are you with each plan? Very well satisfied? Fairly well satisfied? Not very well satisfied? Or very much dissatisfied?" The answers given by the physicians for the various agencies are shown in Table 44. Of those who answered in Ontario, all were at least "fairly well satisfied" with Blue Cross and Windsor Medical Services; and only 1 man was "not very well satisfied" with the Workmen's Compensation Board of Ontario, with which 68 per cent of the entire group were "very well satisfied." In Nova Scotia, on the other hand, 26 per cent of those who answered were either "not very well satisfied" or "very much dissatisfied" with Blue Cross and 24 per cent with the Workmen's Compensa-

TABLE 44

DEGREE OF SATISFACTION OF PHYSICIANS WITH VARIOUS PLANS
OF PAYMENT FOR SERVICES

| Plan | Degree of satisfaction | | | | |
|---|---|---|---|---|---|
| | Very well satisfied | Fairly well satisfied | Not very well satisfied | Very much dissatisfied | Total number answering* |
| A. *Ontario* | | | | | |
| Blue Cross | 22 | 18 | 0 | 0 | 40 |
| Physicians' Services Incorporated | 13 | 18 | 10 | 3 | 44 |
| Windsor Medical Services | 3 | 2 | 0 | 0 | 5 |
| Commercial insurance companies | 7† | 15 | 12 | 4 | 38‡ |
| Workmen's Compensation Board | 30 | 10 | 1 | 0 | 41 |
| Medical Welfare Plan | 11 | 16 | 9 | 4 | 40 |
| B. *Nova Scotia* | | | | | |
| Blue Cross | 7 | 19 | 6 | 3 | 35 |
| Maritime Medical Care | 8 | 18 | 9 | 3 | 38 |
| Commercial insurance companies | 9 | 18 | 8 | 3 | 38 |
| Workmen's Compensation Board | 13 | 15 | 7 | 2 | 37 |
| Social assistance medical care programme | 18 | 9 | 5 | 1 | 33 |

*Individual parts of the question were not answered by physicians who had had no experience with the particular item. Four Nova Scotia physicians failed to answer any of the subdivisions of this question. Three of these did not answer, because, as salaried employees of other physicians, they did not feel competent to answer; the reason for the fourth physician's failure to answer is unknown.

†One of these physicians qualified his statement with "one company tries to get out of its obligations."

‡Not included are 3 physicians who were "fairly well satisfied" with some companies but "very much dissatisfied" with others and 1 physician who was "fairly well satisfied" with some companies but "not very well satisfied" with others.

tion Board. Both of these percentages are significantly higher than the corresponding percentages in Ontario ($p < 0.01$).

With Physicians' Services Incorporated, approximately 7 per cent of the Ontario physicians were "very much dissatisfied," 23 per cent "not very well satisfied," 41 per cent "fairly well satisfied," and 30 per cent "very well satisfied." Physicians of different ages and in communities of different sizes did not differ significantly in the answers that they gave about Physicians' Services Incorporated. All of the physicians who were either very well or fairly well satisfied with Physicians' Services Incorporated were participating physicians. On the other hand, of those who were not very well satisfied or who were very much dissatisfied, 38 per cent were non-participating, i.e., instead of being paid by Physicians' Services Incorporated, they were paid by the patient, who then sought reimbursement of the applicable portion of the fee from Physicians' Services Incorporated.

Although only 30 per cent were either "not very well satisfied" or "very much dissatisfied," 59 per cent of all the physicians made one or more adverse comments about Physicians' Services Incorporated. The amounts paid by the company were the cause of dissatisfaction on the part of 50 per cent of the men. Eighteen per cent were quite specific in saying that they objected to the company's practice of deducting 10 per cent from *all* accounts. Some pointed out that this practice had been accepted by the participating physicians, at the time when Physicians' Services Incorporated came into being, in order that the company might build up a surplus, but on the understanding that the practice would be discontinued when the company had become soundly established. Eight or nine years later, they said, not only was the 10 per cent still being deducted, but there was no longer any talk of discontinuing the deduction.* It was repeatedly stated that the deduction was wrong in principle, as it meant that the doctors were subsidizing the plan, which should be run on a business-like basis.

Another 9 per cent of the doctors complained that Physicians' Services Incorporated often made further deductions from their accounts, in addition to the routine 10 per cent. Still another 16 per cent of the doctors, without specifying whether they had in mind the 10 per cent deduction or the additional deductions, said that the tariff was "too low." One doctor pointed out that the Ontario Medical Association set a fair schedule of fees, but that Physicians' Services Incorporated, the offspring of the Ontario Medical Association, had a lower schedule; and he warned that, when a government plan came into being, it would use the lower tariff. Another doctor summed the matter up with the statement that "PSI makes a constant attempt to pare payments to the bone—their attitude is 'when in doubt, cut it.' "

Several men were dissatisfied because, they said, the company, having set a fee for a full history and examination of a patient, would arbitrarily decide, without investigation, that the visit had been a routine office call and would then cut the fee in half, in addition to casting doubt on the physician's honesty. This complaint, which was made by several very competent physicians, is of some importance

*At the time of writing, Physicians' Services Incorporated has been in operation for thirteen years and the deduction is still being made.

because of its bearing on the quality of medical care. These men pointed out that, if the doctor knew from previous experience with Physicians' Services Incorporated that he would not be paid for the extra time that he took to investigate a case thoroughly, he would tend, through sheer economic necessity, to do only the less time-consuming and less thorough work for which he was being paid. One doctor stated quite definitely that he was not a participating physician of Physicians' Services Incorporated because he knew that the inadequate compensation would force him to lower the standard of his work. Another, whose income was pitifully inadequate in relation to the high quality of service that he was giving his patients, expressed grave doubts whether, with the existing schedule of fees, one could both practise first-rate medicine and make a reasonable living, unless one included in one's practice surgery, which he thought should be left to those with special training.

Another charge brought against Physicians' Services Incorporated and having to do with quality of care was that the company made decisions that showed a poor understanding of medicine. One doctor, for example, who had a patient in hospital for investigation of vaginal bleeding and thought that the cervix looked abnormal requested a surgeon to do a biopsy. Physicians' Services Incorporated insisted, according to the practitioner, that, from then on, the patient must belong to the surgeon, though the surgeon had merely performed a technical procedure.

Other complaints of lesser importance were that Physicians' Services Incorporated was slow in paying the physicians' accounts, that they paid nothing for medicine that was given the patient, that they paid nothing for milage, which was a sizable expense in some practices, and that the intervention of a "third party" between doctor and patient was undesirable or even unethical. The general attitude of the company was described by one man as "brusque and discourteous," and by another as "suspicious." The latter suggested that Physicians' Services Incorporated should adopt a plan that one of the railroads had introduced. According to him, at the end of the patient's visit, the doctor filled out a form, on which he included the amount charged, and both he and the patient signed the form.

Not all the comments made about Physicians' Services Incorporated were unfavourable. Eleven per cent of the physicians attributed various merits to it. One of the main advantages was said to be that a doctor could give a patient better service because he was not worried about the *direct* cost to the patient. It was said, also, that Physicians' Services

Incorporated, which was being run more efficiently than any government service could be, was the answer to the public's demand for "socialized medicine." Finally, it was recognized by some men as an advantage that they could count on the patients' accounts being paid. One man suggested that, if hard times should come, this would be an even greater advantage, though this is questionable since there is no assurance that the payment of the premiums would be continued in bad times. Just as some of the detractors of Physicians' Services Incorporated were outspoken in their criticism, so some of its supporters were most enthusiastic in expressing their belief that Physicians' Services Incorporated was a satisfactory answer to the demand for a prepaid medical service.

In Nova Scotia, 21 per cent of the physicians who answered were "very well satisfied" with Maritime Medical Care, 47 per cent were "fairly well satisfied," 24 per cent "not very well satisfied," and 8 per cent "very much dissatisfied." All, however, were participating physicians. There was no significant difference between the percentages of Nova Scotia physicians giving the various answers regarding Maritime Medical Care and the percentages of Ontario physicians who gave the corresponding answers about Physicians' Services Incorporated (Table 44, on page 197). Physicians in different age groups and physicians in communities of different sizes did not differ significantly in the opinions that they expressed about Maritime Medical Care. More than two-thirds of the Nova Scotia physicians who expressed an opinion on Maritime Medical Care pointed out that the regularity of the payments was a distinct advantage. Some mentioned, also, that the account had only to be submitted once, instead of repeatedly as was necessary when some patients were being billed privately, and that the physician's book-keeping was greatly simplified. On the other hand, as in Ontario, at least half of the practitioners expressed dissatisfaction with the payments that they received for their services. The complaint heard repeatedly was that the accounts were prorated. There were some complaints, also, of accounts' being disallowed in an arbitrary manner. One physician, for instance, said that Maritime Medical Care tended to regard as "overservicing" any attention to patients in excess of one or two visits. Another said that Maritime Medical Care had a schedule of set fees and tended to disregard the extra work that was involved in the management of cases that developed complications.

About the commercial insurance companies, some of the practitioners either expressed no opinion or were ambivalent in their answers. Of the remainder, who gave unequivocal answers, 58 per cent in Ontario and 71 per cent in Nova Scotia declared themselves either "very well satisfied" or "fairly well satisfied," whereas 42 per cent in Ontario and 29 per cent in Nova Scotia were either "not very well satisfied" or "very much dissatisfied" (Table 44).

More than half of the doctors in each province found fault with the commercial insurance companies on at least one score. Frequent complaints were that their forms were too long, varied, and confusing. In view of the frequent demand for a standardized form, it is gratifying to report that recently, as a "result of two years of cooperative effort between the insurance industry and the Canadian Medical Association," forms have been worked out which "will be used by insurance companies representing approximately 95% of the Accident and Sickness Insurance sold in Canada."*

Another major criticism was that certain of the commercial companies were "crooked." One man said, "Private insurance companies don't play fair with patients. Usually I get paid, but the patients don't know what they are buying." He mentioned one company that put on a "sales blitz" each year. They would send in a new agent who would say, "This year it's different." Some patients "got stung" more than once. The doctor said that it did not harm him but that he objected to his patients' being victimized. From the fact that repeatedly the same one or two companies were named, it appeared that the sharp practices complained of were confined to a small segment of the insurance industry. A few doctors objected, also, to the fact that, in their contracts, the companies included clauses that gave them the right to refuse to continue the insurance after the insured had had one illness.

Perhaps the most serious cause of dissatisfaction with the commercial companies was the fact that they did not make clear to the insured the nature of the coverage. Patients assumed that their insurance covered *all* medical expenses, when, in fact, it did not. For example, one physician had a patient whom he had not seen before and who required hospitalization for a serious illness. He chose to be admitted to a semi-public bed, which meant that he had virtually the same accommodation as a public ward patient but was under the care of his own private physician instead of being cared for by the hospital staff. The physician did not make any inquiry about his financial status, but the patient volunteered the information that he was well covered by insurance. The patient recovered completely and expressed

*Canadian Medical Association Journal, 83: 611, 1960.

himself as well satisfied with the treatment that he had received. When the physician submitted his account, however, seventy dollars for services rendered almost daily over a period of several weeks, it turned out that the patient's insurance covered only surgical conditions. Because the patient's illness had been non-surgical and because the patient either could not or would not pay, the doctor received for his services not a cent. In other cases reported to us, the payment made by the insurance company covered only part of the physician's fee. In order to collect the remainder of his fee, the physician had to explain to the patient that the amount paid by the insurance company is a matter between the patient and the company, but that the fee charged for the medical care is determined by the doctor, not by the insurance company. The difficulty is that the patient tends to resent the unexpected expense; but he directs his resentment against the doctor instead of against the insurance company, which, when issuing the policy, either did not make clear what it covered or may have deliberately misled him. The serious consequence of this situation is its deleterious effect on the trust that should exist between doctor and patient.

The Medical Welfare Plan in Ontario was another type of prepaid plan that was the subject of comment. Sixty-eight per cent of those who answered said that they were either "very well satisfied" or "fairly well satisfied," whereas 32 per cent were either "not very well satisfied" or "very much dissatisfied." A significantly larger percentage of the younger than of the older doctors were either not very well satisfied or very much dissatisfied. Those who gave one or other of these two replies constituted 17 per cent of the doctors over forty-five years of age, 27 per cent of those between thirty-six and forty-five years of age, but 55 per cent of those up to thirty-five years of age ($p < 0.05$).

In order that the physicians' objections to the Medical Welfare Plan may be clear, we shall quote Malcolm G. Taylor's description of the plan. He says, "Five provincial governments have established tax-supported programs to provide a varying range of medical services for certain specified indigent groups of the population. . . . The Ontario program is limited to physicians' calls in office or home and certain laboratory procedures. Hospital care remains a responsibility of the municipality, and medical or surgical care in hospital is obtained in the public ward as a responsibility of the medical staff."[*]

One or more aspects of the Medical Welfare Plan called forth cen-

---

[*]Malcolm G. Taylor: The Administration of Health Insurance in Canada (Toronto: Oxford University Press, 1956), p. 8.

sure from 36 per cent of the Ontario practitioners. The two objections most frequently raised were that the payments were too low and that there was no remuneration for the care given to the patients in hospital. Several physicians pointed out that, not only were the payments so small that they barely covered the cost of the paper work involved, but the provincial government was getting the credit for providing the service, while any criticism from a patient was directed against the individual doctor. One doctor, who claimed that the major portion of the cost of the care given to the patients under the Medical Welfare Plan was borne by the doctors, felt that "the government is exploiting the medical profession in pretending that it is supplying full medical care, when it is the *doctors* who are providing it." Those who spoke in these terms said that, if the government was not prepared to cover the cost completely, they would prefer to give their services to the patient for nothing, as then the patient would know the situation. The occasional doctor referred to these patients as "extremely demanding"; on the other hand, they were occasionally described as "grateful and nice to treat." A complaint heard from a few doctors was that people who were well-to-do, or whose families were well-to-do, were receiving care under the Medical Welfare Plan.

In Nova Scotia, 82 per cent of those who answered were either "very well satisfied" or "fairly well satisfied" with the way in which they were paid for giving medical care to indigent patients, and 18 per cent were either "not very well satisfied" or "very much dissatisfied." It is to be noted, however, that 95 per cent of the practitioners up to forty-five years of age, but only 73 per cent of those over forty-five years of age, were either very well, or fairly well, satisfied ($p < 0.05$).

The complaints made about the various plans or agencies from which the physicians received payment might have meant more had we known what proportions of the practitioners' incomes came from the various sources. We attempted to obtain information on this, but, since we were not prepared to make a detailed analysis of the doctors' financial records—this was outside our province—the doctors' answers could only be guesses. When it became apparent that many of the men had not the least idea what proportion of their income was received from various sources, we discarded these data as quite unreliable.

In both provinces, the practitioners were asked, "What percentage of the fees billed privately are collected?" Ninety-three per cent of the Ontario, and 95 per cent of the Nova Scotia, physicians were able to reply. The figures given by the Ontario physicians ranged from 50 per cent to 99 per cent, with a mean of 81 per cent. In Nova Scotia, the answers ranged from 20 per cent to 90 per cent, with a mean of 65 per cent. The difference between the means is significant ($p <$ 0.01). Twenty-one per cent of the Nova Scotia physicians who replied to this question said that they collected 50 per cent or *less* of the fees that they billed privately. The reliability of these figures may be questioned, but they do indicate that collections in Ontario were thought to be quite good at the time when the Survey was conducted, whereas in Nova Scotia they were thought to vary from good to very unsatisfactory. An additional question was asked of the Ontario physicians only: "What percentage of the fees billed through a prepayment plan are collected?" The mean percentage named was 91 per cent. Apparently, the Ontario physicians believed that collections of the amounts billed were about 10 per cent better with the prepaid plans, though it must be remembered that some had said that it was useless to bill Physicians' Services Incorporated for all the work that they had done because the accounts were arbitrarily scaled down (see page 198).

From the specific prepayment plans, we went on to try to obtain the doctors' opinions, in more general terms, on the way in which medical care is paid for and should be paid for. The doctors were asked, first, whether the present system of paying for medical care, i.e. the combination of private payment, prepaid insurance plans, and public assistance and voluntary medical care for the indigent, was satisfactory to the doctor. Twenty per cent of the Ontario, and 36 per cent of the Nova Scotia, physicians gave negative answers. The difference is not statistically significant.

The doctors were next asked, regarding the present system of paying for medical care, "Do you think that *the majority of patients* are satisfied with the present arrangements?" Eighty-six per cent of the Ontario doctors and 90 per cent of those in Nova Scotia gave affirmative answers. Those who thought that the majority of patients were not satisfied said that the public felt that the cost of medical care was too high and that it wished a prepaid plan, either private or government-sponsored.

Thirdly, we asked, "Do you think that any other system of paying for medical care would result in a higher quality of medical care?" Twenty-three per cent in Ontario and 17 per cent in Nova Scotia replied that they thought it would, 73 per cent and 79 per cent in the two provinces, respectively, gave a negative answer, and the remainder could not answer. Half of those in Ontario who answered in the affirmative, i.e. 11 per cent of the entire Ontario sample of doctors, advocated a universal prepaid health insurance plan. A few others were in favour of wider coverage than at present, but did not suggest that it should be universal. It was thought that such a plan would allow the doctor to give better care than at present, because he would be able to give more time to patients and would not hesitate to order whatever tests or treatment might be necessary. Though we were frequently told that, when his patient was covered by health insurance, the doctor was relieved of worry about the patient's finances, seldom did we hear any mention of the fact that it would be the doctor's responsibility to consider the financial resources of the plan, i.e. that the doctor would still have the responsibility of deciding whether a particular measure was justified in a particular case. In Nova Scotia, also, some of those who thought that another system of paying for medical care would result in a higher quality of care said that the principle of prepayment should be applied to a greater proportion of the population.

One subject that we deliberately planned to avoid raising ourselves in our discussion, because we felt that its contentiousness might stir up such feelings as to interfere with the attainment of the major objectives of the Survey, was fee-splitting. This practice, which consists of the giving by a consultant, usually a surgeon, of part of his fee to the doctor by whom the patient was referred, is condemned, by both the Canadian Medical Association and the Royal College of Physicians and Surgeons of Canada, as unethical. Accordingly, we were surprised when several Ontario practitioners brought the practice into the discussion and defended it. (The subject never came up in Nova Scotia.) One man, expressing dissatisfaction with the teaching hospitals to which he referred patients, said, "I work the case up and then I'm right out of it. I lose the patient. It's hard to make a living." When asked how this deficiency could be rectified, he replied, "I see nothing wrong with fee-splitting, as long as the surgeon is top notch." It was apparent that he either did not see, or refused to admit, the possibility that unscrupulous surgeons might bid against one another for referrals and that tremendous economic pressure would be brought to bear on even the most high-principled surgeons in a community in which the practice prevailed. His complaint, however, that without fee-splitting the general practitioner sometimes received nothing at all while the surgeon "gets a hundred dollars for fifteen minutes' work" is food for thought. We shall return to this presently.

Another man practised in an area where, according to him, fee-splitting occurred. His patients were admitted to a large hospital, in which he was not permitted to do surgery. He said that, if fee-splitting were stopped, he would send his patients to a smaller hospital, where he would be permitted to operate himself. His argument was that, since it was better for the patient to be operated on by a qualified surgeon than by him, this was an adequate reason for perpetuating the practice of fee-splitting. On the surface, it appears that his patient benefits from the practice of fee-splitting; but this is so only because of a defect in the doctor's attitude. For whether the doctor recognized it or not and whether or not he would actually do as he said, his stated attitude, at least in regard to surgery, was that he would do what was best for the patient only as long as it did not hurt him (the doctor) economically, or, in other words, that he put his own economic welfare before the patient's physical welfare. Perhaps the physician concerned had not recognized the implication of his own words; but, if he did not realize what he was saying, then there is a great need that the meaning of his words be made quite clear to him and to any others who may hold the same opinion as he about fee-splitting.

It is our understanding that the College of General Practice has no official policy on fee-splitting because it regards this as a purely economic matter and, as such, beyond its purview. It is obvious, however, from the foregoing story that economics, ethics, and the standard of medical care, which *is* an acknowledged concern of the College (see page 151), are inextricably connected. In view of this, we suggest that, if the College of General Practice, in emulation of its sister-institution, the Royal College of Physicians and Surgeons of Canada (which also is concerned with education and with standards rather than with economics), were to adopt an uncompromising attitude towards fee-splitting, it would be making a positive contribution to the improvement of medical care in this country. Moreover, if another practitioner was correct when he said that fee-splitting had played a part in producing "the general practitioner's inferiority complex plus guilt feelings" and that it made the surgeons feel too superior when they "virtually tip" the general practitioner, then a stand taken by the College of General Practice against fee-splitting might do much to improve the standing of general practitioners in the eyes of the public, in the eyes of the specialists, and, most important, in their own eyes.

So much for the ethics of fee-splitting. Both of the general practitioners whom we have quoted as defending fee-splitting referred also to economic aspects of this practice, which call for comment. Each of these men implied that surgical work was more profitable than non-surgical work; but one was comparing his own remuneration for non-surgical work with the remuneration of a qualified surgeon for surgery, whereas the other was, by implication, comparing what *he* himself would receive for surgical work with what he received for non-surgical work.

In view of what was said by these men, we submit for consideration four propositions. First, a physician, whether he be a general practitioner or a specialist, depends for his livelihood upon selling* his time and his skill, the latter being based on knowledge and technical training.† It is self-evident that without both the professional skill of a physician and time in which to exercise that skill, he would not be able to earn his living *as a physician.*

Secondly, unless surgical procedures are very much more demanding on the skill of a general practitioner than is non-surgical work, we can see no reason why he should be paid more for an hour of his time spent in the operating-room than for the same amount of his time given to house calls, office work, or hospital rounds. If general practitioners claim that surgical work *does* make a greater demand than non-surgical work on their skill, we must reply that we have repeatedly heard some general practitioners, when objecting to the possibility of their surgery being limited, say how "simple" it is to do an appendectomy or a hernial repair; we must also point out that only 16 per cent of the Ontario, and 19 per cent of the Nova Scotia, physicians had

---

*If anyone should object to the use of the word "selling," on the ground that it connotes commercialism, we would say three things in reply. First, as long as a physician sets a fee for his services—instead of imitating the clergyman and leaving it to the patient to reward him or not as the patient sees fit—he *is* selling his services, regardless of what euphemism may be employed to cloak this fact. Secondly, a physician need not be ashamed to admit that he sells his services, provided that he gives good value for what he receives, since, however high-minded he may be, he still must have the necessities of life for himself and he fails in a primary responsibility if he neglects his family, while he lives, or leaves them destitute, when he dies. Finally, the fact that a physician sells to those who can afford to buy does not in any way preclude his giving his services without charge to those who need them but cannot afford to pay for them. There is a great deal of confused thinking, on the part both of the doctors and of the public, on this subject of remuneration, which has a detrimental effect on the relationships between different segments of the profession and between the profession and the public.

†It is true that some physicians also sell drugs to their patients; but, though this may be necessary and commendable in certain circumstances, these men are not, strictly speaking, functioning as physicians while they are engaged in this activity.

had over 6 months of postgraduate training in surgery, and that only 7 per cent and 12 per cent, in the two provinces respectively, had had more than 12 months;* and finally we would quote one older general practitioner, who did a good deal of surgery and who said that he enjoyed it because "surgery is easier than medicine" and that he found the general run of medical diseases (including such problems as diabetes, hypertension, and emotional problems) distasteful, because they "take a lot of time." On the other hand, there is a positive argument in favour of the same remuneration for medical work and for surgical work requiring the same amounts of time: that the physician who is doing both medical and surgical work, in deciding between medical and surgical treatment of a patient, will be free from any economic prejudice.

Thirdly, although what follows is not strictly germane, because it does not directly concern general practitioners, nevertheless, because it is related to the quality of medical care available to the population, we submit, as a parallel proposition to the preceding one, that, unless the work of a qualified specialist in surgery makes greater demands on *his* skill than does non-surgical work on the skill of a qualified specialist in internal medicine or in paediatrics, then a paediatrician or an internist should be paid the same amount as a surgeon for an hour of his time. Perhaps a qualified specialist in surgery may insist that his work *is* more demanding than the work of an internist or paediatrician. In answer to this, we would admit without hesitation that certain standard operations, such as gastrectomy, cholecystectomy, or abdominoperineal resection, call for great skill, but we would contend that such non-surgical conditions as coronary thrombosis, meningitis, and severe diarrhoea in infancy are equally demanding.

The preceding paragraph applies only to those specialists who are following the well-worn trail, whether in medicine or in surgery. The trail-blazer, the man who is courageous enough to enter unknown territory, where a misstep may mean disaster, may well claim that his work makes special, and perhaps exorbitant, demands on his skill. We refer to such men as the cardiac surgeons, who, for example, in devising methods of dealing with lesions in areas heretofore considered inaccessible, bear the heavy burden of deciding whether the disease or the high mortality rate of a new operation carries the greater risk for a particular patient. These physicians we hold in the greatest respect; and we do not presume to suggest how their remuneration should

*These figures include time spent in non-teaching hospitals as well as teaching hospitals.

compare with that of the specialists to whom our third proposition applied.

Fourthly, we hold that a man who has spent years in studying a particular branch of medicine and who, if the present specialist qualifications have any meaning, has greater skill than a general practitioner in that particular field is entitled to greater remuneration per hour for his services than the man who has not submitted himself to the discipline and the deprivation involved in such extended training. This principle is so generally accepted in our society that we make no comment on it.

To recapitulate the four propositions that we have stated, we submit that a medical practitioner depends for his livelihood on selling his time and his professional skill; that specialists, by virtue of their greater skill and the sacrifices that they have made to attain that greater skill, are entitled to a higher remuneration per unit of time than are general practitioners; but that the rate of remuneration either of a general practitioner or of a specialist should be independent of the clinical branch of medicine (in the broad sense of the word) to which the patient's condition belongs. (We have exempted from this those who are pioneering in certain fields.)

From the remarks made by several practitioners about the economics of fee-splitting, it is apparent that they were dissatisfied with the gap that they thought existed between the remuneration for surgical work and that for non-surgical work, i.e. that they believed that the fees for surgical procedures were too high or the fees for non-surgical work were too low or both. Whether surgical work is *really* more remunerative, per hour of work, than non-surgical work, we do not know. It may be that it merely appears to be so because non-surgical work is usually charged for by the visit, whereas for much of surgical work there is a single charge to cover not only the operation but also the pre- and post-operative care. However, in view of the strength of the opinions expressed by the practitioners we have quoted and in view of the increasingly firm stand that two professional organizations have taken against fee-splitting in recent years, we suggest that there is a need to investigate this matter from the economic point of view. In any such investigation, the four propositions that we have set forth above would, it seems to us, be basic. We would hope that a comparative study of the earnings accruing from surgical work and from non-surgical work and whatever adjustments of fees might be necessary to bring these into line with each other would do much to bring an end to fee-splitting, to improve the quality of medical care, and to better the relationship between general practitioners and surgical specialists.

After this long discussion of fee-splitting, which was prompted by the remarks made by certain practitioners who chose to bring the matter up and to argue in favour of it, it is pleasant to be able to report that other physicians, both in Ontario and in Nova Scotia, left no doubt in our minds that they placed their patients' welfare before their own economic interests. One young man said, "I refer a lot of patients. This is being fair to them. I'm content with what is left." An older man said that at one time he had done some major surgery but that several years previously he had stopped because he felt that younger men, with specialist qualifications in surgery, were better equipped for this work and that therefore it was in the patients' best interests to have them operate.

Before leaving the topic of fee-splitting, we must state quite explicitly that our discussion of it is not to be interpreted as indicating that the practice is prevalent. It would be interesting to know how common it is and whether, as rumour has it, it is confined to certain geographical areas. On these points, however, we have no information. We do know, as we have stated, that fee-splitting occurs in Ontario; whether it occurs in Nova Scotia, we do not know, since the subject did not come up.

The remaining question to be considered in this chapter is what provision the practitioner makes for the future. To be told by one of the older doctors in the group, a man who appeared tired and was not in particularly good health, that he had been unable to save anything, that he would not be able to retire without taking the cash surrender value of his life insurance, and that even then he would be poor, was a saddening experience. We heard more than one such statement, though just how often such a situation as this occurs, we do not know. Because doctors are reputed to be poor business men, we included in our questionnaire a few questions that we hoped would show what the situation really was. Our first question was, "How do you think a doctor can best provide for his old age and for his dependents?" This evoked conflicting statements about the relative merits of mortgages, real estate, bonds, shares, annuities, and insurance. More than 90 per cent of the doctors in Ontario and a little over 75 per cent in Nova Scotia mentioned life insurance. A few had read one or another of the books that make clear the real costs of various types of insurance. These men were unanimous in recommending insurance as protection, but not as a means of saving. Many of the doctors, however, gave little or no evidence of having any sound knowledge of insurance. Though some spoke of the high cost of the insurance they were carrying, they showed no awareness that there was any alternative. Several doctors stated quite frankly that they knew little about investments and other financial matters. Occasionally, a doctor would describe himself as "a babe in the woods." One man's entire answer was that one "shouldn't worry about it." Another, who was in his mid forties said, "It's a problem that I haven't managed to solve yet." On the other hand, a small number of doctors gave answers that suggested that they thought about the problem in a systematic way. For instance, one man divided our question into its two parts and said that he would provide for his old age with annuities and for his dependents with renewable term insurance. Another doctor advised having family income insurance during the earlier years, lessening the insurance and replacing it with annuities in the later years (when the need for protection would be less), and supplementing these two methods with other investments. Our reason for giving these examples is not that they are "correct" ways of providing for one's old age and one's dependents, because we believe that each man's plan must be determined by his own circumstances and needs, so that what is correct for one man may be quite the wrong thing for another. Rather, we have given these examples because they show how some of the physicians have approached the problem of making provision for the future.

It was not until the field work in Ontario was well along towards completion that the law relating to income tax was changed to allow self-employed persons to contribute to a pension plan as do employees. Because there was no such provision when the Survey was commenced, the Ontario doctors were asked, "Would you like to be able to contribute to a pension plan?" More than 85 per cent replied in the affirmative. The few who did not were either too old to benefit from such a provision or were men who did not wish their money to be tied up or beyond their own control. The Nova Scotia physicians were asked, "Do you contribute to a registered pension plan?" Forty-three per cent replied that they did, 57 per cent that they did not. Those who gave affirmative answers constituted 50 per cent of the doctors up to thirty-five years of age, 47 per cent of those between thirty-six and forty-five, and 33 per cent of those over forty-five years of age.

In order to obtain more specific information, we asked a group of three questions: "With regard to investments (stocks, bonds, real estate, etc.), (1) do you enjoy handling investments? (2) Do you find that you have adequate time to devote to your invesment problems? (3) Do you find that you are able to handle your investments to your own satisfaction?" In Ontario each of the three questions, and in Nova Scotia the two questions regarding time and ability, were answered in the affirmative by less than 50 per cent of the physicians. When the answers relating to time and to ability were combined, we found that 41 per cent of the Ontario, and 43 per cent of the Nova Scotia, doctors said that they had neither the time nor the ability to manage their investments; 27 per cent of the Ontario, and 29 per cent of the Nova Scotia, doctors said that they had both; 27 per cent and 21 per cent in the two provinces, respectively, lacked one or other of the two; and the remaining few men in Nova Scotia did not answer because they had no investments.

Our final question on this subject was, "What do you think are the best sources of information and advice on financial matters?" Sixteen per cent of the Ontario doctors and 14 per cent of those in Nova Scotia were unable to make any suggestions. One man said, "I'm a poor financier, I always was." Another said, "I'd like to know. When you find out let me know." The remainder named friends and relatives, bankers, lawyers, accountants, trust companies, investment dealers, and various publications. In the last-named category, the two most frequently mentioned were the *Financial Post* and the articles on financial matters in the *Ontario Medical Review*. Only 32 per cent of the Ontario doctors and 12 per cent of those in Nova Scotia made any reference to reading material, and the only one who suggested reading of a type that would make the doctor aware of the existence and of the advantages and disadvantages of various types of investment was one Nova Scotia doctor who referred to the University of Toronto's extension course on "How To Invest Your Money."

Our impression, over all, was that a large percentage of the doctors visited by us, both in Ontario and in Nova Scotia, had comparatively little knowledge of business matters. Having worked hard for their income, they did not know how to conserve the surplus for the years when they would no longer be able, or would no longer wish, to work.

In dealing with the financial problems that are encountered by the medical student and the practising physician, we are well aware that we have just scratched the surface. It was not the purpose of this study to collect detailed information on these problems; and the available figures are too indefinite to allow us to proceed further than we have. The very meagreness of the data, however, suggests the need for more definitive studies of the economic aspects of medical education and medical practice. In chapters 23 (especially pages 434–439) and 24 (especially pages 469–477), we shall consider certain relationships between economics and quality of medical care.

# 14 / The General Practitioner as a Person

At the opening of chapter 3, we set for ourselves the task of giving a picture of the general practitioner, as a prerequisite to an understanding of the problems of general practice. Up to this point we have described what training he has had, we have examined the arrangements that he has made for carrying on his practice, and we have presented him as a member of the medical community and of the general community. Before we go on to examine what his work comprises and how well he does it, it remains for us to picture him in his home, with his family and his friends, in his leisure activities, and finally as an individual possessing certain characteristics—in short, to consider him as a person.

In order to find out what the physician's leisure activities were, we listed nine types of activity and asked, for each one, whether the physician engaged in that activity frequently, occasionally, or not at all and whether participation was limited to his vacations. The list consisted of going to movies, watching television, reading of a non-medical nature, listening to music, playing a musical instrument, watching sports, participating in sports, spending social evenings with friends, and playing bridge. In addition, the physician was asked to name any other hobbies or activities. Initially, we tried to obtain an estimate of the number of hours per week that were spent on these activities, but this attempt was abandoned as impracticable.

Of the nine types of activity listed, the one named most often in Ontario (by 55 per cent of the physicians) as a frequent activity was the spending of social evenings with friends (Table 45). On the other hand, this was a frequent activity of only 29 per cent of the Nova

TABLE 45

FREQUENCY WITH WHICH ONTARIO AND NOVA SCOTIA PHYSICIANS
PARTICIPATED IN VARIOUS RECREATIONAL ACTIVITIES

| | Ontario | | | | Nova Scotia | | | |
|---|---|---|---|---|---|---|---|---|
| | Number of physicians participating | | | | Number of physicians participating | | | |
| Activity | Fre-quently | Occasion-ally | During vacations only | Not at all* | Fre-quently | Occasion-ally | During vacations only | Not at all* |
| Movies | 1 | 21 | 0 | 22 | 5 | 23 | 11 | 3 |
| Television | 21 | 17 | 1† | 5 | 19 | 23 | 0 | 0 |
| Non-medical reading | 22 | 16 | 2 | 4 | 23 | 18 | 1 | 0 |
| Listening to music | 15 | 23 | 0 | 6 | 16 | 23 | 2 | 1 |
| Playing a musical instrument | 2 | 5 | 0 | 37‡ | 0 | 7 | 0 | 35 |
| Watching sports | 17 | 16 | 0 | 11 | 19 | 22 | 0 | 1 |
| Participating in sports | 23 | 4 | 5 | 12 | 20 | 8 | 0 | 14 |
| Social evening with friends | 24 | 17 | 0 | 3§ | 12 | 26 | 3 | 1 |
| Playing bridge | 13 | 16 | 0 | 15 | 3 | 21 | 5 | 13 |
| Other hobbies or activities | 26 | 8 | 1 | 9 | 14 | 11 | 0 | 17 |
| Total number of physicians visited by the Survey | 44 | | | | 42 | | | |

*Some of these physicians said "very rarely" or "almost never."

†There was no television in this physician's community.

‡One of these physicians had had voice training and sang in a quartet.

§One of these physicians said that he and his wife would be all ready to go out, when he would be called to see a patient.

Scotia practitioners. The difference between the two provinces is statistically significant ($p < 0.05$).* Reading, participating in sports, watching sports, watching television, and listening to music were activities each of which was frequently engaged in by approximately one-third to one-half of the practitioners who were visited in each province. Only a small percentage of the doctors in either province showed interest in playing a musical instrument or in going to the movies. Playing bridge was a frequent activity of 30 per cent of the Ontario, but of only 7 per cent of the Nova Scotia, doctors ($p < 0.05$). Again, frequent participation in hobbies or activities other than the nine specifically inquired about was indicated by 59 per cent of the Ontario physicians, but by only 33 per cent of those in Nova Scotia ($p < 0.05$). Since social evenings and bridge both involve making commitments to other people and since hobbies are probably more demanding of time than reading, listening to music, or watching television—to each of which it is possible to turn in quite a desultory manner—it is interesting to speculate whether the differences noted between the replies of the

*This is explained on pages 32–33.

Ontario, and the Nova Scotia, physicians were a reflection of the longer hours of work (see page 102) of the general practitioners in Nova Scotia.

The physicians who named non-medical reading as one of their activities were asked to state what types of material they liked to read. On examining the answers of those physicians who said that they read *frequently,* our findings were: 32 per cent of all the Ontario physicians who were visited and 29 per cent of those in Nova Scotia referred to newspapers and magazines; 18 per cent in Ontario and 29 per cent in Nova Scotia named such subjects as archaeology, biography, geology, history, philosophy, physics, seamanship, and travel; and 18 per cent and 21 per cent, in the two provinces respectively, mentioned fiction. Those who frequently listened to music were questioned about their preferences. In Ontario, 20 per cent of the doctors said that they listened frequently to classical music; semiclassical music, jazz, general and popular music, folk music, and the operas of Gilbert and Sullivan were each named by less than 10 per cent. In Nova Scotia, 21 per cent listened frequently to general and popular music, 18 per cent to classical music, and 14 per cent to semiclassical; jazz, opera, and sacred music were each listed by less than 10 per cent of the doctors.

The four sports in which the greatest number of Ontario practitioners said they *participated* were golf, fishing, hunting, and curling, each of which was named, though not necessarily as a *frequent* activity, by between 20 and 36 per cent of the doctors. Other sports, which were less often named, were bowling, shooting, swimming, boating, badminton, tennis, flying, and tramping in the woods. In Nova Scotia, swimming was mentioned by 24 per cent of the doctors; golf, fishing, and hunting were each named by about 20 per cent; and sports that were less frequently listed were boating, badminton, tennis, curling, bowling, shooting, flying, baseball, hockey, volleyball, skating, skiing, and walking.

In addition to the nine activities about which the physicians were questioned specifically, other activities were named by 80 per cent of the Ontario men and by 60 per cent of those in Nova Scotia, and, as we have already noted, were frequently engaged in by 59 per cent and 33 per cent in the two provinces, respectively. These interests were so diverse as to include photography, stock market transactions, squaredancing, talking to alcoholics, and growing Christmas trees, to name only a few. The three most popular among those mentioned appeared to be woodworking, gardening, and—especially in Ontario, where it was named by 25 per cent of the doctors—photography.

As to the doctor's friendships, we were interested in learning whether his close friends were drawn entirely from the ranks of the medical profession or whether they included non-medical persons. The question asked was, "Think of the five people, apart from your immediate family, whom you regard as your five closest friends, regardless of whether they live in your own community or at a distance. How many of these five are members of the medical profession?" Those who answered that less than five were members of the profession were asked, "In what types of work are the remainder engaged?" The number of medical persons among the five closest friends varied from 0 to 5 in each province, with a mean of approximately 2 in each province (Table 46). The other friends were engaged

TABLE 46

NUMBER OF MEMBERS OF THE MEDICAL PROFESSION AMONG THE FIVE
CLOSEST FRIENDS OF THE ONTARIO AND NOVA SCOTIA PHYSICIANS

| Number of medical persons among five closest friends | Ontario physicians | | Nova Scotia physicians | |
|---|---|---|---|---|
| | Number | % | Number | % |
| None | 4 | 9.1 | 7 | 16.7 |
| One | 15 | 34.1 | 8 | 19.0 |
| Two | 12 | 27.3 | 18 | 42.9 |
| Three | 8 | 18.2 | 7 | 16.7 |
| Four | 3 | 6.8 | 0 | 0.0 |
| Five | 2 | 4.5 | 2 | 4.8 |
| Total | 44 | 100 | 42 | 100 |

in a very great variety of occupations, including many professions, trades, and businesses. One doctor stated that he tended to "grow away from" his non-medical friends. The occasional man was encountered who apparently had few, if any, close friends. One man, for example, had no close friends in the medical profession and was obviously embarrassed when asked in what activities his friends were engaged. When given the opportunity to let the question go unanswered, he looked relieved and said that that would be best and that "we don't have too much social intercourse." Another man, who said that he had three close friends in the profession, declined to name two other friends and said that he was "gregarious—not the buddy-buddy type."

All but one of the Ontario doctors were married. Of those who were married, all but two had children. The number of children varied from 1 to 8, the average, including adopted children, being slightly over 2½ per household. In Nova Scotia, 3 of the doctors were single, 1 divorced, and 38 married at the time of our visit. Of the last group, 2 were married for the second time, one following a divorce, the other having been left a widower. All but three of those who had been married had children. The number of children ranged from 2 to 7, with a mean of approximately 3½.

For a number of reasons, no attempt was made to interview the practitioners' wives. It is unfortunate that it was not possible to do this, since there can be little doubt that the wives' attitudes have some effect on the practices and that the wives, having a different view of their husbands' practices, could have contributed a great deal of valuable information. However, from things said by the wives during meals, from remarks made by the doctors themselves, and from observations made by the members of the Survey team during their many visits to the doctors' homes, impressions were gained of the physicians' homes and family relationships.

A minority of the physicians did not invite us to their homes. Of those who did, few had homes that were luxurious, most varied between being comfortably housed and being rather cramped, and the occasional man lived in remarkably poor quarters. Permanent domestic help was very rarely encountered, especially in the homes where it was most needed, namely, where the wives had young children with whom, because of their husbands' long and irregular hours, they had to cope almost single-handed.

The atmosphere in those homes that we saw varied greatly. A few had to bear the burden of chronic illness or were split by sordid squabbling. In others, in which relationships appeared to be most harmonious, it was obvious that the practitioner derived great happiness from his family life. In still others, beneath a placid surface ran detectable currents of distrust or of selfishness. It was sad, for example, to hear a man who had been in practice for many years say that he had never had a nurse or secretary because he knew that his wife would not be pleased. Another cause of wifely complaint, according to several of the doctors, was that the doctor devoted so much time to his practice that he had little left for his wife and children. One man repeatedly expressed regret that he had "neglected" his family, with serious consequences. Another said that his wife often complained of his work habits, but he gave no indication that he attached any importance to her complaints. Yet another spoke of his wife's objecting to the relatively little time he spent at home, but said that he often felt restless at home because he liked to be "doing things."

Some of the wives spoke to the observers about how little time their husbands had for family life. It was apparent, from observation, that in some cases the doctor's work did leave him little time for his family. In other cases, pressure of work was pleaded as an excuse for what really amounted to thoughtlessness. Thus, when one doctor and his wife had been invited to dine with the observer and the time had been set to suit the doctor, for no good reason he kept himself and the observer an hour late and then, because of the demands of his office, postponed the dinner for another hour and a half. When he and the observer finally met the wife, the doctor showed no concern over the fact that his wife, who had dressed for the occasion, had sat waiting for more than two and a half hours.

The importance, in a physician's life, of the division of time between work and family is shown by the remarks made by several men about their postgraduate training. One said that he had gone into general practice, instead of training in a specialty, in order to be able to marry and start raising a family; he did not wish to leave his wife to "a lonely existence," in which she would be by herself day after day, evening after evening, and night after night, while her husband worked and slept in a hospital. Two others, one at the insistence of his wife, the other because he felt that he must not impose further on his wife, had given up their specialty training before it was completed in order to be able to live with their families, instead of living at a great distance and seeing them rarely.

We shall have more to say later (pages 465 ff.) about the problem of time in a doctor's life; but it is appropriate to report, at this point, the answers to one question. Each doctor was asked what he thought about the amount of time that he was able to devote to his family, whether he had "ample time, just enough time, not enough time, or little or no time." Four per cent in Ontario and 21 per cent in Nova Scotia replied that they had "little or no time," and another 73 per cent and 50 per cent, in the two provinces respectively, that they had "not enough time" for their families. The answers of the remaining 23 per cent in Ontario and 29 per cent in Nova Scotia were divided almost equally between "ample time" and "just enough time."

Throughout the past dozen chapters, we have sought to make clear how greatly the physicians differed in many respects—in their training, in the arrangements for their practices, and in their relationships to one another and to their communities. Nowhere were the divergences more apparent than in those general qualities that, taken together, constitute personality and character. Since such qualities as sincerity, conscientiousness, honesty, and their opposites, to name only a few, do not lend themselves to quantitative measurement and since often it is not possible to state with any degree of certainty whether one or another quality is present or is lacking in a person, we did not attempt to investigate these in any systematic way. Nevertheless, certain characteristics obtruded themselves so forcibly upon our notice that failure to mention them would be a distortion on our part and would leave the description of the practitioners even more incomplete than it must necessarily be.

The fact that a man has taken the medical course and is engaged in the practice of medicine might be thought to presuppose an interest in medicine. Whether this *is* the reason for taking the medical course we shall consider in a later chapter (pages 334–335). As we saw the physicians carrying on their practices, however, we were impressed with the fact that some were obviously deeply interested but that others, just as obviously, had little or no interest in medicine. Of some doctors' interest, or lack of it, we could not form any worthwhile estimate. This is as one would expect, since, between those with strong interest and those with weak interest, are probably men whose different degrees of interest form a continuum. Most, but not all, of those who seemed to be lacking in interest were over forty-five years of age. In the occasional case, poor health seemed to be at least a contributing cause. One man, who freely admitted his lack of enthusiasm, attributed it to geographic isolation and advancing age.

Some took pleasure in carrying on a medical practice, i.e. they enjoyed the busyness and the rushing about that were part of practice and they delighted in meeting people and in engaging in conversation, but they lacked interest in the real nature of their patients' maladies. Such was one young practitioner who spoke fairly slowly and intelligibly to his patients when he was chatting about local affairs but who, in taking a medical history, spoke very rapidly and often gave the patient little or no time to answer before he asked the next question. He often complained to the observer of lack of time and gave this as the reason for the speed with which he questioned and examined patients. In actual fact, conversing with patients interested him; taking their histories and examining them did not.

One man who did appear to be interested in medicine said that he thought that he was probably becoming "slipshod" and that he spent too little time listening to patients and examining them and too much time talking himself. Observation confirmed what he said. He enjoyed talking, whereas examining patients and listening carefully to what *they* said required real self-discipline.

In some cases, lack of interest in medicine and lack of self-confidence appeared together. Whether they were related, and if so what the relationship was, we do not know. One doctor's lack of confidence in his own ability and his refusal to accept any great amount of responsibility were expressed in a number of such unequivocal statements as, "I don't accept any responsibility for sick patients. If they're sick, I ship them off at once to a specialist. I believe in calling in someone who knows a particular subject. I'm only a general practitioner." When he sent a boy with a fractured clavicle to a surgeon to have a figure-of-eight bandage applied, he said that, a few years before, he would have done this himself but that now he preferred to "get out from under." Another man's lack of self-confidence was apparent in his unwillingness to commit himself to a definite opinion, except when he was able to bolster it by referring to what "they say" or to what Osler or some other eminent authority "said." The importance to him of being certain was shown in his statement that "it is nice to know all there is to know about a condition and be on sure ground, rather than have a smattering of knowledge as a G.P. has." His lack of self-confidence caused him frequent difficulty in the conduct of his practice. He was vague in talking to patients and in giving them instructions; he had a nervous laugh, which came out at most inappropriate times, as, for example, when he was discussing with a patient the possibility of cancer as a complication of gastric ulcer; and frequently, having told a patient what course of action he had decided was best, he proceeded to talk himself out of it and to adopt precisely the opposite course.

Both in their manner of answering our questionnaire and in their questioning of their own patients, the practitioners showed great variation in their ability to think systematically. Some men seemed to have much difficulty with this. One man, for example, even in answering questions that called for a straight "yes" or "no," introduced a great deal of irrelevant material as he groped for an answer. Another, who often started to answer a question before the interrogator had finished asking it, would talk quickly and often irrelevantly for a few minutes and then suddenly stop and ask, "What was that question again?" When he did understand the question, his answer would often be verbose and indefinite, and sometimes would be changed to the reverse of what he at first had said. Inability of another man to follow a clear line of thought led, in his history-taking, to a great deal of dithering, the omitting of important questions, back-tracking, and, in general, the wasting of much time. On the other hand, others repeatedly demonstrated their ability to grasp quickly the meaning of a question or of a patient's statement and to strike straight at the heart of a problem. This faculty was a major contributor to the high quality of care given by many practitioners.

A sense of responsibility was another attribute whose presence or absence was manifested in a variety of ways. One physician showed his lack of respect for the law when he recounted with relish and obvious approval the indignity inflicted upon a member of the local police force when he attempted to quell rowdyism. This was the only case that we encountered of overt contempt for the maintenance of physical order in the community. Several men, however, in the two provinces, behaved in an irresponsible way towards the Survey itself. One, who had had the study explained to him and who had shown no reluctance to taking part, failed to meet the observer at the agreed time, kept him waiting for five hours, though within one hour he had been informed by his office of the observer's arrival, and then refused to take part in the study. Apart from the discourtesy involved in his not notifying us of his decision, the cost to the Survey was approximately one hundred miles of driving, the complete loss of one day, and the loss, as far as field work was concerned, of one week. Another man agreed readily to participate, and a mutually convenient date was set for the observer's visit. For some reason, perhaps because he was going to have to drive two hundred and fifty miles over a winding highway, the observer was prompted, just before setting out, to check with the doctor by telephone. This saved the Survey and the observer five hundred miles of driving, because in the interval since the initial contact the doctor had moved to another province. When the observer reached him by telephone in order to confirm that the move was permanent, the doctor offered no apology for failing to notify the Survey and seemed quite oblivious that he had assumed a responsibility when he agreed with the Director of the Survey to take part. These incidents were nothing more than minor irritations to the Survey, but there is the disturbing possibility that these men's irresponsible attitude may extend to their practices.

Another physician who agreed to take part but changed his mind adopted the responsible course of writing to inform us of this. Although we regretted his decision, we felt that he had treated us in a very straightforward manner. Still others, who later told us that they were quite apprehensive about taking part, agreed to participate out of a sense of duty to their profession. The courage that this required in certain cases was worthy of great admiration. Despite the examples we have given of startlingly irresponsible behaviour, it was our impression that the majority of the doctors were conscientious, and many of them extremely so.

Gross dishonesty, reprehensible in anyone, is especially so in a medical man, the very foundation of whose relationship with a patient is trust; but we did encounter dishonesty. One physician, complaining that Physicians' Services Incorporated scaled down his fees, said that he had "the edge on them" because he simply arranged to have the patient make more visits. Whether any significant number of practitioners yield to this temptation, which is inherent in any fee-for-service type of prepaid plan, we do not know. We do hope that this doctor is unique in engaging in another, and most repulsive, type of dishonesty, of which he told us quite unashamedly. He boasted that he was grossly overcharging a patient who, because of his condition, was unable to keep track of the number of visits that the physician made. Perhaps some faint awareness of his own baseness prompted him to add, as though in justification, "Anyway, he's loaded." Again, a practitioner in Nova Scotia, who could not find the time that was necessary to do the continuing study that the College of General Practice of Canada demanded as a condition for membership, told us that some of his colleagues had said that he should just say, as they had, that he had done the required amount of study. Our informant chose to preserve his own integrity rather than to follow the advice given.

A difficulty that besets doctors as it does other men is alcoholism. The only evidence that we had that this was a problem to any of the doctors at the time of our visit was the statement of one man that he drank a bit too much and that on a slow day in the office, had the observer not been there, he would probably have gone off for a drink "with the boys." Several other practitioners told us that alcoholism had been a serious problem to them in the past. These men appeared to have been successful in giving up alcohol completely.

In view of the many differences that we have noted, it is not surprising to find that one practitioner varied markedly from another in his manner of dealing with patients. One older doctor was calm, dignified, reserved, and courteous—what many people perhaps picture as the family doctor of forty or fifty years ago. Others called most patients by their first names, bantered them, and even subjected them to humorous insults. Sometimes such an approach was effective in relaxing a tense, worried-looking patient, though occasionally the language used exceeded the bounds of good taste. One man who was kindly and interested in his patients had a tendency to lapse into baby-talk, not only with children but with women. Though this was well received by the children, it was noted that several of his adult patients were ill at ease when he talked in this way. Another doctor did not really seem to enjoy dealing with patients; and the personal aspects of medical problems seemed to be a particular nuisance to him. This, together with the fact that he enjoyed the organizational aspects of practice, caused us to doubt whether he was temperamentally suited for the practice of medicine and to wonder whether he might have been happier in some type of administrative work. Other men had an impersonal, even a cold, attitude towards patients. One, who said that he used to spend a good deal of time talking to "neurotics" and had found that this helped them, could not "be bothered now with their damn nonsense," and he laughed as he said it. Another repeatedly used a word with a curiously mechanical connotation, when he talked of "fixing" patients. One doctor was proud of his ability to appear relaxed before patients and said that he acted as though he had "all the time in world" with the result, he said, that very few of them noticed that he spent only about two minutes with them on the average. On the other hand, others not only gave the impression of not being rushed and of having time for the patient, but actually spent as much time as was necessary. One such man allowed twenty minutes for each appointment, but sometimes devoted a good deal longer than that to the patient.

Finally, what was the general practitioner's outlook on life? We were unable, in many cases, to obtain a unified picture, which is perhaps not to be wondered at, in view of the relative shortness of our visit. A few men, however, who obviously had given much thought to their lives, shared with us the results of their thinking. One man, approaching middle age, had long hours and did a great deal of driving on the highway. Yet, with him, the observer had no feeling of rush. His dealings with his patients in his office and in their homes were unhurried; and the observer always felt safe in his car, which he did not with many other doctors. This absence of great pressure was not accidental; it was the result of a deliberate policy. The doctor said that in his early years in practice he had been overworked. He had decided that he either had to control his practice where he was or go elsewhere. Though his colleagues believed that it could not be done, he had controlled his practice instead of letting his practice control him. It was quite apparent that to have adequate time, to do good work, and to enjoy the practice of medicine were all linked together. Another, somewhat younger, man had an over-all plan for living that included his wife and his children and that called for a balance, made possible by routine and flexibility, between self, practice, and family.

The time available to us was too short for the amount of information that we wished to obtain from the doctors we met, although, with few exceptions, they did their best to answer our questions and to give us a full picture of their lives. As a result, many fascinating conversations had to be curtailed to meet the needs of the Survey, when our own inclination would have been to ignore both the clock and the questionnaire and to let the discussion take its natural course while we enjoyed it to the full.

# THE WORK OF THE
# GENERAL PRACTITIONER

# 15 / The Content of the
## General Practitioner's Work

In the chapters of the preceding section, we have tried to create a picture of the men who are engaged in general practice; in particular we have laid emphasis on the endless variation that we encountered in the Survey. Though we have spoken repeatedly of "the general practitioner" because it has been convenient to do so, in fact there is no such man as *the* general practitioner. There are general practitioners, as many different ones as there are men doing general practice.

From the general practitioners, the men who do the work of general practice, we turn now to consider the work itself. In succeeding chapters of this section, we shall examine the quality of general practice as we saw it; in this present chapter, we shall see first what the work comprises. We shall start with a broad outline of general practice and then consider some of the details.

Ninety-five per cent of the Ontario practitioners and 98 per cent of those in Nova Scotia included in their practices adult medicine, paediatrics, obstetrics, and minor surgery (Table 47). Three men carried on more circumscribed practices. One of these, who practised in a large city but who neither possessed specialist qualifications nor professed to be a consultant, confined his practice to adult medicine. He saw patients in his office and in their homes, but did no paediatrics, obstetrics, major or minor surgery, or anaesthesia. One man restricted his practice to adult medicine, obstetrics, and minor surgery, and did no paediatrics or major surgery and little or no general anaesthesia. The third did adult medicine and paediatrics, but no obstetrics, anaesthesia, or surgery.

TABLE 47

Major Categories* of Work Undertaken by the Ontario
and Nova Scotia Physicians

| | Ontario physicians | | Nova Scotia physicians | |
|---|---|---|---|---|
| Work undertaken | Number | % | Number | % |
| Medicine, paediatrics, obstetrics, and minor surgery | 22 | 50.0 | 12† ‡ | 28.6 |
| Medicine, paediatrics, obstetrics, minor surgery, and abdominal surgery (with or without other major surgery) | 14 | 31.8 | 15 | 35.7 |
| Medicine, paediatrics, obstetrics, minor surgery, abdominal surgery (with or without other major surgery), and more than occasional general anaesthesia | 0 | 0.0 | 9§ | 21.4 |
| Medicine, paediatrics, obstetrics, minor surgery, and more than occasional general anaesthesia | 6 | 13.6 | 5‡ § ‖ | 11.9 |
| Medicine, obstetrics, and minor surgery | 1 | 2.3 | 0 | 0.0 |
| Medicine and paediatrics | 0 | 0.0 | 1 | 2.4 |
| Medicine (adult) only | 1 | 2.3 | 0 | 0.0 |
| Total | 44 | 100 | 42 | 100 |

*Psychiatry is not included in this table, for the reason given on page 231 of the text.

†The minor surgery named by 3 of these physicians included only such procedures as the suturing of lacerations and the removal of cysts; the other 9 included one or more of the reduction of simple fractures, the removal of tonsils and adenoids, and uterine curettage.

‡One physician in each of these groups said that he would do an appendectomy in an emergency.

§In each of these groups were 2 physicians whose anaesthetic work was more than occasional but probably only of moderate volume.

‖All of these physicians specified that they included in their surgery the reduction of simple fractures, 1 that he repaired extensor tendons, and 1 that he removed tonsils and adenoids.

Thirty-two per cent of the Ontario, and 57 per cent of the Nova Scotia, general practitioners visited by us did abdominal surgery. The remainder did no abdominal surgery, except occasionally as assistants. The difference between the two provinces was statistically significant ($p < 0.05$).* Those in Ontario and in Nova Scotia who did do abdominal surgery were distributed, by age and by size of community, as shown in Tables 48 and 49 respectively. In Ontario, the age groups did not differ significantly in the percentages doing abdominal surgery. In Nova Scotia, on the other hand, a significantly smaller proportion of the younger, than of the older, practitioners were doing such

*This is explained on pages 32–33.

TABLE 48

ONTARIO AND NOVA SCOTIA PHYSICIANS OF VARIOUS AGES WHO
UNDERTOOK ABDOMINAL SURGERY

|  | Ontario physicians | | Nova Scotia physicians | |
|---|---|---|---|---|
| Age of physician | Number | % | Number | % |
| Up to 35 | 5 | 45.5 | 2 | 25.0 |
| 36–45 | 4 | 26.7 | 10* | 52.6 |
| 46 and over | 5 | 27.8 | 12 | 80.0 |
| Total | 14 | 31.8 | 24 | 57.1 |

*Two other physicians said that they would perform an appendectomy
in an emergency only.

TABLE 49

ONTARIO AND NOVA SCOTIA PHYSICIANS IN COMMUNITIES OF VARIOUS
POPULATIONS WHO UNDERTOOK ABDOMINAL SURGERY

|  | Ontario physicians | | Nova Scotia physicians | |
|---|---|---|---|---|
| Population of community | Number | % | Number | % |
| Over 500,000 | 0 | 0.0 | — | — |
| 100,001 to 500,000 | 1 | 25.0 | 0 | 0.0 |
| 10,001 to 100,000 | 7 | 46.7 | 7 | 87.5 |
| 1,001 to 10,000 | 5 | 35.7 | 14 | 82.4 |
| 1,000 and under | 1 | 25.0 | 3* | 37.5 |
| Total | 14 | 31.8 | 24 | 57.1 |

*Two other physicians said that they would perform an appendectomy
in an emergency only.

surgery ($p < 0.05$). Comparison of the age groups in one province
with the corresponding groups in the other showed a significant
difference only between the groups of practitioners over forty-five
years of age ($p < 0.01$).

Turning to communities of various sizes, we found that more than
80 per cent of the Nova Scotia practitioners in communities of between
1,000 and 100,000 said that they did abdominal surgery, in contrast
with none in Halifax, the one city of over 100,000 ($p < 0.001$), and
in contrast with 37.5 per cent in the communities of 1,000 or less
($p < 0.05$). In Ontario, the percentage of the practitioners in communities of between 1,000 and 100,000 who were doing abdominal
surgery was somewhat greater than the percentages in cities of over
100,000 or in communities of less than 1,000; but the differences were
not statistically significant. On the other hand, the percentage of practitioners doing abdominal surgery in communities of between 1,000
and 100,000 in Ontario was less than the percentage in Nova Scotia.

In the case of the communities of between 1,000 and 10,000, the difference is statistically significant ($p < 0.05$); in the case of communities of between 10,000 and 100,00, the difference does not reach the level of statistical significance, but is nonetheless suggestive. It appears, then, that, with respect to the percentage of general practitioners doing abdominal surgery, the communities of between 1,000 and 100,000 in Ontario occupy a position between communities of the same size in Nova Scotia, on the one hand, and, on the other hand, communities of under 1,000 and of over 100,000 in both provinces. It is likely that hospital restrictions, especially those in the teaching hospitals, are the reason why few general practitioners do major surgery in the large cities and that lack of hospital facilities and of professional assistance is the inhibiting factor in the smallest places. The interesting question is why there is a difference (providing that it is a real difference) between the middle-sized communities in Ontario and those in Nova Scotia. Though we cannot be certain, the answer may be that the general practitioners in Ontario tend to believe, to a greater extent than their colleagues in Nova Scotia, that major surgery should be done by those who are specially trained in surgery. This is suggested by the fact that, when the practitioners were asked what surgery the future general practitioner should be trained to do, the Ontario physicians were more conservative in their answers than were those in Nova Scotia (see page 511 and Table 104).

Some of those who undertook abdominal surgery did such operations as Caesarean section, hysterectomy, and cholecystectomy, whereas others limited themselves to such operations as appendectomy and hernial repair. Many of the men who did no abdominal surgery, except occasionally as assistants, did do excisions of tonsils and adenoids and uterine curettage. The occasional doctor was interested in orthopaedic surgery and performed such operations as open reductions of fractures and nailing of the neck of the femur. Though the doctors were not specifically asked whether they were doing as much surgery as formerly, almost 15 per cent of the Ontario men stated that they had reduced the amount of their surgical work or had given it up completely. One older practitioner who, because of the great distance of the nearest hospital, had operated in former years either in his own home or in his patients' homes had ceased to do surgery. Others had stopped operating now that there were qualified surgeons in their communities.

Anaesthesia was a particular interest of 14 per cent of the Ontario practitioners, who usually adminstered several general anaesthetics each week. These were men of all ages, who were not concentrated in communities of any particular sizes. In Nova Scotia, 33 per cent of the practitioners gave more than occasional general anaesthetics. As we shall see (Table 52), however, only 10 per cent professed a particular interest in anaesthesia. Both those who included this type of work in their practices and those who had a particular interest in it were of various ages and were located in communities of various sizes. Other men in each province gave only occasional general anaesthetics.

All but one of the doctors visited in each province did some obstetrics, though the volume varied greatly from one practice to another. Twenty-five of those in Ontario and all of those in Nova Scotia were asked how many deliveries they did per year, on the average. In Ontario, the replies ranged from 0 to 120; in Nova Scotia, from 0 to 225. The median was 69 in Ontario, and 67.5 in Nova Scotia (Table 50).

TABLE 50

DISTRIBUTION OF ONTARIO AND NOVA SCOTIA PHYSICIANS ACCORDING TO THE NUMBER OF OBSTETRICAL DELIVERIES PER YEAR

| Number of deliveries said to be done per year | Ontario physicians | | Nova Scotia physicians | |
|---|---|---|---|---|
| | Number | % | Number | % |
| 0–19 | 1 | 4.0 | 2 | 4.8 |
| 20–39 | 4 | 16.0 | 7 | 16.7 |
| 40–59 | 2 | 8.0 | 9 | 21.4 |
| 60–79 | 6 | 24.0 | 10 | 23.8 |
| 80–99 | 6 | 24.0 | 3 | 7.1 |
| 100–119 | 5 | 20.0 | 8 | 19.0 |
| 120–139 | 1 | 4.0 | 1 | 2.4 |
| ×××. | — | — | — | — |
| 200 and over | 0 | 0.0 | 2 | 4.8 |
| Total physicians | 25* | 100 | 42 | 100 |

*The other 19 Ontario physicians were not asked about the volume of their obstetrical work.

It was impossible to form a clear picture of the volume of psychiatric work done in general practice. Very few patients who were overtly either psychotic or severely psychoneurotic were seen during the Survey. The patients with less overt mental disturbances could not be identified by us with any degree of certainty. The reasons for this and the type of psychotherapy that was done will be discussed in later chapters (see pages 286 and 306). Only one doctor mentioned that he used insulin shock.

Four of the Ontario general practitioners had been granted specialist certificates by the Royal College of Physicians and Surgeons of Canada, one in medicine, one in obstetrics, one in general surgery, and one in anaesthesia. In Nova Scotia, 2 of the practitioners held specialist certificates of the Royal College in general surgery. Each of these 6 men demonstrated a special, but not exclusive, interest in his specialty.

In order to obtain some idea of the likes and dislikes of the men in practice, we made up a list of thirteen types of problem, some specific, some more general, which might be expected to occur relatively commonly in a general practice, and asked the practitioners whether they found some of these "definitely enjoyable to handle" and some "definitely distasteful." We emphasized to the doctors that we did not expect them to assign every one of the thirteen items to one or other category but wished them to indicate only those about which they felt strongly one way or the other. The thirteen items, in the order in which they were listed, were non-traumatic surgical cases, the general run of medical diseases, feeding problems in infancy, traumatic surgical cases, problems of old age, alcoholism, diabetes, behaviour problems in children, neurological diseases, obstetrical cases, emotional problems, hypertension, and marital problems. Each of three items was called definitely enjoyable by at least 50 per cent of the practitioners in each province: obstetrical cases, which apparently were the most favoured, non-traumatic surgical cases, and the general

TABLE 51

NUMBERS OF ONTARIO AND NOVA SCOTIA PHYSICIANS WHO FOUND VARIOUS TYPES OF CLINICAL PROBLEM DEFINITELY ENJOYABLE OR DEFINITELY DISTASTEFUL

| | Ontario | | Nova Scotia | |
|---|---|---|---|---|
| | Number of physicians answering: | | Number of physicians answering: | |
| Problem | Enjoyable | Distasteful | Enjoyable | Distasteful |
| Obstetrical cases | 36 | 1 | 35 | 1 |
| Non-traumatic surgical cases | 31 | 1 | 34 | 1 |
| General run of medical diseases | 22 | 1 | 37 | 0 |
| Traumatic surgical cases | 16 | 9 | 26 | 2 |
| Hypertension | 14 | 5 | 23 | 3 |
| Diabetes | 15 | 6 | 18 | 12 |
| Neurological diseases | 15 | 6 | 14 | 8 |
| Emotional problems | 12 | 13 | 12 | 15 |
| Feeding problems in infancy | 7 | 8 | 13 | 11 |
| Problems of old age | 8 | 8 | 8 | 9 |
| Marital problems | 6 | 17 | 10 | 14 |
| Behaviour problems in children | 4 | 15 | 8 | 19 |
| Alcoholism | 2 | 31 | 3 | 35 |
| Total number of physicians visited | 44 | | 42 | |

run of medical diseases (Table 51). Traumatic surgical cases and cases of hypertension were called definitely enjoyable by more than 50 per cent of the Nova Scotia doctors. Though the last two were definitely enjoyable to less than 50 per cent in Ontario, they were more often called enjoyable than distasteful, as were also diabetes and neurological diseases in both provinces. Feeding problems in infancy and problems of old age were liked and disliked by about the same numbers of doctors. In each province, emotional problems, marital problems, behaviour problems in children, and alcoholism were all called distasteful more often than they were called enjoyable. All of these last four items were distasteful to more than 25 per cent of the 86 doctors; and 77 per cent disliked dealing with cases of alcoholism.

Two doctors explained that they enjoyed dealing with problems of old age because they liked old people. Two referred to neurological diseases as a diagnostic challenge, which they enjoyed. One doctor, who liked handling patients with emotional problems, said, "It's up to me to get them to a psychiatrist." In cases of diabetes, one doctor enjoyed making the diagnosis, another enjoyed the therapeutic aspects, but a third felt frustrated because of the difficulty he had in working out a satisfactory regimen for the patient. One doctor said, regarding his dislike of emotional problems, that he used to spend hours listening to these patients but never "got anywhere with them," that he had "had enough of it" and now suggested that they find another doctor. Another man said that modern medicine had become a business, that, though the patient should be treated as an individual, the doctor could not be the emotional supporter of the patient as the old-fashioned doctor was said to have been. In his words, "That's outdated."

The reasons for the likes and dislikes of other problems are not known to us. It is to be noted that there were no significant differences between the two provinces in the percentages of doctors who disliked the various items. A significantly higher percentage, however, of Nova Scotia, than of Ontario physicians, answered that the general run of medical diseases and traumatic surgical cases were definitely enjoyable to handle. The reason for these two differences is unknown. The likes and dislikes of practitioners, or of medical students, might be a fruitful area for further study.

Each of the physicians was asked also, "Is there any field of medicine in which you are *particularly* interested?" Twenty per cent in Ontario and 14 per cent in Nova Scotia replied in the negative; each of the remaining practitioners named one, two, or three fields that particularly interested him. As in answer to the previous question, obstetrics was named most frequently, by 32 per cent of the Ontario doctors and by 36 per cent of those in Nova Scotia (Table 52). In view of the previously voiced likes and dislikes, it is not surprising that emotional problems were a particular interest of only 7 per cent of the men in each province. That only 2 per cent in Ontario and only 14 per cent in Nova Scotia expressed a particular interest in paediatrics, however, *is* surprising, when one considers how many of a general practitioner's

TABLE 52

NUMBERS OF ONTARIO AND NOVA SCOTIA PHYSICIANS PROFESSING
PARTICULAR INTEREST IN VARIOUS FIELDS OF MEDICINE

|  | Ontario physicians | | Nova Scotia physicians | |
|---|---|---|---|---|
| Particular interest | Number* | % | Number* | % |
| Obstetrics | 14 | 31.8 | 15 | 35.7 |
| Surgery | 10 | 22.7 | 12 | 28.6 |
| Medicine | 6 | 13.6 | 5 | 11.9 |
| Anaesthesia | 6 | 13.6 | 4 | 9.5 |
| Paediatrics | 1 | 2.3 | 6 | 14.3 |
| Emotional problems | 3 | 6.8 | 3 | 7.1 |
| Cardiovascular diseases | 1 | 2.3 | 3 | 7.1 |
| Diagnosis | 3 | 6.8 | 1 | 2.4 |
| Gynaecology | 3 | 6.8 | 1 | 2.4 |
| Dermatology | 2 | 4.5 | 0 | 0.0 |
| Preventive medicine | 1 | 2.3 | 0 | 0.0 |
| Others† | — | — | — | — |
| None | 9 | 20.5 | 6 | 14.3 |
| Total number of physicians visited | 44 | | 42 | |

*Some men named more than one particular interest and therefore are included in more than one of the first eleven categories.

†Other particular interests, each of which was named by a single doctor, were alcoholism, allergy, anticoagulants, diabetes, endocrinology, geriatrics, haematology, industrial medicine, military medicine, nutrition, pathology, and problems of middle age.

patients are children (see Table 58, on page 242). Preventive medicine was named only once. The slight show of interest in paediatrics and in preventive medicine may be related, since so much of paediatrics today is preventive in nature. The possible importance of these findings lies in the fact that paediatrics is often described, by general practitioners and by some at least of the paediatricians, as "general practice among children," and one hears the demand made by some general practitioners (see page 160) and the suggestion put forward by some eminent paediatricians that the paediatricians confine their work to consultations on referred cases. During the past several decades, an increasing amount of paediatric care has been given by physicians specially trained for the purpose. Before steps are taken to reverse this trend, it might be advisable that further study be given to the comparative interests and abilities of general practitioners and paediatricians in the care of children.

The other particular interests named by the practitioners are shown in Table 52.

The laboratory work done in the practitioners' offices was, as we stated earlier (page 61), of the simplest kind, seldom extending beyond haemoglobin determinations and urinalyses. Regarding diagnostic radiology, each physician was asked what procedures he carried out himself. Seventy-seven per cent of the Ontario men and 98 per cent in Nova Scotia replied that they neither took films nor did fluoroscopy themselves. The procedure performed by the largest number of general practitioners, by 20 per cent of those in Ontario, was fluoroscopy. One physician, who had had a considerable amount of training in radiology, even did barium swallows in cases of mitral stenosis. Films of the chest and of long bones were taken by between 10 and 20 per cent of the Ontario doctors and by the one Nova Scotia doctor who used X-ray equipment himself. Less than 10 per cent in Ontario took films of such other areas as the nasal sinuses, the urinary tract, the alimentary tract, and the gall bladder. The communities of different sizes in Ontario did not differ significantly in the percentages of general practitioners who carried out radiological procedures.

The practitioners were asked, also, how much of the *interpretation* of the films they had done by a radiologist, whether they made use of a radiologist for this purpose "never," "occasionally," "quite often," or whether "most of the films" were read by a radiologist. In Ontario, 9 per cent replied "occasionally." The other 91 per cent said that "most of the films" were read by a radiologist; and 68 per cent of all the Ontario doctors made their answer even more specific by volunteering that *all* of their films were seen by a radiologist. The majority of those who only occasionally had films interpreted by a radiologist were located at great distances from radiologists. In Nova Scotia, 69 per cent of the practitioners said that all of their films, and the remainder that "most of the films," were read by a radiologist. In at least one case, however, the "radiologist," though doing the radiology for his hospital, was not certificated and did general practice in addition to radiology.

In addition to private practice, 25 of the 44 Ontario physicians and 26 of the 42 Nova Scotia physicians undertook various types of part-time salaried work. In Ontario, 7 were medical officers of health for their own, or for neighbouring, municipalities, 6 did salaried industrial work, and 3 did both of these types of work. In Nova Scotia, 6 were paid medical officers of health (2 other Nova Scotia physicians were medical officers of health but received no remuneration), 3 did industrial work, and 1 served in both capacities. Some doctors held such other appointments as those of coroner, physician to the local home for the aged, reserve army medical officer, school physician, physician to the local Children's Aid Society, and life insurance medical officer. The amount of time given to salaried work varied, in each province, from a "negligible"* amount to between 18 and 20 hours per week. The average, for the men who did any salaried work, was between 6 and 7 hours per week in Ontario and about 3 hours per week in Nova Scotia.

This, in broad outline, was the work done by the general practitioners. We come now to a more detailed examination of the patients and their reasons for seeking the physicians' services. In an earlier chapter (see page 15), we described the lists that the practitioners were asked to keep of the patients seen by them during a period of seven days. In addition to asking the patient's age and sex, we sought four other items of information: whether the illness was a new illness or an old one, where the patient was seen (whether in home, office, hospital, or elsewhere), the diagnosis, and the method of payment (see page 195). A "new illness" was defined as one for which this doctor had never seen the patient before, even though the doctor might have seen this patient many times for other reasons. In other words, "new illness" is not synonymous with "new patient." The corollary of this was that any visit subsequent to the initial visit for a particular illness was to be listed as having been made for an "old illness." If, for example, a patient whom a doctor treated six months ago for a fracture becomes acutely ill today with pneumonia and is seen by the doctor, the pneumonia is listed as a new illness; but, when the doctor visits the patient again tomorrow, his illness will then be classed as an old illness.

If the doctor did not arrive at a diagnosis, he was asked to give the

*This reply was given by an Ontario physician who received $250 a year to act as medical officer of health. Because of the meagreness of the salary, he regarded the position as little more than a nominal one and made plain that he accepted the appointment because the municipality was required by law to have a medical officer of health and was unable to obtain the services of any other physician. In Nova Scotia, one medical officer of health said that he gave about 5 minutes a week to this work.

most probable diagnosis, or, failing that, the nature of the illness, for example, "abdominal pain, not yet diagnosed." If the reason for the visit was an operation, an obstetrical delivery, or the giving of an anaesthetic, this was to be entered on the form. Again, if the patient came in for such a purpose as to have a pre-camp or pre-employment examination or to have the doctor fill out an insurance form, rather than because of an illness, the doctor was to indicate this.

Forty-three of the 44 physicians visited in Ontario and all of the 42 in Nova Scotia returned records of various degrees of completeness. Office, home, and other non-hospital visits were reported for all seven days of the week by 35 of the Ontario, and by 27 of the Nova Scotia, practitioners. The remaining lists were less complete, usually omitting one or more of the days of the week. Hospital visits, however, were recorded for all seven days of the week by only 27 of the men in each province.

In all the records, three types of error are probably present to some extent. In the first place, some patients may have been omitted. This is most likely to have occurred in the case of hospital visits, because these were often recorded after a series of patients had been seen. Indeed, the reason why fewer records were submitted of hospital visits than of non-hospital visits was that some men, including some with very busy practices, found it impossible to keep track of their hospital visits for us. Some home visits, also, may occasionally have been omitted, though these, involving more time and effort than hospital visits, are less likely to have been forgotten. Omission of office visits from the lists probably occurred least frequently, since the data on these patients were usually recorded at the completion of each visit. Secondly, errors in diagnosis are bound to occur, and the proportion of such errors probably varies considerably from physician to physician. The extent of either of these two types of error cannot be estimated. Thirdly, so few of the doctors kept a record of those persons who came in, not for professional advice, but for renewal of a prescription or for the filling out of an insurance form, that, in analysing the records, we have been obliged to exclude the few such entries that were made. Though a few doctors said that the records should include the telephone calls too, because, as they pointed out, these took up a great deal of time, we did not consider it feasible to ask the doctors to keep a list of their telephone calls.

One cannot but wonder whether or not the practices of the physicians who reported for the seven days of the week are similar to the practices of the men whose records covered only part of the week.

Any comparison of the two groups must be very rough, since the number of patients reported by one doctor for one day of the week cannot be taken as comparable with the number reported by another doctor for a different day of the week. Yet, when those who reported for all seven days of the week were compared with those who reported for less than a week, we found that, in Ontario, the mean number of visits (hospital and non-hospital combined) per day was 19.1 for the former group and 18.9 for the latter group; nor was there any appreciable disparity between the groups with respect to the means for office visits, home visits, or hospital visits. Thus we have no reason to believe that either the 35 Ontario physicians who sent us records of their non-hospital visits, or the 27 who sent us records of their hospital visits, for a full week are different from the remainder of the Ontario sample. In Nova Scotia, on the other hand, the mean numbers of the visits (hospital and non-hospital) of the 27 physicians who sent us records for the full week and of the 15 who sent us records for less than the full week were 17.8 and 28.4 per day respectively; and, between the two groups, a disparity of approximately the same magnitude was found with respect to office visits, home visits, and hospital visits. Though, as we have said, the comparison is a rough one, there appears to be a strong possibility that the Nova Scotia doctors who sent in records for the full week were less busy than the rest of the doctors whom we visited.

Since, in what follows, we shall speak repeatedly of the numbers of visits made by the practitioners, it is desirable that we define the word, "visit." The word is used by us to refer to any occasion upon which professional service was rendered to a patient by a physician in his office, in hospital, in the patient's home, or elsewhere. Thus the word, "visit," is used regardless of whether the patient came to the physician or the physician went to the patient. A physician who went to a home and rendered professional service to two, or more, of the occupants is regarded as having made two, or more, visits. Similarly, in reporting the various diseases dealt with by the physicians, we shall state the numbers of visits (as defined above) that were made because of a particular disease rather than the number of separate patients who were treated for that disease. For example, if one patient with pneumonia was seen three times by the doctor, this work would appear in our tables, not as one case of pneumonia, but as three visits for pneumonia. We have chosen to report the number of visits rather than the number of patients, because the former is probably a better indicator of the doctor's work load; and it is with the doctor's work, rather than with the prevalence of one or another disease in the population, that we are concerned.

The numbers of non-hospital visits listed by the 35 Ontario, and by the 27 Nova Scotia, practitioners whose records covered the seven days of the week ranged, in Ontario, from 44 to 397 and, in Nova Scotia, from 36 to 150, for the seven-day period (Table 53). The median

TABLE 53

NUMBERS OF OFFICE, HOME, AND OTHER NON-HOSPITAL VISITS OF ONTARIO AND NOVA SCOTIA PHYSICIANS DURING A COMPLETE WEEK

| Number of of visits | Ontario physicians | | Nova Scotia physicians | |
|---|---|---|---|---|
| | Number | Percentage of those reporting | Number | Percentage of those reporting |
| Less than 50 | 2 | 5.7 | 4 | 14.8 |
| 50–69 | 10 | 28.6 | 4 | 14.8 |
| 70–89 | 8 | 22.9 | 8 | 29.6 |
| 90–109 | 6 | 17.1 | 4 | 14.8 |
| 110–129 | 3 | 8.6 | 5 | 18.5 |
| 130–149 | 2 | 5.7 | 1 | 3.7 |
| 150–199 | 1 | 2.9 | 1 | 3.7 |
| 200–249 | 1 | 2.9 | 0 | 0.0 |
| 250–299 | 1 | 2.9 | 0 | 0.0 |
| 300–349 | 0 | 0.0 | 0 | 0.0 |
| 350–399 | 1 | 2.9 | 0 | 0.0 |
| Not known | 9 | — | 15 | — |

number of visits in each province was 86, but, as stated above, there is some reason to believe that the Nova Scotia figure may be on the low side. It will be seen that office visits greatly outnumbered home and other non-hospital visits in each province (Tables 54 and 55), the median numbers of office visits for the seven days being 74 and 65 in

TABLE 54

NUMBERS OF OFFICE VISITS OF ONTARIO AND NOVA SCOTIA PHYSICIANS DURING A COMPLETE WEEK

| Number of visits | Ontario physicians | | Nova Scotia physicians | |
|---|---|---|---|---|
| | Number | Percentage of those reporting | Number | Percentage of those reporting |
| Less than 40 | 3 | 8.6 | 5 | 18.5 |
| 40–59 | 10 | 28.6 | 8 | 29.6 |
| 60–79 | 8 | 22.9 | 7 | 25.9 |
| 80–99 | 7 | 20.0 | 6 | 22.2 |
| 100–149 | 5 | 14.3 | 1 | 3.7 |
| 150–199 | 0 | 0.0 | 0 | 0.0 |
| 200–299 | 1 | 2.9 | 0 | 0.0 |
| 300–309 | 1 | 2.9 | 0 | 0.0 |
| Not known | 9 | — | 15 | — |

TABLE 55

NUMBERS OF HOME VISITS* OF ONTARIO AND NOVA SCOTIA PHYSICIANS
DURING A COMPLETE WEEK

| Number of visits | Ontario physicians | | Nova Scotia physicians | |
|---|---|---|---|---|
| | Number | Percentage of those reporting | Number | Percentage of those reporting |
| 0–4 | 6 | 17.1 | 1 | 3.7 |
| 5–9 | 4 | 11.4 | 1 | 3.7 |
| 10–14 | 11 | 31.4 | 3 | 11.1 |
| 15–19 | 5 | 14.3 | 5 | 18.5 |
| 20–29 | 5 | 14.3 | 7 | 25.9 |
| 30–39 | 1 | 2.9 | 8 | 29.6 |
| 40–49 | 2 | 5.7 | 0 | 0.0 |
| 50–59 | 0 | 0.0 | 2 | 7.4 |
| 60–69 | 1 | 2.9 | 0 | 0.0 |
| Not known | 9 | — | 15 | — |

*Included with the home visits are non-hospital visits (10 in Ontario and 28 in Nova Scotia) made in places other than the physician's office or the patient's home.

Ontario and Nova Scotia, respectively, and the median numbers of home plus other non-hospital visits being 12 and 25 in the two provinces, respectively. In Table 56 are shown the median numbers of office visits and of home visits reported by the physicians in the various age groups in each province. It is noteworthy that the median number

TABLE 56

MEDIAN NUMBER OF NON-HOSPITAL VISITS PER WEEK OF
PHYSICIANS OF VARIOUS AGES

| Age of physician | Physicians reporting | | Median number of visits | | |
|---|---|---|---|---|---|
| | Number | % of total | Office visits | Home* visits | All non-hospital visits |
| A. *Ontario* | | | | | |
| 31–35 | 10 | 90.9 | 77.0 | 15.5 | 90.5 |
| 36–45 | 12 | 80.0 | 90.0 | 15.0 | 100.0 |
| 46–61 | 13 | 72.2 | 59.0 | 10.0 | 66.0 |
| Total | 35 | 79.5 | 74.0 | 12.0 | 86.0 |
| B. *Nova Scotia* | | | | | |
| 28–35 | 6 | 75.0 | 68.0 | 32.5 | 97.5 |
| 36–45 | 12 | 63.2 | 61.5 | 21.0 | 84.0 |
| 46–60 | 9 | 60.0 | 55.0 | 21.0 | 74.0 |
| Total | 27 | 64.3 | 65.0 | 25.0 | 86.0 |

*Included with the home visits are non-hospital visits (10 in Ontario and 28 in Nova Scotia) made in places other than the physician's office or the patient's home.

of home visits reported by each age group was higher in Nova Scotia than in Ontario.

The numbers of *hospital* visits, which, as we have said, were reported for all seven days of the week by only 27 of the practitioners in each province, varied, in Ontario, between 2 and 75 per week, with a median of 29 visits, and varied, in Nova Scotia, between 0 and 111 per week, with a median of 35 visits (Table 57).

TABLE 57

NUMBERS OF HOSPITAL VISITS OF ONTARIO AND NOVA SCOTIA
PHYSICIANS DURING A COMPLETE WEEK

| Number of visits | Ontario physicians | | Nova Scotia physicians | |
|---|---|---|---|---|
| | Number | Percentage of those reporting | Number | Percentage of those reporting |
| 0–9 | 5 | 18.5 | 5 | 18.5 |
| 10–19 | 6 | 22.2 | 4 | 14.8 |
| 20–29 | 4 | 14.8 | 2 | 7.4 |
| 30–39 | 4 | 14.8 | 4 | 14.8 |
| 40–49 | 2 | 7.4 | 5 | 18.5 |
| 50–59 | 3 | 11.1 | 2 | 7.4 |
| 60–69 | 1 | 3.7 | 0 | 0.0 |
| 70–79 | 2 | 7.4 | 2 | 7.4 |
| 80–89 | 0 | 0.0 | 2 | 7.4 |
| 90–99 | 0 | 0.0 | 0 | 0.0 |
| 100–109 | 0 | 0.0 | 0 | 0.0 |
| 110–119 | 0 | 0.0 | 1 | 3.7 |
| Not known | 17 | — | 15 | — |

From the numbers of visits made by the physicians, we pass on to a consideration of the patients' ages and sexes and whether they were seen for new illnesses or for old illnesses. In Ontario, 43 physicians submitted records of the non-hospital visits made by them on a total of 290 days; and 41 submitted records of hospital visits made on a total of 275 days.* In Nova Scotia, all of the 42 physicians submitted records of both the non-hospital visits and the hospital visits made by them on a total of 253 days.

The records of office visits, of home visits,† and of hospital visits

*In considering, previously, the numbers of visits made during seven days, we made use of the records of those physicians only whose records covered all seven days of the week. Now, however, in classifying the patients according to age, sex, and reason for seeking the doctor's services, we are able to use also the data supplied by those men whose records covered fewer than seven days, since there is no reason to suppose that patients of a certain sex, or of a certain age, or with a certain condition, would be more numerous on one day than on another.

†Wherever the term "home visit" is used, it is to be understood to include all non-hospital visits that were not office visits. Twelve of these in Ontario (1.8 per cent) and 52 in Nova Scotia (4.7 per cent) were made elsewhere than in the homes,

showed a preponderance of female patients in each province (Table 58). Comparison of the patients and the population at large, in the matter of age distribution, shows that there were relatively few home visits for the groups in Ontario between 5 and 54 years of age and for the groups in Nova Scotia between 5 and 44 years of age. In each province, the lowest demand relatively was between 15 and 24 years of age, and visits to patients 65 years of age or over were relatively numerous (Table 58). A rough idea of the disparity may be conveyed if we say that, for every home visit required by the individual between 15 and 24 years of age, the average number of home visits required by

TABLE 58

NUMBERS OF OFFICE VISITS, OF HOME VISITS, AND OF HOSPITAL
VISITS REPORTED BY THE PHYSICIANS

(Grouped according to patient's sex, according to patient's age,
and according to whether the visit was for a new illness or an old illness)

A. *Ontario*

| | Office visits (43 physicians) (290 days) | | Home visits† (43 physicians) (290 days) | | Hospital visits (41 physicians) (275 days) | | Canada Census Ontario 1956 | |
|---|---|---|---|---|---|---|---|---|
| | Number | %* | Number | %* | Number | %* | Number | % |
| *Sex* | | | | | | | | |
| Male | 1597 | 43.8 | 292 | 44.2 | 524 | 47.1 | 2,721,519 | 50.4 |
| Female | 2047 | 56.2 | 369 | 55.8 | 588 | 52.9 | 2,683,414 | 49.6 |
| Not recorded | 4 | — | — | — | 12 | — | — | — |
| Total | 3648 | | 661 | | 1124 | | 5,404,933 | |
| *Age* | | | | | | | | |
| Under 1 yr. | 150 | 4.4 | 11 | 1.7 | 49 | 4.5 | } 628,825 | 11.6 |
| 1–4 | 261 | 7.6 | 64 | 10.1 | 83 | 7.6 | | |
| 5–14 | 276 | 8.1 | 82 | 13.0 | 84 | 7.7 | 989,600 | 18.3 |
| 15–24 | 515 | 15.1 | 36 | 5.7 | 94 | 8.6 | 712,010 | 13.2 |
| 25–34 | 719 | 21.1 | 54 | 8.5 | 176 | 16.1 | 856,108 | 15.8 |
| 35–44 | 491 | 14.4 | 54 | 8.5 | 148 | 13.6 | 751,882 | 13.9 |
| 45–54 | 374 | 11.0 | 51 | 8.1 | 99 | 9.1 | 581,506 | 10.8 |
| 55–64 | 277 | 8.1 | 70 | 11.1 | 97 | 8.9 | 430,627 | 8.0 |
| 65–74 | 238 | 7.0 | 87 | 13.8 | 138 | 12.7 | } 454,375 | 8.4 |
| 75 and over | 105 | 3.1 | 123 | 19.5 | 122 | 11.2 | | |
| Not recorded | 242 | — | 29 | — | 34 | — | — | — |
| Total | 3648 | | 661 | | 1124 | | 5,404,933 | |
| *Illness* | | | | | | | | |
| New illness | 1612 | 44.3 | 322 | 48.7 | 243 | 21.7 | | |
| Old illness | 2023 | 55.7 | 339 | 51.3 | 877 | 78.3 | | |
| Not recorded | 13 | — | — | — | 4 | — | | |
| Total | 3648 | | 661 | | 1124 | | | |

*The percentages shown are percentages of those visits for which the particular item of information was reported.
†Included are 12 visits made in places other than home, office, or hospital.

TABLE 58 (*Continued*)

B. *Nova Scotia*

| | Office visits (42 physicians) (253 days) | | Home visits† (42 physicians) (253 days) | | Hospital visits (42 physicians) (253 days) | | Canada Census Nova Scotia 1956 | |
|---|---|---|---|---|---|---|---|---|
| | Number | %* | Number | %* | Number | %* | Number | % |
| *Sex* | | | | | | | | |
| Male | 1035 | 41.8 | 458 | 41.6 | 633 | 39.8 | 353,182 | 50.8 |
| Female | 1441 | 58.2 | 644 | 58.4 | 957 | 60.2 | 341,535 | 49.2 |
| Not recorded | 5 | — | — | — | 1 | — | — | — |
| Total | 2481 | | 1102 | | 1591 | | 694,717 | |
| *Age* | | | | | | | | |
| Under 1 yr. | 106 | 4.3 | 59 | 5.4 | 102 | 6.4 | 85,972 | 12.4 |
| 1–4 | 146 | 5.9 | 113 | 10.3 | 66 | 4.2 | | |
| 5–14 | 312 | 12.6 | 165 | 15.1 | 136 | 8.6 | 149,599 | 21.5 |
| 15–24 | 404 | 16.4 | 87 | 7.9 | 176 | 11.1 | 105,395 | 15.2 |
| 25–34 | 423 | 17.1 | 97 | 8.9 | 194 | 12.2 | 90,428 | 13.0 |
| 35–44 | 374 | 15.1 | 110 | 10.0 | 156 | 9.8 | 89,889 | 12.9 |
| 45–54 | 295 | 11.9 | 118 | 10.8 | 211 | 13.3 | 65,755 | 9.5 |
| 55–64 | 208 | 8.4 | 102 | 9.3 | 150 | 9.5 | 48,772 | 7.0 |
| 65–74 | 146 | 5.9 | 123 | 11.2 | 211 | 13.3 | 58,907 | 8.5 |
| 75 and over | 55 | 2.2 | 122 | 11.1 | 183 | 11.5 | | |
| Not recorded | 12 | — | 6 | — | 6 | — | — | — |
| Total | 2481 | | 1102 | | 1591 | | 694,717 | |
| *Illness* | | | | | | | | |
| New illness | 1418 | 57.4 | 615 | 56.4 | 217 | 13.7 | | |
| Old illness | 1052 | 42.6 | 475 | 43.6 | 1372 | 86.3 | | |
| Not recorded | 11 | — | 12 | — | 2 | — | | |
| Total | 2481 | | 1102 | | 1591 | | | |

*The percentages shown are percentages of those visits for which the particular item of information was reported.

†Included are 52 visits made in places other than home, office, or hospital.

the individual of 65 or over was approximately nine in Ontario and approximately five in Nova Scotia. Office visits were least in demand by the group between 5 and 14 years of age, inasmuch as, for each visit required by the individual in this age group, the child below 5 years of age and the individual of 15 or over, in Ontario, required two to three visits, and, in Nova Scotia, one and a half to two visits. The patients over 65 years of age did not account for a disproportionate number of office visits, except in Ontario in relation to one age group, namely the group between 5 and 14 years of age. Hospital visits, however, were in greatest demand by the individual of 65 or over, his requirement, in each province, being more than twice as great as that of the individual in *any* other age group and being more than six times as great as that of the child between 5 and 14 years of age.

These differences between the age groups are understandable in terms of the tendency of older persons to have more illness than younger persons. A more interesting finding is the difference between the two provinces in the division of visits between office, home, and hospital. The difference is most marked in the case of the home visits. In Ontario, 661 home visits were reported during a total of 290 days (i.e., 2.3 visits per day on the average), whereas, in Nova Scotia, 1,102 home visits were reported during a total of 253 days (i.e., 4.4 visits per day on the average) (Table 58). Hospital visits, also, were more numerous in Nova Scotia (1,591 in 253 days; i.e., 6.3 visits per day) than in Ontario (1,124 in 275 days; i.e., 4.1 visits per day). The number of office visits, on the other hand, was greater in Ontario

TABLE 59

RELATIVE FREQUENCIES (PERCENTAGES) OF OFFICE VISITS,
HOME VISITS, AND HOSPITAL VISITS FOR PATIENTS IN VARIOUS AGE GROUPS

| | Age of patient (years) | | | | | | | | | | |
|---|---|---|---|---|---|---|---|---|---|---|---|
| | Under 1 | 1–4 | 5–14 | 15–24 | 25–34 | 35–44 | 45–54 | 55–64 | 65–74 | 75 and over | All ages |
| Place of visit | Percentages of visits | | | | | | | | | | |
| *A. Ontario* | | | | | | | | | | | |
| Office | 71.4 | 63.9 | 62.4 | 79.8 | 75.7 | 70.9 | 71.4 | 62.4 | 51.4 | 30.0 | 67.1 |
| Home | 5.2 | 15.7 | 18.5 | 5.6 | 5.7 | 7.8 | 9.7 | 15.8 | 18.8 | 35.1 | 12.1 |
| Hospital | 23.3 | 20.3 | 19.0 | 14.6 | 18.5 | 21.4 | 18.9 | 21.8 | 29.8 | 34.9 | 20.7 |
| Total | 100 | 100 | 100 | 100 | 100 | 100 | 100 | 100 | 100 | 100 | 100 |
| *B. Nova Scotia* | | | | | | | | | | | |
| Office | 39.7 | 44.9 | 50.9 | 60.6 | 59.2 | 58.4 | 47.3 | 45.2 | 30.4 | 15.3 | 48.0 |
| Home | 22.1 | 34.8 | 26.9 | 13.0 | 13.6 | 17.2 | 18.9 | 22.2 | 25.6 | 33.9 | 21.3 |
| Hospital | 38.2 | 20.3 | 22.2 | 26.4 | 27.2 | 24.4 | 33.8 | 32.6 | 44.0 | 50.8 | 30.7 |
| Total | 100 | 100 | 100 | 100 | 100 | 100 | 100 | 100 | 100 | 100 | 100 |

(3,648 during 290 days or 12.6 visits per day) than in Nova Scotia (2,481 in 253 days or 9.8 visits per day). If these figures are turned into percentages (Table 59), we find that office visits made up 67 per cent of the visits reported from Ontario, but only 48 per cent of those reported from Nova Scotia; that house calls made up 12 per cent of the visits in Ontario, but 21 per cent of those in Nova Scotia; and that hospital visits made up 21 per cent and 31 per cent of the visits in Ontario and in Nova Scotia, respectively.

The relative frequencies of office visits, home visits, and hospital visits were worked out, also, for each of ten age groups in each province (Table 59). In Ontario, in each of the age groups up to the age of 64, between 60 and 80 per cent of the visits were office visits, whereas, for the group between 65 and 74 years of age, only 51 per cent were office visits, and, for the group 75 years of age or over, only 30 per cent were office visits. The Nova Scotia figures are roughly parallel to those in Ontario but are lower throughout. Thus, in each of the groups up to the age of 64, between approximately 40 per cent and 60 per cent of the visits were office visits, whereas, between 65 and 74 years of age, only 30 per cent were office visits, and, for those 74 years of age or older, only 15 per cent were office visits. In Ontario, the percentage representing home visits was 5 per cent for patients under 1 year of age, increased to between 15 and 20 per cent for the patients between 1 and 14 years of age, fell back to between 5 and 6 per cent for the next two decades, and then rose steadily until, at 75 years of age and over, home visits constituted 35 per cent of the visits. In Nova Scotia, the figures for home visits show a similar pattern but at a higher level. Starting at 22 per cent in the first year, they increase to 35 per cent between 1 and 4 years of age, decrease to 13 per cent between 15 and 24 years of age, and then rise to 34 per cent, almost the same percentage as in Ontario, for the oldest group. For hospital visits, the parallelism between the provinces is not as close, though, in each province, the figure is higher at the two extremes than for the intervening ages.

Whereas new illnesses and old illnesses accounted for approximately equal numbers of *home* visits and of *office* visits (Table 58), only 22 per cent of the *hospital* visits in Ontario and 13 per cent of the hospital visits in Nova Scotia were for new illnesses, the remainder being visits subsequent to the first visit for the particular illness. Though there was apparently confusion in the minds of some physicians over the terms, "new illness" and "old illness," the figures presented above are probably reasonably accurate.

The diagnoses or reasons for visits, as recorded in Ontario by the 43 physicians who returned records of non-hospital visits and the 41 who returned records of hospital visits and as recorded in Nova Scotia by the 42 who returned records of both non-hospital and hospital visits, have been coded according to the detailed list of three-digit categories of the World Health Organization's International Classification of Diseases (Seventh Revision, 1955). The reasons for the non-hospital visits fall into 378 categories in Ontario and 370 in Nova

Scotia, and those for the hospital visits into 176 categories in Ontario and 226 in Nova Scotia. These are listed in Appendix A. The most frequent reasons, however, for non-hospital and hospital visits, in Ontario and in Nova Scotia, are shown in Tables 60, 61, 62, and 63.

TABLE 60

NON-HOSPITAL VISITS OF ONTARIO PHYSICIANS*

(Incidences ofthose categories that occurred at a rate
of one or more visits in every two hundred)†

| Three-digit numbers | Category | Ontario | | Nova Scotia rate per 100 visits |
|---|---|---|---|---|
| | | No. of visits | Rate per 100 visits | |
| Y06 | Prenatal care (without abnormal symptoms) | 311 | 7.2 | 6.3 |
| 470–475‡ | Acute upper respiratory infections | 279 | 6.5 | 5.9 |
| 780–795 | Symptoms, senility, and ill-defined conditions | 234 | 5.4 | 5.5 |
| Y02 | Persons receiving prophylactic inoculation and vaccination§ | 230 | 5.3 | 5.6 |
| 690–698 | Infections of skin and subcutaneous tissue | 142 | 3.3 | 3.2 |
| 310–318 | Psychoneurotic disorders | 138 | 3.2 | 2.5 |
| 444 | Essential benign hypertension | 130 | 3.0 | 3.8 |
| 480–483 | Influenza | 119 | 2.8 | 5.6 |
| Y00.0⎫ Y00.3⎭ | General medical or laboratory examination (without complaint or finding indicating need of observation or medical care) | 102 | 2.4 | 2.1 |
| 420 | Arteriosclerotic heart disease, including coronary disease | 98 | 2.3 | 1.8 |
| N870–N908 | Laceration and open wound‖ | 89 | 2.1 | 1.9 |
| 501 | Bronchitis unqualified | 65 | 1.5 | 1.7 |
| 241 | Asthma | 63 | 1.5 | 0.8 |
| N840–N848 | Sprains and strains of joints and adjacent muscles | 63 | 1.5 | 1.3 |
| 293 | Anaemia of unspecified type | 58 | 1.3 | 1.2 |
| Y00.5 | Well baby and child care§ | 58 | 1.3 | 1.0 |
| 260 | Diabetes mellitus | 57 | 1.3 | 0.9 |
| 391–393 | Otitis media and mastoiditis | 57 | 1.3 | 1.8 |
| N800–N829 | Fractures | 54 | 1.3 | 1.4 |
| N910–N929 | Superficial injury and contusion | 52 | 1.2 | 1.3 |
| 490–493 | Pneumonia | 50 | 1.2 | 2.5 |
| 287 | Obesity, not specified as of endocrine origin | 48 | 1.1 | 0.5 |
| 571 | Gastro-enteritis and colitis, except ulcerative, age 4 weeks and over | 48 | 1.1 | 1.2 |
| 540–541 | Ulcer of stomach and duodenum | 46 | 1.1 | 0.4 |
| Y07 | Postpartum observation (without abnormal symptoms) | 43 | 1.0 | 0.6 |
| 635 | Menopausal symptoms | 42 | 1.0 | 0.4 |
| 290 | Pernicious and other hyperchromic anaemias | 40 | 0.9 | 0.5 |
| 500 | Acute bronchitis | 40 | 0.9 | 1.0 |
| 240 | Hay fever | 39 | 0.9 | 0.03 |
| 726 | Muscular rheumatism | 39 | 0.9 | 1.1 |
| 630 | Infective disease of uterus, vagina, and vulva | 33 | 0.8 | 0.7 |
| 634 | Disorders of menstruation | 29 | 0.7 | 0.5 |
| 741–742 | Synovitis, bursitis, and tenosynovitis | 29 | 0.7 | 0.8 |
| 605 | Cystitis | 25 | 0.6 | 1.2 |
| 085 | Measles | 23 | 0.5 | 0.2 |
| 330–334 | Vascular lesions affecting central nervous system | 23 | 0.5 | 0.6 |
| 530–535 | Diseases of teeth and supporting structures | 22 | 0.5 | 1.3 |
| 560–561 | Hernia of abdominal cavity | 22 | 0.5 | 0.3 |
| N940–N949 | Burns | 22 | 0.5 | 0.2 |
| 725 | Arthritis, unspecified | 21 | 0.5 | 0.5 |
| — | Other categories# | 1226 | 28.5 | 28.8 |
| | Total | 4309 | 100 | |

*4,309 office, home, and other non-hospital visits made by 43 physicians during a total of 290 days.
†International Classification of Diseases, 1955 Revision: World Health Organization, Palais des Nations, Geneva, 1957.
‡The individual categories are listed in Appendix A.
§Prophylactic inoculations and vaccinations in infants and children are entered under Y02 rather than Y00.5.
‖Wounds of scalp are not included. See Appendix A, N850.
#Some of these categories bear such non-specific titles as "other diseases of . . ." or "other and unspecified diseases of. . . ." With the exception of these non-specific categories, each category accounted for less than 0.5 per cent of the visits. The individual categories are listed in Appendix A.

TABLE 61

Hospital Visits of Ontario Physicians*

(Incidences of those categories that occurred at a rate
of one or more visits in every two hundred)†

| Three-digit numbers | Category | Ontario No. of visits | Ontario Rate per 100 visits | Nova Scotia rate per 100 visits |
|---|---|---|---|---|
| Y07 | Postpartum observation (without abnormal symptoms) | 82 | 7.3 | 7.5 |
| N800–N829‡ | Fractures | 80 | 7.1 | 6.3 |
| 420 | Arteriosclerotic heart disease, including coronary disease | 67 | 6.0 | 5.3 |
| 260 | Diabetes mellitus | 49 | 4.4 | 2.7 |
| 550–552 | Appendicitis | 43 | 3.8 | 2.4 |
| 510 | Hypertrophy of tonsils and adenoids | 38 | 3.4 | 1.3 |
| 780–795 | Symptoms, senility, and ill-defined conditions | 38 | 3.4 | 4.1 |
| 660 | Delivery without mention of complication§ | 35 | 3.1 | 2.3 |
| 540–541 | Ulcer of stomach and duodenum | 31 | 2.8 | 1.4 |
| 560–561 | Hernia of abdominal cavity | 31 | 2.8 | 1.0 |
| 490–493 | Pneumonia | 25 | 2.2 | 6.0 |
| 470–475 | Acute upper respiratory infections | 21 | 1.9 | 0.8 |
| 241 | Asthma | 19 | 1.7 | 0.9 |
| 571 | Gastro-enteritis and colitis, except ulcerative, age 4 weeks and over | 17 | 1.5 | 1.4 |
| N870–N908 | Laceration and open wound‖ | 17 | 1.5 | 1.1 |
| 310–318 | Psychoneurotic disorders | 17 | 1.5 | 1.3 |
| 391–393 | Otitis media and mastoiditis | 15 | 1.3 | 0.9 |
| 444 | Essential benign hypertension | 15 | 1.3 | 0.5 |
| 690–698 | Infections of skin and subcutaneous tissue | 15 | 1.3 | 0.5 |
| 584–585 | Cholelithiasis, cholecystitis, and cholangitis | 14 | 1.2 | 0.7 |
| 330–334 | Vascular lesions affecting central nervous system | 12 | 1.1 | 1.9 |
| 650 | Abortion without mention of sepsis or toxaemia | 11 | 1.0 | 0.4 |
| 735 | Displacement of intervertebral disc | 11 | 1.0 | 0.6 |
| 450 | General arteriosclerosis | 10 | 0.9 | 0.4 |
| 461 | Haemorrhoids | 10 | 0.9 | 0.9 |
| 776 | Immaturity, unqualified (early infancy) | 9 | 0.8 | 0.7 |
| 153–154 | Malignant neoplasm of large intestine | 8 | 0.7 | 0.4 |
| 605 | Cystitis | 8 | 0.7 | 0.4 |
| 303 | Sciatica | 7 | 0.6 | 0.0 |
| 460 | Varicose veins of lower extremities | 7 | 0.6 | 1.6 |
| 463–464 | Phlebitis and thrombophlebitis | 7 | 0.6 | 0.0 |
| 610 | Hyperplasia of prostate | 7 | 0.6 | 1.6 |
| 642 | Toxaemias of pregnancy | 7 | 0.6 | 0.1 |
| 704 | Pemphigus | 7 | 0.6 | 0.0 |
| 157 | Malignant neoplasm of pancreas | 6 | 0.5 | 0.0 |
| 400 | Rheumatic fever without mention of heart involvement | 6 | 0.5 | 0.0 |
| 453 | Peripheral vascular disease | 6 | 0.5 | 0.3 |
| 519 | Pleurisy | 6 | 0.5 | 0.1 |
| 543 | Gastritis and duodenitis | 6 | 0.5 | 0.7 |
| 570 | Intestinal obstruction without mention of hernia | 6 | 0.5 | 0.4 |
| 631 | Uterovaginal prolapse | 6 | 0.5 | 0.6 |
| 755 | Cleft palate and harelip | 6 | 0.5 | 0.0 |
| N850–N856 | Head injury (excluding skull fracture) | 6 | 0.5 | 0.5 |
| — | Other categories# | 284 | 25.3 | 34.3 |
| | Total | 1124 | 100 | |

*1,124 visits made by 41 physicians during a total of 275 days.
†International Classification of Diseases, 1955 Revision: World Health Organization, Palais des Nations, Geneva, 1957.
‡The individual categories are listed in Appendix A.
§Caesarean section without complication is included in this category.
‖Wounds of scalp are not included. See Appendix A, N850.
#Some of these categories bear such non-specific titles as "other diseases of ..." or "other and unspecified diseases of. ..." With the exception of these non-specific categories, each category accounted for less than 0.5 per cent of the visits. The individual categories are listed in Appendix A.

In these tables, it should be noted, we have arbitrarily grouped together certain conditions under one heading, when we have felt that to do so would give a clearer picture of the work done in practice. Fractures, for example, instead of being assigned to a number of

TABLE 62

NON-HOSPITAL VISITS OF NOVA SCOTIA PHYSICIANS*

(Incidences of those categories that occurred at a rate
of one or more visits in every two hundred)†

| Three-digit numbers | Category | Nova Scotia | | Ontario rate per 100 visits |
|---|---|---|---|---|
| | | No. of visits | Rate per 100 visits | |
| Y06 | Prenatal care (without abnormal symptoms) | 226 | 6.3 | 7.2 |
| 470–475‡ | Acute upper respiratory infections | 211 | 5.9 | 6.5 |
| Y02 | Persons receiving prophylactic inoculation and vaccination§ | 201 | 5.6 | 5.3 |
| 480–483 | Influenza | 200 | 5.6 | 2.8 |
| 780–795 | Symptoms, senility, and ill-defined conditions | 196 | 5.5 | 5.4 |
| 444 | Essential benign hypertension | 135 | 3.8 | 3.0 |
| 690–698 | Infections of skin and subcutaneous tissue | 114 | 3.2 | 3.3 |
| 310–318 | Psychoneurotic disorders | 91 | 2.5 | 3.2 |
| 490–493 | Pneumonia | 89 | 2.5 | 1.2 |
| Y00.0 Y00.3 | General medical or laboratory examination (without complaint or finding indicating need of observation or medical care) | 74 | 2.1 | 2.4 |
| N870–N908 | Laceration and open wound ‖ | 68 | 1.9 | 2.1 |
| 391–393 | Otitis media and mastoiditis | 63 | 1.8 | 1.3 |
| 420 | Arteriosclerotic heart disease, including coronary disease | 63 | 1.8 | 2.3 |
| 501 | Bronchitis unqualified | 62 | 1.7 | 1.5 |
| N800–N829 | Fractures | 50 | 1.4 | 1.3 |
| 530–535 | Diseases of teeth and supporting structures | 46 | 1.3 | 0.5 |
| N840–N848 | Sprains and strains of joints and adjacent muscles | 46 | 1.3 | 1.5 |
| N910–N929 | Superficial injury and contusion | 45 | 1.3 | 1.2 |
| 293 | Anaemia of unspecified type | 44 | 1.2 | 1.3 |
| 571 | Gastro-enteritis and colitis, except ulcerative, age 4 weeks and over | 44 | 1.2 | 1.1 |
| 605 | Cystitis | 43 | 1.2 | 0.6 |
| 726 | Muscular rheumatism | 41 | 1.1 | 0.9 |
| 500 | Acute bronchitis | 36 | 1.0 | 0.9 |
| Y00.5 | Well baby and child care‡ | 35 | 1.0 | 1.3 |
| 051 | Streptococcal sore throat | 32 | 0.9 | 0.2 |
| 260 | Diabetes mellitus | 31 | 0.9 | 1.3 |
| 241 | Asthma | 30 | 0.8 | 1.5 |
| 741–742 | Synovitis, bursitis, and tenosynovitis | 30 | 0.8 | 0.7 |
| 630 | Infective disease of uterus, vagina, and vulva | 24 | 0.7 | 0.8 |
| 330–334 | Vascular lesions affecting central nervous system | 23 | 0.6 | 0.5 |
| Y07 | Postpartum observation (without abnormal symptoms) | 23 | 0.6 | 1.0 |
| 287 | Obesity, not specified as of endocrine origin | 18 | 0.5 | 1.1 |
| 290 | Pernicious and other hyperchromic anaemias | 18 | 0.5 | 0.9 |
| 584–585 | Cholelithiasis, cholecystitis, and cholangitis | 18 | 0.5 | 0.0 |
| 634 | Disorders of menstruation | 18 | 0.5 | 0.7 |
| 092 | Infectious hepatitis | 17 | 0.5 | 0.0 |
| 725 | Arthritis, unspecified | 17 | 0.5 | 0.5 |
| 735 | Displacement of intervertebral disc | 17 | 0.5 | 0.2 |
| N850–N856 | Head injury (excluding skull fracture) | 17 | 0.5 | 0.3 |
| —— | Other categories# | 1033 | 28.8 | 28.5 |
| | Total | 3583 | 100 | |

*3,583 office, home, and other non-hospital visits made by 42 physicians during a total of 253 days.
†International Classification of Diseases, 1955 Revision: World Health Organization, Palais des Nations, Geneva, 1957.
‡The individual categories are listed in Appendix A.
§Prophylactic inoculations and vaccinations in infants and children are entered under Y02 rather than Y00.5.
‖Wounds of scalp are not included. See Appendix A, N850.
#Some of these categories bear such non-specific titles as "other diseases of . . ." or "other and unspecified diseases of. . . ." With the exception of these non-specific categories, each category accounted for less than 0.5 per cent of the visits. The individual categories are listed in Appendix A.

categories according to the site of the fracture, are shown as a single
item. A glance at the left-hand column of any of these tables will
make clear whether more than one of the original categories have
been combined; and the reader who wishes to break down such a

combination into the constituent categories may do so by consulting the appendix. The items in the four tables are listed in decreasing order of frequency, and each item accounts for at least 0.5 per cent of the non-hospital or hospital visits, as the case may be. Taken together, the items listed in each of these tables account for between 65 and 75 per cent of the visits. The right-hand column of each table gives the

TABLE 63

HOSPITAL VISITS OF NOVA SCOTIA PHYSICIANS*
(Incidences of those categories that occurred at a rate
of one or more visits in every two hundred)†

| Three-digit numbers | Category | Nova Scotia | | Ontario rate per 100 visits |
|---|---|---|---|---|
| | | No. of visits | Rate per 100 visits | |
| Y07 | Postpartum observation (without abnormal symptoms) | 119 | 7.5 | 7.3 |
| N800–N829‡ | Fractures | 100 | 6.3 | 7.1 |
| 100 493 | Pneumonia | 95 | 6.0 | 2.2 |
| 420 | Arteriosclerotic heart disease, including coronary disease | 85 | 5.3 | 6.0 |
| 780–795 | Symptoms, senility, and ill-defined conditions | 65 | 4.1 | 3.4 |
| 260 | Diabetes mellitus | 43 | 2.7 | 4.4 |
| 550–552 | Appendicitis | 38 | 2.4 | 3.8 |
| 660 | Delivery without mention of complication§ | 36 | 2.3 | 3.1 |
| 330–334 | Vascular lesions affecting central nervous system | 31 | 1.9 | 1.1 |
| 460 | Varicose veins of lower extremities | 25 | 1.6 | 0.6 |
| 610 | Hyperplasia of prostate | 25 | 1.6 | 0.6 |
| 480–483 | Influenza | 23 | 1.4 | 0.1 |
| 540–541 | Ulcer of stomach and duodenum | 23 | 1.4 | 2.8 |
| Y00.5 | Well baby and child care | 23 | 1.4 | 0.4 |
| 571 | Gastro-enteritis and colitis, except ulcerative, age 4 weeks and over | 22 | 1.4 | 1.5 |
| 310–318 | Psychoneurotic disorders | 21 | 1.3 | 1.5 |
| 510 | Hypertrophy of tonsils and adenoids | 20 | 1.3 | 3.4 |
| N870–N908 | Laceration and open wound‖ | 18 | 1.1 | 1.5 |
| 560–561 | Hernia of abdominal cavity | 16 | 1.0 | 2.8 |
| 391–393 | Otitis media and mastoiditis | 15 | 0.9 | 1.3 |
| N940–N949 | Burns | 15 | 0.9 | 0.3 |
| 151 | Malignant neoplasm of stomach | 14 | 0.9 | 0.0 |
| 241 | Asthma | 14 | 0.9 | 1.7 |
| 461 | Haemorrhoids | 14 | 0.9 | 0.9 |
| 470–475 | Acute upper respiratory infections | 13 | 0.8 | 1.9 |
| 572 | Chronic enteritis and ulcerative colitis | 12 | 0.8 | 0.0 |
| 725 | Arthritis, unspecified | 12 | 0.8 | 0.0 |
| 543 | Gastritis and duodenitis | 11 | 0.7 | 0.5 |
| 584–585 | Cholelithiasis, cholecystitis, and cholangitis | 11 | 0.7 | 1.2 |
| 776 | Immaturity, unqualified (early infancy) | 11 | 0.7 | 0.8 |
| 221 | Pilonidal cyst | 10 | 0.6 | 0.1 |
| 501 | Bronchitis unqualified | 10 | 0.6 | 0.2 |
| 600 | Infections of kidney | 10 | 0.6 | 0.1 |
| 735 | Displacement of intervertebral disc | 10 | 0.6 | 1.0 |
| 631 | Uterovaginal prolapse | 9 | 0.6 | 0.5 |
| 444 | Essential benign hypertension | 8 | 0.5 | 1.3 |
| 500 | Acute bronchitis | 8 | 0.5 | 0.1 |
| 690–698 | Infections of skin and subcutaneous tissue | 8 | 0.5 | 1.3 |
| 730 | Osteomyelitis and periostitis | 8 | 0.5 | 0.0 |
| N850–N856 | Head injury (excluding skull fracture) | 8 | 0.5 | 0.5 |
| — | Other categories# | 545 | 34.3 | 25.3 |
| | Total | 1591 | 100 | |

*1,591 visits made by 42 physicians during a total of 253 days.
†International Classification of Diseases, 1955 Revision: World Health Organization, Palais des Nations, Geneva, 1957.
‡The individual categories are listed in Appendix A.
§Caesarean section without complication is included in this category.
‖Wounds of scalp are not included. See Appendix A, N850.
#Some of these categories bear such non-specific titles as "other diseases of . . ." or "other and unspecified diseases of. . . ." With the exception of these non-specific categories, each category accounted for less than 0.5 per cent of the visits. The individual categories are listed in Appendix A.

corresponding percentage for the other province, for ease of comparison.

The most frequent reason for non-hospital visits in each province was prenatal care without abnormal symptoms. This accounted for 7.2 per cent of the 4,309 non-hospital visits in Ontario and for 6.3 per cent of the 3,583 non-hospital visits in Nova Scotia. Since the median number of non-hospital visits per physician per week was 86 in each province (see page 239), it may be said that the "average" general practitioner saw, on the average, approximately one prenatal patient per day.

The most frequent disease category for the non-hospital visits in each province was, not surprisingly, acute upper respiratory infection. This category, which constituted 6.5 per cent of the non-hospital visits in Ontario and 5.9 per cent of those in Nova Scotia, includes the common cold and acute infections of the sinuses, pharynx, tonsils, larynx, and trachea.

Skin diseases, excluding wounds, accounted for 6.8 per cent of the non-hospital visits in Ontario and 6.4 per cent of those in Nova Scotia.* This is of interest and importance in view of the fact that many physicians expressed dissatisfaction with their training in dermatology (see page 348).

The incidence of essential hypertension, 3.0 per cent of the non-hospital visits in Ontario and 3.8 per cent in Nova Scotia, is probably overstated. Some physicians appeared to make this diagnosis on the basis of a solitary determination of blood pressure; and some based the diagnosis on the systolic pressure without regard for the diastolic pressure. Relatively few men used the ophthalmoscope as an aid in assessing the significance of elevated blood pressure.

It is to be noted that, in each province, "anaemia of unspecified type" was more frequently recorded (58 visits in Ontario, 44 in Nova Scotia) than either pernicious anaemia (40 visits in Ontario, 18 in Nova Scotia) or iron deficiency anaemia (14 visits in Ontario, 8 in Nova Scotia). Some physicians appeared to make no effort to determine the specific type of anaemia encountered, and some appeared to make or to accept the diagnosis of pernicious anaemia on little or no evidence.

The non-diagnostic category termed "symptoms, senility, and ill-defined conditions" accounts for 5.4 per cent of the non-hospital visits

*In arriving at this percentage, we have taken into account not only the items whose three-digit numbers are 690–716 (diseases of the skin and cellular tissue), but also numbers 131 (dermatophytosis), 135 (scabies), 243 (urticaria), and 244 (allergic eczema). (See Appendix A.) We have regarded all of these as skin diseases, because it is in this guise that they are seen by the practitioner.

in Ontario and 5.5 per cent in Nova Scotia. How far this was owing to unavoidable diagnostic failure and how far to lack of adequate investigation or medical knowledge or both, it is not possible to say. The observers had the impression that some physicians were singularly lacking in intellectual curiosity and, having made little or no effort to reach a diagnosis, seemed quite content to employ symptomatic therapy.

The total number of *hospital* visits reported was 1,124 in Ontario and 1,591 in Nova Scotia (Tables 61 and 63 and Appendix A). An operation performed by the doctor or attended by him either as assistant-surgeon or as anaesthetist was counted as one visit. The conditions most frequently encountered in hospital practice were, as would be expected, different from those that occurred most commonly in home and office practice.

Of all the hospital visits, 3.1 per cent in Ontario and 2.3 per cent in Nova Scotia were for the purpose of delivering obstetrical patients. Several postpartum visits were made to each mother, and postpartum observation, accounting for 7.3 per cent in Ontario and 7.5 per cent in Nova Scotia, was the most frequent single reason for hospital visits (Tables 61 and 63).

Accounting for almost as many visits as postpartum care were fractures. Many of the patients with fractures had been in hospital for protracted periods, so that, of the total number of visits shown, a relatively small proportion was for freshly sustained fractures.

The relative frequencies of most of the conditions listed in Tables 61 and 63 require no comment; but it does seem rather surprising that "psychoneurotic disorders" account for more than 1 per cent of the hospital visits. With regard to "essential benign hypertension," which accounts for 1.3 per cent of the hospital visits in Ontario and for 0.5 per cent in Nova Scotia, we must point out, lest the title of the category mislead the reader, that, in the International Classification of Diseases, this category includes cases recorded simply as "hypertension." It is possible that some of the physicians neglected to record clinical features, such as hypertensive heart disease, congestive heart failure, myocardial infarction, or even cerebro-vascular accident, any one of which would have led to inclusion of such cases in categories with titles of more serious import than "essential benign hypertension."

A word of explanation is required, also, in the case of the category called "hypertrophy of tonsils and adenoids," which is shown as the reason for 3.4 per cent of the Ontario, and 1.3 per cent of the Nova Scotia, visits. The International Classification of Diseases includes in this category "chronic tonsillitis," "enlargement of tonsils (and adenoids)," and "tonsils (and adenoids)—diseased," but not "acute or unspecified tonsillitis."

Examination of Tables 60, 61, 62, and 63, shows that, both for non-hospital visits and for hospital visits, the relative frequencies in Ontario were very similar to the corresponding frequencies in Nova Scotia for a considerable proportion of the diagnostic categories. There were certain notable exceptions, however. The most outstanding of these was hay fever, for which 39 non-hospital visits were recorded in Ontario, but only 1 in Nova Scotia. Some of the other diagnostic categories accounting for at least twice as great a percentage of the non-hospital visits in Ontario as in Nova Scotia included obesity, not specified as of endocrine origin, ulcer of stomach and duodenum, and menopausal symptoms. On the other hand, the percentage of non-hospital visits was at least twice as great in Nova Scotia as in Ontario for each of a number of categories, including influenza, pneumonia, cystitis, streptococcal sore throat, and diseases of teeth and supporting structures. Similarly, hospital visits were more numerous, relatively, in Ontario than in Nova Scotia for certain conditions, including hypertrophy of tonsils and adenoids, ulcer of stomach and duodenum, hernia of abdominal cavity, and acute upper respiratory infections, whereas, for other conditions, including pneumonia and influenza, hospital visits were more numerous, relatively, in Nova Scotia than in Ontario.

There are several possible explanations for these differences between the two provinces. First, there may have been a difference between the incidence of the particular disease in the population of the one province and its incidence in the population of the other province. Secondly, the populations of the two provinces may differ in their tendency to seek medical attention for a particular condition. Thirdly, the general practitioners in one province may tend to make more visits than those in the other province to a patient who has a particular condition. Finally, the differences may be due to diagnostic failure on the part of the practitioners. We know, for example, from observation, that some physicians used the terms "influenza" and "flu" to describe any acute febrile illness that had few or no localizing signs or symptoms. The result of this was that the incidence of cases of influenza is shown as higher than it actually was, not only in Nova Scotia, but also in Ontario.* It is not possible, from our data, to assess the relative importance of these various factors in producing the differences that we have noted between Ontario and Nova Scotia.

In Table 64, the reasons for the visits are classified in broad groups provided by the International Classification of Diseases.

TABLE 64

ONTARIO AND NOVA SCOTIA PHYSICIANS' NON-HOSPITAL AND HOSPITAL
VISITS CLASSIFIED ACCORDING TO MAJOR GROUPS OF DISEASES
OR OF OTHER REASONS FOR VISITS*

| Section number | Three-digit numbers | Section | Number of visits | | | |
|---|---|---|---|---|---|---|
| | | | Ontario | | Nova Scotia | |
| | | | Office, home, and other non-hospital visits | Hospital visits | Office, home, and other non-hospital visits | Hospital visits |
| I | 001–138 | Infective and parasitic diseases | 119 | 4 | 153 | 40 |
| II | 140–239 | Neoplasms | 65 | 38 | 46 | 92 |
| III | 240–245 250–289 | Allergic disorders Endocrine, metabolic, and nutritional diseases | 150 148 | 21 52 | 51 72 | 14 48 |
| IV | 290–299 | Diseases of the blood and blood-forming organs | 116 | 1 | 71 | 13 |
| V | 300–326 | Mental, psychoneurotic, and personality disorders | 159 | 21 | 113 | 31 |
| VI | 330–398 | Diseases of the nervous system and sense organs | 220 | 59 | 193 | 57 |
| VII | 400–468 | Diseases of the circulatory system | 378 | 160 | 327 | 196 |
| VIII | 470–527 | Diseases of the respiratory system | 648 | 102 | 695 | 200 |
| IX | 530–587 | Diseases of the digestive system | 248 | 174 | 226 | 230 |
| X | 590–637 | Diseases of the genito-urinary system | 229 | 91 | 179 | 126 |
| XI | 640–689 | Deliveries and complications of pregnancy, childbirth, and the puerperium | 24 | 71 | 36 | 57 |
| XII | 690–716 | Diseases of the skin and cellular tissue | 263 | 26 | 204 | 17 |
| XIII | 720–749 | Diseases of the bones and organs of movement | 148 | 19 | 134 | 46 |
| XIV | 750–759 | Congenital malformations | 4 | 6 | 4 | 8 |
| XV | 760–776 | Certain diseases of early infancy | 17 | 10 | 6 | 30 |
| XVI | 780–795 | Symptoms, senility, and ill-defined conditions | 234 | 38 | 196 | 65 |
| XVII | N800–N999 | Accidents, poisonings, and violence | 386 | 133 | 301 | 165 |

*International Classification of Diseases, 1955 Revision: World Health Organization, Palais des Nations, Geneva, 1957.

TABLE 64 (*Continued*)

| Section number | Three-digit numbers | Section | Ontario Office, home, and other non-hospital visits | Ontario Hospital visits | Nova Scotia Office, home, and other non-hospital visits | Nova Scotia Hospital visits |
|---|---|---|---|---|---|---|
| Special conditions and examinations without sickness | Y00.0 Y00.3 | General medical examination or laboratory examination | 102 | 0 | 74 | 1 |
| | Y00.5 | Well baby and child care | 58 | 4 | 35 | 23 |
| | Y01 | Skin immunity and sensitization tests | 3 | 0 | 3 | 0 |
| | Y02 | Persons receiving prophylactic inoculation and vaccination | 230 | 0 | 201 | 0 |
| | Y06 | Prenatal care | 311 | 1 | 226 | 6 |
| | Y07 | Postpartum observation | 43 | 82 | 23 | 119 |
| | Y09 | Other person without complaint or sickness† | 6 | 11 | 5 | 7 |
| | | Total number of visits | 4309 | 1124 | 3583 | 1591 |
| | | Total number of days | 290 | 275 | 253 | 253 |
| | | Number of physicians | 43 | 41 | 42 | 42 |

†The majority of these visits were either for circumcision or for contraceptive advice.

We have already reported (page 228) the percentages of practitioners who were doing anaesthesia and surgery in each province. It remains for us to report what work of these two types was actually done during the days on which the doctors kept records of their work for us. In Ontario, there were only 11 physicians, 25 per cent of the entire group, who gave any general anaesthetics. Six of these were those who had indicated to us that they had a particular interest in anaesthesia. Their records covered a total of 40 week-days, during which they gave a total of 64 general anaesthetics. The other 5 who reported the giving of any anaesthetics gave a total of 10 general anaesthetics during a total of 28 week-days (no anaesthetics were given on Sundays). In Nova Scotia, the 4 physicians who professed a particular interest in anaesthesia gave a total of 22 general anaesthetics during a total of 22 week-days; 10 physicians who said that they did more than occasional general anaesthesia but who did not name anaesthesia as a particular interest gave 20 anaesthetics during 48 week-days; and 6 physicians who said that they gave only occasional anaes-

*In addition, the figure for Ontario may have been raised to an unusual height by the fact that a few of the physicians were visited by us at a time when influenza was epidemic.

thetics gave 4 anaesthetics during 30 week-days (again, no anaesthetics were given on Sundays).

The surgical procedures are listed in Table 65, where it is indicated, also, whether the practitioner being visited by us was the principal operator or was assisting. Because of certain obscurities in the records that were returned for the days following our departure, we have included in this table only the surgical work done during the days of our visit to the doctor. We have excluded all fractures except those for which special procedures were used and all skin wounds that did not involve deeper structures such as tendons or nerves. With these exclusions, we find that, in each province, about two-fifths of the practitioners did no surgery during our visit, one-third carried out one or more surgical procedures themselves, and the remainder acted as assistants. If we exclude also circumcisions and excisions of tonsils and adenoids, those physicians who acted as principal operators are reduced to approximately one-quarter of the total group in each province.

It is probable that the practitioners ordinarily did a larger volume of surgical work than they did during our visit, inasmuch as some of them made plain that, as a courtesy to us, they had deliberately postponed surgical work that was not urgent, in order to leave more time available for us. We had not intended that they should do this, since we wished to see their practices as they were normally carried on; and the fact that they did defer some of their work has resulted in a somewhat distorted picture of the surgical portion of their practices. On the other hand, we probably gained as much as we lost, since the postponement of major surgical procedures made more time available for discussion and allowed us to see a wider range of home and office practice.

At this point the reader may ask whether our picture of the non-surgical portion of the doctor's practice was similarly distorted. We think that it was not. To postpone a procedure that one knows will take at least an hour, or perhaps two or three hours, is one thing. To put off a large number of appointments, each of a few minutes' duration, is quite another matter, much more difficult and purposeless; and those men who see patients as they come, i.e. without appointments, would find it virtually impossible to rearrange their office work. We must admit that, when the week first suggested by us for our visit was inconvenient for a particular doctor—usually because he planned to be away either on vacation or at a medical meeting—we always chose another week for our visit. Because we did make such changes instead of simply recording that no work was done by the doctor during the time first suggested by us, it is not possible from the

TABLE 65

SURGICAL OPERATIONS PERFORMED DURING THE VISITS OF THE SURVEY
TO ONTARIO AND NOVA SCOTIA PHYSICIANS*

| | Ontario | | Nova Scotia | |
|---|---|---|---|---|
| | Number of operations at which the physician being visited by the Survey was: | | | |
| Operation | Assistant | Principal operator† | Assistant | Principal operator§ |
| Circumcision | — | 2 | — | 4§ |
| Uterine curettage | — | 2 | — | 3 |
| Tonsillectomy and/or adenoidectomy | — | 4 | — | — |
| Appendectomy | — | 2 | 2 | 1 |
| Extraction of teeth | — | — | — | 3§ |
| Incision and drainage of abscess | — | 1 | — | 2 |
| Caesarean section | — | — | — | 2‖ |
| Repair of hernia (a) inguinal | 1 | 2 | — | — |
| (b) umbilical | 1 | — | — | — |
| Excision of sebaceous cyst | — | 2 | — | — |
| Amputation, mid-thigh | — | 1 | — | — |
| Cystoscopic examination | — | — | — | 1 |
| Elevation of nasal fracture | — | 1 | — | — |
| Excision of callus of foot | — | — | — | 1 |
| Excision of coccyx | — | 1 | — | — |
| Excision of ganglion of hand | — | 1 | — | — |
| Excision of lipoma from axilla | — | 1 | — | — |
| Hysterectomy | — | 1 | — | — |
| Insertion of pin through tibia for traction in case of fracture of femur | — | 1 | — | — |
| Repair of cystocoele and rectocoele and amputation of cervix | — | 1 | — | — |
| Suturing of extensor tendon of finger | — | 1 | — | — |
| Uterine curettage, repair of cystocoele, and haemorrhoidectomy | — | — | — | 1 |
| Cholecystectomy | 1 | — | 1 | — |
| Excision of calcaneal spur | — | — | 1 | — |
| Number of physicians performing at least one of the above-listed operations as principal operator | | 14‡ | | 14# |
| Number of physicians assisting but not performing any of the above-listed operations as principal operator | | 4 | | 3 |
| Number of physicians not taking part in any of the listed operations | | 26 | | 25 |

*Skin wounds are not listed, unless their repair involved such deeper structures as tendons or nerves. Fractures are not included, except those involving the use of special procedures.

†Since none of the Ontario physicians performed the same type of operation twice during the Survey's visit, the figures in this column indicate not only the numbers of each type of operation but also how many physicians performed each type of operation during the Survey's visit.

‡Three of these physicians did not take part in any of the operations listed, except excision of tonsils and adenoids or circumcision or both. Another physician did only an excision of tonsils and adenoids as principal operator but also assisted with a cholecystectomy.

§One physician circumcised 2 patients; another extracted teeth from 2 patients. The figures shown in this column for all other items indicate, not only the numbers of each type of operation, but also how many physicians performed each type of operation during the Survey's visit.

‖One of these physicians had a certificated surgeon be present during the operation.

♯Three of these physicians did not take part in any of the operations listed except circumcision.

---

records of the cases seen to indicate with complete accuracy the work that would be done by the "average" general practitioner during such a long period as, say, six months or a year. There is no reason to believe, however, that, because we made some visits a week or two earlier or later than we had planned, the relative incidences of the various conditions or of the sexes and ages of patients were altered. In short, after allowance has been made for the possible errors that we have discussed earlier (pages 237–238), and with the possible exception of surgery (the volume of which may have been underestimated), the data that we have reported are believed by us to give a reasonably accurate picture of the work of the general practitioners.

In order to gain some impression of what the practitioners themselves thought of the volume of the work that they were doing, we asked each one to state how many patients he saw per week-day on the average and then to say whether this number was "too few," "satisfactory," or "too many." Seven per cent of the Ontario group and 12 per cent of the Nova Scotia group thought that they were seeing too few patients. Sixty-one per cent in Ontario and 60 per cent in Nova Scotia were satisfied with the number of patients that they were seeing; and 32 per cent and 29 per cent, respectively, said that they were seeing too many patients per day. The doctors' replies about the number of patients being seen by them per day are shown in Table 66. The figures suggest that the practitioners believe that the

TABLE 66

ESTIMATES OF ONTARIO AND NOVA SCOTIA PHYSICIANS OF NUMBER OF PATIENTS SEEN BY THEM ON THE AVERAGE WEEK-DAY AND THEIR OPINIONS ON THIS NUMBER

| Physician's opinion of number of patients seen by him | Ontario | | | Nova Scotia | | |
|---|---|---|---|---|---|---|
| | Number of physicians | Physician's estimate of number of patients seen per week-day | | Number of physicians | Physician's estimate of number of patients seen per week-day | |
| | | Range | Median | | Range | Median |
| Too few | 3 | 6–12 | 10.0 | 5 | 15–30 | 25.0 |
| Satisfactory | 27 | 13–45 | 23.8 | 25 | 9–72 | 24.0 |
| Too many | 13* | 27–100 | 38.8 | 12 | 20–75 | 30.0 |
| Unknown | 1 | — | — | — | — | — |

*One of these 13 did not give an estimate of the number of patients seen by him.

optimum number of patients per day is in the neighbourhood of from 20 to 30.

The presentation that we have given of the work done by the general practitioners has an obvious defect. Since no one man's practice can be taken as typical, it has been necessary to put together the records kept for us by 43 doctors in Ontario and by 42 in Nova Scotia. We could wish that we were magician enough that, having mixed all of our ingredients in the cauldron, we could now bring forth the typical practice. Unfortunately, we find that, if we try to accomplish this by dividing the cases evenly among the practitioners, the "typical" practice that emerges is such a grotesque monster as to consist of such-and-such a fraction of a case of one type of disease per day (or per week) and a different fraction of a case of another type and so on. Such a picture of practice is quite meaningless. Our failure to perform the feat of magic is, of course, inherent in the subject of our study. Just as there is no such thing as a typical general practitioner, so there is no such thing as a typical general practice. Since we cannot give a picture of what work this non-existent individual does in a certain period, we can only report, as we have already, what a representative group of general practitioners (i.e., our randomly selected sample) did on a number of days and give a few sample days as illustrations. In Tables 67, 68, 69 are shown the cases seen during three days of practice, one day in the life of each of three different general practitioners. One day has been selected from a very light practice, one from a very

TABLE 67

ONE DAY'S WORK IN A LIGHT PRACTICE

| Sex | Age | Illness | | Seen in | | | Diagnosis, operation, or delivery (or reason for visit) |
| --- | --- | --- | --- | --- | --- | --- | --- |
| | | New | Old | Office | Home | Hospital | |
| F | 10 | | X | | | X | Acute appendicitis (post-operative) |
| F | 34 | | X | | | X | Hysterectomy (postoperative) |
| F | 33 | | X | | | X | Not yet diagnosed—Anxiety state |
| F | 40 | X | | X | | | Paronychia |
| F | 39 | X | | X | | | Neurodermatitis |
| M | 70 | X | | X | | | Postural hypotension |
| F | 36 | X | | X | | | Prescription only |
| F | 10 | X | | X | | | Subacute appendicitis |
| F | 78 | | X | X | | | Essential hypertension |
| M | 74 | | X | X | | | Diabetes mellitus |
| M | 15 | | X | X | | | Acute tonsillitis |
| M | 52 | X | | X | | | Acute bronchitis |
| F | 36 | X | | X | | | Acute cystitis |
| F | 42 | | X | X | | | Prescription only |

TABLE 68

ONE DAY'S WORK IN A HEAVY PRACTICE

| Sex | Age | Illness | | Seen in | | | Diagnosis, operation, or delivery (or reason for visit) |
|---|---|---|---|---|---|---|---|
| | | New | Old | Office | Home | Hospital | |
| M | 14 | X | | | X | | Acute bronchitis |
| M | 76 | | X | | X | | Coronary insufficiency |
| M | 80 | X | | | X | | Chronic arthritis |
| M | 65 | | X | | X | | Pneumonia-Pleurisy |
| F | 82 | | X | | X | | Hypostatic pneumonia |
| M | 3 mos | X | | | X | | Acute bronchiolitis |
| M | 30 | | X | | X | | Crush injury of foot |
| M | 7 | X | | | X | | Acute bronchitis and pneumonitis |
| F | 73 | | X | | | X | Acute right heart failure |
| F | 76 | | X | | | X | Carcinomatosis |
| F | 68 | | X | | | X | Thrombophlebitis |
| F | 65 | | X | | | X | Diabetes mellitus |
| M | 53 | | X | | | X | Herniorrhaphy |
| F | 73 | | X | | | X | Hysterectomy (post-operative) |
| F | 78 | | X | | | X | Cerebral accident |
| F | 88 | | X | | | X | Diabetes mellitus |
| F | 34 | X | | | | X | Obstetrical delivery |
| M | 78 | | X | X | | | Abdominoperineal for carcinoma of rectum (post-operative) |
| F | 28 | | X | X | | | Pregnancy |
| F | 60 | | X | X | | | Secondary anaemia |
| F | 8 | X | | X | | | Acute tonsillitis |
| M | 12 | | X | X | | | Chronic bronchial asthma (bacterial vaccine) |
| F | 84 | | X | X | | | Pernicious anaemia |
| F | 65 | | X | X | | | Secondary anaemia |
| F | 78 | | X | X | | | Hypertensive cardiovascular disease |
| F | 64 | | X | X | | | Hypotension |
| M | 12 | | X | X | | | Ringworm of arms |
| M | 14 | | X | X | | | Chronic bronchial asthma (bacterial vaccine) |
| M | 70 | X | | X | | | Infection of hand |
| F | 65 | | X | X | | | Acute bronchitis |
| F | 34 | X | | X | | | Cystic mastitis |
| M | 50 | X | | X | | | Recurrent gastritis |
| M | 78 | X | | X | | | Acute bronchitis |
| M | 10 | X | | X | | | Injury of hand—fracture? |
| { M | 24 | | X | X | | | Diabetes mellitus a.c. and |
| { M | 24 | | X | X | | | p.c. blood sugars—8.30 a.m. and 4.30 p.m. } |
| M | 26 | X | | X | | | Acute bronchitis |
| M | 45 | X | | X | | | Cyst on wrist |
| F | 30 | | X | X | | | Ulcerative colitis |
| M | 26 | X | | X | | | Infection of hand—adenitis of axilla |
| M | 55 | X | | X | | | Functional chest pain |
| F | 52 | | X | X | | | Pernicious anaemia |
| F | 60 | | X | X | | | Sprain of ankle |
| F | 65 | X | | X | | | Furunculosis of buttock |

TABLE 68 (*Continued*)

| Sex | Age | Illness New | Illness Old | Seen in Office | Seen in Home | Seen in Hospital | Diagnosis, operation, or delivery (or reason for visit) |
|---|---|---|---|---|---|---|---|
| F | 24 | | X | X | | | Pregnancy |
| F | 50 | | X | X | | | Pyelonephritis |
| F | 26 | | X | X | | | Pregnancy |
| M | 20 | | X | X | | | Chronic bronchial asthma (bacterial vaccine) |
| M | 48 | X | | X | | | Functional eye disturbance (?) |
| M | 48 | | X | X | | | Post-influenza fatigue |
| F | 26 | | X | X | | | Post-miscarriage check |
| M | 55 | | X | X | | | Lumbar disc |
| F | 28 | | X | X | | | Pregnancy |
| M | 22 | | X | X | | | Post-infection fatigue |
| M | 48 | | X | X | | | Injury of thumb |
| M | 25 | | X | X | | | Multiple abrasions and contusions |
| M | 58 | X | | X | | | Life insurance examination |

TABLE 69

One Day's Work in a Practice That was Neither Light nor Heavy

| Sex | Age | Illness New | Illness Old | Seen in Office | Seen in Home | Seen in Hospital | Diagnosis, operation, or delivery (or reason for visit) |
|---|---|---|---|---|---|---|---|
| F | 38 | X | | | | X | Uterine dilatation and curettage and amputation of cervix |
| F | 36 | | X | X | | | Arterial hypertension |
| F | 23 | | X | X | | | Prenatal examination |
| F | 28 | | X | X | | | Prenatal examination |
| F | 33 | | X | X | | | Prenatal examination |
| F | 23 | | X | X | | | Bartholin abscess |
| F | 28 | | X | X | | | Acute retroflexion of uterus— insert pessary |
| F | 28 | | X | X | | | Prenatal examination |
| F | 52 | X | | X | | | Cervical erosion—biopsy |
| F | 40 | | X | X | | | Nervous exhaustion |
| F | 72 | | X | X | | | Arterial hypertension |
| M | 44 | | X | | | X | Fracture of tibia and fibula |
| M | 10 mos | | X | | | X | Acute mastoiditis |
| F | 68 | | X | | | X | Hemiplegia |
| M | 73 | | X | | | X | Diabetes mellitus |
| M | 61 | | X | | | X | Coronary thrombosis |
| F | 25 | X | | | | X | Delivery |
| F | 26 | X | | X | | | Prenatal examination |
| F | 22 | | X | X | | | Prenatal examination |
| F | 24 | | X | X | | | Prenatal examination |
| F | 28 | | X | X | | | Postnatal examination |
| M | 33 | X | | X | | | Insurance examination |
| M | 19 | X | | X | | | Foreign body in eye |
| F | 22 | X | | X | | | Acute pharyngitis |
| M | 24 | X | | X | | | Gross haematuria |
| M | 47 | X | | | | X | Admitted for partial gastrectomy for duodenal ulcer |

heavy practice, and one from a practice that was neither very light nor very heavy.

If we look at Table 69, we find that this practitioner began his day's work at the hospital, where he performed a gynaecological operation. Then he saw 10 patients in his office, 1 with a new condition, a gynaecological lesion from which he took a biopsy for examination, and 9 whom he had been following: 4 prenatal patients, 2 patients with gynaecological conditions, 2 with hypertension, and 1 whose disorder was mental. Next came 6 more hospital visits, including an obstetrical delivery and follow-up visits to patients with two different types of surgical condition and three different types of medical condition. Then there were 8 more office patients: 1 new and 2 old prenatal patients, 1 for a postpartum examination, 1 for removal of a foreign body from the eye, 2 with different types of medical condition for which they had not previously been seen, and 1 for an insurance examination. The day ended with a visit to a patient admitted to hospital for an operation. On this particular day, this practitioner made no house calls. The day's work represented in Table 67 comprised only about half as many visits, and that shown in Table 68 consisted of more than twice as many visits, as the day's work that we have just described. Of the three days, the one that has been described comes closest to the mythical typical practice in *volume* of work; but, as the tables show, the *type* of work varies so widely that it is impossible to describe a typical day of general practice.

# 16 / The Quality of General Practice
## *Method of Assessment*

Of the several objectives of the Survey of General Practice (described on pages 7–8), one of the most important, if not *the* most important, was to determine the *quality* of the work being done by the general practitioners. In describing the origin of the study, we mentioned (pages 4–5) the emphasis that was laid upon this objective by the Steering Committee and by those members of the College of General Practice of Canada whose thought and action brought the Survey into being. We remind the reader, also, that the Steering Committee, though allowing us great freedom in the carrying out of the study, was quite explicit in one requirement: that the practitioners' work should be observed and should be assessed according to the method developed by Peterson° (see pages 5, 10 above).

Because it is essential that we make quite clear how the assessments of quality were made, we shall devote this chapter to a detailed description of the method, before going on, in the next chapter, to a report of our findings. It is not enough that we merely reproduce the rating scale that we used. As anyone familiar with clinical medicine will at once realize, no method of assessment can foresee, and lay down rules to meet, every eventuality. The situations that may be expected to occur in the assessment of any group of practices are myriad. Since we had to make many decisions and since the validity of the results depends on the soundness of our decisions, the way in which we made our assessments of the practices will be illustrated with clinical examples.

°O. L. Peterson *et al.*: Journal of Medical Education, *31*, No. 12, Part 2: 1–165, 1956.

In an earlier chapter, we described how the observer accompanied the general practitioner as he carried on his practice (pages 13–15). To repeat the important points, each of the observers was a physician,* who both saw and heard how the practitioners practised in office, home, and hospital during a period, usually, of three days' duration. On the basis of this direct observation of the practitioner's management of a large number of cases, points were assigned, according to pre-determined criteria, for history-taking, for many items of physical examination, for certain items of laboratory work, treatment, obstetrical care, and preventive medicine, and for keeping clinical records.

On some of the items, every one of 85[†] practitioners could be assessed; on other items, one or more practitioners could not be assessed. For example, only 3 out of the 43 Ontario practitioners and 6 out of the 42 in Nova Scotia could be assessed on the item, spinal tap, because, during our visits, these were the only doctors who had patients whose conditions required spinal taps. On the other hand, the taking of temperature could be assessed in 84 of the 85 practices. The one physician who could not be assessed on the taking of temperature did not take the temperature of any patient during the course of our visit, but neither did he see any patient whose temperature we could reasonably have expected him to take; and one of the basic principles by which we were guided in making our assessments was that we should compare what was done by the physician with what the patient needed rather than with any arbitrary or inflexible academic standard.

In computing the final scores of the practitioners, we had to decide whether or not to include those items on which some, but not all, of the practitioners had been assessed. If all of these items were excluded, all of the physicians would then be compared on the basis of the same group of items; but to insist on uniformity to the extent of excluding even those items on which just a few physicians, or perhaps just one, had not been assessed would narrow considerably our basis of comparison. It seemed ridiculous, for example, to exclude the taking of temperature, on which 84 doctors had been assessed, simply because we had not had the opportunity to assess 1 man on this item. Conversely, it seemed unrealistic to include the item, spinal tap, in the rating scale, when only 9 men had been assessed on it. Our final decision was to retain in the rating scale all items on which we had been able to assess at least 75 per cent of the practitioners visited in

*The observers' qualifications have been discussed on pages 24–26.
†Because of technical difficulties, 1 of the 44 Ontario practitioners visited was not assessed at all.

each of the two provinces and on which we had been able to assess at least 80 per cent of the two groups combined.

The items that were excluded by this compromise are listed in Table 70. Mainly they were items of laboratory work and of obstetrical care. Though they were not used in the calculation of the practitioners' scores, we shall have more to say later about some of them.

TABLE 70

ITEMS OF PRACTICE ON WHICH OBSERVATIONS WERE MADE, BUT WHICH WERE NOT USED IN THE COMPUTATION OF THE PHYSICIANS' SCORES*

| Category | Item |
|---|---|
| Physical examination | Ears—hearing |
| | Paranasal sinuses |
| | Lungs—fremitus |
| | Peripheral pulses |
| | Back |
| Laboratory work | White blood cell count |
| | Blood smears and differentials |
| | Stools |
| | Bacteriology |
| | Blood glucose |
| | Blood urea nitrogen or non-protein nitrogen |
| | Serological test for syphilis |
| | Tuberculin test |
| | Spinal tap |
| | Biopsy or Papanicolaou smear |
| | Electrocardiogram |
| | Miscellaneous |
| Therapy | Anaemia |
| | Hypertension |
| | Cardiac failure |
| Obstetrics | Initial history |
| | Initial examination |
| | Initial laboratory work |
| | Complications |
| | Labour |
| | Forceps |
| | Episiotomy |
| | Management of the baby |
| | Consultations |
| | Special skill |
| Preventive medicine | Checkups |

*The reason for not using these items is discussed above.

The points assigned for the items that were retained in the rating scale totalled 80; but, since we were not able to assess every practitioner on every one of the items, it follows that some of the practitioners were scored out of less than 80. For this reason, every score was expressed as a percentage of the total number of points that were assignable for the items on which that particular doctor was assessed. In Ontario, the lowest number of points out of which any doctor was scored was 67 (i.e., 84 per cent of the full rating scale); the corresponding figure for Nova Scotia was 71 points (i.e., 89 per cent of the full rating scale). However, 86 per cent of the Nova Scotia doctors and 81 per cent of the Ontario doctors were scored out of 76 or more of the 80 points; in each province 95 per cent of the doctors were scored out of 72 or more of the 80 points; and in each province the mean number of points out of which the doctors were scored was 77.7 (Table 71).

TABLE 71

DISTRIBUTIONS OF ONTARIO PHYSICIANS AND OF NOVA
SCOTIA PHYSICIANS ACCORDING TO THE TOTAL NUMBER
OF POINTS OUT OF WHICH THEY WERE SCORED

| Number of points assignable for the items on which the physician could be assessed | Number of physicians | |
|---|---|---|
| | Ontario | Nova Scotia |
| 80 (the total for all the items in the rating scale) | 14 | 10 |
| 79 | 10 | 10 |
| 78 | 6 | 8 |
| 77 | 1 | 5 |
| 76 | 4 | 3 |
| 75 | 4 | 2 |
| 74 | 0 | 1 |
| 73 | 0 | 0 |
| 72 | 2 | 1 |
| 71 | 1 | 2 |
| 70 | 0 | 0 |
| 69 | 0 | 0 |
| 68 | 0 | 0 |
| 67 | 1 | 0 |
| Total number of physicians | 43 | 42 |

The rating scale (a modification of the scale devised by Peterson in his study of general practice in North Carolina; see his page 154), various parts of which will be explained and illustrated later, is now reproduced in full:

SCALE FOR ASSESSING QUALITY OF WORK

To be applied to *new patients*, patients with *new illnesses*, patients requesting a checkup, or patients whose complaint, history, appearance, or attitude would indicate the *need* for careful history and examination.

Credit should be given for good regional examinations when these are clearly indicated and when the doctor's previous contacts with the patient have been sufficiently frequent or recent to justify a partial history or physical examination.

When specific tests are omitted by the physician for good reason, NA (not assessable) should be entered in the margin beside the procedure. The doctor, for example, who does no obstetrics or whose obstetrical practice is not observed, should not be graded on the obstetrics items. The reason for writing NA should be given.

## I  HISTORY

| Item | Points to be assigned | |
|---|---|---|
| | 0–10 | If the history is limited to the presenting complaint or the involved organ. If no history is taken, 0 should be assigned. Questions as to periodicity, duration, severity, and location, and other questions largely limited to the patient's presenting complaint may increase the points to a maximum of 10. |
| | 11–20 | For fair histories. Histories in this class should indicate that the doctor is giving attention to the organ involved and to the possible diagnoses and complications. Some questions as to past history and the major organ systems should be asked. Incompleteness, lack of knowledge, and lack of interviewing skill serve to distinguish histories in this class from those in the next higher. |
| | 21–30 | For very good histories. Histories in this class should give evidence that the doctor is thinking in terms of the organ involved and the possible complications. There should be evidence that the doctor is thinking of all possible diagnoses and is trying to assess these by his questioning. Classification in this group should be limited to doctors who elicit some past history and who determine the presence or absence of symptoms in the major organ systems other than that involved in the presenting complaint. Skill in interviewing should be given credit here. Clinical knowledge is evident in history-taking, and credit should be given where such knowledge is obviously extensive. |

## II  PHYSICAL EXAMINATION

| | | |
|---|---|---|
| 1. Disrobing | 0 | Examination performed with the patient dressed or almost completely dressed. |
| | 1 | Patient sufficiently undressed to allow easy access to parts being examined. |
| 2. Temperature | 0 | Not taken when indicated. |
| | 1 | Taken when indicated. |

| Item | Points to be assigned | |
|---|---|---|
| 3. Skin | 0 | Not examined when indicated. |
| | 1 | Careful examination of whole skin surface when indicated. |
| 4. Eyes<br>(*a*) ophthalmoscopic examination | 0 | Not done when indicated. |
| | 1 | Performed with frequency indicated by clinical conditions presenting. |
| (*b*) other | 0 | No examination or examination of conjunctivae only. |
| | 1 | Examination of conjunctivae with occasional determination of visual fields or pupillary reactions or extraocular movements or visual acuity. |
| 5. Ears | 0 | Not examined with otoscope. |
| | 1 | Examined with otoscope. |
| 6. Nose | 0 | Not examined when indicated. |
| | 1 | Examined. |
| 7. Mouth and throat | 0 | Inspection of tonsils or throat only. |
| | 1 | Complete inspection of tonsils, throat and mouth, including teeth, gums, and tongue. |
| 8. Neck | 0 | Not examined. |
| | 1 | Examination is limited to submaxillary nodes. |
| | 2 | Examination includes thyroid, mobility of neck, etc., when such examination is indicated. |
| 9. Lymph nodes (cervical, axillary, and inguinal) | 0 | Never examined or submaxillary only. |
| | 1 | Examined in part as indicated. |
| | 2 | Examined completely. |
| 10. Breasts | 0 | Not examined routinely. |
| | 1 | Examined as part of a general physical examination. |
| 11. Lungs<br>(*a*) percussion | 0 | Not done or chest thumped perfunctorily. |
| | 1 | Percussion over all major lobes, or determination of diaphragmatic movements, etc. |
| (*b*) auscultation | 0 | Not done, or performed through clothes. |
| | 1 | Only part of chest auscultated (e.g., a single area in front or back). |
| | 2 | All lobes auscultated with apparent care. |
| 12. Heart | 0 | Auscultation of base or other single area of the heart. |
| | 1 | Adequate auscultation of all areas. |

| Item | Points to be assigned | |
|---|---|---|
| | 2 | Good complete examination including auscultation and either palpation or percussion. |
| 13. Blood pressure | 0 | Systolic measurement only. |
| | 1 | Careful systolic and diastolic measurements. |
| 14. Abdomen | 0 | No examination, or examination with the patient sitting up. |
| | 1 | Examination with the patient lying down, but done perfunctorily. |
| | 2 | Examination with careful palpation of liver and spleen and of all areas; eliciting of costovertebral tenderness when present; percussion and auscultation when indicated. |
| | 3 | Above plus examination of genitals (in males) and palpation of inguinal rings (in males). |
| 15. Extremities | 0 | No examination although indicated. |
| | 1 | Adequate inspection, palpation, and movement. |
| 16. Nervous system | 0 | No neurological examination when indicated. |
| | 1 | Partial neurological examination either in neurological cases or in the course of routine physical examination. In neurological cases, some items of importance omitted. |
| | 2 | Skilled use of neurological tests. |
| 17. Rectum | 0 | Not examined when indicated. |
| | 1 | Examined when indicated by symptoms or by age (over 40). |
| 18. Vagina | 0 | Not examined when indicated. |
| | 1 | Bimanual examination including use of speculum. |
| 19. Over-all skill | 0–3 | In the foregoing assessment of the physical examination, it may be just to revise the score up or down. Up to 3 points may be added to the score for general excellence, as evidenced by the frequent performance of complete examinations, by the use of nasopharyngeal or laryngeal mirrors or proctoscope, or by other diagnostic procedures. *The reason for giving extra points should be stated.* |
| | | Conversely, points may be withheld, when this seems to be the more realistic course. For example, the doctor who continues to talk while he auscultates a |

| Item | Points to be assigned | |
|------|------|------|

chest or who misses a clear abnormality in performing his examination should not receive credit for such work, even though he is going through the form of a complete examination. *Where such downgrading is done, it should be noted and the reason stated in the margin beside the examination involved.*

## III  LABORATORY PROCEDURES

The following refers to procedures which are done in the doctor's office or for which the doctor refers the patient elsewhere. If the referral is made for good indications, credit should be given for this.

| | | |
|---|---|---|
| 1. Haemoglobin | 0 | No haemoglobin determinations or Tallqvist method only. |
| | 1 | Done when indicated, by Sahli or other acceptable method. |
| 2. Urine | | |
| (a) chemical tests | 0 | Not done or done rarely or omission of protein or sugar. |
| | 1 | Frequent protein and sugar examinations. |
| (b) microscopic examination | 0 | Not done when indicated. |
| | 1 | Done when indicated. |
| 3. Diagnostic X-ray | 0 | No use of X-ray, no referral for X-ray, or unskilled use of X-ray and fluoroscopy (as indicated by improper operation of the machine, performance of procedures beyond the doctor's training and skill, or ordering of X-ray procedures in grossly inappropriate circumstances). |
| | 1 | Appropriate referrals for X-ray, proper operation of X-ray or fluoroscope, limitations on scope of work performed. |
| 4. Sterile technique | 0 | Breaks in technique; inadequate sterilization, as with alcohol or merthiolate; use of unsterilized needles, syringes, or stylettes. |
| | 1 | As below but instruments and hands not cleaned or syringe not sterilized between intracutaneous injections. |
| | 2 | Adequate boiling (15–30 minutes) or autoclaving of syringes, needles, and stylettes. Appropriate cleaning of other instruments and of hands. No gross breaks in technique. |

## IV  THERAPY

| | | |
|---|---|---|
| 1. Antibiotics and sulphonamides | 0 | Lack of knowledge of general principles for use of these drugs; indiscriminate use, inadequate dosage, inadequate duration of treatment, etc. |

| *Item* | *Points to be assigned* | |
|---|---|---|
| | 1 | Fair knowledge of general principles. |
| | 2 | Skilled use of these drugs, as evidenced by decisions regarding their use, dosage, duration, combinations of drugs, dangers of toxicity, emergence of resistant strains, etc. |
| 2. Obesity | 0 | Failure to recognize as a clinical problem; dietary advice inadequate. |
| | 1 | Recognized as a clinical problem and treated by adequate dietary explanation and support of morale. |
| 3. Potentially dangerous medications | 0 | No effort made to avoid drug reactions or complications. |
| | 1 | Awareness of possible toxicity of a drug. Inquiry about previous penicillin injections and reactions. Inquiry and testing before antitetanus serum. Proper supervision and advice with propylthiouracil, adrenocorticotrophic hormone, cortisone, chlorpromazine, etc. |
| 4. General therapeutic measures | 0 | Seldom or never advises regarding diet, bed rest, remaining indoors, etc. |
| | 1 | Consistent attention to these aspects of treatment. |

## V   OBSTETRICS*

| | | |
|---|---|---|
| 1. Follow-up schedule | 0 | If the doctor has no schedule of visits or makes no effort to have the patient make antenatal visits regularly and attend for a postnatal check. |
| | 1 | If more frequent visits near term or postnatal visit or both are omitted. |
| | 2 | If the doctor has an acceptable schedule of prenatal and postnatal visits and if the doctor makes an effort to convince the patient of the necessity for such visits. An acceptable schedule would be one visit per month until about the 28th week, visits at intervals of two to three weeks until about the 36th week, weekly visits thereafter until term, and a postnatal visit about six weeks after delivery. |
| 2. Follow-up investigation (i.e., at visits subsequent to the initial prenatal visit) | 0 | If blood pressure, urine, and weight are not examined at each visit. |
| | 1 | If, at each visit, blood pressure, urine, and weight are examined. |
| | 2 | If, at each visit: blood pressure, urine, and weight are examined; the uterus is pal- |

*Obstetrical items on which some observations were made but which could not be included in the rating scale have been listed in Table 70.

| *Item* | *Points to be assigned* | |
|---|---|---|

pated; later in pregnancy the foetal heart is auscultated; the patient is questioned about vaginal bleeding and symptoms of toxaemia.

## VI PREVENTIVE MEDICINE

1. Well-child care

0    No effort is made to educate parents as to need for immunization.

1    Has a schedule for immunizations. Makes an attempt to get children immunized. Preventive work is limited to immunization.

2    Superior preventive care. This should include a schedule of well-child examination and immunization, education of the parents, employment of special tests such as serological test for syphilis and tuberculin test when indicated, and routine inquiry about prior immunization and about diet in the case of new patients.

2. Health education

0    No effort is made to inculcate into patients a knowledge of general principles of maintenance of health.

1    Patients are advised regarding rest, diet, exercise, hobbies, advisability of periodic checkups, etc.

## VII RECORDS

0    If the only information recorded is medication, fees, or isolated data such as blood pressure in normotensive patients.

1    For scant records with minimal information about positive findings and medications.

2    For very good records. These should include all positive items of history and physical examination, including blood pressure and weight, results of laboratory work, and medications and other treatment. Special files on obstetric, paediatric, or other patients. Well-filled check sheets would tend to place a doctor in this group.

Table 72, in which the items of the rating scale are gathered together without the criteria for scoring, shows that 75 per cent of the points were for history-taking and physical examination, 7.5 per cent for laboratory work, 15 per cent for prevention and treatment, and 2.5 per cent for the keeping of clinical records. Because Peterson, in computing the scores of the North Carolina practitioners whom he studied,

TABLE 72

SCALE FOR RATING QUALITY OF PRACTICE

| Category | Item | Points | Percentage of total score |
|---|---|---|---|
| History-taking | | 30 | 37.50 |
| Physical examination | Disrobing | 1 | |
| | Temperature | 1 | |
| | Skin | 1 | |
| | Eyes—ophthalmoscopic | 1 | |
| | —other | 1 | |
| | Ears—otoscopic | 1 | |
| | Nose | 1 | |
| | Mouth and throat | 1 | |
| | Neck | 2 | |
| | Lymph nodes | 2 | |
| | Breasts | 1 | 30 | 37.50 |
| | Lungs—percussion | 1 | |
| | —auscultation | 2 | |
| | Heart | 2 | |
| | Blood pressure | 1 | |
| | Abdomen | 3 | |
| | Extremities | 1 | |
| | Nervous system | 2 | |
| | Rectum | 1 | |
| | Vagina | 1 | |
| | Over-all skill | 3 | |
| Laboratory work | Haemoglobin | 1 | |
| | Urine—chemical | 1 | |
| | —miscroscopic | 1 | 6 | 7.50 |
| | X-ray | 1 | |
| | Sterile technique | 2 | |
| Therapy | Antibiotics and sulphonamides | 2 | |
| | Obesity | 1 | |
| | Potentially dangerous medications | 1 | 5 | 6.25 |
| | General therapeutic measures | 1 | |
| Obstetrics | Follow-up schedule | 2 | |
| | Follow-up investigation | 2 | 4 | 5.00 |
| Preventive medicine | Well-child care | 2 | |
| | Health education | 1 | 3 | 3.75 |
| Records | | | 2 | 2.50 |
| Total points | | 80 | 100.00 |

did not exclude any of the items on which he was unable to assess some of the practitioners, our scale differs from his in the distribution of points among the three categories, history-taking, physical examination, and laboratory work. Peterson assigned 28 per cent, 32 per cent, and 24 per cent of the points, respectively, for these three categories (see his page 14), whereas, in our scale, history-taking and physical examination each received 37.5 per cent of the points but laboratory work only 7.5 per cent. The smaller percentage of points assigned for laboratory work is, in our opinion, a more accurate reflection of the importance of laboratory work in general practice in this country than is the percentage in Peterson's scale. Though some cases undoubtedly call for such tests as blood glucose determination, spinal tap, or bacteriological investigation of one sort or another, the vast majority of cases seen in the office and in the home require no laboratory tests other than haemoglobin determination, urinalysis, and diagnostic X-ray. Indeed, it was for this very reason that we were unable to assess so many practitioners on many of the other laboratory items. However, when the three categories, history-taking, physical examination, and laboratory work, are combined, we see that in each scale, Peterson's and ours, the combination of the three categories was given approximately the same percentage of the points.

Explaining the emphasis that was put on diagnosis, Peterson says (his pages 13–14):

A physician's first responsibility to his patient is to make a diagnosis. The well-tried methods for reaching this goal are by taking a history, performing a physical examination and the indicated laboratory work. These were accordingly used as the major criteria for classifying each practice. . . . Greatest importance was attached to the process of arriving at a diagnosis since, without a diagnosis, therapy cannot be rational. Furthermore, therapy is in the process of constant change, while the form of history and physical examination has changed very little over the years.

Peterson's statement that "without a diagnosis, therapy cannot be rational" must not, of course, be taken too literally, since sometimes it is necessary to prescribe symptomatic treatment before the cause of the symptoms is known, and the causes of some symptoms are never discovered. These exceptions to Peterson's statement were borne in mind, as the practices were being observed and assessed. In general, however, we may say that diagnosis is a prerequisite of rational therapy.

So essential is an understanding of this principle both to the carrying on of a practice of good quality and to a valid assessment of the quality of practice, that it is worthwhile to consider a clinical example. Headache, a very common complaint, may result from any one of a number of causes. Among these are eye strain, which is annoying but not a threat to a patient's life, and various types of brain tumour, which are of much more serious import. Though it may be possible in each of these cases to relieve the headache before its cause is known, the important thing is to discover and, if possible, to remove the cause of the symptom, i.e. to remove the tumour or to banish the eye strain by means of appropriate glasses. A patient himself is able to deal, on a purely symptomatic level, with many of his headaches. He takes acetylsalicylic acid or some other mild analgesic, which relieves the symptom but has no effect on the cause of it. This type of first aid or of "home medicine" amounts to gambling that the condition is not serious. For a patient to take such an approach to his own symptoms is quite natural, since many of his symptoms are relatively inconsequential. However, if a physician to whom the patient goes for professional advice adopts the same attitude, this can only be regarded as poor medicine. The physician has no right to gamble that the patient's symptom is due to some trivial cause. It is the physician's responsibility to make an effort to discover what is causing the symptom and in particular to satisfy himself that the patient is not suffering from one of the more serious causes of the particular symptom.

What we have just said is so fundamental and may seem so obvious that we may be accused of being either naive or condescending in making so explicit a statement of a physician's responsibility. Yet the fact is that repeatedly we saw practitioners making either an inadequate attempt or no attempt to discover the cause of a patient's complaint. For example, a young woman who complained of headache was asked one question, the location of the headache. When she replied that it was in the forehead, the doctor, without further questions and without *any* examination, said that she had acute sinusitis. This may well have been so, but it was not established by the doctor with any degree of certainty.

Another patient, a woman thirty-two years of age, complained that she tired easily. She had made her own "diagnosis" of anaemia and asked for "iron pills." She looked healthy and of good colour to the observer. The doctor took no history, did no examination, and did not do a haemoglobin determination. He gave her the "iron pills" but did not arrange for any follow-up visit. Whether this woman had anaemia and, if so, whether it was an iron-deficiency anaemia, we did not know. Nor did the practitioner know, because he did not carry out the investigation that was necessary if he was either to establish or to exclude the diagnosis of iron-deficiency anaemia. The medication given *may* have been the correct one—but only by chance—or the patient's symptom may have been the result of any one of a number of causes, physical or psychological, that would be unresponsive to iron.

Thus, although Peterson's dictum, quoted above, that "without a diagnosis, therapy cannot be rational," seems so basic as not to need labouring, it is evident from our examples that some practitioners are so little aware of the importance of diagnosis that they prescribe treatment with only a token attempt, or even with no attempt, to reach a diagnosis. When the treatment is correct by chance, credit for practising medicine of good quality should be given, not to the doctor, but to chance. On the other hand, to a physician whose treatment follows logically from adequate investigation of a patient's complaint, great credit is due for practising medicine of a high calibre. By now, it should be clear that the main reason for attaching more importance to a physician's diagnostic efforts than to treatment is that the latter is dependent on the former. An additional reason, important in a rating scale of this type, is that there is much more room for controversy about treatment, even when the diagnosis is certain, than about the long-established methods of diagnosis.

The assessing of the practices must now be considered in more detail. In the first paragraph of the rating scale, it is stated that the scale is "to be applied to *new patients*, patients with *new illnesses*, patients requesting a checkup, or patients whose complaint, history, appearance, or attitude would indicate the *need* for careful history and examination." Emphasis is put on the word "new" because it is in new illnesses, and especially with new patients, that a good history and a thorough examination are needed. With a patient who was seen last week or yesterday, there is no need, except in special circumstances, to repeat the history, and often only certain parts of the examination need be repeated. Another reason why the word "new" is emphasized at the head of the rating scale is that, in withholding points for important omissions, we had to be certain that the item of investigation or treatment had not been performed in the recent past. Part of what we said in chapter 2 (page 19) in our general description of the method we consider sufficiently important to repeat:

Whenever there was any reasonable doubt, we refused to use that particular case in arriving at the score; and, if the discarded evidence was all that we had on which to evaluate the doctor's practice in regard to a certain item, we marked that item "Not assessable." Because of these difficulties, we attached the greatest importance, in the scoring, to new illnesses or, even better, to new patients, since in these cases we were on an even footing with the doctor.

The other word that is stressed in the instructions at the head of the rating scale is the word, "need." We pointed out earlier at some length (pages 20–21) that, in assessing what a doctor did, we were guided by the need of his patient. Thus we did not require that a comprehensive history and general physical examination should be done when a patient came in with a broken finger or a dermatitis caused by poison ivy. Rather, we considered what was required in each case if the cause of the patient's symptoms were to be discovered and the proper treatment to be instituted.

When an examination was confined to one region, credit was given for the examination if it was satisfactory. For example, if a patient presented himself with an injury of the hand, and the doctor examined for fractures, dislocations, and the various soft tissue injuries, the doctor was given credit for his examination under the item, extremities. In such a case, examination of other parts was not required, unless there was some definite reason for such further examination. There was, however, one type of circumstance in which credit was not given for examination of a single part of the body, namely, when a patient was so specific in his request that the fact that the doctor performed the examination gave no information about the quality of his practice. For example, when a mother says, "Please look in Johnnie's ear. I think he's put something in it," and the doctor complies, he is not demonstrating any knowledge of medicine. On the other hand, when the mother says, "Johnnie has a cold," and the doctor says, "I want to have at look at his ears," he is demonstrating his awareness of infection of the middle ear as a complication of upper respiratory infections. Again, though the patient (mentioned above) with the injured hand indicates the part he wishes examined, the details of the examination are left to the physician, who is thereby afforded an opportunity to demonstrate his knowledge and skill.

Certain parts of a physician's work can safely be delegated to persons who are not trained as physicians. When a patient was referred to a hospital laboratory for a particular test, we gave credit for the item (provided that it was ordered in appropriate circumstances), on the assumption that the hospital's technician was adequately qualified for the work. When the laboratory work was delegated to a member of the doctor's office staff, we observed her way of doing the work just as we observed the doctor when he did the laboratory work himself. Again, if temperatures were taken by a nurse or secretary and reported to the doctor, credit was given just as though the practitioner himself had taken the temperature.

Because we were not entirely satisfied with the part of the scale that had to do with history-taking (see page 266), we attempted to break this down into a number of constituent items and to assess the practitioner's proficiency in each of these. These items were history of present complaint, possible diagnoses, complications, functional inquiry, past history, family history, and unusual skill or thoroughness. Because of the overlapping of the various items, this method did not prove satisfactory by itself, but it served as a useful check on the scores that were assigned by the method described above.

We cannot illustrate all the grades of history-taking that existed between the poorest and the best, but we shall give examples of the three broad categories described in the rating scale. Before doing so, we must make clear that each of these histories is the history of only one of the many patients seen by the doctor during our visit and that, in assigning the score for history-taking, we took into account all the examples of the doctor's history-taking that were observed by us. Some men almost always did a functional inquiry and asked about past history and family illnesses; others almost never asked about these things. Between, there were intermediate grades. There were men who usually made these inquiries or some of them but, at times, omitted them; and there were others who usually did not make such inquiries but did now and then. In assigning the scores, we bore in mind the frequency with which the various inquiries were made and the relative importance of the information in the cases in which inquiry was made and in the cases in which inquiry was not made. From these comments, it must be apparent that this method of assessing history-taking is by no means precise. Yet, as the following histories will show, history-taking varied so greatly in quality that this method is thought to give a reasonable measure of a physician's ability to take histories.

A man in his mid-fifties was seen in a practitioner's office. He had been seen by this doctor in the past but not for his present symptoms. He complained of a cough and of numbness and tingling in the lower limbs. Each symptom had been present for three months. The doctor first asked questions designed to bring forth information about the cough. He discovered that the patient had had a cough for years—the patient called it "smoker's cough," attributed it to the fact that he smoked one and a half packages of cigarettes daily, and said that it occurred mainly in the morning. But the cough for which he sought the doctor's advice was different. Its onset had been gradual, unaccompanied by anything resembling either "a cold" or "flu." It had become worse, until now the patient was wakened at night and was racked throughout the day by paroxysms of coughing. There was no pain associated with the cough, but the area beneath the sternum "felt raw." The cough was productive of yellow sputum, about a cupful daily, without any blood in it. There was no shortness of breath at night or on exertion. The patient had had no night sweats. He had lost eight pounds in the previous two months. He had never had any chest disease before. In the patient's family, there was no history of chest disease, including tuberculosis about which the doctor inquired specifically. Questioning brought to light the fact that the patient's occupation exposed him to a great deal of silica dust, that ventilation in the work area was poor, and that a mask was not worn. One man in the same establishment was said to have died of tuberculosis and silicosis.

Then, turning his attention to the patient's complaint of numbness and tingling in the lower extremities, the doctor asked whether both limbs were affected equally and was told that they were. The tingling was present only at times and showed no particular pattern. The feet were never cold, nor did the limbs ever feel very hot. Walking produced no pain in the calves. There had never been any sharp pain in the limbs. There had been no previous trouble with the limbs.

The history was concluded with questions about headache, sleep, chest pain on exertion, swelling of the lower limbs, diet, regularity of bowel function, colour and consistency of stools, ease and frequency of urination, colour of urine, past illnesses, and current illness of other persons in the patient's home. From this the doctor went on to physical examination and other forms of investigation. This excellent history, taken by a doctor whose score for history-taking was between 21 and 30 points, i.e. in the top third of the range, illustrates the systematic type of approach that brings out the important facts quickly and reduces the risk of the physician's missing information of importance.

In marked contrast with this was the history obtained by another physician in another new case. The patient was a girl in her teens, who said that she had been sent by her mother because she felt tired and had lost three pounds recently. The doctor did not ask any questions, did not make an examination, and did not carry out any laboratory work. He prescribed a "tonic." The histories taken by this physician, though not all of the calibre of the one just reported, were consistently poor, dealing in an inadequate manner with the presenting complaint and only occasionally including one or two other questions. The score assigned was between 0 and 10 points.

Another example of a history belonging to the bottom third of the scale concerns a three-month-old baby, whose mother said that the baby had not slept the previous night and had been vomiting. The doctor asked one question, whether the vomiting was projectile.

On being told that it was, he did not make sure that the mother understood what he meant by this word, did not ask how long the vomiting had gone on and whether it was related to the intake of food, and did not inquire about any associated symptoms, such as constipation or diarrhoea, loss of appetite, irritability, nasal discharge, cough, etc. The mother volunteered that the baby had lost one pound in the previous month. After a perfunctory examination of the abdomen and in spite of not finding the pyloric tumour for which he was searching, the doctor continued to talk of the possibility of pyloric stenosis and gave no evidence of considering any other diagnosis. His treatment was a change of formula and a prescription for phenobarbitone and atropine. He made no provision for seeing this patient again.

Our next history is of the type for which a score of between 11 and 20 points would be given. The patient, an elderly man, complained that for about a year he had had episodes of dizziness and of falling. In answer to a question, he said that the episodes of falling had come on "more recently" than the dizziness. The attacks of dizziness sometimes came on while the patient was working. They might occur while the patient was standing, sitting, or lying down. The doctor elicited the fact that, by "dizziness," the patient did not mean light-headedness but a sensation that he was whirling around in relation to his external environment. The doctor inquired about ringing in the ears and was told that there had not been any. No questions were asked about the frequency of either of the symptoms, about the severity or duration of the dizziness, or whether there was a tendency to fall in one particular direction. No inquiry was made about headache, vomiting, weakness or paralysis, abnormal sensations (other than dizziness), unconsciousness, convulsions, visual disturbances, disorientation, or other disorders of mental function. No questions were asked about the other major organ systems or about past illnesses, though the latter may have been known to the doctor. In this case, more information was obtained than in either of the two preceding cases, but so many pertinent questions were left unasked that the picture of the patient's disorder remained very incomplete.

The value of questioning a patient more than once, if it seemed necessary, was brought out by a doctor who had a young man in hospital for investigation of tarry stools. The doctor questioned him in detail each morning, though he had taken a history in his office before the patient was admitted to hospital. His repeated questions had to do with previous "indigestion." Finally, on the third morning, the patient said that, after the previous day's visit, he had recalled that, about two years previously, he had had troublesome indigestion for about a week; and, without being asked any leading questions, he volunteered the information that he would take a glass of milk and the pain would go away for about two hours. Going down the corridor, the doctor remarked, "See, it pays to go over the history again and again. He didn't tell me that in the office, and he didn't tell me that here until today." X-rays showed evidence of a duodenal ulcer. Because the radiographic finding reduced the importance of the history in this particular case, it must not be supposed that history-taking in general is not as important as this doctor believed, since in this same case X-ray examination might have failed to disclose the ulcer and in another case the information sought by questioning might not be obtainable by any other method.

The items of physical examination and of laboratory work on which the practitioners were assessed are listed in Table 72, and the criteria on which the assessments were based have already been stated (pages 266–269). It is not necessary to discuss these criteria in detail, except to make one thing clear, namely, the circumstances in which we expected a particular item of examination or of laboratory work to be done. We have already given an example—an injury of the hand—of a case in which a localized examination would be considered adequate. We shall now give additional examples of circumstances in which it would be considered that one or another of the items of investigation should be performed.

It was not expected that the temperature of every patient would be taken, since in many cases this information would be of no value whatever to the doctor, either in making his diagnosis or in following the course of the patient's condition. It did seem reasonable, however, to expect that temperatures would be taken in cases of infection of various sorts, except those that were obviously localized.

The commonest reason for which the point for ophthalmoscopic examination was withheld was failure of the practitioner to use the ophthalmoscope on his hypertensive patients. Since a patient who had been seen by the doctor a short time before our visit might have had an ophthalmoscopic examination at that time, we based our assessment of this item on new patients or on old patients who were said not to have been seen for a long time. There were other circumstances, also, in which we thought it reasonable to expect an ophthalmoscopic examination to be performed, for example when there was any question of a space-occupying lesion causing intracranial pressure.

Examination of the ears with the otoscope was expected in the case of an adult complaining of earache, and in the case of a young child with respiratory infection because of the frequency of infection of the middle ear as a complication of respiratory infections in this age group.

Examination of the several groups of lymph nodes was considered to be indicated in cases in which there was any question of such diseases as leukaemia or infectious mononucleosis. On the other hand, in cases of localized infection or malignancy, examination of the nodes related to that particular region was accepted as sufficient.

Examination of the breasts was required as a routine when a general physical examination was performed, because cancer of the breast is of such common occurrence and yet, in many cases, can be detected while still quite small without the use of any equipment other than the physician's own eyes and hands. Similarly, because of the frequent occurrence of cancer of the rectum and of the cervix, rectal and vaginal examinations were considered to be indicated in patients over forty of years of age when a general physical examination was being done. It is hardly necessary to specify that we did not expect these examinations to be done if a patient came in for treatment of some minor complaint that did not call for a general physical examination.

When the physician did not auscultate the chest at all, in circumstances that called for auscultation, or when he attempted to auscultate through the patient's clothing, his score was 0. One practitioner, though commonly examining the front of a patient's chest, never in a period of three days examined the back of the chest, even though one of his patients was suffering from pneumonia. He was given 1 point, out of 2, for partial auscultation of the lungs.

The point for determining blood pressure was given unless the practitioner omitted to do this examination in circumstances in which it was definitely of importance, or unless he carried out the procedure in such a rapid, or otherwise unsatisfactory, manner that it was obvious that he could not have obtained accurate systolic and diastolic readings, or unless he indicated, by recording only the systolic pressure, that he was not interested in the diastolic pressure.

The point for disrobing was withheld only if the physician, habitually or in particularly important circumstances, attempted to carry out an examination with the part so inadequately exposed that a proper examination was impossible. For example, a woman of seventy-six complained of swelling of the feet, towards the end of each day, and shortness of breath. Though the doctor remarked to the observer that he should have examined, not only the heart, but also the lungs and the liver, he confined himself to auscultation of the heart with the stethoscope pushed down between the patient's chest and tightly-fitting clothing. By this method it is almost impossible to reach all the valve areas with the stethoscope; and the auscultation of the small area that can be reached is usually unsatisfactory because of the adventitious noises that are caused by the patient's clothing rubbing on the tubing of the stethoscope.

Haemoglobin determinations and urinalyses were not demanded as a routine; but, when the appropriate tests were not carried out on patients possibly suffering from such conditions as anaemia, diabetes, or urinary tract infections, the point was withheld because one or another of these tests is specifically needed in the investigation of patients with these conditions.

The point for diagnostic X-ray would be withheld if the practitioner failed to order films to be taken in cases in which fractures seemed likely. One doctor saw a man who had dropped a heavy block of wood on his great toe. The toe was greatly swollen, blue, and tender. No X-ray was ordered, and the patient was told to continue to walk on his foot. The same physician saw another man whose car had overturned and dropped ten feet off the highway. Two other occupants of the car had landed on the patient. The patient complained of tenderness in the supraclavicular and infraclavicular fossae and marked limitation of movements at the shoulder. No X-ray was ordered at the first visit and a diagnosis of a "cracked first rib" was made. When the patient returned the next day and complained that he was no better, an X-ray was ordered. The physician was marked 0 for X-ray, because it was apparent that only reluctantly did he make use of X-ray, even for patients with quite severe injuries, which could well be fractures.

In certain situations, it was considered that the use of diagnostic X-ray was not justified. For example, a girl in her teens complained of severe constipation of gradual onset and of three months' duration. Laxatives, of unstated type, had been used. They had been effective at first, but their effectiveness had decreased. The bowels had last moved five days previously, when a "small, hard motion" was passed. No inquiry was made regarding abdominal pain or distention, pain on passage of the stools, the presence of blood in the stools, or vomiting. There were no questions about diet, about toilet habits, about previous difficulty of this or any other type, or about psychological factors. The doctor examined the abdomen and performed a rectal examination. The abdomen was not distended. The large bowel, from the middle of the transverse colon down to, and including, the rectum, was found to be filled with hard masses of faeces. This patient was admitted to hospital to have the bowel cleaned out and to have a barium enema and radiological examination of the large bowel. So eminent an authority as Nelson, in discussing constipation in children, says, "Roentgenologic examinations are rarely necessary. . . . A simple enema may be all that is necessary in acute constipation. If the feces are hard or if there is impaction, . . . mineral oil may first be injected and allowed to remain for a few hours. . . . In the treatment of chronic constipation attention should be given to the cause, which is usually a faulty diet or faulty bowel habits."*

Another physician told us that, in all cases in which *any* type of radiological investigation was indicated for an abdominal symptom, he had a gastro-intestinal series, a barium enema, and a gallbladder series done. He said that he did this even though the history seemed typical of duodenal ulcer in a young man. In his practice, we saw all three types of examination ordered for just such a patient, a man in his late twenties who had a *proven* duodenal ulcer. The doctor's reason for doing this was to avoid missing something. He mentioned, also, that the hospital had a special reduced rate if all three examinations were ordered at the same time.

Each of these two physicians was given 0 for X-ray. Leaving out of consideration the unnecessary expense for the patient, we believed that each of the patients was being exposed unnecessarily to radiation, particularly in view of the relatively long exposure that is inevitable since the fluoroscope is used in the examination of the gastro-intestinal tract.

In the matter of sterile technique, our attention was directed mainly to whether the syringes and needles were adequately sterilized. We expected that they would be boiled or autoclaved. When the doctor removed a syringe from a case containing alcohol, gave the patient an injection, rinsed the syringe with tap water, put it back in the alcohol, and then used it for another patient, his score for sterile technique was automatically 0. In some cases, the doctors may have been unaware of the danger of transmitting the serum hepatitis virus. Others, however, told us that they were aware of the possibility but were willing to take the risk, by which they meant that they were willing to subject their patients to an unnecessary risk. Again, if the doctor used an ear speculum on a patient whose ear was discharging

*Waldo E. Nelson: Textbook of Pediatrics (7th ed., Philadelphia and London: W. B. Saunders Company, 1959), p. 653.

pus and then, without cleansing the speculum, used it in other patients' ears, we gave the intermediate score of 1 point. We reduced the score from 2 points to 1, also, when any physician used his oral thermometer on successive patients with no attempt to cleanse it other than by wiping it on the patient's sheets. On the other hand, we considered it unrealistic to deduct any points because a practitioner did not daub the skin with alcohol, or some other "disinfectant," before he removed sutures, even though this is standard procedure in some hospitals.

It was possible to include in the diagnostic part of the rating scale a large proportion of the commonly used procedures, but this was not possible with the therapeutic part of the scale. With a dozen different cases, though the emphasis placed on the different methods of investigation may vary from case to case, a physician's diagnostic approach is *basically* the same—the taking of a history, the examination of the patient, and laboratory investigation. On the other hand, each one of the twelve cases may present quite a different problem from the point of view of treatment. For this reason, no scale could possibly anticipate all the therapeutic problems that even one physician might encounter in two or three days, nor is it possible to pick a large number of problems and be certain that they will occur in every practice, or even in the majority of the practices, during the observation period of three days. This is illustrated by the fact that even such common conditions as anaemia, hypertension, and cardiac failure, on the handling of which we attempted to assess the practitioners, did not occur in enough of the practices for us to retain them in the rating scale when we were computing the doctors' scores.

Each of the four items of therapeutics that were included in the definitive rating scale had to do with a different aspect of treatment. The items called "antibiotics and sulphonamides" and "potentially dangerous medications" were both tests of specific, detailed knowledge; but, with the former item, we were concerned mainly with the doctor's ability to use certain drugs effectively, whereas, with the latter, we considered whether he made an effort to avoid causing trouble by his use of drugs. The other two items, "general therapeutic measures" and "obesity," gave us an opportunity to observe whether the doctor paid attention to those aspects of treatment that seem less precise, more diffuse, and perhaps less easy to describe to a patient than the specific details of drug therapy. The one item, "obesity," was concerned with a specific problem; the other, "general therapeutic measures," was included because we felt that sometimes, in this era of *specific* therapeutic agents, the *non-specific* aspects of treatment, such as advice on diet, rest, remaining indoors, etc., are forgotten or ignored.

In considering the use of antibiotics and sulphonamides, we did not demand any arbitrary routine. We tried, instead, to determine whether the physician was aware of, and was guided by, the generally accepted principles in his use of these agents. One physician, for instance, ordered these drugs in adequate dosages and usually for a reasonable duration, but gave them for certain conditions on which they would have no effect. Thus, he gave a dose of penicillin to a young adult the morning following what he diagnosed, probably correctly, as acute food poisoning. He had given penicillin, also, for an undiagnosed infection in a child of about two years of age; and, when the patient's temperature subsided and a rash, which the doctor recognized as that of roseola infantum, appeared, he continued the penicillin. Because he showed a knowledge of some of the principles but used these drugs for conditions for which they could not be effective, he was given 1 point out of 2.

Another doctor saw two patients for whom he prescribed drugs of this type. One was a girl of eight with sore throat, earache, and a temperature of 100°F. She was given an intramuscular injection of penicillin and streptomycin. The next day, her temperature was normal, and no further medication was given. The other patient, a man of twenty-five, complained of sore throat and difficulty in swallowing and talking. His temperature was 101°F. He was given an injection of penicillin and streptomycin intramuscularly; and tablets of triple sulphonamide were prescribed, without a loading dose. The patient was seen again two days later, was given another injection of the two antibiotics, and was told to continue to take the sulphonamide. The doctor said that he should have come the day before to give the second injection but had been busy and "frankly" had forgotten. This practitioner's use of these drugs illustrates several errors. He frequently used combinations of two or three drugs for conditions for which one drug, at the most, was required. In the former of the two cases, if he was correct in using an antimicrobial agent, then he was wrong in discontinuing treatment after one day, merely because the temperature had returned to normal. With the second patient he showed a casualness that was incongruous with his use of three drugs at the same time. For these reasons, he was given a score of 0 out of 2 points for his use of sulphonamides and antibiotics.

The remaining portions of the rating scale—obstetrics, preventive medicine, and records—do not call for any comment beyond the criteria of assessment that have already been stated (pages 270–271), but a few words must be said about surgery and psychiatry. No attempt was made to include surgical items in the rating scale, both because we expected—correctly, as it turned out—that we should not see enough surgery in three days to enable us to assess it and because we did not consider ourselves competent to assess the finer details of surgical technique. The few observations that we were able to make will be described in the next chapter. In an attempt to evaluate the practitioner's handling of psychiatric problems, we sought advice from a number of qualified psychiatrists and made up a rating scale that we hoped would give a reasonable measure of the practitioner's ability; but our attempt to evaluate this part of the physician's work was unsuccessful. Our lack of success we attribute partly to the diffuseness of psychiatry, partly to the fact that the observers' training in, and experience with, psychiatry were inadequate to allow assessments to be made with sufficient accuracy to justify their inclusion in the rating scale, and partly to the observers' lack of information about the particular patients. Some general observations were made and will be discussed in the next chapter.

In describing our method of assessing the doctors' practices, we have not been able to deal with all the situations that we met, because these were numberless. We have given examples, however, to indicate the way in which we approached the problem of assigning the scores and to make clear the standard with which we compared the practices.

In addition to assigning scores for the individual items in the rating scale, we classified the practitioners into five groups on the basis of our over-all opinions of the quality of their practices. To those in the group that was the poorest in quality we gave 1 point; to those with practices that we regarded as excellent we gave 5 points; and to those between the two extremes, either 2, 3, or 4 points. In every case, these points were assigned before we knew what the physician's total score was on the detailed rating scale. These 5 points were thus a completely separate method of rating. We chose, however, to use the scores obtained by the detailed rating scale because, with this method, many different grades of work are distinguished, whereas, since the scores based on over-all impression allow only five grades, the individual score may be in error by a greater amount than with the more detailed method of scoring. Our reason for referring at all to the five-point method is that in each province, Ontario and Nova Scotia, the correlation between the total scores assigned according to the rating scale and the scores assigned according to our over-all impression is very high, the correlation coefficients being 0.956 in the case of Ontario and 0.947 in the case of Nova Scotia.*

In our general description, in chapter 2, of the assessment of the quality of practice, we enunciated certain principles to which we adhered in applying the rating scale (see pages 17–21). Since these principles constituted an integral part of the method, it is essential that the reader have them in mind when he comes, in the next chapter, to consider our observations on quality of practice. Briefly restated, the principles were that our object was to discover, not what the practitioner *could* do under special or artificial circumstances, but what he was actually doing in his practice; that, in deciding doubtful points, we gave the benefit of the doubt to the practitioner; that we made every effort to keep our standard of assessment as unvarying as possible; and that, in making our evaluations of quality of practice, we compared what the physician did, not with any arbitrary or artificial standard of academic medicine, but with what was required for the welfare of the patient.

*A correlation coefficient of 1.0 would indicate a perfect correlation.

# 17 / The Quality of General Practice
## *Observations*

The present chapter, to which all the preceding ones have led up and from which, in turn, the succeeding ones will follow, presupposes that the reader has a clear picture of the method that was used to assess the quality of practice. The method has been described in general terms in chapter 2 and in detail in chapter 16. It is suggested that any reader who may, for one or another reason, have omitted these chapters read them now, before he continues with the present chapter, unless he is willing to take the latter on trust.

In reporting our observations on the quality of general practice, we shall, as far as it is practicable, follow the order in which the items are grouped in the rating scale (pages 265–271): history-taking, physical examination, laboratory work, therapy, obstetrics, preventive medicine, and records. The great variation that we encountered in history-taking is indicated by the fact that, in Ontario, the lowest score for this was 5 points out of 30 (i.e., 17 per cent of the points) and the highest score was 30 points (i.e., 100 per cent) and, in Nova Scotia, the lowest and highest were 3 points (10 per cent) and 28 points (93 per cent), respectively. Every one of the doctors took some history, though some men's history-taking was of such extremely poor calibre as to be almost worthless. Of this type of history and of the high degree of excellence at the other end of the scale, we have given examples in the preceding chapter. Our observations on history-taking are summarized in Table 73. In Ontario, 44 per cent of the practitioners had scores of more than 60 per cent for history-taking, 19 per cent had scores of between 41 and 60 per cent, and the remaining 37 per cent had scores of 40 per

TABLE 73

SCORES OF ONTARIO AND NOVA SCOTIA PHYSICIANS FOR HISTORY-TAKING

| Score assigned for history-taking (percentage of total points for history-taking) | Ontario physicians | | Nova Scotia physicians | |
|---|---|---|---|---|
| | Number | % | Number | % |
| 0–20 | 6 | 14.0 | 16 | 38.1 |
| 21–40 | 10 | 23.3 | 8 | 19.0 |
| 41–60 | 8 | 18.6 | 6 | 14.3 |
| 61–80 | 13 | 30.2 | 7 | 16.7 |
| 81–100 | 6 | 14.0 | 5 | 11.9 |
| Total physicians | 43 | 100 | 42 | 100 |

cent or less. In Nova Scotia, 29 per cent had scores of more than 60 per cent, 14 per cent had scores of between 41 and 60 per cent, and 57 per cent had scores of 40 per cent or less for history-taking. Those who had scores of more than 60 per cent were all considered satisfactory as far as history-taking was concerned. Some of them, especially the 14 per cent in Ontario and the 12 per cent in Nova Scotia whose scores were over 80 per cent, were excellent. Those whose scores were 40 per cent or less were regarded as unsatisfactory. It may be that some of these men took poor histories because of lack of time. In many practices, however, the cause of the poor history-taking appeared to be either that the doctors had never learnt *how* to take an adequate history (some men were obviously bewildered as to what question to ask next, and one physician, who complained repeatedly about having to complete the records on his hospital cases, said that he did not know what was meant by the terms, "functional inquiry" and "psychic," which appeared on the hospital's history forms) or had never truly learnt, i.e. had never accepted in more than a superficial way, the *necessity* of taking a good history. The history-taking ability of those whose scores were between 41 and 60 per cent lay in the no man's land between what was definitely satisfactory and what was definitely unsatisfactory.

On physical examination, the doctors' scores were as shown in Tables 74, 75, and 76 (see page 292). In Tables 74 and 75, which deal with Ontario and Nova Scotia respectively, the items are listed in decreasing order of the percentage of doctors receiving the full score for the particular item. Thus at the head of the list, in each table, is the item, blood pressure, the taking of which was satisfactory in 98 per cent of the Ontario practices and in 86 per cent of the Nova Scotia practices, and at the bottom of the list of specific items in each table is an item for which only 9 or 10 per cent of the practitioners received the full

TABLE 74

Scores of Ontario Physicians for Individual Items of Physical Examination

| Item of examination | Number assessed | Physicians | | |
|---|---|---|---|---|
| | | Percentage of those assessed who were awarded: | | |
| | | No points | Partial score (where applicable) | Full score |
| Blood pressure | 43 | 2.3 | — | 97.7 |
| Temperature | 42 | 2.4 | — | 97.6 |
| Ears—otoscopic | 43 | 4.7 | — | 95.3 |
| Vagina | 35 | 11.4 | — | 88.6 |
| Disrobing | 43 | 16.3 | — | 83.7 |
| Extremities | 38 | 18.4 | — | 81.6 |
| Nose | 38 | 23.7 | — | 76.3 |
| Lungs—auscultation | 43 | 11.6 | 18.6 | 69.8 |
| Mouth and throat | 43 | 39.5 | — | 60.5 |
| Skin | 39 | 41.0 | — | 59.0 |
| Abdomen—other than inguinal rings and external genitalia | 43 | 14.0 | 39.5 | 46.5 |
| Rectum | 34 | 58.8 | — | 41.2 |
| Eyes—other than ophthalmoscopic | 43 | 62.8 | — | 37.2 |
| —ophthalmoscopic | 43 | 69.8 | — | 30.2 |
| Lungs—percussion | 43 | 69.8 | — | 30.2 |
| Breasts | 40 | 70.0 | — | 30.0 |
| Neck | 42 | 9.5 | 66.7 | 23.8 |
| Nervous system | 43 | 55.8 | 23.3 | 20.9* |
| Abdomen—inguinal rings and external genitalia (male) | 41 | 82.9 | — | 17.1 |
| Heart | 43 | 32.6 | 55.8 | 11.6 |
| Lymph nodes | 43 | 51.2 | 39.5 | 9.3 |
| Over-all skill | 43 | 67.4 | 32.6† | 0.0 |

*These 9 physicians include 3 who could be assessed only on the lst of the 2 points.
†Of these physicians, half received 1 point, the other half 2 points, out of the 3 points that were possible.

score. On examining Tables 74 and 75, one is struck by the fact that, in Ontario and in Nova Scotia, only about one-half and one-third, respectively, of the items of physical examination were performed satisfactorily by 50 per cent or more of the doctors visited. These items were, both in Ontario and in Nova Scotia, the taking of blood pressure and of temperature, disrobing of the patient, examination of the ears with the otoscope, examination of the vagina, and examination of the extremities; in Ontario but not in Nova Scotia, examination of the nose, mouth and throat, and skin, and auscultation of the lungs; and, in Nova Scotia but not in Ontario, the examination of the neck. Those items that were done unsatisfactorily by more than 50 per cent of the doctors included, in each province, abdominal examination, rectal

TABLE 75

| | | Physicians | | |
| | | Percentage of those assessed who were awarded: | | |
| Item of examination | Number assessed | No points | Partial score (where applicable) | Full score |
|---|---|---|---|---|
| Blood pressure | 42 | 14.3 | — | 85.7 |
| Disrobing | 42 | 33.3 | — | 66.7 |
| Extremities | 40 | 35.0 | — | 65.0 |
| Ears—otoscopic | 42 | 35.7 | — | 64.3 |
| Vagina | 36 | 38.9 | — | 61.1 |
| Neck | 42 | 14.3* | 28.6 | 57.1† |
| Temperature | 42 | 42.9 | — | 57.1 |
| Nose | 39 | 51.3 | — | 48.7 |
| Rectum | 34 | 55.9 | — | 44.1 |
| Lungs—auscultation | 42 | 14.3 | 42.9 | 42.9 |
| Mouth and throat | 42 | 59.5 | — | 40.5 |
| Abdomen—other than inguinal rings and external genitalia | 42 | 19.0 | 42.9 | 38.1 |
| Lungs—percussion | 42 | 61.9 | — | 38.1 |
| Eyes—other than ophthalmoscopic | 41 | 63.4 | — | 36.6 |
| Heart | 42 | 35.7 | 35.7 | 28.6 |
| Skin | 32 | 71.9 | — | 28.1 |
| Nervous system | 39 | 61.5‡ | 17.9 | 20.5 |
| Lymph nodes | 42 | 33.3 | 50.0 | 16.7‡ |
| Abdomen—inguinal rings and external genitalia (male) | 40 | 85.0 | — | 15.0 |
| Breasts | 38 | 89.5 | — | 10.5 |
| Eyes—ophthalmoscopic | 41 | 90.2 | — | 9.8 |
| Over-all skill | 42 | 78.6 | 19.0§ | 2.4 |

*These physicians include 2 who could be assessed only on the first of the 2 points.
†These physicians include 4 who could be assessed only on the first of the 2 points.
‡These physicians include 1 who could be assessed only on the first of the 2 points.
§Of these 8 physicians, 5 received 1 point and the other 3 received 2 points out of the 3 points that were possible.

examination, percussion of the lungs, the examination of breasts, lymph nodes, and nervous system, and the examination (both ophthalmoscopic and other) of the eyes; in Ontario, the examination of the neck; and, in Nova Scotia, auscultation of the lungs and examination of the nose, mouth and throat, and skin. It will be noted that, though only 12 per cent of the Ontario doctors and 29 per cent of the Nova Scotia doctors were awarded 2 points for examination of the heart, 67 per cent in Ontario and 64 per cent in Nova Scotia received at least 1 point. Since 1 point was given for auscultating at all the valve areas, whereas 2 points called for the use of percussion or palpation in

TABLE 76

SCORES OF ONTARIO AND NOVA SCOTIA PHYSICIANS FOR
PHYSICAL EXAMINATION

| Score assigned for physical examination (percentage of total points on which the physician was assessed)* | Ontario physicians | | Nova Scotia physicians | |
|---|---|---|---|---|
| | Number | % | Number | % |
| 0–20 | 3 | 7.0 | 4 | 9.5 |
| 21–40 | 11 | 25.6 | 20 | 47.6 |
| 41–60 | 14 | 32.6 | 9 | 21.4 |
| 61–80 | 11 | 25.6 | 3 | 7.1 |
| 81–100 | 4 | 9.3 | 6 | 14.3 |
| Total physicians | 43 | 100 | 42 | 100 |

*In Ontario, 23 doctors were scored out of the full 30 points, 9 doctors out of 29 points, 4 doctors out of 28 points, 4 doctors out of 27 points, 2 doctors out of 26 points, and 1 doctor out of 25 points. In Nova Scotia, 14 doctors were scored out of the full 30 points, 14 doctors out of 29 points, 7 doctors out of 28 points, 6 doctors out of 27 points, and 1 doctor out of 25 points.

addition to auscultation, the situation in respect of cardiac examination, though leaving a good deal to be desired, was not as unsatisfactory as the small percentage awarded 2 points might, at first sight, suggest.

A few words are in order about the partial scores that were awarded for other items of physical examination. In the case of abdominal examination, 1 point was given for a perfunctory examination on a reclining patient. Since the assessments were based on observations of cases in which thorough abdominal examinations were indicated, we believe that the percentages (47 in Ontario and 38 in Nova Scotia) shown for those who received 2 points for abdominal examination (other than inguinal rings and external genitalia) indicate fairly the percentages of doctors who performed satisfactory examinations of the abdomen. Since neck examination was given 1 point when examination was limited to the submaxillary lymph nodes, the 67 per cent in Ontario and the 29 per cent in Nova Scotia who are shown as receiving a partial score for neck examination should probably not be regarded as having done even half-satisfactory examinations of the neck. Since 2 points were given for lymph node examinations only if the practitioners gave attention, at one time or another, to all the palpable groups (except the submaxillary nodes, which were included with neck examination), 1 point given for examination of the lymph nodes represents a more positive activity on the doctor's part than does a partial score for examination of either the abdomen or the neck. One point was given for auscultation of the lungs when only part of the chest was auscultated. This procedure might be of some value or of no value, according as the doctor was or was not lucky enough to hit upon an area in which the abnormal findings were audible. Sometimes, the area auscultated was chosen for no reason that was apparent to the observer or that was suggested by the patient's history.

It is interesting to note that the physicians differed in the attention that they paid to the several parts of the examination of the ear-nose-throat system. In Ontario, examination of the ears with the otoscope was satisfactory in 95 per cent of the practices. Hearing, on the other hand, seldom received attention, even when it was called for. Though the tonsils were given a perfunctory glance more often than Table 74 indicates, satisfactory examinations of the structures of the mouth and throat were observed in only 60 per cent of the practices. The practitioners were not required to use laryngeal or nasopharyngeal mirrors in order to obtain credit for a satisfactory examination of the throat, but it was a pleasure to observe that the occasional doctor used them both frequently and adroitly. Credit was given more often for examination of the nose than for examination of the mouth and throat. This was probably because less was demanded of the doctor in the examination of the nose, since the point was given if he usually looked for nasal bleeding or nasal discharge in cases in which this examination was indicated. In Nova Scotia, a similar pattern was observed. The item in the ear-nose-throat examination that was performed satisfactorily by the largest percentage of practitioners was examination of the ear with the otoscope, which was judged satisfactory in 64 per cent of the practices. This was followed, in decreasing order, by examination of the nose, examination of the mouth and throat, and examination of hearing, which were satisfactory in 49 per cent, 40 per cent, and 22 per cent of the practices, respectively. Examination of the paranasal sinuses, the assessment of which was possible in too few practices to permit of its inclusion in the final rating scale, was performed satisfactorily in 61 per cent of the Ontario, and 52 per cent of the Nova Scotia, practices in which it could be assessed.

Auscultation of the lungs was considered adequate in 70 per cent of the Ontario practices and in 43 per cent of those in Nova Scotia. Percussion of the lungs was performed in a satisfactory manner in 30 per cent and 38 per cent of the practices in Ontario and Nova Scotia, respectively. It was disturbing to discover in how many practices such important examinations as auscultation and percussion of the lungs either were not done when indicated or were done so perfunctorily as to be of little or no value. We must point out, also, that, when we say that auscultation was satisfactory in a certain percentage of the practices, we mean that this examination was performed when it seemed to be called for by the circumstances of the particular case and that the examination *appeared* to us to have been performed in a satisfactory manner. Sometimes, however, the physician would ask the observer to listen to the chest. On more than one such occasion, though the practitioner stated that the chest was "full of rales" or "full of rhonchi," the observer heard nothing but normal breath sounds. Lest the reader think that perhaps the observer was taken in by a practical joke on the doctor's part, we must add that the latter's treatment was based on the alleged abnormal findings.* These physicians' failure to recognize what they heard with the stethoscope illustrates a defect in our method: that except when we were invited to check the findings we had no way of knowing whether they were correct. This defect was not confined to auscultation; it applied to palpation of the abdomen, breasts, and lymph nodes, to rectal and vaginal examinations, and to examinations with the ophthalmoscope and the otoscope. How often this type of defect, which always operated in the doctor's favour, introduced error into the scores, i.e. how often credit was given for an examination that appeared adequate but was not, we do not know. Certainly, there were other occasions on which we were asked to check an interesting finding and were impressed by the fact that something that might easily have been missed, such as a faint cardiac murmur, had not escaped the doctor's notice.

In Ontario, our observations on vaginal examination and rectal examination showed a rather strange contrast, in that credit was given for the former in 89 per cent of the 35 practices assessed, whereas rectal examination was judged satisfactory in only 41 per cent of the 34 practices assessed. The reason for this difference, which is statistically significant ($p < 0.01$),† is unknown, though a possible explanation of our finding is that the indications for vaginal examination, especially vaginal bleeding, vaginal discharge, and pregnancy, are more definite than are some of the indications for rectal examination. This explanation is consistent with our finding that, on the average, the obstetrical part of the Ontario practitioners' work was the part that was most capably handled (see pages 302–303). In Nova Scotia, vaginal examinations were regarded as satisfactory in 61 per cent of

*Such instances of incorrect treatment resulting from the physician's diagnostic failure are further evidence of the correctness of giving more weight, in the rating scale, to diagnosis than to treament. This has been discussed on pages 273–275.
†The meaning of this is explained on pages 32–33.

the practices, and rectal examinations in 44 per cent. The difference is not statistically significant.

Satisfactory examinations of the skin were observed in 59 per cent of the 39 Ontario practices in which this item could be assessed and in 28 per cent of the 32 Nova Scotia practices in which it could be assessed. Those doctors from whom the point was withheld tended to confine their examination to the exposed parts and to show no interest in seeing the rest of the skin. This was observed both when it was important to know how extensive the lesions were and when the doctor had not reached a diagnosis and might have been aided by seeing another lesion in a different stage of its development.

Every one of the 85 doctors was assessed on whether he had his patients disrobe adequately to enable him to carry out a satisfactory examination of whatever parts he was attempting to examine. Eighty-four per cent of the Ontario doctors and 67 per cent of those in Nova Scotia were given the point for this item. Those whose practices were considered unsatisfactory in this respect might place the stethoscope over the clothing or attempt to auscultate the heart or lungs by putting the stethoscope down between the patient's body and tight articles of clothing, or they might palpate the abdomen with the patient fully clothed and perhaps sitting up or standing. In the preceding chapter (page 281), we cited the case of an elderly lady whose heart was examined inadequately and whose lungs and liver were not examined at all, though the doctor recognized the necessity for examination. It was apparent, in this case and with other female patients seen by this same practitioner, that an adequate examination was not done because he was embarrassed about insisting that the chest and the abdomen be exposed sufficiently to enable him to perform the necessary items of examination. This doctor was one of several who did not attempt to examine male patients through their clothing but did not appear to be sufficiently comfortable with their female patients to ask for adequate exposure of the parts being examined. In view of the infrequency with which the breasts were examined—this examination was judged satisfactory in only 30 per cent of the Ontario, and 11 per cent of the Nova Scotia, practices—it may be that the percentage of doctors who are not too comfortable with female patients is higher than the observations on disrobing suggest.

Though one may sympathize with a physician's embarrassment, yet to fail to insist on proper exposure is to fail in one of his responsibilities as a physician, since, if a physician does not insist on what he knows should be done, his patient has no way of knowing that it is important.

Indeed, the very fact that the doctor does not insist on doing a thorough examination may well lead the patient to suppose that such an examination is actually *un*necessary. Not only is this detrimental to the patient at the time; in the future, also, it may make it more difficult for any other physician to bring that patient to believe that adequate examination *is* a real necessity.

We found it interesting that the Ontario doctors whose patients were not adequately disrobed had a mean total score (i.e., for history-taking, physical examination, laboratory work, etc.) of 29.4 per cent, whereas the Ontario physicians whose patients were adequately disrobed had a mean score of 62.7 per cent. The difference between the mean scores of the two groups is significant ($p < 0.01$). For the corresponding Nova Scotia groups, the mean scores were 34.1 per cent and 48.5 per cent, respectively ($p < 0.05$). These findings, though interesting, are not surprising. Indeed, it would have been most surprising if we had found that practitioners who omitted something as basic as having their patients disrobe adequately for examination were, on the whole, practising medicine of satisfactory quality. On the other hand, the fact that patients are adequately undressed does not by itself indicate that the quality of the particular practice is satisfactory, as is shown by the fact that 14 per cent of those Ontario, and 46 per cent of those Nova Scotia, doctors who were given credit for requesting disrobing had over-all scores of less than 40 per cent. We come back to what we have said previously, that diagnosis, based on the proper performance of the various diagnostic procedures, is the root of good medicine.

In Table 76 are shown the doctors' scores for physical examination as a whole. The items of this part of the rating scale totalled 30 points. Because not every doctor could be assessed on every one of the items (see footnote to table), each doctor's score has been expressed as a percentage of the total number of points out of which he was scored. As the table shows, approximately one-third of the Ontario doctors had scores of 40 per cent or less for physical examination, one-third had scores of between 41 and 60 per cent, and one-third had scores of 61 per cent or more. In Nova Scotia, slightly less than three-fifths of the doctors had scores of 40 per cent or less, a little over one-fifth had scores of between 41 and 60 per cent, and a little over one-fifth had scores of 61 per cent or more for physical examination. It is to be noted that some of the doctors had very high scores, even extending into the nineties. In each province, there was a close correspondence be-

TABLE 77

SCORES OF ONTARIO AND NOVA SCOTIA PHYSICIANS FOR
INDIVIDUAL ITEMS OF LABORATORY WORK

| Item of laboratory work | Ontario physicians | | | | Nova Scotia physicians | | | |
| --- | --- | --- | --- | --- | --- | --- | --- | --- |
| | | Percentage of those assessed who were awarded | | | | Percentage of those assessed who were awarded | | |
| | Number assessed | No points | Partial score (where applicable) | Full score | Number assessed | No points | Partial score (where applicable) | Full score |
| Haemoglobin | 43 | 18.6 | — | 81.4 | 42 | 42.9 | — | 57.1 |
| Urine—chemical | 43 | 18.6 | — | 81.4 | 42 | 64.3 | — | 35.7 |
| Urine—microscopic | 43 | 65.1 | — | 34.9 | 40 | 60.0 | — | 40.0 |
| X-ray | 42 | 9.5 | — | 90.5 | 42 | 16.7 | — | 83.3 |
| Sterile technique | 42 | 9.5 | 7.1 | 83.3 | 41 | 46.3 | 22.0 | 31.7 |

tween the scores obtained for history-taking and those for physical examination.

Of the five items of laboratory work that formed part of the rating scale, four were judged to be satisfactory in more than 80 per cent of the Ontario practices (Table 77). These were haemoglobin determinations, examination of urine for sugar and protein, X-ray, and sterile technique. In Nova Scotia, the use of X-ray was satisfatcory in more than 80 per cent of the practices, haemoglobin determinations in almost 60 per cent, examination of the urine for protein and sugar in 36 per cent, and sterile technique in 32 per cent. In only 35 per cent of the Ontario, and 40 per cent of the Nova Scotia, practices was microscopic examination of the urine done as often as it was indicated; and, in some of the practices, it was never done. A frequent observation was that infection of the urinary tract was diagnosed and treatment started without any examination of the urine. We remind the reader that, for each of these laboratory procedures, the doctor was given credit even if he had the examination done by someone else, i.e. we did not require that he do it himself in order to receive credit for the examination.

Those doctors, 10 per cent of the Ontario sample and 46 per cent of the Nova Scotia sample, who were given 0 for sterile technique used techniques that were grossly defective. One man, for example, both in his office and in patients' homes, used the same syringe and needle for successive patients. After an injection given in the office, the syringe and needle were rinsed twice in cold water and then placed in a hot-water sterilizer. Sometimes the water in the sterilizer was brought to the boil before the syringe was used for the next injection, but more often it was not. In a patient's home, the doctor would ask for a cup of hot water, in which he would rinse the syringe and needle before and after the injection. This was repeated in each home in which an injection was given. Another practitioner would insert the needle into a vial without wiping off the rubber cap of the vial. This was probably of minor importance, however, in comparison with his use of the same syringe and needle, without sterilization, on one patient after another. We could conclude only that these doctors were either ignorant or reckless of the dangers inherent in their poor technique.

On those five items of laboratory work that were included in the rating scale, 74 per cent of the Ontario doctors had scores of 61 per cent or more, and only 9 per cent of the doctors had scores of 40 per cent or less. The corresponding figures for Nova Scotia were 45 per cent and 40 per cent, respectively.

Observations were made on a number of other items of laboratory work, which were not included in the rating scale because too few practices could be assessed on them. In each province, the use of blood glucose determinations, of electrocardiograms, and of the serological test for syphilis was satisfactory in more than 75 per cent of the practices that could be assessed on the particular item. The use of the white blood cell count was assessed in more than half of the practices in Ontario and in Nova Scotia; in each province, it was found to be unsatisfactory in about one-third of those that could be assessed. Failure to examine blood films, in cases calling for this procedure, was noted in 55 per cent of the 22 Ontario practices, and in 57 per cent of the 28 Nova Scotia practices, in which there were opportunities to assess this. The examination of stools, which was assessable in not quite half of the practices in each province, was satisfactory in only 25 per cent of those assessed in Ontario and 15 per cent of those assessed in Nova Scotia. The test for occult blood, especially, was greatly neglected.

It was somewhat surprising to observe how little use was made of the tuberculin test, either by the intracutaneous, or by the patch, method. It was used in 5 of the 7 Ontario practices, and in 5 of the 33 Nova Scotia practices, in which there was a definite need for this test in specific cases. In the remaining practices, definite indications for tuberculin testing did not occur during the days of our visits; and there was no evidence, in any of these practices, that the test was used as a screening procedure.

No practice was encountered, in Ontario, in which either a biopsy or a spinal tap was indicated but was not done; but only a small percentage of the practices could be assessed on these two items. In Nova Scotia, a few practices were observed in which biopsies and spinal taps were not done when they were indicated. The difference between Ontario and Nova Scotia, with respect to each of these items, was not statistically significant.

Urinalysis seldom extended beyond microscopic examination and tests for sugar and protein, our observations on which have already been reported (see page 297). The measuring of specific gravity and the use of chemical tests for blood, acetone, or bilirubin were observed in only a small percentage of the practices in which there were definite indications for them.

The observation that impressed us most, as far as laboratory work was concerned, was that very few doctors, in either province, showed any *interest* in doing laboratory work themselves. For this reason, apparently, the practitioners tended to make better use of those items of laboratory work which they could order than of those which they had to perform themselves. In view of this lack of interest, it would seem that, as technicians become more widely available, the medical schools and the teaching hospitals might well decrease their emphasis on these purely technical aspects of medicine. In fact, it might be better if students and young doctors were actively encouraged *not* to do their own laboratory work (except the simplest procedures), in the interest of accuracy. Since there can be no doubt, for example, that the well-trained technician who is examining one blood smear after another is more proficient and can give a more reliable opinion about the smear than the doctor who does this type of examination only sporadically (and most doctors fall into this group), it is probably preferable that the doctor make use of a reliable technician, whenever possible, rather than attempt to do this type of work himself. These remarks can be applied equally well to many other laboratory procedures.

The scores assigned for the treatment items in the rating scale are shown in Table 78. Of those men who could be assessed, 83 per cent in Ontario and 45 per cent in Nova Scotia took proper precautions in the use of dangerous drugs. Those physicians whose practices were unsatisfactory in this particular tended, though with a few exceptions, to practise medicine of poor quality generally. This is evident in the mean over-all scores (32.2 per cent in Ontario, and 34.6 per cent in Nova Scotia) of those physicians who failed to take proper precautions. These scores were significantly lower than the mean scores (61.4 per

TABLE 78

SCORES OF ONTARIO AND NOVA SCOTIA PHYSICIANS FOR
INDIVIDUAL ITEMS OF THERAPY

| | Ontario physicians | | | | Nova Scotia physicians | | | |
| | Percentage of those assessed who were awarded | | | | Percentage of those assessed who were awarded | | | |
| Item of therapy | Number assessed | No points | Partial score (where applicable) | Full score | Number assessed | No points | Partial score (where applicable) | Full Score |
|---|---|---|---|---|---|---|---|---|
| Antibiotics and sulphonamides | 41 | 26.8 | 31.7 | 41.5 | 42 | 45.2 | 42.9 | 11.9 |
| Obesity | 37 | 43.2 | — | 56.8 | 35 | 60.0 | — | 40.0 |
| Potentially dangerous medications | 36 | 16.7 | — | 83.3 | 40 | 55.0 | — | 45.0 |
| General therapeutic measures | 42 | 38.1 | — | 61.9 | 42 | 42.9 | — | 57.1 |

cent in Ontario, and 55.9 per cent in Nova Scotia) of those who did take proper precautions in the use of dangerous drugs ($p < 0.01$). Among those doctors whose practices were considered unsatisfatcory in this respect, it was common to give patients penicillin without making any inquiry whether the patient had ever had a reaction to it. Corticosteroids, also, were used without due caution. One doctor, for example, handed a patient a box containing 1-milligram, 2-milligram, and 4-milligram tablets, but gave neither instructions about dosage nor any warning about the manifestations of overdosage.

Adequate directions about such general items of treatment as bed rest, remaining indoors, fluid requirements, and type of diet were given by 62 per cent of the Ontario doctors and by 57 per cent of those in Nova Scotia. The remainder appeared to be oblivious of any need to instruct their patients in these matters. Obesity was recognized as a problem, and adequate advice was given, by 57 per cent of the Ontario, and by 40 per cent of the Nova Scotia, doctors; the remainder either gave no sign of recognizing the existence of the problem or gave such vague advice as to be useless.

Approximately 27 per cent of the Ontario doctors demonstrated so little knowledge of the general principles involved in the use of antibiotics and sulphonamides that they were given 0; 41 per cent were skilled in their use; and the remaining 32 per cent occupied an intermediate position. The corresponding figures for Nova Scotia were 45 per cent, 12 per cent, and 43 per cent. The individual doses seemed generally to be adequate, as far as they could be determined by the observers; but, in respect of duration of therapy, the use of combinations of drugs, awareness of the danger of toxicity and of emergence of resistant strains of organisms, and ability to differentiate between conditions that should and conditions that should not be treated with these drugs, there were frequent departures from the generally accepted principles.

For the items of therapy taken together, 49 per cent of the Ontario doctors had scores of 61 per cent or more, and 33 per cent had scores of 40 per cent or less. The corresponding figures for Nova Scotia were 12 per cent and 60 per cent.

Observations were made on three items of treatment that were not included in the rating scale: the management of cardiac failure, of hypertension, and of anaemia. Cardiac failure, on which 20 of the Ontario physicians were assessed, was handled well by 40 per cent of them, poorly by 15 per cent, and with an intermediate degree of skill by 45 per cent. Of the 15 practitioners who were assessed on this in Nova Scotia, 33 per cent handled their cases well, 60 per cent poorly, and the remaining physician showed an intermediate degree of skill. Points that were considered when the handling of cardiac failure was being assessed included salt restriction, weight reduction, the use of digitalis and diuretics, and the adequacy of the instructions that the patients were given.

The management of hypertension was assessed in 32 of the Ontario, and in 34 of the Nova Scotia, practices. The observations were disappointing, in that, in each province, approximately 75 per cent of the doctors who were assessed appeared to limit their interest to the blood pressure itself and showed little or no concern for, or even awareness of, the important complications. Anaemia, the handling of which could be assessed in 22 of the Ontario, and in 19 of the Nova Scotia, practices, was managed adequately by 55 per cent of those assessed in Ontario and by 32 per cent of those in Nova Scotia. The two errors most commonly observed were the prescribing of several, or many, therapeutic agents in combination, without the doctor's having determined the cause of the anaemia, and failure to search for a site of bleeding in adult males in whom a diagnosis of iron-deficiency anaemia had been made. In these latter cases, many of the physicians obviously were satisfied with the diagnosis of iron-deficiency anaemia and did not consider the possibility of peptic ulcer or of malignancy.

Though attention was, of necessity, focused on a small number of therapeutic problems and though no one of these was encountered in every practice, yet the variety was sufficiently great, and the problems were seen in enough practices, to warrant a few general comments. Our over-all impression was that the therapeutic efforts of the general practitioners constituted a service of great value to the people of their communities but, as the observations on the specific items showed, left much room for improvement. The inadequacies that were noted in therapeutics appeared to spring much less from lack of knowledge of details than from lack of awareness of, or from failure to apply, basic principles.

Obstetrical representation in the rating scale was limited to two items, the schedule for pre- and postnatal visits and the follow-up investigation, i.e. the combination of history-taking, physical examination, and laboratory work at prenatal visits subsequent to the initial one (see pages 270–271). Ninety-two per cent of the 38 Ontario practitioners who were assessed on their schedule for visits were given 2 points, the remainder 1 point. Of the 38 Nova Scotia practitioners assessed on this, 84 per cent were given 2 points, 8 per cent 1 point, and 8 per cent 0. Of the 36 Ontario practitioners assessed on their follow-up investigation, 72 per cent were given 2 points, 22 per cent 1 point, and 6 per cent 0. For the 35 physicians in Nova Scotia who were assessed on this, the corresponding figures were 20 per cent, 43 per cent, and 37 per cent. Those who were given the intermediate score limited their examinations to urinalysis and measurements of blood pressure and weight, and showed no interest in determining foetal position, auscultating the foetal heart, or asking questions referable to such complications as toxaemia or haemorrhage. Those practitioners who were given 0 omitted such basic items of prenatal care as blood pressure determinations, weight determinations, and examination of the urine for protein. The remaining physicians did follow-up examinations that varied from good to excellent.

As a great deal of the obstetrical work in Ontario and in Nova Scotia, especially in the small communities, is done by general practitioners, we had hoped to assess the practitioners on a number of other items: their history-taking at the initial visit of the obstetrical patient, the initial examination, the initial laboratory work, awareness of complications, the use of consultants, the care with which the practitioner followed the progress of labour, his use of forceps and of episiotomy, and his handling of the baby immediately after delivery. Because deliveries and complications occurred very seldom during the observers' visits, the observations were too few to support any conclusions about these parts of obstetrical practice. Twenty-two of the

43 Ontario doctors, however, were assessed on every one of initial history, initial physical examination, initial laboratory work, schedule for pre- and postnatal visits, and follow-up investigation. Of these 22, 86 per cent scored 61 per cent or more on these five items of obstetrics, and 50 per cent of them had scores of over 80 per cent. Only 4.5 per cent of the doctors scored 40 per cent or lower on these five items. Only 14 of the Nova Scotia doctors could be assessed on every one of these five items of obstetrics. One-half of these had scores of 40 per cent or less on these items; the remainder were divided almost evenly between scores of between 41 and 60 per cent and scores of 61 per cent or more.

Our observations on those obstetrical items that were not included in the rating scale suggest a few further comments. One of the greatest deficiencies observed was in the matter of history-taking when the obstetrical patient first presented herself. Thirty-five per cent of the 23 Ontario doctors who could be assessed and 31 per cent of the 16 in Nova Scotia took a good general medical history from their obstetrical patients, 39 per cent in Ontario and 13 per cent in Nova Scotia took a fair history, but 26 per cent and 56 per cent in the two provinces, respectively, confined their history-taking entirely to obstetrical symptoms. Sixty-seven per cent of the 24 Ontario doctors who were assessed on their initial examinations of obstetrical patients performed a general physical examination, 25 per cent limited themselves to a pelvic examination, and 8 per cent did no examination. The corresponding figures for the 16 Nova Scotia practitioners who could be assessed were 19 per cent, 25 per cent, and 56 per cent, respectively. Initial laboratory work included haemoglobin estimation, Rh typing, and a serological test for syphilis in 80 per cent of the 30 Ontario practices that were assessed on this. The situation with respect to Rh typing by itself was even more satisfactory, in that this test was ordered by 97 per cent of the 37 Ontario doctors whose practices we were able to evaluate. In Nova Scotia, Rh typing was ordered by 93 per cent of the 30 practitioners who were assessed on this. Haemoglobin and Rh typing were both done in 57 per cent of 28 Nova Scotia practices; and, in 39 per cent of these 28, a serological test for syphilis, also, was ordered.

In summary, our assessment of obstetrical care was limited by force of circumstances to pre- and postnatal care. Both in Ontario and in Nova Scotia, obstetrics, perhaps because of the limited nature of the work, appeared to be handled more capably, on the average, than the rest of the general practitioner's work.

Of the preventive medicine items (see page 271), the immunization portion of well-child care was observed to be the best practised. Probably because of the great emphasis that has been put upon this in recent years and because this is a definite, clear-cut procedure, 97 per cent of the 39 Ontario doctors assessed had satisfactory immunization programmes. Well-child care extending beyond this, however, was found to be satisfactory in only 47 per cent of the 36 Ontario practices in which this could be assessed. Similarly, only 38 per cent of the 42 Ontario doctors assessed received credit for making an attempt to instruct their patients in general principles of maintenance of health. In Nova Scotia, satisfactory immunization programmes were observed in 63 per cent of 41 practices assessed; well-child care extending beyond this was satisfactory in 18 per cent of 34 practices assessed; and instruction of patients in principles of maintenance of health was encountered in 12 per cent of the 42 practices. These three items were included in the rating scale. The one other item on which observations were made, the quality of checkups, was not included in the rating scale. These were less than satisfactory in 62 per cent of the 39 Ontario practices assessed and in 86 per cent of the 28 that could be assessed in Nova Scotia; and, in some practices, the checkups were almost worthless.

It is our belief that much more of a preventive nature could be done by the practitioners than was being done when we visited them. For example, it was only on the rare occasion that the doctor, on making a house call, gave any attention to possible hazards. It appeared that the physicians were just not accustomed to thinking along these lines. Again, one man, who did most of the work of the medical officer of health in his community, made a house call, diagnosed measles, and prescribed penicillin. In spite of the highly contagious nature of the disease, the doctor had the patient brought to his office that day for an injection of penicillin and to the hospital the next day for re-examination and another injection.

For clinical records, 35 per cent of the Ontario doctors were given 0, 30 per cent 1 point, and 35 per cent 2 points. The mean over-all scores of these three groups were 47 per cent, 53 per cent, and 71 per cent, respectively. In Nova Scotia, 62 per cent of the doctors had scores of 0, 19 per cent 1 point, and 19 per cent 2 points, for clinical records. The mean over-all scores of these three groups were 38 per cent, 34 per cent, and 71 per cent, respectively. Of the doctors who were given 2 points for records, 87 per cent in Ontario and 75 per cent in Nova Scotia had over-all scores of 61 per cent or more. On the other hand, lack of adequate records is not incompatible with practice of a good, or even an excellent, quality, inasmuch as a considerable number of the doctors who were given 0 for records had over-all scores of 61 per cent or more and a few had over-all scores that were above 80 per cent.

Little need be said about the good records; they included enough detail about positive findings and important negative findings, about diagnosis, and about the management of the problem to give a clear picture of the case. Other records might consist of whole pages of dates and systolic blood pressure readings, with only an occasional word of other findings or of symptoms. These records were so superficial as to be all but useless. Some men either kept no records or kept their records in such a way that they were inaccessible. One physician, for example, who kept good records on his obstetric and paediatric patients, had no records of other patients except notes, made by his nurse, of the patient's name, the medication, and the fee. As these notes were filed, not alphabetically, but chronologically, they would have been very difficult to ferret out and put together into a continuous record for a particular patient. Other men kept literally no records, except the names and addresses of those patients who did not pay cash at the time of the visit. These constituted 20 per cent of the Ontario doctors visited and 38 per cent of those in Nova Scotia; and an additional 7 per cent and 14 per cent in the two provinces, respectively, kept no clinical records except on their obstetric, or occasionally their paediatric, cases.

Some physicians, as we have said, were able to carry on a practice of good quality, even though they kept no records. Others, however, who could not remember what their findings had been or what treatment they had prescribed on previous occasions, were obviously handicapped by their lack of adequate records. Quite apart from the fact that few men have sufficiently infallible memories to carry on their practices without the aid of records, failure to keep records struck us as an act of foolhardiness, from the medico-legal point of view, especially on the part of those men whose practices were of unsatisfactory quality.

The number of surgical procedures done during our visits to the practitioners was so small (see page 255 and Table 65) that the quality of the surgical work could not be assessed. One practitioner, in the middle of a gynaecological operation, admitted that he was somewhat confused as to the placing of some of the sutures; but, with the advice of the colleague who was assisting him, he worked out a technique that satisfied him and that appeared satisfactory to the observer. All the other surgical procedures *observed** by us appeared to be done competently, except for occasional slackness in sterile technique. We repeat, however, that the amount of operative work observed by us was too little to allow its quality to be estimated with any degree of reliability.

The quality of the anaesthetic work being done by the general practitioners could not be assessed, because of the small number of cases seen by us and the highly technical nature of this work. Radiography, either fluoroscopy or the taking of films, was done by less than one-quarter of the Ontario doctors and by only one of those in Nova Scotia (see page 235). We were unable to determine whether the machines were used properly except in the cases of two men, who, by not wearing gloves and an apron, exposed themselves unnecessarily to the risk of excessive radiation.

We mentioned in the preceding chapter (page 286) that an attempt was made to evaluate the practitioners' handling of psychiatric problems but that it was unsuccessful. In fact, the detailed rating that we attempted was so unsatisfactory that to report it would be an act of irresponsibility. Certain general comments, however, we do think are warranted. It was apparent, from discussion with the practitioners, that they believed that patients with serious mental illnesses should be referred to psychiatrists as soon as possible; but, whether these illnesses were generally recognized, we are unable to say. After observing the handling of many patients, we were left with the impression that the general practitioners, in dealing with their patients' emotional problems, were basing their practice on their personal experience rather than on any professional preparation that they had had for such practice (see page 399). Extremely rare was the physician who attempted to gain a clear picture of the particular situation and to explore the underlying causes in more than the most superficial way. Therapy comprised sedative drugs and brief, direct advice. It appeared that, apart from advice about physical matters, a clergyman or a lawyer, if he had been as well disposed as was the doctor and if he had had as many years of experience with human problems, would have been able to counsel as effectively as most of the practitioners; and some psychiatric social workers are probably a good deal more effec-

*Another man, who did not have specialist qualifications in surgery, *told* us that he had given up doing surgery since the day when he had become so confused, while repairing a hernia, that he had had to ask his assistant, who was a certificated specialist in surgery, to take over and complete the operation.

tive at this. In brief, the general practitioners' handling of emotional or psychological problems appeared to be based on personal, rather than professional, qualifications. The vast majority of the practitioners gave the impression that they attempted to deal with these problems, not because of interest in them, but because the problems were wished upon them and were inescapable (see page 233).

One doctor, who was aware of his lack of success in helping patients with emotional problems, usually asked numerous questions, which were specific and often leading. He would say, for example, "Do you have any pounding headache over your eyes or any feeling of pressure on your head?" Several times, the observer thought that the patient might have said something significant if the doctor, instead of asking, "Does your job bother you?" had said "Tell me about your job." With one man who complained of "nerves," the doctor asked a series of specific questions, including, "Are you worried about your health?" "Do you and your wife get along alright?" and "Do you like your job?" Whenever a patient paused in his replies to questions, the doctor would ask another question. Because the doctor never sat back and allowed the patient to talk on unhindered, the patient never got down to talking about what was really bothering him. This doctor's approach to emotional problems is typical of what was seen in many offices.

In the course of the visit to each doctor, the observer tried to determine how the doctor usually regarded his patients. Seventy-five per cent in Ontario and 76 per cent in Nova Scotia were thought to regard their patients as individuals, 5 per cent and 10 per cent in Ontario and Nova Scotia, respectively, as disease entities mainly, and the attitudes of the remainder were not clear to the observer. In many practices, there were opportunities to observe how the physician handled certain situations. We were impressed with the fact that most of the men were skilful in dealing with children on whom it was necessary to do a painful procedure. When a patient had an emotional outburst such as anyone may have on occasion, this was usually handled with gentleness and sympathy. Now and then, however, a physician showed himself tactless and lacking in feeling. We observed this in connection with a boy with enuresis (bed-wetting), who showed both embarrassment and antagonism towards his mother and the doctor during discussion of the problem. Neither during the physical examination nor at any other time did the doctor see the boy apart from the mother. The doctor not only did not attempt to discover any emotional problem that might have been the cause of the symptom, enuresis, but did not even try to deal with the boy's natural feelings of embarrassment.

Occasionally, also, patients with serious or irremediable conditions were handled in ways that betrayed a lack of understanding on the doctor's part; but this was uncommon.

No examination of quality of practice can be regarded as complete, unless it takes into consideration the referrals that the practitioner makes. The *availability* of consultants has been considered in an earlier chapter (pages 90–91). Our concern now is with two questions, whether referrals were made in those cases that seemed to require the services of a physician who possessed greater knowledge or skill and whether the consultants to whom referrals were made were adequately qualified. To determine the quality of the practice of the consultants was obviously beyond the scope of our study; but many of the consultants named by the practitioners were physicians with very high reputations. Though others were not so eminent, we were not aware that any referrals were being made to physicians whose qualifications were known to be inadequate.

Turning to the question whether referrals were made as often as they should have been (see also page 125), we are faced with the difficulty of establishing criteria on which to base our assessment of this aspect of practice. In fact, it is impossible to say that such-and-such a case should be referred by general practitioners but that another type of case is within their competence to handle, because the case that, in one doctor's hands, cries out for referral may be dealt with most skilfully by another general practitioner. For this reason, in deciding whether a case should have been referred to a specialist, we were reduced to using the need of that particular patient as our criterion. Some of the practices were so extremely poor that we should have preferred to see patient after patient in the hands of another doctor. We refer, of course, to those practices in which little or no history was taken and in which examinations were perfunctory and incomplete. Though many of the cases seen in these practices were inadequately investigated and thus neither we nor the practitioner had enough information to know what sort of management was required, we did not list these as cases that should have been referred unless they were obviously serious cases. Even with this very conservative approach to the problem, in 30 per cent of the Ontario practices and in 31 per cent of the Nova Scotia practices we saw patients whom the practitioner should have referred but whom he did not either refer or apparently seriously consider referring. Because this is a matter of importance, we shall give a few examples of the type of case in which referral seemed indicated.

A man, 60 years of age, complained of steady, aching pain in the right costovertebral region. The patient said, and his appearance suggested, that the pain was severe. It was not affected by a change in posture. The man also stated that he had had mild pain on urination, that the urine was yellow and cloudy, and that he had recently passed blood at the beginning of urination. In answer to a question, he said that the costovertebral pain did not radiate. The patient had been seen by the practitioner a year earlier because of suprapubic pain and difficulty in voiding. He had been referred to a urologist who had done a transurethral resection of the prostate for benign prostatic hyperplasia and had removed a stone from the bladder. The patient had been well until a few days before the present visit. The doctor, who usually examined an abdomen with the patient sitting in a chair and fully dressed, had this patient lie down while he examined the right side only of the abdomen. The urine was not examined chemically or microscopically but was merely inspected with the naked eye. Pyelonephritis was diagnosed, and tablets of triple sulphonamide were prescribed. No mention was made of the possibility of another stone or of urinary tract obstruction. The patient was sent home. No suggestion was made of a referral for a more intensive investigation.

Another patient, a woman of middle age, who had rheumatic heart disease with auricular fibrillation, had had a stroke several weeks previously. This the doctor attributed to an embolus originating in the heart. It was thought by the observer that this patient should have been referred for further investigation; but it was apparent, from the doctor's remarks, that he was unaware of valvotomy as a possible means of preventing further embolic episodes.

Another doctor saw a patient who had ripped two of his fingers badly with a power saw. Though the doctor remarked that, if he had belonged to a group that included a surgeon, he would have had the surgeon see this patient, he did not make any attempt to obtain a second opinion in this case. In view of the severity of the injury and the economic importance of the fingers to the patient, the observer was strongly of the opinion that the practitioner owed it to the patient to have expert advice.

Yet another patient, an elderly man, was seriously injured in an accident. The doctor made an incomplete examination. He recognized that the patient was in shock and that he had sustained a fracture of one of the major long bones. He did not consider the possibility of internal abdominal injuries. Having splinted the limb and started an intravenous infusion of dextran, he left while the patient was still in shock. He was called back to the hospital two hours later because the patient was unconscious. When the observer suggested that perhaps there were other injuries, the doctor appeared surprised at the suggestion. Before further action could be taken, the patient died. Autopsy disclosed internal injuries and unsuspected fractures of such severity that it is unlikely that the patient could have been saved. However, there was little doubt in this case that the practitioner should have called for expert assistance as soon as the patient came under his care.

Another case, not as dramatic, but potentially as serious, was that of a man of middle age who complained of substernal aching pain of ten days' duration. It had no relation to breathing or to effort. It was sometimes worse after the ingestion of solid food. The patient had not lost weight, and his appetite was good. The history-taking and examination took about an hour, most of which was spent on unsystematic questions and aimless chatter on the part of the doctor. The doctor said that he heard "sticky rales" in the right side of the chest, laterally. The observer listened but did not hear them; and the doctor, listening again, said that they had disappeared. The chest was not percussed. The doctor decided that an oesophageal lesion was unlikely because there had been no vomiting, and that the heart was not likely the cause of the complaint because there had been no shortness of breath. He diagnosed pleurisy. No laboratory work was done. The patient's remark that he had had "a lot of stomach trouble for years" was not followed up. The observer suggested a chest X-ray and a barium swallow, but the doctor considered these unnecessary. Finally, however, he told the patient to get a miniature X-ray of the chest when the next survey was made in the area. At the patient's request for a "shot," the doctor gave an intravenous injection of vitamin B complex. The observer thought that the case called for a better history and physical examination, a full-size chest X-ray, and a barium examination of the oseophagus, stomach, and duodenum. This case is a good illustration of the type of case that would undoubtedly have been handled very competently by some of the general practitioners whom we visited but that called for greater skill than this particular practitioner possessed.

The 13 Ontario practitioners who failed to refer patients who seemed to need referral had a mean over-all score of 41.5 per cent; the remaining 30 Ontario practitioners had a mean over-all score of 64.1 per cent. The difference is significant ($p < 0.01$). In Nova Scotia, the 13 doctors who were observed not to seek a consultant's help when it was needed had a mean over-all score of 36.5 per cent; the mean over-all score of the rest of the Nova Scotia practitioners was 46.9 per cent. The difference between these two mean scores is not statistically significant.

In some cases in which referrals were made, it appeared that the referring doctor waited longer than he should have before he made the referral. One doctor admitted to hospital a patient who had vomited dark brown fluid. The doctor suspected that this was blood, but did not test either the vomitus or the stool for blood. Though the patient continued to vomit the same type of material at frequent intervals and was becoming very weak and though the hospital had no blood bank, the doctor allowed twenty-four hours to elapse before he had the patient transferred to the care of an internist (i.e., a specialist in internal medicine) in another hospital, a few miles away, where facilities were available for transfusion.

Another physician, who saw a patient as an emergency and made a diagnosis of leukaemia, referred the patient to an internist without delay. The internist confirmed the diagnosis; he did not order treatment himself but made suggestions to the referring doctor. He told the observer that the referring doctor and most of the other general practitioners in the area seldom asked a consultant to look after a patient but merely to advise on treatment. There could be little doubt that a patient as seriously ill as this one, suffering from acute leukaemia with a deficiency of platelets and severe haemorrhage, should have been under the *direct* care of the consultant rather than under the care of the general practitioner, whose experience with this type of case was limited and who was beset by the demands of a busy practice.

Another problem, and one on which doctors differed, was the *choice* of consultants. One physician saw a female baby with a harelip. Without asking the mother's wishes, he telephoned a certificated surgeon and arranged for admission of the child to hospital. The mother asked whether it might not be better to take the child to the Hospital for Sick Children in Toronto, where she had heard that "they do a good job." The doctor replied that the local surgeon had done many of these operations and that he did a "good job" too. Without giving her any opportunity to discuss the matter further, he asked her to take the child to the local hospital that same evening. What experience the surgeon had had with harelips, we do not know. He may have been highly competent. We are critical, however, of the referring doctor because he virtually deprived the mother of her right to decide where the operation should be done. On the other hand, another physician, in referring a patient to an otolaryngologist, asked the patient her preference and then made an appointment for her with the specialist whom she had named. The doctor told the observer that he always asked a patient to name the specialist to whom he wished to be referred. If the patient asked his advice, he gave it. If the patient named a consultant whom the doctor did not think capable of dealing with the situation, he would tell the patient that the consultant for whom he had asked was a good physician but that his work had not involved cases of this type. In other words, this practitioner guided the patient away from consultants whom he did not regard as competent to deal with the case, but left the patient free to choose among those consultants who were adequately qualified.

In densely populated areas, there is little difficulty about referring a patient to a specialist if the general practitioner recognizes the need for referral. In more sparsely settled areas, a referral may be more of a problem. Yet, with improvements in highways and in transportation by air, a referral from an isolated area is less of a problem today than it used to be, provided that an imaginative approach is taken. One young physician, practising several hundred miles from Toronto, told us of a young man who had sustained very severe injuries. The doctor treated him for shock and performed an emergency operation, but he recognized that a further operation, which was beyond his ability and beyond the facilities of his hospital, was needed with a minimum of delay. Putting the patient into an ambulance, he accompanied him to Toronto. Each time they approached a town that had a hospital, the doctor checked the patient's condition, in case it might be necessary to stop at a hospital before they reached Toronto. The patient reached his destination safely.

We have been critical of certain general practitioners for failing to call for a consultation, for not calling for it early enough, and for not giving the consultant a free enough hand in the management of the case. Other practitioners appeared to us to have a much clearer picture of their responsibility in this regard. One doctor, for example, who felt a polyp on rectal examination and found blood in the stool, by the benzidine test, referred the patient to a surgeon for sigmoidoscopic examination and either removal of the polyp or whatever other treatment the surgeon should advise. Another practitioner had a patient who had had recurrent nosebleeds. Having taken a good history and done a general physical examination to rule out various systemic diseases, the doctor was satisfied that the cause of the bleeding was a local one. He referred the patient to an otolaryngologist for cauterization of the area. He told the observer that he could have done this

himself, but that he was convinced that it would be done more satisfactorily by someone who was more experienced in this type of work.

From the examples that we have given, it should be clear that the
problem of how much responsibility a physician should accept himself
and how soon he should seek help from someone more expert is a large
problem and one that is inextricably bound up with the problem of
quality of practice. We shall say more about this in chapters 25 and 26.

We have described the quality of various parts of the practitioners'
work, namely, history-taking, physical examination, laboratory work,
therapy, obstetrics, preventive medicine, records, and referrals. It remains now for us to report the over-all scores, which were based on
all the items mentioned in the preceding sentence, except referrals.
The scores of the Ontario physicians ranged from 14.7 per cent to
97.5 per cent, with a mean of 57.3 per cent; the scores of the Nova
Scotia physicians ranged from 13.9 per cent to 86.3 per cent, with a
mean of 43.7 per cent. The scores are summarized in Table 79. It will

TABLE 79
OVER-ALL SCORES OF ONTARIO AND NOVA SCOTIA PHYSICIANS

|  | Ontario physicians | | Nova Scotia physicians | |
| --- | --- | --- | --- | --- |
| Score | Number | % | Number | % |
| 0–20 | 1 | 2.3 | 5 | 11.9 |
| 21–40 | 11 | 25.6 | 17 | 40.5 |
| 41–60 | 9 | 20.9 | 9 | 21.4 |
| 61–80 | 18 | 41.9 | 8 | 19.0 |
| 81–100 | 4 | 9.3 | 3 | 7.1 |
| Total physicians | 43 | 100 | 42 | 100 |

be noted that 51 per cent of the Ontario doctors who were visited and
26 per cent of those in Nova Scotia had scores of 61 per cent or more,
that 28 per cent in Ontario and 52 per cent in Nova Scotia had scores
of 40 per cent or less, and that the remaining 21 per cent in each
province had scores that fell between 41 and 60 per cent.

The question facing us at this point is what these numbers mean.
It is the opinion of the observers that those doctors, 51 per cent of
the Ontario sample and 26 per cent of the Nova Scotia sample, whose
scores were 61 per cent or over were, on the average, practising
medicine of a satisfactory quality. It appeared that the deficiencies of
these men were not likely to have serious consequences for their
patients, especially as they were likely to seek the help of a specialist

when the gaps in their own knowledge were of greater importance to the patient. As the scores indicate, some of these practices were of outstanding quality. On the other hand, those doctors, 28 per cent of the Ontario, and 52 per cent of the Nova Scotia, sample, whose scores were 40 per cent or less caused the observers grave misgivings. The deficiencies in these men's practices were thought likely to expose their patients to serious risk. The remaining doctors, the 21 per cent in each province whose scores lay between 41 and 60 per cent, constituted a group about whom the observers were in some doubt. These practices could not be labelled unequivocally either as satisfactory or as unsatisfactory.

It is important to note that these percentages are based on relatively small samples, so that they may differ considerably from the values that would have been obtained from a complete survey. This can readily be seen from the magnitude of their 95 per cent confidence intervals.* In the case of Ontario, the true percentage of practitioners with scores of 40 per cent or less is likely to lie between 15 and 44 per cent. Similarly, in the case of Nova Scotia, the true percentage of practitioners with scores of 40 per cent or less is likely to lie between 40 and 71 per cent. While the estimates, then, are not particularly reliable, it does seem likely that *at least* 15 per cent of those Ontario practitioners, and *at least* 40 per cent of those Nova Scotia practitioners, from whom the two samples were drawn† would have scores of 40 per cent or less.

Our finding that a substantial proportion of the practitioners in each of the two samples were practising medicine of unsatisfactory quality is consistent with the opinions expressed by some of the men whom we visited (see pages 157, 172) and vindicates those members of the College of General Practice of Canada who instituted the Survey because they had doubts about the quality of the work being done by some general practitioners (see page 5).

Since the Survey was carried out in two provinces, the reader may tend to compare our findings in the two provinces and to ask whether they differ significantly. The mean over-all scores of the two groups of physicians do differ significantly ($p < 0.01$). Before the reader accepts this statement at face value, however, he must be aware that the difference may be an artifact resulting from either of two possible occurrences. First, it may be that either the Ontario sample of doctors

*This term has been explained on page 32.
†See pages 28–29 and 31 for a statement of those practitioners who were excluded before the drawing of the sample and the reasons for their exclusion.

or the Nova Scotia sample was atypical of the larger body of general practitioners from which it was drawn. This is the risk involved in any study that has to be limited to a sample. Secondly, it is conceivable that our standard of scoring differed appreciably between the two provinces. Though this possibility cannot be excluded, we consider it unlikely in view of the determined effort that we made to maintain as unvarying a standard as possible (see page 19). Whether the observed difference was due to either of the two possible occurrences that we have mentioned or whether there was a real difference between the two provinces is of minor importance, however, in comparison with the fact that, in each province, Ontario and Nova Scotia alike, the quality of a substantial proportion of the practices fell short of what could be considered satisfactory. It is to this gap between what was hoped for and what was observed that we shall turn our attention in the remaining chapters.

In case our examination of the details of the quality of practice may have obscured the over-all view, it is well that we recapitulate our findings. First of all, we may say that, both in Ontario and in Nova Scotia, much excellent work is being done by general practitioners. Indeed, in some practices, as the very high scores achieved by some of the physicians indicate, we should be hard pressed to suggest any improvements. However, the figures and the clinical examples that we have given make clear that an appreciable percentage of the practices visited in each of the two provinces were seriously deficient in quality. We must emphasize that the deficiencies to which we refer were *not* lack of knowledge of the details of recently discovered drugs or lack of familiarity with the abstruse complexities of rare diseases. The deficiencies were in the fundamentals of clinical medicine—failure to take an adequate history, i.e. failure to gather, and to make use of, the information that the patient himself could provide about his disorder; failure to perform an adequate physical examination, and, in some cases, inability to distinguish between normal and abnormal physical findings; failure, in the investigation and the treatment of cases, to think in terms of basic principles of biochemistry, physiology, pathology, microbiology, and pharmacology.* The former group of physicians, those whom we found doing satisfactory work, may well be the pride of the medical profession; the latter group, the deficient group, is perhaps the more important, inasmuch as it is the challenge to the profession.

*For the comment of a general practitioner on this subject, see page 357.

# 18 / The Quality of General Practice
## *Its Relationship to Age, Education and Other Factors*

Why is one physician's practice so excellent in quality, but another's so poor? That is the question to which we must attempt to find an answer. We have already seen how greatly the physicians differ from one another in many respects. We should be unrealistically optimistic, then, if we were to expect to find a single factor accounting for the great variety of ways in which they react in a situation as complex as a general medical practice. Rather, we must expect that the phenomena reported in the preceding chapter result from the interaction of many factors. If we can elucidate even a few of these, we shall be fortunate; many of them we can expect to elude us.

In this chapter, we shall deal with some of the direct comparisons we made of the physicians' scores (as a measure of the quality of their practices) with other data we had collected about them. The relationships we examined were many, and most of the examinations showed nothing of significance. To list all the items that we examined without finding any significant relationships would be pointless; but a few of them are reported here, both because they are thought to be interesting in themselves and because they illustrate the diversity of the items that we considered in our search for factors that might have a bearing on the quality of practice (other items showing no significant relationship to physician's score will be encountered in later chapters):

1. The population of the place of practice (chapter 2).
2. Whether or not the physician's father was a physician (chapter 3).

3. Whether the physician practised alone or as a member of a group (chapter 8).
4. The number of professional societies to which the physician belonged (chapter 10).
5. Membership in the College of General Practice of Canada (chapter 10).
6. The degree of difficulty that the physician had experienced in financing his undergraduate medical education (chapter 13).
7. The part that financial difficulties had played in terminating the physician's postgraduate training (chapter 13).
8. The choice of career that the physician would have made if it had not been for financial difficulties (chapter 13).
9. The physician's opinion on whether the present system of paying for medical care is satisfactory from the physician's point of view (chapter 13).
10. The number of physicians among the physician's five closest friends (chapter 14).
11. Whether or not the physician's practice included surgery (chapter 15).

It is interesting to note that, both in Ontario and in Nova Scotia, there were, on the average, no significant differences in quality of practice between physicians whose fathers had been physicians and those whose fathers had not been physicians, between physicians practising in communities of different sizes, or between physicians whose practices included surgery and those who did no surgery. Nor did the number of professional societies to which the physician belonged appear to be related in any significant way to the quality of his practice.

When the physicians were divided into those who had found it either "very difficult" or "fairly difficult" to finance their undergraduate medical education and those who had found it either "not very difficult" or "not at all difficult," the difference between the mean scores of the two groups was not significant in either province. Again, there was no significant difference between the mean score of those who said that financial difficulties had been the determining factor in the termination of their postgraduate training, the mean score of those who said that it had been a contributing factor only, and the mean score of those who said that financial difficulties had played no part in terminating their training. Finally, we found no significant difference, either in Ontario or in Nova Scotia, between the mean scores of those men who were general practitioners out of preference and those who would have chosen a specialty in preference to general practice had it not been for financial difficulties.

TABLE 80

<small>SCORES OF THOSE ONTARIO AND NOVA SCOTIA PHYSICIANS IN SOLO PRACTICE
AND THOSE PRACTISING AS MEMBERS OF GROUPS OF TWO OR MORE</small>

|  | Ontario | | Nova Scotia | |
|---|---|---|---|---|
| Type of practice | Number of physicians | Mean score % | Number of physicians | Mean score % |
| Solo | 29 | 54.6 | 28 | 42.4 |
| Group of two or more | 14 | 62.8 | 14 | 46.2 |
| Total physicians | 43 | 57.3 | 42 | 43.7 |

The mean scores of those men who were practising alone and of those who were practising as members of groups of two or more are shown in Table 80. In neither province was there a significant difference. There appeared to be no relationship, either, between the quality of practice and the number of visits made by the physicians per week.

Because of the concern of the College of General Practice of Canada with quality of practice, it was of particular interest to compare the quality of those men in our sample who were members of the College and those who were not members. The mean scores of the two groups did not differ significantly in Ontario or in Nova Scotia (Table 81).

TABLE 81

<small>MEMBERSHIP IN THE COLLEGE OF GENERAL PRACTICE OF CANADA
AND SCORES OF PHYSICIANS OF VARIOUS AGES</small>

|  | Member of College of General Practice | | Non-member of College of General Practice | |
|---|---|---|---|---|
| Age of physician | Number of physicians | Mean score % | Number of physicians | Mean score % |
| A. *Ontario* | | | | |
| Up to 35 | 3 | 75.8 | 7 | 69.3 |
| 36–45 | 5 | 57.6 | 10 | 59.9 |
| 46–60* | 6 | 49.8 | 12 | 47.2 |
| Totals | 14 | 58.1 | 29 | 56.9 |
| B. *Nova Scotia* | | | | |
| Up to 35 | 4 | 43.2 | 4 | 52.2 |
| 36–45 | 9 | 58.9 | 10 | 43.5 |
| 46–60 | 4 | 22.5 | 11 | 36.2 |
| Totals | 17 | 46.6 | 25 | 41.7 |

*One physician was 61 by the time of the Survey's visit.

When the men were divided into three age groups, though the age groups showed noteworthy differences, which we shall discuss presently, the mean scores of the members and of the non-members of the College of General Practice did not differ significantly within any one of the three age groups in either province. In examining the scores, we found that some men with practices of good, or even excellent, quality, did not belong to the College and that some men who were members of the College were practising medicine of doubtful, or even obviously unsatisfactory, quality. Since the College of General Practice demands that applicants for membership in the College measure up to certain standards, our finding is of significance, in that it makes clear that, even with as careful a check as the College carries out on its members both initially and at intervals, it is very difficult in many cases, and in some cases probably impossible, to determine the quality of a physician's practice except by direct observation. We shall refer to this again in chapter 26 when we consider the future of medical practice.

TABLE 82

DISTRIBUTION OF PHYSICIANS BY AGE AND SCORE

| Age of physician | Score | | | Total physicians | Mean Score % |
|---|---|---|---|---|---|
| | 0–40 % | 41–60 % | 61–100 % | | |
| A. *Ontario* | | | | | |
| Up to 35 | 1 | 1 | 8 | 10 | 71.2 |
| 36–45 | 2 | 4 | 9 | 15 | 59.1 |
| 46–60* | 9 | 4 | 5 | 18 | 48.1 |
| Total physicians | 12 | 9 | 22 | 43 | 57.3 |
| Mean age | 49.2 | 44.6 | 40.7 | 43.9 | |
| B. *Nova Scotia* | | | | | |
| Up to 35 | 3 | 3 | 2 | 8 | 47.7 |
| 36–45 | 8 | 3 | 8 | 19 | 50.8 |
| 46–60 | 11 | 3 | 1 | 15 | 32.5 |
| Total physicians | 22 | 9 | 11 | 42 | 43.7 |
| Mean age | 45.6 | 40.7 | 39.3 | 42.9 | |

*One physician was 61 by the time of the Survey's visit.

We turn now to those items that did appear to be related in some way to quality of practice. As we examined the scores, we were struck by the relationship between quality of practice and age of physician. With increasing age, there was a tendency for practice to be of poorer quality. The inverse correlation was significant both in Ontario ($p < 0.01$) and in Nova Scotia ($p < 0.05$).* Table 82 shows the mean scores of the three age groups in Ontario decreasing progressively from the youngest to the oldest group, whereas in Nova Scotia the difference appears to have been mainly between those physicians up to forty-five years of age and those over forty-five. In chapter 16 (pages 273–275), we pointed out that the assessment of quality of practice was based mainly on diagnostic procedures, especially history-taking and physical examination, rather than on therapeutic procedures. We need not discuss again the reasons for this. The point of importance is that the physicians' scores did not depend on their knowledge of recent advances—except to a slight degree[†]—but were determined by their use of, or their failure to use, the long-established, basic procedures of clinical medicine. From this, it follows that the higher scores achieved by the younger men can*not* be attributed to the fact that the rating scale was composed of items in which the younger men, but not the older men, would have been instructed in medical school, since this was not the case.

Why, then, did practice tend to be of poorer quality with increasing age? The reason for this may be that individual physicians tend to do poorer work as they become older or that the older physicians visited by us have always practised medicine of poorer quality, on the average, than the present group of younger doctors or that both factors are involved. If the younger doctors whom we visited were practising medicine of a higher quality than the older doctors had practised in their younger days, then the difference may have been the result of differences in the type of person entering upon the study of medicine or of changes in the quality of medical training, undergraduate, postgraduate, or both. Though it is interesting to speculate on the causes of the observed differences in quality, all that we can say with certainty is that, in each province, the younger doctors were practising medicine of significantly higher quality, on the average, than the older doctors. It must be emphasized that we are speaking of averages and that, among the doctors visited, there were certain older doctors with practices of very high quality and certain younger ones whose work was of quite inferior quality.

Because of Peterson's conclusions that "the better medical student

*The meaning of this statement is explained on pages 32–33.

†For example, the assessment took into account the way in which antibiotics were used and the doctors' awareness of the dangers of any drugs that they elected to use.

tends to become a better physician" and that "the more training a physician has received in internal medicine the more likely he is to become a good physician,"* we were especially interested in the relationships between the physician's academic record and the duration and the type of his postgraduate training, on the one hand, and, on the other, the quality of his practice. The academic records of all the doctors whose records were requested were made available, on a strictly confidential basis, through the kind co-operation of the deans of the medical schools. When the records from the various schools were compared, it was at once apparent that many of them did not give the student's standing in his class, which might have been the most suitable basis for comparison, and that, in the information that they did contain, they differed so greatly that they could not satisfactorily be combined. For this reason, our examination of the relationship between academic marks and quality of practice in Ontario was limited to 23 graduates of the University of Toronto, for each of whom both a score and a complete academic record were available. In the Nova Scotia sample, there were 39 graduates of Dalhousie University for each of whom we had both a score and an academic record.

The large number of individual entries on each man's medical school record could have been combined in an almost endless variety of ways. Arbitrarily, we chose, as the measure of the doctor's academic ability, the mean† of all the marks recorded for the 4 major clinical subjects, i.e. medicine, surgery, obstetrics, and paediatrics. It is to this mean that we shall be referring, whenever we use the word "marks" in the course of our discussion of the relationship between academic record and quality of practice.

When the relationship between academic marks and quality of practice, as indicated by score, was examined (Table 83), it was found

*O. L. Peterson *et al.*: Journal of Medical Education, *31*, No. 12, Part 2: 1–165, 1956; see p. 143. It is to be noted that Peterson, in speaking of training in internal medicine, is referring to postgraduate training. Peterson's work has been described on pages 5 and 10–11, above.

†For all but one of the Ontario doctors, this was the mean of 3 marks for medicine (i.e., the mark at the end of his third-last year, the mark at the end of his second-last year, and the mark at the end of his final year), 3 marks for surgery, 2 for obstetrics, and 1 for paediatrics. In the case of 1 man, owing to a reorganization of the medical course, there were only 2 marks recorded, instead of 3, for each of medicine and surgery. For this reason, the mark for this doctor was the mean of 7 marks. In Nova Scotia, all the academic records contained 3 marks for medicine and 3 marks for surgery; but for obstetrics there were 3 marks entered on some records and 2 on others, and the number of entries for paediatrics was either 2 or 1, except on one record which contained no paediatric mark.

TABLE 83

ACADEMIC MARKS AND SCORES OF THOSE ONTARIO PHYSICIANS WHO WERE
GRADUATES OF THE UNIVERSITY OF TORONTO AND OF THOSE NOVA SCOTIA
PHYSICIANS WHO WERE GRADUATES OF DALHOUSIE UNIVERSITY

| Academic marks*<br>% | Ontario physicians | | Nova Scotia physicians | |
|---|---|---|---|---|
| | Number | Mean score<br>% | Number | Mean score<br>% |
| 66.6 and over | 5 | 69.4 | 13 | 51.3 |
| 63.3–66.5 | 6 | 67.8 | 10 | 44.9 |
| 60.0–63.2 | 7 | 49.5 | 8 | 45.4 |
| Under 60.0 | 5 | 37.3 | 8 | 36.9 |
| Total physicians | 23 | 56.0 | 39 | 45.5 |

*The mean of all the marks recorded for medicine, surgery, obstetrics, and paediatrics.

TABLE 84

ACADEMIC MARKS OF VARIOUS AGE GROUPS OF THOSE
ONTARIO PHYSICIANS WHO WERE GRADUATES OF THE
UNIVERSITY OF TORONTO

| Age of physician | Number of<br>physicians | Mean academic mark<br>% |
|---|---|---|
| 31–35 | 5 | 66.6 |
| 36–45 | 9 | 63.9 |
| 46–61 | 9 | 60.2 |
| Total physicians | 23 | 63.0 |

that, in Ontario, a significant correlation existed ($r = 0.557$, $r_{0.01} = 0.526$), i.e. the men with the better marks had higher scores, on the average, than those with poorer marks, though certain physicians who had good marks had low scores and others with poorer marks had relatively high scores. Because we had already found that younger doctors practised medicine of better quality, on the average, than older doctors,* it was necessary to examine also the relationship between age of physician and academic marks. Between these two also, there turned out to be a significant negative correlation (Table 84), i.e. the younger doctors had had higher marks, on the average, than the older doctors ($r = -0.527$, $r_{0.01} = 0.526$).† Thus, for the Ontario prac-

*This was so, not only for the total Ontario sample, but also for the University of Toronto graduates, i.e. for the physicians with whose academic records we were dealing. When the University of Toronto graduates were divided into those up to 35 years of age, those between 36 and 45, and those between 46 and 61 years of age, the mean scores for the 3 groups were, respectively, 73.5 per cent, 58.6 per cent, and 42.3 per cent.

†To investigate the cause of this was beyond the scope of the present study.

titioners, we ended up with three relationships that were statistically significant: that the older doctors (on the average) were practising medicine of poorer quality than the younger doctors, that the older doctors (on the average) had had lower marks in medical school than the younger doctors, and that the doctors with lower medical school marks were (on the average) practising medicine of poorer quality than those who had had higher marks. *

Three explanations of these relationships suggest themselves as possibilities. First, it may be that the correlation between marks and quality of practice is merely a reflection of two unrelated facts: that deterioration in quality of practice occurs as a result of the aging process (which is stated not as a proven fact but merely as a possibility) and that the older doctors had lower marks than the group of younger doctors whom we visited. In this case, marks could not be expected to be of any value to us in predicting quality of practice. Secondly, it may be that the correlation between academic marks and quality of practice occurred because each variable was a measure of such specific qualifications for practice as possession of a body of professional knowledge and skill in applying it. Finally, the correlation between marks and quality of practice may have been the result of characteristics that determined both marks and quality of practice but that were less specific than professional knowledge and specific training in its application. One might consider such characteristics as interest in medicine, intelligence, intellectual curiosity, studiousness, meticulousness, and many others. Which of these explanations, if any, is the correct one remains undetermined.

In short, although, for the Ontario physicians who were graduates of the University of Toronto, a significant correlation existed between medical school marks and quality of practice, it was not possible to determine the basis of this relationship. The effect of the other variable, age, in obscuring the relationship between academic marks and quality of practice illustrates only too well the difficulty that one may encounter when one attempts to interpret "statistically significant" findings that involve a number of variables.

*If, instead of using medical school marks as our measure of academic ability, we divide the Ontario doctors into those who had had either to repeat a year or to write supplemental examinations and those who had had no such difficulties, the findings are similar to the findings that we obtained when we used marks as a measure of academic ability, namely, that those who had had academic difficulties had a mean score of 47.6 per cent, whereas those without academic difficulties had a mean score of 64.5 per cent, but that the former group was older, with a mean age of 45.7 years, than the latter group, whose mean age was 41.9 years.

In the case of the Nova Scotia physicians, there appeared to be some tendency for the practitioners who had had the higher marks at medical school to be practising medicine of a better quality, on the average, than those who had had poorer academic marks (Table 83); but the correlation was not statistically significant: $r = 0.245$, $r_{0.05} = 0.316$. On the other hand, when the practitioners were divided into those who had had either to repeat a year or to write supplemental examinations and those who had had no such difficulties, the mean scores, which were 38.9 per cent and 53.9 per cent respectively, differed significantly ($p < 0.05$). As in Ontario, however, the significance of this finding is obscured by the fact that those who had had academic difficulties had a mean age of 46.1 years, whereas those who had not had difficulties had a mean age of 38.9 years.

When we came to examine the relationships between quality of practice, as indicated by the physician's score, and postgraduate training, the situation proved even more complicated and confusing. For those who may be interested in the details, our examination of the Ontario data is described in Appendix B. We see no point, however, in burdening the general reader with a description of an analysis from which, because of the number of variables and the multiplicity of interrelationships among them, few firm conclusions emerged. Suffice it to say that we examined the relationships between quality of practice, on the one hand, and, on the other, duration of postgraduate training in non-teaching hospitals, in teaching* hospitals, and on each of the 4 major clinical services (medicine, surgery, paediatrics, and obstetrics) in teaching hospitals and that our conclusions for the Ontario doctors were as follows:

There was a significant correlation between *total* duration of postgraduate training (i.e., time spent in teaching hospitals plus time spent in non-teaching hospitals) and quality of practice. There was no evidence, however, of a significant relationship between duration of training in *non-teaching* hospitals and quality of practice. On the other hand, the practice of those physicians who had had at least some of their postgraduate training in *teaching* hospitals was, on the average, of significantly higher quality than the practice of those whose

---

*Teaching hospitals are defined, for the purposes of this study, as those hospitals in which medical students (i.e., undergraduates) are continually receiving instruction in general medicine, surgery, obstetrics, or paediatrics. Those hospitals whose activities are narrowly limited within the major fields (e.g., infectious diseases hospitals) are not counted as teaching hospitals, except when the physician was sent to such a hospital for a short period in order to round out the rotation of a major teaching hospital.

postgraduate training had been entirely in *non-teaching* hospitals, the mean scores of the two groups being 64.3 per cent and 46.3 per cent respectively ($p < 0.01$). It was not possible, however, to determine whether this difference resulted from the difference that existed between the mean ages of the two groups or from superiority of the teaching hospitals as training institutions or from a tendency on the part of the teaching hospitals to give training opportunities to the men with the better academic records or to differences in personal qualities that caused the men to choose one type of hospital for their postgraduate training in preference to the other.

The Ontario doctors whose postgraduate training time in *internal medicine* in teaching hospitals and whose *total* postgraduate training time in teaching hospitals had both been prolonged showed a tendency to carry on practices of better quality than those whose postgraduate training in teaching hospitals had been of shorter duration. It was not possible, however, to discover whether the factor determining the better quality of practice was ( *a* ) the longer *total* duration of teaching hospital postgraduate training or ( *b* ) the longer duration of teaching hospital postgraduate training in *internal medicine*—the training, in either case, showing its effect after a long latent period—or ( *c* ) qualities possessed by the doctor that induced him to prolong either his total postgraduate training or its medical component.

It must be emphasized that the results stated in the preceding paragraphs are averages and that certain individual doctors, though they had had no postgraduate training in teaching hospitals, were practising medicine of a high quality and that certain others were practising medicine of poor quality although they had had postgraduate training in teaching hospitals. From this we must conclude that individual qualities affect the quality of practice in other ways than through whatever effect they may have in influencing the individual in his choice of training hospital.

In Nova Scotia, there was no significant relationship between quality of practice and either *total* duration of postgraduate training or duration of postgraduate training in *non-teaching* hospitals.

The Nova Scotia doctors who had had some of their postgraduate training in teaching hospitals did not, as a group, differ significantly in quality of practice from those whose postgraduate training had been taken entirely in non-teaching hospitals, the mean scores of the two groups being 44.3 per cent and 42.3 per cent, respectively, and the former group being approximately four years younger, on the average, than the latter group. Our failure to find a difference between the mean scores of these two groups of Nova Scotia practitioners is in contrast with our finding in Ontario that the practitioners who had had some teaching hospital postgraduate training had a significantly higher mean score than those whose postgraduate training had been entirely in non-teaching hospitals. We must point out, however, that the Ontario and the Nova Scotia findings are not really comparable inasmuch as most of the Ontario physicians had spent the entire duration of their junior interneship in one hospital, either a teaching hospital or a non-teaching hospital, whereas the junior interneship of many of the Nova Scotia physicians had been divided between a teaching hospital and affiliated non-teaching hospitals.

In Nova Scotia, as in Ontario, the practitioners who had had prolonged postgraduate training in teaching hospitals had a considerably higher mean score than those who had had shorter periods of postgraduate training in teaching hospitals; but the difference, in Nova Scotia, did not reach the level of statistical significance.

It was not possible to examine the result of prolonged teaching hospital training in internal medicine, since only one of the Nova Scotia practitioners had had more than six months of such training. On the other hand, five doctors who had had more than twelve months of teaching hospital postgraduate training in surgery had a mean score of 60.6 per cent, whereas the mean score of the remaining practitioners was 41.4 per cent. The mean ages of the two groups differed by only one year. The difference between the scores of the two groups was not statistically significant but was, nevertheless, great enough to suggest that whatever merit may be inherent in prolonged teaching hospital training in internal medicine may be inherent also in similarly prolonged teaching hospital training in surgery. It may be, of course, that the factor determining quality of practice is not the particular clinical subject, either medicine or surgery, but is either the duration of the training or qualities that induce the physician to prolong his training.

In summary, our findings are too indefinite either to confirm or to contradict Peterson's conclusions that "the better medical student tends to become a better physician" and that "the more training a physician has received in internal medicine the more likely he is to become a good physician."

In Table 85 are listed several other items that were compared with the physicians' scores. In Ontario, our findings were that those who had no nursing or secretarial assistance were practising poorer medicine, on the average, than those who had such assistance; that those who had no hospital responsibilities were practising medicine of poorer quality, on the average, than those who had hospital responsi-

TABLE 85

ONTARIO AND NOVA SCOTIA PHYSICIANS' SCORES COMPARED
WITH VARIOUS OTHER ITEMS

| Item on which physicians were compared | Groups compared | Ontario physicians | | | Nova Scotia physicians | | |
|---|---|---|---|---|---|---|---|
| | | Number of physicians | Mean score % | Mean age yrs. | Number of physicians | Mean score % | Mean age yrs. |
| Nursing or secretarial assistance | None | 9 | 43.1 | 46.7 | 17 | 38.7 | 44.2 |
| | Some | 34 | 61.1 | 43.1 | 25 | 47.1 | 42.0 |
| Hospital responsibilities | None | 11 | 46.7 | 47.4 | 13 | 42.5 | 42.5 |
| | Some | 32 | 61.0 | 42.8 | 29 | 44.2 | 43.1 |
| Number of hours of work per week | Less than 36 hours | 4 | 35.3 | 49.0 | 0 | — | — |
| | 36–45 hours | 8 | 45.6 | 47.0 | 8 | 37.4 | 43.8 |
| | 46–55 hours | 16 | 61.1 | 42.9 | 9 | 39.8 | 42.9 |
| | 56–65 hours | 7 | 67.8 | 40.7 | 10 | 42.0 | 43.2 |
| | Over 65 hours | 8 | 63.3 | 43.0 | 15 | 50.4 | 42.3 |
| Appointment system | None or partial | 17 | 42.5 | 46.5 | 32 | 37.6 | 44.5 |
| | Complete | 26 | 67.0 | 42.2 | 10 | 63.2 | 37.8 |

bilities; that those who worked a smaller number of hours per week tended to practise medicine of poorer quality than those who worked a greater number; and that those who had no appointment system or only a partial one were practising poorer medicine, on the average, than those who had a complete appointment system (see page 71). In the case of every item, the Ontario results were significant ($p < 0.05$).

In the case of the Nova Scotia physicians, there were no significant differences between the scores of the groups that were based on assistance in the office or on hospital responsibilities. There appears to have been a tendency for the scores to increase as the number of hours of work per week increased, but the finding did not prove to be statistically significant. In Nova Scotia, however, as in Ontario, the physicians who had a complete appointment system had a mean score significantly higher than the mean score of those who had no appointment system or only a partial one ($p < 0.01$ for each province).

Unfortunately, in the case of every one of the "significant" differences that we have reported in the preceding paragraph, the physicians with the higher mean score were several years younger, on the average, than those with the lower mean score. Because we have already found that there was a significant negative correlation between age of physician and quality of practice, i.e. that the younger doctors practised better medicine, on the average, than the older doctors, we cannot draw any conclusions about the relationships between quality of practice and the items listed in Table 85. Even if age were not a complicating factor, the results would have to be interpreted with caution. For example, we should still not know whether Ontario physicians working more hours per week were practising medicine of better quality because of their more concentrated experience or whether the patients' recognition of the quality, good or poor, of the doctor's practice determined the demand, great or little, made for his services or whether personal qualities of the physician—perhaps interest in medicine, to name only one—determined both the quality of his practice and the amount of time given by him to his work. Similarly, the other relationships shown in Table 85 admit of more than one explanation, but it is not worthwhile to consider these in view of the uncertainty that is introduced into every one of the other relationships by the relationship that we know existed between quality of practice and age of physician.

Of the items with which we compared quality of practice, the final one that we shall mention in this chapter is the time of the physician's marriage. Prior to World War II, it was almost unheard of for an interne, let alone a medical student, to marry; but, as we have already pointed out, in recent years there has been a tendency for the doctor to marry both at an earlier age and earlier in his career (see page 40 and Tables 5, 6). In former years, the young doctor, especially if he aspired to a career as a specialist, was commonly advised to delay marriage, to put his "emotions in cold storage" for a few years. The trend towards earlier marriages, though accepted today as part

TABLE 86

AGES AT MARRIAGE AND SCORES OF PHYSICIANS UP TO
45 YEARS OF AGE AND BETWEEN 46 AND 60 YEARS OF AGE

| | Age at time of Survey's visit | | | | | |
|---|---|---|---|---|---|---|
| | Up to 45 | | 46–60* | | Total physicians | |
| Age at marriage | Number of physicians | Mean score % | Number of physicians | Mean score % | Number of physicians | Mean score % |
| A. *Ontario* | | | | | | |
| Under 30 | 21 | 66.7 | 8 | 53.4 | 29 | 63.0 |
| 30 and over | 4 | 49.6 | 9 | 38.4 | 13 | 41.9 |
| B. *Nova Scotia* | | | | | | |
| Under 30 | 20 | 52.9 | 8 | 31.9 | 28 | 46.9 |
| 30 and over | 4 | 47.5 | 7 | 33.3 | 11 | 38.5 |

*One Ontario physician was 61 by the time of the Survey's visit.

of the present order, still calls forth sporadic expressions of dismay and even of indignation on the part of some of the older men in the profession. In view of this, the scores achieved by the physicians were compared with their ages at the time of marriage (Table 86) and with the number of years between graduation from medicine and marriage (Table 87). Though these tables do not provide an answer

TABLE 87

NUMBER OF YEARS BETWEEN GRADUATION FROM MEDICAL SCHOOL
AND MARRIAGE, AND SCORES OF ONTARIO AND NOVA SCOTIA PHYSICIANS

| Number of years between graduation and marriage | Ontario physicians | | | Nova Scotia physicians | | |
|---|---|---|---|---|---|---|
| | Number | Mean score % | Mean age yrs. | Number | Mean score % | Mean age yrs. |
| — (1 or more)* | 7 | 64.9 | 39.6 | 12 | 53.2 | 39.2 |
| 0 | 7 | 56.3 | 38.0 | 4 | 44.0 | 43.8 |
| 1 to 5 | 22 | 59.9 | 45.8 | 17 | 41.6 | 43.3 |
| Over 5 | 6 | 34.3 | 48.2 | 6 | 36.0 | 54.3 |

*The minus sign indicates that marriage preceded graduation.

to the question whether a physician is wise or unwise to marry before the completion of his training, they do make clear that, on the average, general practice may be of at least as good quality after early marriage as after later marriage. Consistent with our finding is the statement of John R. Ellis, Sub-Dean of London Hospital Medical College, who, commenting on the fact that approximately a third of their medical students "are married before qualification or just after," says, "I have never seen any evidence that marriage affects the student's work."[*]

In this chapter, we have reported what we found on comparing quality of practice, as represented by the practitioners' scores, with the data available to us on a number of other matters. In brief, though we were able to demonstrate statistically significant relationships between the quality of the physician's practice, on the one hand, and, on the other, his age, his academic record in medical school, certain aspects of his postgraduate training, and several of his practice arrangements, we found it impossible, because of the number of variables involved, to distinguish those relationships that were merely secondary phenomena from those, if any, that were of fundamental importance. It is clear that, in seeking to explain the variation that we observed in quality of practice, we must look beyond mere statistical comparisons. This we shall do in the chapters of the next section.

[*]J. R. Ellis: Journal of Medical Education, 33, No. 10, Part 2: 239, 1958.

PROBLEMS OF MEDICAL

EDUCATION AND OF

MEDICAL PRACTICE

# 19 / Counselling of Medical Students and Young Graduates

The frontal attack made in the preceding chapter did not bring us to an understanding of the great variation that exists in the quality of general practice. In the remaining chapters, we shall take a more indirect path. The search to discover why some practices are of satisfactory and some of unsatisfactory quality requires examination of the structure of medicine, from medical education, which is the foundation of good care, up to the organization of medical practice, which is the superstructure, important in its function but unable to stand without support. It is necessary to consider what the practitioners themselves told us of their medical education and of their experience of practice and what we observed in the course of our visits to them. Our task will be to try to draw together the facts—some that we have already reported in our systematic examination of the practitioners and their work, and some that we shall be presenting for the first time—in such a way as to make clear what changes, in medical education and in the organization of medical practice, appear to be required if the quality of general medical practice is to be improved.

In the next few chapters, we shall consider problems of medical education, both undergraduate and postgraduate. First of all, it is appropriate to consider why the student chooses to seek admission to the medical course and whether he receives adequate advice both prior to starting his medical studies and throughout the course of his undergraduate and postgraduate education. His decision to become a doctor, rather than to enter on some other line of endeavour, is one that will affect the whole of the rest of his life and is also one of a series of decisions that he will have to make regarding his medical career. Though one would suppose that decisions of such importance would be based upon the soundest advice available and would be made only after careful consideration of the factors involved, the evidence indicates that in too many cases this is not so.

As we tried to form a picture of the circumstances surrounding a student's entry into the medical course, the first question that we asked each of the Ontario men about this was, "At what age did you decide to study medicine?" The earliest age given in reply to this question was three years. The doctor who gave this answer said that he was seen by a doctor at that age, when he had a sore throat. He remembered the "cool, soothing hands" on his neck, and from then on he always wished to be a doctor. The most advanced age at which any of the Ontario men made the decision to study medicine was twenty-five years. The decision was said by 11 per cent of the men to have been made before eleven years of age, by 25 per cent between eleven and fourteen years of age, by 48 per cent between fifteen and eighteen years of age, and by the remaining 16 per cent over eighteen years of age. There was no significant relationship between the age at which this decision was made and the quality of practice at the time of our visit.

Because of the very early ages stated by some of the Ontario practitioners, we divided the question into two parts in Nova Scotia and asked, "At what age did you first think of being a doctor?" and "At what age did you decide definitely to study medicine?" Approximately 26 per cent said that they had first thought of being a doctor before the age of eleven years, 26 per cent between eleven and fourteen, 26 per cent between fifteen and eighteen, and 21 per cent over eighteen years of age. The decision was said to have been made definitely by 5 per cent before the age of eleven, by 7 per cent between eleven and fourteen, by 48 per cent between fifteen and eighteen, and by 40 per cent over eighteen years of age. The earliest age at which being a doctor was first thought of was said to be five years; the most advanced age at which the definite decision to study medicine was made was thirty-one years. There was no clear relationship between the quality of practice and either the age at which the first thought was given to being a doctor or the age at which the definite decision was made.

The reasons given by the doctors for their choice of medicine as a career varied greatly in both provinces. One man said, "I was always interested in science, always curious about nature. Father had a good book collection. This led to an interest in man." Another said, "I was interested in biology at high school, and my mother was a nurse." Yet another's grandfather had been a doctor and had told interesting stories, from which our informant concluded that medicine would be "a satisfying life." Quite different were the answers of two other practitioners, one of whom said, "Mother decided for me"—and what mother's reason was he did not know—while the other said that he had chosen medicine "by the process of elimination. An older brother had first place in the family business. I felt unsuited for law as a career." Another decision that was reached in what seemed to have been a roundabout way was that of a doctor who decided not to be a farmer, because, as he said with a laugh, he was too lazy for farming, but to be a professional man, "either a lawyer, a preacher, or a doctor." The first two of these three alternatives were eliminated because he was "shy and not gabby."

Some of the doctors' answers, as exemplified by "Mother decided for me," showed no constructive element, whereas others mentioned such motives as intellectual interest and desire to be of service. Because of the vagueness of some of the answers, it was not possible to classify all of them into those that did, and those that did not, give some indication of constructive motivation, but a very conservative estimate of the percentage of answers that lacked any constructive element is 20 per cent of the total both in Ontario and in Nova Scotia. As the answers were given years after the event—many years, in some cases—it is possible that they may have represented the doctor's thinking at the time of the administration of the questionnaire rather than what he remembered from the time of his entry to medical school. However, though men who had no constructive motivation when they entered medical school might have thought that they had had when they answered our question, it is not too likely that men who *were* constructively motivated when they made their choice would either have forgotten this or have chosen to conceal it. It appears, then, that an appreciable percentage of the men in each sample were able to enter medical school with little or no thought about the step that they were taking.

Several questions were asked to find out what advice the doctors had had before entering medical school. In answer to the question, "When you were considering whether or not to enter medicine, did you have advice from members of medical school or teaching hospital staffs?" 95 per cent in each province replied in the negative. When they were asked, "Did you receive advice from others?" 43 per cent in Ontario and 62 per cent in Nova Scotia replied in the negative, the remainder in the affirmative. Various sources of advice were named by the doctors, some of whom, as might be expected, had had advice from several sources. Parents were mentioned as advisers by only 23 per cent of the Ontario doctors and 14 per cent of those in Nova Scotia, and other relatives by the occasional doctor. Forty-one per cent in Ontario and 21 per cent in Nova Scotia were advised by physicians, including fathers and other relatives who were physicians, whereas 59 per cent and 81 per cent in the two provinces, respectively, had no advice from members of the medical profession. Clergymen and teachers were consulted in a few cases; but one doctor's only source of advice was a non-medical friend, who was two years his senior. From the information that we received, it appears, also, that the more recent graduates and those who graduated further in the past did not differ significantly in the percentage who had entered medicine without advice, either from a physician or from any source at all.

The doctors were asked, "Do you think that the advice that you received before entering medical school was (1) sufficient? (2) sound?" In Ontario, 41 per cent thought that they had had insufficient advice, 29.5 per cent had had advice that they regarded as sufficient, and 29.5 per cent had had no advice but regarded this as sufficient. In Nova Scotia, the corresponding figures were 38 per cent, 26 per cent, and 36 per cent. Eighty per cent of those doctors in Ontario, and 94 per cent of those in Nova Scotia, who had had advice regarded it as sound; but those doctors who had had advice that they regarded as sound comprised only 45 per cent of the total Ontario sample and 36 per cent of the total Nova Scotia sample. Finally, only 27 per cent of the Ontario sample and 26 per cent of the Nova Scotia sample had had advice and regarded it as both sufficient and sound.

In an effort to throw more light on how adequately the advice had met the needs of the student as he was making his decision to study medicine, the interrogator asked the physician, "When you *entered* medical school, had you obtained a reasonably accurate picture of (1) the duration of undergraduate medical training? (2) the cost of undergraduate medical training? (3) the duration of postgraduate training? (4) the cost of postgraduate training? and (5) the life of the average medical practitioner?" Only one doctor was encountered in Ontario, and two in Nova Scotia, who had not had an accurate picture of the duration of the undergraduate medical course on which they were embarking, and 91 per cent in Ontario and 81 per cent in Nova Scotia had had an accurate picture of the cost of the undergraduate training. The duration of postgraduate training, however, had been known to only 55 per cent of the men in Ontario and 52 per cent in

Nova Scotia, and its cost to only 43 per cent and 40 per cent in the two provinces, respectively. Only 45 per cent of the Ontario practitioners, but 76 per cent of those in Nova Scotia, had been aware of the type of life led by the average medical practitioner ($p < 0.01$).* These findings indicate a need for a great deal more information to be brought to the attention of the would-be entrant to medicine. The answers given by doctors of different ages did not give us any reason to believe that the more recent graduates were better informed when they entered medicine than their predecessors had been.

In Table 88, those doctors who had had advice from physicians and

TABLE 88

THE PHYSICIANS' PICTURE OF MEDICINE ON ENTERING MEDICAL SCHOOL

Whether the physicians had obtained a reasonably accurate picture, when they entered medical school, of the duration and the cost of undergraduate and postgraduate training and a reasonably accurate picture of the life of the average medical practitioner—answers of those who had had advice from physicians and of those who had not had advice from physicians

| Whether he had obtained a reasonably accurate picture of: | Of those who had had advice from physicians, number answering: | | Of those who had not had advice from physicians, number answering: | |
|---|---|---|---|---|
| | Yes | No | Yes | No |
| A. *Ontario* | | | | |
| The duration of undergraduate medical training | 17 | 1 | 26 | 0 |
| The cost of undergraduate training | 18 | 0 | 23 | 3 |
| The duration of postgraduate training | 10 | 8 | 14 | 12 |
| The cost of postgraduate training | 7 | 11 | 12 | 14 |
| The life of the average medical practitioner | 8 | 10 | 12 | 14 |
| Total number of physicians | 18 | | 26 | |
| B. *Nova Scotia* | | | | |
| The duration of undergraduate medical training | 9 | 0 | 31 | 2 |
| The cost of undergraduate training | 6 | 3 | 28 | 5 |
| The duration of postgraduate training | 7 | 2 | 15 | 18 |
| The cost of postgraduate training | 5 | 4 | 12 | 21 |
| The life of the average medical practitioner | 9 | 0 | 23 | 10 |
| Total number of physicians | 9 | | 33 | |

those who had had no advice from physicians are compared in respect of the proportions of each group that had a reasonably accurate picture of the five items listed in the preceding paragraph. In respect of

*This is explained on pages 32–33.

every one of the items, there was no significant difference, in either province, between those who had had, and those who had not had, advice from physicians before they entered medical school.

A student's need for adequate advice about problems having to do with his career does not end when he is admitted to medical school. It continues throughout his years of undergraduate and postgraduate education. When questioned about their years in medical school, 30 per cent of the Ontario physicians and 50 per cent of those in Nova Scotia said that adequate advice had not been available. The Nova Scotia men did not elaborate upon their answers. In Ontario, the two commonest complaints were that, though advice might have been available, the student did not know where to seek it and that the members of the staff were "unapproachable." One doctor referred to a particular professor who was the "class adviser" but gave students "the brush off." Another said, "I didn't feel there was anyone who was accessible to students for advice. All advice was given by senior students to junior students." A graduate of another medical school attributed the coldness and inaccessibility of the faculty members to the fact that there were "too many of us" and added that "the bright students got the attention." Some eminent men were named as willing to advise students, but just as many who were equally highly placed were criticized for their coldness and lack of interest in students and their problems.

In the period of postgraduate training, 16 per cent of the Ontario doctors had found that adequate advice was not available, 77 per cent that it was available, and the remainder did not answer either way. In Nova Scotia, 60 per cent said that adequate advice had not been available, and 38 per cent that it had been available, after they had graduated; one doctor was unable to answer. A few of the Ontario men indicated that as internes they had found it easier to seek advice, since they were coming in closer contact with the attending staff on the wards, than when they had been undergraduate students.

The scores* achieved by the physicians were examined in relation to their answers about the adequacy of the counselling available to them. The difference between the mean scores of those who had had, and of those who had not had, advice from physicians before their entry to medical school was not statistically significant either in Ontario or in Nova Scotia. Nor was there a significant difference either between the mean scores of those who said that adequate advice had been available in medical school and those who said that it had

*For score as a measure of quality of practice, see chapters 16 and 17.

not been or between the mean scores of those who said that adequate advice had been available in the period of postgraduate training and those who said that it had not been. In other words, there is no *statistical* evidence of a relationship, in either province, between quality of practice and the adequacy of the advice that was available to the medical student or young graduate. The facts that we have reported make clear, however, that the doctors who were interviewed[*] needed much more advice, both before they entered medical school and while they were in medical school, than was made available to them. It seems reasonable, also, to suppose that, in some cases at least, the quality of the man's work would have been improved if he had had help with his problems.

There may be those who will say that it should not be necessary to take a university student by the hand, that he must learn to stand on his own feet. When the matter is considered with an eye to the quality of a student's future practice, however, when it is remembered that we found men, in practice, who were taking inadequate histories, who were doing inadequate examinations, who were uncertain how to approach clinical problems, who were unable to distinguish between normal and abnormal findings, it might be worthwhile to ask whether more attention to a student's problems, however insignificant they might seem to the teaching staff, would not help him to stand on his own feet and to lay a more substantial foundation on which to build a practice of good quality. Boyd, in the preface to his *Textbook of Pathology*, says, "The medical student who steps from the laboratory into the clinical years is apt to find himself in a very unfamiliar country where for a time he may be lost to a degree little guessed by his clinical teachers."[†] We suspect that the student or recent graduate is "lost" at other times than when he passes into the clinical years, that he is lost when he enters university in the first place and again when he begins his interneship. It may well be, too, that he is lost in other situations than when he is first confronted with clinical work. He may be lost in dealing with patients, in taking histories from those who are unwilling to co-operate because he is "only a student," in

---

[*]The most recent graduates in the Ontario sample and in the Nova Scotia sample were the graduates of 1951 and of 1955, respectively. Whether medical students and applicants for admission to the medical course have their needs met more adequately today, we do not know, though such sporadic comments as we have heard in more recent years from undergraduate and postgraduate students have led us to believe that the counselling may still be inadequate.

[†]William Boyd: Textbook of Pathology (6th ed.; Philadelphia: Lea and Febiger, 1953), p. 7.

asking questions about personal matters, especially those relating to sex, in deciding whether to do a full examination or cut corners with a patient who seems likely to bring the examination to an abrupt end. He may be at a loss to know how to cope with those nurses—few, but immensely important if the student must have frequent contact with them—who tyrannize over their wards. It is not necessary to list all the situations in which the student may feel "lost." The point is that, though many students may take these situations in their stride, others probably react in ways that are detrimental to their learning of medicine. For example, we know that a nurse was allowed for years to remain in charge of an important ward in a large teaching hospital, although she was notorious for her rudeness and general unpleasantness, with the result that many medical students spent as little time as possible on the ward—an unhealthy influence, surely, from the point of view of medical education. Again, a student who is uncomfortable with his patients cannot give more than half-hearted attention to their medical problems.

We do not for a moment think that more effective counselling of medical students will put an end to the problem of inferior quality of practice. We do suggest, however, that this approach to the problem should not be overlooked, and that through better counselling much valuable information might be obtained. Why, for example, do young people choose medicine as a career? The answers reported above suggest that this needs further investigation. Why do some young people consider medicine but choose some other career? Is the reason the length of the medical course? the cost of the medical course? the length and cost of postgraduate training? the excessively long hours? or the fear of socialized medicine? Why does a medical student or recent graduate choose general practice, or one or another of the pecialties, or research, or administration, as his career? Are these choices soundly based? We have offered a few examples of the type of problem that we think might be tackled by better counselling of medical students. It is conceivable that both the advice given individual students, if it were adequate, and an increased knowledge of the factors that influence medical students in their career decisions might have a beneficial effect on the quality of medical practice.

# 20 / Undergraduate Medical Education
## *The Problem of Cost*

In chapter 13, we discussed the cost of medical education; and, at that time, we looked at the problem entirely from the point of view of a student or a young physician. In the intervening chapters, we have examined the work of general practitioners and have described the excellences and the deficiencies that we found in the practices we visited. Now, when we are considering the various ways in which the quality of practice might be improved, it is appropriate that we consider certain of the economic aspects further. Since our concern is no longer limited to the physician who provides the medical care but extends to society as a whole, which expects, justifiably, to obtain care of the highest quality possible, we must take a broader view and consider the problem of the economics of medical education, not merely as one to be solved by the individual concerned, but as one that places responsibilities on society itself.

The economic problems connected with the period of postgraduate training will be discussed in chapter 23. In this chapter, we shall confine ourselves to the period of undergraduate medical education. We have estimated, in chapter 13 (page 177), that the real cost to a student of his undergraduate medical education is at least $14,000, and probably more than this. Counts and Stalnaker found that, in 1952–1953, about one-third of the medical students in twenty-six medical schools in the United States expected to be in debt when they graduated, that the median value of the debt was $3,500, and that 3 per cent of the students expected a debt of more than $10,000.*

*S. Counts and J. M. Stalnaker: Journal of Medical Education, 29: 2, 22–23, 1954.

Whiting and his associates, on the basis of replies received from 4,899 out of 6,827 final-year medical students in the United States to whom a questionnaire was sent in the spring of 1959, say that 47 per cent of the students were in debt and that 67 per cent were working to earn money during the academic year.[*] Speaking of the financial difficulties of medical students, J. A. MacFarlane, as Dean of the Faculty of Medicine of the University of Toronto, said:

> The work of the Committee on Loans and Bursaries of the Faculty has steadily increased in the past few years . . . there is no question that many students are hard put to find money to continue with their course. In other reports I referred to the fact that a certain number of bright students fail to reach the university because of finance. Certainly, others who are able to come with only limited support put medicine at the bottom of the list because of the costs which extend over six or seven years. If Canadians really set some store by higher education, if they truly believe that gifted young men and women are more likely to assume positions of leadership and contribute to the well-being of the nation through the best education that is available in our universities, surely there is some way of assuring them reasonable financial support other than through this social welfare effort in which all faculties and schools must engage, in an attempt to see that the funds available are reaching those who are most deserving. In the meantime, the University finds no other way to balance its budget but by an increase in fees (Medicine is now $650 plus $57 incidental) which comes into effect at the opening of the autumn session.[†]

In a recent article entitled, "Wanted: More and Better Medical Students: The Facts and Figures on Medical Education," James S. Thompson, Secretary of the Association of Canadian Medical Colleges, expresses concern over the number and the quality of the students who are now applying for admission to the medical schools of this country.[‡] About quality, he says:

> . . . it appears that Canadian schools are accepting about 19% of their students with premedical averages in the "C" category. (This is based on an A, B, C scale, C being the lowest level assigned to those who pass.) Only 15% of successful applicants are in the "A" category and the rest are "B." Surely a field so vital to the well-being of a country deserves more than one student in six who could be classified as very good.

About the number of students applying for medicine, Thompson goes on to say:

> . . . Canadian medical schools could have enrolled 78 more first-year students without changing existing medical school facilities and it is expected that,

[*]J. F. Whiting *et al.*: Journal of Medical Education, *36*: 751, 757, 759, 1961.
[†]President's Report for the Year Ended June 1960, University of Toronto, pp. 40, 41.
[‡]J. S. Thompson: Canadian Medical Association Journal, *84*: 689–91, 1961.

with only minor changes, in a few years existing schools could (and would be prepared to) accommodate between 200 and 225 more medical students than they did in 1959–60. Clearly the failure to produce more Canadian-trained doctors lies not in the capacity of Canadian medical schools, at the present moment, but in the lack of suitable applicants.

Similarly, the Association of American Medical Colleges reports that "the total number of applicants" for admission to United States medical schools in the academic year, 1960–1961, showed "the fourth . . . decrease in numbers since 1956–57, and a loss of approximately 4 per cent from 1959–60."*

Thompson points to three reasons for the lack of suitable applicants for medicine: "the problem of high expenses coupled with short summers in which to earn money"; "the long haul of two premedical years, plus four medical years, plus a year of compulsory internship before an individual may obtain a licence to practise (and beyond this there may be the many years needed for specialty training)"; and the fact that "members of the medical profession work long hours and no longer enjoy the tremendous public respect they once had."

The amount that must be spent by a student during the four medical years alone is estimated by Thompson to be in the vicinity of eight or nine thousand dollars. Such a sum, as he points out, the student cannot hope to earn by summer employment. MacFarlane, also, speaking of summer employment, says in the report quoted above:

It is doubtful whether in the last two long vacations of a professional course they [i.e., the students] are adding much to their future in medicine if they spend four months at some job completely divorced from scientific effort. . . . I believe firmly that at least in the last long vacation, and preferably also during the period between his second and third year, the student should be doing work in a hospital or a research laboratory.

Thompson, comparing the student working towards a doctor's degree in medicine with a student proceeding to a doctorate in some other field, says, "It is clear that when fellowships, lower fees, etc., are considered, a student proceeding to a Ph.D. degree has a tremendous financial advantage over one proceeding to an M.D."

Though there may be other factors, such as the length of the total training in medicine, the type of life led by the doctor in practice, and a fear that the medical profession may be nationalized, which play a part in deterring ambitious and intellectually able students from entering medicine, there can be no doubt that the present high cost of undergraduate medical education is a serious problem. Thompson

*Association of American Medical Colleges, Datagrams, Vol. 3, No. 5, 1961.

344   *The General Practitioner*

suggests that, "In order to ensure an increase in the number of applications for medical school, especially among the better students, it may well be necessary to stop penalizing the individual financially because he decides to become a medical student." He adds a warning, which, in view of the poor quality of medicine that we observed being practised by some physicians, we consider very timely, namely, that unless an attempt is made to deal with the problem "Canada may be faced with an inadequate supply of doctors, many of low ability, at a time when an increased supply is essential and when men of the highest calibre are needed."

The question facing society is whether it is prepared to make available the money that is necessary to ensure an adequate supply of doctors of high calibre or whether it is going to allow those who cannot afford the high cost of a medical education to be drawn into other equally attractive but less expensive fields. We would suggest that the finances of medical students should be studied in some detail. What percentage of students are in debt when they graduate and how great is their indebtedness? What are they doing with their summer vacations and are any significant proportion of them trying to carry on jobs during the academic year? Finally—and this we consider of great importance—how many students are considering medicine but deciding, for financial reasons, in favour of other university courses? And what is the calibre of these students who consider, but reject, medicine? There may be those who will say that the student who is considering several alternatives at the end of high school does not *really* wish to be a doctor. We suspect that, while there are some students whose sole interest, in the way of a career, is medicine, there are others who possess both the intellectual ability and the idealism that are desirable in a physician but who consider several careers in which they could derive satisfaction from giving service, and that these men, weighing medicine against the other possibilities, find medicine less inviting. To obtain the answers to these questions is not merely a matter of academic interest; it is of great importance to the future quality of medical practice.

# 21 / Medical Education as Preparation for General Practice
## *Undergraduate Education*

In this chapter and the next, we shall record what the practitioners of the Survey said of their medical education. Though medical educators, with their background of long experience in educating physicians, have probably a clearer perception than a general practitioner of certain educational problems, yet some faculty members have had no experience of medical practice of any sort—indeed, some members of preclinical departments are not themselves physicians —and many have had no experience of *general* practice. On the other hand, though the general practitioner may be quite unaware of some of his educational needs, he may, as he faces the problems of practice, be more acutely conscious of others than are his teachers. The fact that we report the criticisms and recommendations of the doctors is not to be taken as indicating in itself that we are in agreement with them; but it is mandatory that we present the practitioners' criticisms and that those who desire to improve the quality of practice consider them without prejudice.

The physicians were asked whether their premedical education had been a worthwhile experience. Sixty-four per cent in Ontario and 90 per cent in Nova Scotia said that it had been; 30 per cent and 7 per cent, respectively, said that it had not been; and the remainder did not answer. The statements that were made in explanation of these answers were, in the main, vague and platitudinous. However, when the doctors were given a list of subjects—English literature, English composition, history, philosophy, anthropology, modern languages, and economics—and were asked to name any of these or any other subjects (except physics, chemistry, and biology, which were to be taken for granted) that they thought should be included in a doctor's premedical education after high school, their replies contained a few points that call for comment.

Of special interest was the fact that a little over one-quarter of the doctors who were visited in each of the two provinces made a plea for instruction, either in the premedical year or in the final medical year, in what many of them called "practical economics," i.e. business methods. As the inclusion of economics in the premedical curriculum was advocated by an additional 50 per cent of the Ontario doctors and by an additional 55 per cent of the Nova Scotia doctors, most of whom did not specify that they meant academic economics, it may be also that some of those who did not specify really meant "practical economics." At all events, it is apparent, not only that the practitioners desired to know more about matters economic, but that a significant proportion of them felt a need on a very practical level. Similarly, Schumacher and Gee, of the Association of American Medical Colleges, after analysing the replies to a questionnaire that was sent to 2,594 physicians (a 50 per cent random sample of the physicians who graduated from United States medical schools in 1950) and that was returned by 75 per cent of the sample, report that "The economics of medical practice have obviously created problems for about two-thirds of the 1950 graduates" and that 71 per cent of those who were general practitioners "felt that this area should be given greater emphasis during medical school."[*]

Having seen examples of gross inefficiency in the mechanics of carrying on a practice, which we have described in earlier chapters, we concur with the practitioners that the present system of education allows men to go forth inadequately prepared to cope with the business aspects of practice. Since difficulty in dealing with this essential part of his practice wastes a doctor's time and may well cause feelings of frustration, we agree with those men who claimed that too little attention was given to this; and in chapter 26 we shall discuss this further from the practical point of view. We do not think, however, that training in business methods should displace other, more fundamental, subjects from the premedical curriculum; and we doubt

[*]C. F. Schumacher and H. H. Gee: Journal of Medical Education, *36*, No. 4, Part 2: 155, 161, 162, 1961.

whether business methods have any place even in the final medical year (as was suggested), if for no other reason than that the student's own practice still seems so far in the future that he tends at that stage to ignore the details of such a subject since their relevancy is not apparent to him.

A small percentage of the doctors suggested that mathematics be included in the premedical curriculum, because they believed that this subject would test a student's ability to reason and would eliminate those students who, at examinations, were merely reproducing what they had memorized. One of these doctors told us that he had known two men who had been shown by psychometric testing to be "dull normals" but who by memorizing, by writing over and over again such things as "râles occur in pneumonia," had got through the medical course. He was understandably concerned that this was possible. The suggested inclusion of mathematics in the curriculum is based on the assumption that the mind that can cope with mathematical problems can deal readily also with problems of medical diagnosis. Whether this is so we do not know; nor are we aware of its having ever been adequately tested. Possibly such a study, if carefully carried out, might yield worthwhile results.

We pass on from premedical education to undergraduate medical education, about which the practitioners were questioned in some detail and about which they had a good deal to say. It had been our hope to question the doctors about each of the medical school subjects and to obtain their opinions about the amount of time allotted to the subject, about the content of the courses that were given, and about the quality of the instruction. During the preliminary trial of our methods (see page 23), it quickly became obvious that such an amount of detail could not be collected in addition to all the other information we were seeking. The question upon which we finally settled for the Ontario study listed twenty subjects in the approximate order of their appearance in the traditional medical curriculum and asked, "Were your medical school courses in each of the following subjects satisfactory or unsatisafctory *for the purposes of general practice?*" (In Nova Scotia, pathological chemistry was asked about separately from biochemistry, because we had become aware that the answers of the Ontario practitioners to the questions about biochemistry, though almost always referring to the course dealing with the normal chemistry of the body, frequently omitted any mention of the subject of chemical derangements.) The subjects are shown in Tables 89 and 90, where they

TABLE 89

ONTARIO PHYSICIANS WHO REGARDED MEDICAL SCHOOL COURSES AS
UNSATISFACTORY FOR THE PURPOSES OF GENERAL PRACTICE

| Subject | Physicians who were dissatisfied | |
|---|---|---|
| | Number | % |
| Dermatology | 31 | 70.5 |
| Social work | 24 | 54.6 |
| Psychiatry | 22 | 50.0 |
| Ophthalmology and otolaryngology | 20 | 45.5 |
| Fractures | 19 | 43.2 |
| Physiotherapy | 19 | 43.2 |
| Pharmacology | 18 | 40.9 |
| Diagnostic radiology | 18 | 40.9 |
| Biochemistry | 15 | 34.1 |
| Anaesthesia | 15 | 34.1 |
| Paediatrics | 13 | 29.5 |
| Physiology | 9 | 20.5 |
| Surgery | 8 | 18.2 |
| Obstetrics and gynaecology | 6 | 13.6 |
| Basic sciences (physics, chemistry, and biology) | 6 | 13.6 |
| Preventive medicine | 5 | 11.4 |
| Pathology | 3 | 6.8 |
| Medicine, including therapeutics | 3 | 6.8 |
| Anatomy (including histology, embryology, and neuroanatomy) | 3 | 6.8 |
| Bacteriology | 2 | 4.5 |
| Total physicians | 44 | 100 |

have been rearranged in decreasing order of percentage of dissatisfied doctors in Ontario and in Nova Scotia, respectively.

In each province, the percentage expressing dissatisfaction varied widely from one subject to another. A significantly higher percentage of the Nova Scotia, than of the Ontario, physicians expressed dissatisfaction with three subjects: physiotherapy ($p < 0.01$), anaesthesia ($p < 0.01$), and medicine ($p < 0.05$).* The percentages who had found the other subjects unsatisfactory did not differ significantly between the two provinces. Dermatology was regarded as unsatisfactory, for the purposes of general practice, by more than 70 per cent of the group in each province. The only other subject that was called unsatisfactory by 50 per cent or more of each group was social work. In Ontario, 50 per cent asserted that their medical school course in psychiatry had been unsatisfactory, and, in Nova Scotia, physiotherapy, diagnostic radiology, anaesthesia, pathological chemistry (about which the Ontario physicians were not questioned), and ophthalmo-otolaryngo-

*This is explained on pages 32–33.

TABLE 90

Nova Scotia Physicians Who Regarded Medical School Courses
as Unsatisfactory for the Purposes of General Practice

| | Physicians who were dissatisfied | |
|---|---|---|
| Subject | Number | % |
| Physiotherapy | 39 | 92.9 |
| Dermatology | 33 | 78.6 |
| Anaesthesia | 31 | 73.8 |
| Social work | 30 | 71.4 |
| Pathological chemistry | 26 | 66.7* |
| Ophthalmology and otolaryngology | 26 | 61.9 |
| Diagnostic radiology | 25 | 59.5 |
| Psychiatry | 20 | 47.6 |
| Fractures | 17 | 40.5 |
| Paediatrics | 15 | 36.6† |
| Biochemistry | 15 | 35.7 |
| Physiology | 14 | 33.3 |
| Pharmacology | 12 | 29.3† |
| Medicine, including therapeutics | 12 | 28.6 |
| Preventive medicine | 12 | 28.6 |
| Surgery | 12 | 28.6 |
| Anatomy (including histology, embryology, and neuroanatomy) | 7 | 16.7 |
| Basic sciences (physics, chemistry, and biology) | 5 | 11.9 |
| Bacteriology | 4 | 9.5 |
| Obstetrics and gynaecology | 4 | 9.5 |
| Pathology | 4 | 9.5 |
| Total physicians | 42*† | 100 |

*In the case of pathological chemistry, only 39 physicians were able to answer. The percentage shown is the percentage of 39.

†In the cases of pharmacology and of paediatrics, only 41 physicians were able to answer. The percentages shown are percentages of 41.

logy all drew expressions of dissatisfaction from more than 50 per cent of the practitioners.

Because of the great difference in age between the oldest practitioner, who was sixty-one, and the youngest, who was twenty-eight, and because of the possibility that men educated in different eras might hold quite different opinions of their education, we divided the physicians of each province into three groups, those up to thirty-five years of age, those between thirty-six and forty-five, and those over forty-five years, and compared the answers of the three groups about each of the subjects. The only subject with respect to which the groups of Ontario physicians differed significantly in the proportions of satisfied and dissatisfied physicians was biochemistry. This subject was regarded as unsatisfactory, for the purposes of general practice, by 22 per cent of the oldest group and 20 per cent of the middle group, but by 73 per cent of the youngest group ($p < 0.05$). In Nova Scotia, physicians of different ages were found to differ significantly in their answers about three of the subjects. Twenty-seven per cent of the physicians over forty-five years of age, but none of those forty-five years of age or less, were dissatisfied with their undergraduate training in obstetrics ($p < 0.05$). Seventy-three per cent of the men over forty-five years of age and 47 per cent of those between thirty-six and forty-five years of age, but none of those up to thirty-five years of age, had found the undergraduate course in psychiatry unsatisfactory. The oldest group and the middle group did not differ significantly, but the youngest group differed from both the middle group ($p < 0.05$) and the oldest group ($p < 0.01$) in the percentage expressing dissatisfaction. Surgery, on the other hand, evoked expressions of dissatisfaction from 7 per cent of the oldest group, from 32 per cent of the middle group, and from 63 per cent of the youngest group. The percentages of the youngest and the oldest groups who expressed dissatisfaction differed significantly ($p < 0.02$).

It is our good fortune that many of the doctors amplified their answers about the various courses with explanatory remarks. These contribute in two ways to our picture of the problems of undergraduate medical education. First, they show that some men, when forced to choose between calling a subject "satisfactory" and calling it "unsatisfactory," chose the former but still were strongly critical of the subject. In other words, the figures given in Tables 89 and 90 are conservative statements of the percentages of physicians who were critical of their courses. For example, though only 7 per cent of the Ontario practitioners said that the subject, medicine, was unsatisfactory, 4 times as many were adversely critical of this subject in one way or another.

Secondly, the practitioners' comments make clear what they considered to be the major deficiencies of the various courses. The few criticisms that were made of the basic sciences (physics, chemistry, and biology), of anatomy, and of pathology were that the teaching was poor and, except in pathology, that the courses covered too much material or went into too much detail. The vast majority of the doctors, however, described both anatomy and pathology as "good" or "excellent." Biochemistry was criticized on the same grounds, i.e. the quality of the teaching and the amount and the detail of the content, and on the additional ground that it was "too remote" or that it was not closely enough related to pathological chemistry and to clinical medicine. The major complaint about pathological chemistry, on the other hand, was that there had been too little attention given to this subject. We remind the reader that only the Nova Scotia practitioners were questioned about pathological chemistry.

The complaints of the Ontario physicians about physiology were poor teaching, lack of organization of the material taught, and unsatisfactory laboratory courses. Of the laboratory work, which was repeatedly criticized, it was said that a student was expected to accomplish an impossible amount in the time allotted, that his time was wasted on technical procedures, and that, in spite of hard effort, the experiments seldom worked. One of the younger Ontario doctors summed up most of the criticisms that we heard, when he said that physiology was "a hodge-podge as far as teaching went. The demonstrators were nice chaps, but no one knew the object of the lab. The labs did not tie into the course in general. The course was a lot of detached facts. There was no true direction. There was a lack of organization." The Nova Scotia practitioners' criticisms of physiology were too vague to be of any use to us in our consideration of medical education.

Pharmacology, which was classed as unsatisfactory by 41 per cent of the Ontario doctors and by 29 per cent of those in Nova Scotia, was described by a number of the doctors in both provinces as "antiquated," "archaic," or "outdated." It was said that too much time was spent on "pill-rolling" or "old-fashioned pharmacy" and not enough time on the mechanism of action of drugs. There were criticisms, also, of the quality of the instruction.

In connection with the four major clinical subjects, medicine, surgery, obstetrics, and paediatrics, we heard one criticism repeatedly both in Ontario and in Nova Scotia, that there was not enough practical work. Indeed, this was the only criticism of any importance that was made about obstetrics. About surgery, it was said that more emphasis should be put on the techniques of minor surgery, including the use of plaster and the handling of simple fractures. Frequent complaints about medicine and paediatrics were that students did not see enough patients, that common conditions and minor ailments were not covered adequately, and that there was far too much emphasis on rare and obscure conditions. The therapeutic aspect of medicine was also the object of criticism. It is interesting that Peterson reports that "most of the physicians" whom he studied in North Carolina "stated that more clinical training was desirable."* There were few complaints from the Ontario practitioners about the teachers or their ability to teach in

*O. L. Peterson *et al.*: Journal of Medical Education, *31*, No. 12, Part 2: 55, 1956.

either obstetrics or surgery. The teachers of medicine and of paediatrics were more often criticized. Not only were certain ones described as "poor," "dull," or "uninteresting," but we heard a type of criticism that we did not encounter in connection with the preclinical teachers, namely, that some of the clinicians "bullied" students, "frightened" them, "sneered" at them, or were "insufferable" or "domineering." In Nova Scotia, there were complaints about poor teaching in medicine, surgery, and paediatrics. A number of practitioners said that their teachers in these subjects were busy with their own practices and would sometimes fail to turn up for the scheduled hours of instruction. One man said, "Surgeons have to eat. So they can't teach properly at the same time."

The comments that were made about the minor clinical subjects— about anaesthesia, about fractures, about ophthalmology and oto- laryngology, and about dermatology—were the same ones over and over again in both provinces, "not enough" and "no practical ex- perience." The instruction in dermatology, ophthalmology, and oto- laryngology was criticized, by the Ontario practitioners, also as dealing with rarities instead of with the subjects of importance to a general practitioner. One man, to illustrate the unpractical attitude of the department of otolaryngology in his medical school, recalled that the students had been forced to use the head mirror with reflected light instead of the electric auriscope, with which they would have had a better view of the structures under examination. In other words, the short time allotted to otolaryngology had been taken up with coping with a technique that many of the students would never use, rather than with learning to recognize and treat the more common conditions of the ear, nose, and throat.

Psychiatry, which was considered unsatisfactory by 50 per cent of the Ontario general practitioners, was severely criticized. It was said to have been "unpractical," "too remote," "not down to earth," and "over my head." Specifically, it was said that the training was "not adequate to deal with the common neuroses and psychoses" and that the outpatient type of psychiatric work was neglected. One doctor said that the course was "worse than useless" in that it "antagonized us *against* psychiatry." The most significant criticism, because it struck at fundamentals, was that no basic principles of normal and abnormal psychology were taught, that classification and terminology were neglected, and that the teaching comprised demonstrations of already- diagnosed, advanced cases of mental illness. In Nova Scotia, the criticisms had to do with poor organization and inadequate clinical material; but these criticisms were made only by the practitioners who were over thirty-five years of age. Recently, Schumacher and Gee have reported that 48 per cent of the general practitioners in their sample (see page 346, above) of physicians who graduated from United States medical schools in 1950 named "techniques of managing minor psychiatric disorders" as one of the areas that they "thought were in need of greater emphasis during medical school."\*

Social work and physiotherapy both elicited the single comment, that there had been little or no instruction in these subjects and that there should be some instruction. Preventive medicine, which a minority in each province called unsatisfactory, was said to have put too much emphasis on sanitation and vital statistics and not to have paid enough attention to prevention.

The recurrent complaint about diagnostic radiology, both in Ontario and in Nova Scotia, was that there had not been enough of it or there had been little or none. At a later point in the questionnaire, when the physicians were being questioned about the radiological work done by them in practice, those who had stated that the training was unsatisfactory were specifically asked what changes they would suggest. A little over one-third of the Ontario men and one-half of those in Nova Scotia said that there should be more training in reading films, preferably in small classes of the tutorial type. It was suggested, also, that more time could be spent on the films of the patients with whom the students were dealing on the wards. One doctor recalled, as an example of the type of barrier that can be put in a student's path, that he and his contemporaries, as students, were not allowed to see the films on ward patients.† On the other hand, a number of doctors did not advocate more training in radiology, because they were of the opinion that the interpretation of films should be left to men who were well trained in this field. Only the occasional doctor thought that training should be given in the technique of taking films.

Because new drugs have appeared in overwhelming numbers in recent years and physicians have been besieged by detail men and bombarded with advertisements and samples (the physicians' attitudes

---

\*C. F. Schumacher and H. H. Gee: Journal of Medical Education, *36*, No. 4, Part 2: 161–162, 1961.

†We suspect, though we cannot be certain, that this prohibition was intended to force students to make their way towards a diagnosis by means of history-taking and physical examination rather than by the short cut of seeing what the film showed. While we agree, and have repeatedly emphasized in earlier chapters, that history-taking and physical examination are of paramount importance, we wonder whether there are not more positive ways of dealing with those students who are not mature enough to recognize the value of not taking short cuts.

towards these advertising methods have been reported in chapter 11), the doctors were asked, "How well did your medical training prepare you to evaluate the claims made for new drugs? Very well? Fairly well? Or not very well?" In Ontario, 57 per cent replied "Very well," 9 per cent "Fairly well," 32 per cent "Not very well," and one doctor did not answer. The corresponding percentages in Nova Scotia were 26 per cent, 33 per cent, and 40 per cent, respectively. When the doctors were grouped according to age, the groups did not differ significantly in their answers, in either province. Thus there is no indication that the evaluation of new drugs is less of a problem to the younger doctors, who might be expected to be better prepared in this respect, than to the older doctors, whose training preceded the modern therapeutic avalanche.

Those who thought that they had been adequately prepared in this respect told us that they had been encouraged to develop a critical attitude. A number of doctors who chose to specify where this attitude had been fostered made plain that it was not in the department of pharmacology, but in the department of medicine. These comments were intended by the doctors as a criticism of the teaching of pharmacology. Though such criticism may be justified, it is also possible that practical advice was given in the pharmacology course but that, because its applicability was not immediately evident, it fell on deaf ears. In fact, one doctor, one of the younger men, said that pharmacology comes too early in the course so that, by the time of graduation, a student has forgotten the fundamentals of pharmacology and is familiar with proprietary preparations.

Those doctors who regarded their preparation as inadequate said that they had not developed scientific scepticism and that they were "vulnerable" or "wide open" to drug travellers. One doctor, a fairly recent graduate, said: "We were not prepared for general practice therapeutics. The best drugs, the cost of drugs, and what to look for in dealing with drug travellers were not covered." Several doctors, though aware of their own inability to evaluate the claims made for new drugs, did not recognize even the necessity that they be able to do so, as is shown by one doctor's comment, "It didn't matter really that the pharmacology course at —— was no good because you learn all the new stuff from travellers," and by another doctor's statement that he thought that time devoted to teaching medical students to evaluate new drugs would not be well spent "as you use the drug house products anyway." In this connection, we quote from a recent letter written by a member of the College of General Practice of Canada to the Executive Director of the College, "I heard some drug representatives the other day detailing Aldactone. Out of curiosity I asked them how many of the general practitioners they talked to even knew what aldosterone was. Their answer was: 'Not very many.' "*

In addition to the questions about specific subjects, the practitioners were asked a number of other questions relating to their medical school experience. When asked whether, as medical students, they had been given "enough practical clinical experience," 55 per cent of the Ontario physicians said that they had been, 45 per cent that they had not; in Nova Scotia, 21 per cent of the practitioners gave affirmative answers, 79 per cent negative answers. The difference between the two provinces was significant ($p < 0.01$). In neither province, however, did the proportions of affirmative and negative replies differ significantly between the three age groups that were examined. The large number of negative answers was consistent with the repeated statements, made about the various clinical subjects individually, that there was not enough practical work. The few men who commented appeared to attribute the paucity of clinical experience to lack of time and, in one medical school, to lack of clinical material. A few men said that more time spent in the outpatient department and less on the wards would give the student a more useful type of experience.

In answer to the question whether, as medical students, they had been "allowed enough responsibility for patients," 73 per cent in Ontario and 57 per cent in Nova Scotia thought that they had, 27 per cent and 43 per cent in the two provinces, respectively, that they had not. No significant differences in the proportions giving affirmative and negative answers were found either between the Ontario group and the Nova Scotia group or between different age groups within either of the provinces. Many of those who gave affirmative answers went on to say that they had been allowed no responsibility, or very little, but that they did not think that medical students should be allowed to take any responsibility. On the other hand, those who said that they had not been allowed enough responsibility as students thought that students should be allowed to do certain things, especially such procedures as intravenous infusions and spinal taps, under supervision and that there had not been enough of this type of responsibility.

It is of interest to note that so eminent a medical educator as

*J. S. W. Aldis: College of General Practice (Medicine) of Canada, Bulletin, 7: 2, 13, 1960.

Charles A. Janeway, Professor of Pediatrics at Harvard Medical School, in discussing "Student Participation in the Learning Process," says:

> Participation gives the student a kind of motivation for which there is no substitute. It has to be real; it cannot be sham in clinical teaching. I believe that a student's record-keeping should be part of the official record. He must be made to feel that his patient's welfare depends upon his being at a certain place at a certain time, upon his using all the information at his command, and upon his ability to get information from the laboratory and the library for the benefit of his patient. Teachers have a grave responsibility in striking the proper balance (which shifts as the student moves along) between giving the student responsibility and protecting the patient from the student who takes more responsibility than his knowledge and experience justify. But we have to let the student feel he has responsibility at every successive stage in his career once he has begun his real clinical education.[*]

On this same subject, student responsibility, Janeway says also:

> . . . It is quite clear, I think . . . that student responsibility in the care of patients is essential to effective clinical teaching. . . .
>
> It is disturbing to find . . . that in as many as 20 per cent of our teaching hospitals the student's work is not an official part of the records of the hospital where he works, and neither are his laboratory work, his history, nor his physical examination . . . it seemed to most people [attending a medical teaching institute] rather elementary that any kind of teaching with patients that had a make-believe element to it could never be as effective as the real thing. But there are apparently still some differences of opinion on this matter.[†]

We have quoted Janeway because the position that he takes is the opposite of the situation pictured for us by many of the practitioners whom we visited. Even if the latter were incorrect in saying that they were not allowed to take responsibility as students, the important fact still remains that they did not *feel* that they were taking responsibility. The need that the student be required to assume some responsibility for his patients is given added emphasis when it is recalled that we came across certain practitioners who found it difficult to accept responsibility in their practices and some whose behaviour towards the Survey raised doubts about their concepts of responsibility (see pages 220, 221). It appears, then, that further study of the amount of responsibility to be assumed by the medical student might be profitable.

In order to form a rough estimate of the practitioners' enjoyment of their work in medical school, we asked each of them, "In general,

[*]C. A. Janeway: Journal of Medical Education, *34*, No. 10, Part 2: 79, 1959.
[†]C. A. Janeway: Journal of Medical Education, *34*, No. 10, Part 2: 108, 1959.

TABLE 91
PHYSICIAN'S DEGREE OF ENJOYMENT OF PRECLINICAL WORK
AND OF UNDERGRADUATE CLINICAL WORK

| Physician's degree of enjoyment | Preclinical work | | Undergraduate clinical work | |
|---|---|---|---|---|
| | Number of physicians | % | Number of physicians | % |
| A. *Ontario* | | | | |
| Very much | 9 | 20.5 | 35 | 79.5 |
| Moderately | 25 | 56.8 | 8 | 18.2 |
| Not very much | 10 | 22.7 | 1 | 2.3 |
| Total physicians | 44 | 100 | 44 | 100 |
| B. *Nova Scotia* | | | | |
| Very much | 8 | 19.0 | 30 | 71.4 |
| Moderately | 22 | 52.4 | 11 | 26.2 |
| Not very much | 12 | 28.6 | 1 | 2.4 |
| Total physicians | 42 | 100 | 42 | 100 |

thinking of them as subjects and disregarding as much as possible how well they were taught, did you enjoy your preclinical work very much? moderately? or not very much? And your undergraduate clinical work— very much? moderately? or not very much?" The answers are shown in Table 91. The striking thing about these answers is that, whereas 80 per cent of the Ontario physicians and 71 per cent of the Nova Scotia physicians enjoyed their clinical work "very much" and all but one of the remainder in each province enjoyed it "moderately," only about 20 per cent in each province enjoyed their preclinical work "very much," and 23 per cent in Ontario and 29 per cent in Nova Scotia did not enjoy it even "moderately." We did not ask the practitioners how much interest they *now* had in the preclinical subjects or whether they enjoyed learning more about them. As we pointed out in chapter 17, however, it was evident to us that the men whose work was of inferior quality were not basing their practice on the fundamental principles of the various preclinical subjects. That at least some of the general practitioners have little *interest* in these subjects is suggested by the following excerpt from a letter recently received by the Executive Director of the College of General Practice of Canada from a member of the College:

I'm always distressed at the feeling among most* general practitioners that the only type of medical information of any value is so-called "practical"

*Whether the use of the word, "most," is justified, we do not know.

information. The following is an almost verbatim quotation of a comment I overheard in Toronto a year ago:

"I'm not interested in all this theory and scientific stuff—all I want to know is how to treat it."*

In view of this comment and our observations on quality of practice, we may well ask whether there is any relationship between lack of enjoyment of the preclinical work and subsequent performance in practice. On examining the physicians' scores (representing quality of practice), we found that the mean scores of those who enjoyed their preclinical work "very much," "moderately," and "not very much" did not differ significantly either in Ontario or in Nova Scotia.

The Ontario practitioners' opinions on teaching methods were sought in a question asking them to rate as of "great value," of "moderate value," of "slight value," or of "no value" each of four methods, namely, frequent formal lectures covering the whole course, a well-constructed reading list covering the whole course, supplementary group tutorials or seminars (throughout this chapter, this type of instruction, given to small groups, will, for the sake of convenience, be referred to as tutorials), and infrequent lectures on broad aspects of a subject for stimulation and orientation rather than to cover the course. Because a number of the Ontario physicians made a distinction between a reading list that would replace, and a reading list that would supplement, the traditional lecture course, the Nova Scotia physicians were asked to assign a value to each of these uses of the reading list. The question regarding the infrequent lecture for orientation and stimulation was omitted in Nova Scotia. The values assigned to the various methods are shown in Table 92. In Ontario, the percentage (86 per cent) of the physicians who rated frequent lectures covering the whole course as of great value and the percentage (75 per cent) who rated tutorials as of great value did not differ significantly, but the percentage rating each of these methods as of great value was significantly greater than either the percentage (20 per cent) who rated the reading list as of great value or the percentage (32 per cent) who so rated the type of lecture intended for orientation and stimulation ($p < 0.01$). In Nova Scotia, the percentage (26 per cent) of the physicians who rated the lecture course as of great value was significantly smaller than either the percentage (76 per cent) who rated the tutorial as of great value or the percentage (64 per cent) who

*J. S. W. Aldis: College of General Practice (Medicine) of Canada, Bulletin, 7: 2, 13, 1960.

TABLE 92

OPINIONS OF PHYSICIANS ABOUT THE VALUE OF VARIOUS METHODS OF INSTRUCTION

| Method of instruction | Number of physicians who considered the method to be of | | | | Total number of physicians |
|---|---|---|---|---|---|
| | No value | Slight value | Moderate value | Great value | |
| A. *Ontario* | | | | | |
| Frequent formal lectures covering the whole course | 0 | 0 | 6 | 38 | 44 |
| A well-constructed reading list covering the whole course | 6 | 11 | 18 | 9 | 44 |
| Supplementary group tutorials or seminars | 1 | 4 | 6 | 33 | 44 |
| Infrequent lectures on broad aspects of a subject for stimulation and orientation rather than to cover the course | 7 | 10 | 12 | 14 | 43* |
| B. *Nova Scotia* | | | | | |
| Frequent formal lectures covering the whole course | 2 | 8 | 21 | 11 | 42 |
| A well-constructed reading list covering the whole course, instead of a lecture course | 0 | 25 | 14 | 3 | 42 |
| A reading list as a supplement to a lecture course | 1 | 4 | 10 | 27 | 42 |
| Supplementary tutorials and seminars | 0 | 1 | 9 | 32 | 42 |

*The remaining physician said that he did not know.

rated the supplementary reading list as of great value ($p < 0.01$ and $p < 0.05$, respectively), but was significantly greater than the percentage (7 per cent) who so rated the reading list as a replacement of the lecture course ($p < 0.01$).

A few men expressed the opinion that the reading list would be of great value to the "unusual" student, but of little or no value to the "average" student. One doctor, who said that the reading list was of slight value, explained, "You just don't get around to reading. You're young and raise whoopee."

Only about one-quarter of the Ontario doctors commented on the infrequent lecture of the type that we have mentioned. A few of those who regarded it as of great value commended it as giving an "over-all picture" and said that there should be more such lectures by "good, cultured, wise men." On the other hand, a comment that was made by a number of those who considered such lectures of little or no value was that they were of value to graduates but were "wasted" or "lost" on undergraduates, who were "not ready" for them.

The few comments that were made about the formal lecture course merely described it as "indispensable" or an "absolute necessity." The opinions expressed about the seminar or tutorial varied greatly. At one extreme was a doctor who did not know the meaning of either of these words; at the other extreme was a man who described them as "the best of all" the methods, because they separated what was important from what was not important. A few men considered that the seminar was merely another way of doing what the lecture course did, i.e. of "covering the material," with the disadvantage of being much slower.

Another question having to do with learning was put to each of the physicians, namely, "In medical school, do you thing that the faculty gave you enough direction in what to emphasize in your studying?" Only 34 per cent in Ontario and 36 per cent in Nova Scotia replied in the affirmative, 55 per cent in Ontario and 64 per cent in Nova Scotia gave negative answers, and the remainder in Ontario were uncertain. In neither province did the various age groups differ significantly in their answers. It is clear that the ability of more than half of the students to study, at least in respect of deciding where to place the emphasis, fell short of the need that they felt. What is not clear is whether the *real* need of the students was for more specific direction in studying or for more general help in learning to assume responsibility for their own study.

Before going on to examine the postgraduate portion of the physician's education, we shall pause to consider some of our findings about undergraduate medical education in the light of certain principles of pedagogy. These we propound, not by any means as new ideas or as being applicable to the teaching of medicine only, but because the comments made by the practitioners suggest that some medical educators are either unaware, or forgetful, of these principles.

Nathaniel Cantor, of the University of Buffalo, has concerned himself with the question, "What happens, realistically, when living students and living teachers meet together in a classroom in the teaching-learning process?"* In two books entitled, *Dynamics of Learning* and *The Teaching-Learning Process,* he has studied, respectively, "the learning process based on students' written reports and class dis-

*Nathaniel Cantor: Dynamics of Learning (2nd ed.; Buffalo and New York: Foster and Stewart Publishing Corporation, 1950), p. ix.

cussions" and "the same process primarily from the point of view of the teacher."* Talking of the "traditional procedure" in teaching, Cantor says, "The teacher lectures, gives 'answers' to questions not raised by the students. The instructor is supporting the student habit of passive acceptance of the authority of teacher or text."† This is a theme that recurs again and again in Cantor's books on teaching and learning. He points out that, "Until the student himself has struggled with the problems presented in a course, he is not ready to comprehend the problems or to appreciate their resolution. By leaving them alone (with some guidance, however) to find their own way, at their own tempo, the instructor will help the students more quickly to come to grips with the material of the course."‡ He emphasizes strongly that "learning involves more than passive listening or perfunctory talking," that "Learning means that the person synthesizes, integrates and assimilates,"§ and that "*All genuine learning, in the final analysis, is self-education.*"||

Do these quotations from Cantor's writings have any applicability to the medical course? We think that they do have. The majority of medical students come to lectures without having read about the subject beforehand. Because they believe that the lecturer has sifted the material to exclude what is "unimportant" and to include what is "important"—important, that is, for examination purposes—they concentrate on taking down verbatim as much as possible of what the lecturer is saying. Inevitably, even the best note-taker makes some mistakes in what he writes down. Much more important, however, is the fact that the student is so intent on writing down what is being said that he can spare little or no time for thinking about it. In other words, he is not learning but is merely collecting material to be learnt at some later time. Furthermore, because the student has not prepared the material beforehand, because the average lecturer moves too rapidly to allow the student to ponder over material with which he is not familiar, and because the student's note-taking does not leave him time to think, he does not recognize the problems, the difficulties, the possible inconsistencies, until that later time when he does tackle the material himself; and then the lecturer is no longer there to answer his questions.

*Nathaniel Cantor: The Teaching-Learning Process (New York: Dryden Press, 1953), p. 13.
†Cantor: Dynamics of Learning, p. 280.
‡*Ibid.*, p. 221.
§Cantor: The Teaching-Learning Process, pp. 211, 293.
||Cantor: Dynamics of Learning, p. 47.

In short, the traditional lecture course that purports to cover all that the student is required to know appears to do just exactly what Cantor deplores: it provides answers to problems of whose existence the student is not even aware. He is not aware of the problems because he has not had to struggle with the material himself before obtaining assistance. It is true that he *could* have anticipated the lecturer—provided that he knew what the lecturer was going to cover next and that he had sufficient time*—but the student's belief that the lecturer will cover everything that is "important" reinforces his own inertia.

There is another point on which Cantor lays emphasis. In discussing popular fallacies of school teaching, he says, "It is assumed that the teacher is responsible for the pupil's acquiring of knowledge. If the teacher is responsible for the pupil's acquiring of knowledge, then the pupil is not responsible."† This quotation deals with the pre-university phase of education, and the reader may ask whether it is applicable to the medical course. We believe it is. We have heard university colleagues express the fear that, if their students were left to cover the work themselves, too many would fail. Surely this means that the members of the staff feel responsible for the academic success or failure of students. We suggest that the lecture course that "covers" the subject deprives a student of the opportunity to develop the ability to be responsible for his own education. We are reminded of a cartoon that shows two youngsters, one in a high chair, the other at a table, each with his food in front of him, one of whom is saying, "I wish they'd hurry up and start trying to get us to eat. I'm starving." Might it not be better if a medical student, instead of being the object of so much anxious feeding, were left to satisfy his intellectual appetite more on his own?

Another objection that members of medical faculty staffs raise when it is suggested that the students themselves should be responsible for their own success or failure and that strikes us as quite untenable is that the subject-matter is so difficult that it is unreasonable to expect the student to cope with it alone. Some of it *is* very difficult; some is extremely simple. For example, is it necessary to gather students together in a lecture room to tell them the clinical manifestations of congenital hypertrophic pyloric stenosis? When we see what adoles-

*One reason why students do not prepare beforehand may be that, during the day, their time-table contains so few hours, if any, which are not filled with lectures, laboratory work, or clinics, that the evening is barely long enough to deal with what *has* been covered, let alone think of the next day's work. See page 367 for number of hours of scheduled work.

†Cantor: The Teaching-Learning Process, p. 67.

cents are able to learn, on their own, of the workings of motor cycles or motor cars or of the building of radio tuners and amplifiers, it is hard to believe that medical students could not master, by themselves, subjects such as pyloric stenosis (which is very well described in the standard textbooks) and many others, *provided that they are interested.* To quote Cantor again, "The motivation, the drive to learn, must, in the final analysis, come from the learner." He points out that, when students are confronted by problems the answers to which they do not know, "Being involved, they will want to discover, if they can, how to get rid of their dissatisfaction or how to satisfy their curiosity."[*]

We have criticized the traditional lecture course as making it possible for a student to remain blind to problems, since the answers are provided without his recognizing the problems, and as depriving a student of the opportunity to develop the ability to be responsible for his own education. The lecture course, as it is generally constituted, appears, then, to do a student a double *dis*service. The importance of this, it seems to us, lies in the fact that, once in practice, a physician must continue his education throughout the remainder of his career and *on his own initiative.* Anything that tends to inhibit the development of his ability to educate himself appears, in the long run, to be likely to have an injurious effect on the quality of his medical practice; and it is with quality of practice that we are concerned primarily.

Our remarks on the lecture course are not to be interpreted as a suggestion that lectures be abolished. Rather, we suggest that there be less emphasis put on the lecture and more on tutorials. We think that, unless there is a textbook that meets the requirements of a particular course, the student needs guidance in what to read, but that, having been given this guidance and enough unscheduled time in which to do the necessary reading, he should, from the early days of the course, be made increasingly responsible for covering the work himself. The reading should be supplemented by frequent tutorials at which the students would be questioned and would have the opportunity to ask questions on the points that they had not understood when they were reading. To be of value, the tutorials would have to be conducted by instructors who were both interested and quite clear in their own minds about what they were trying to do. Certain pitfalls, in particular, would have to be avoided. First, the tutorial should not be allowed to degenerate into either a verbal free-for-all or a vague platitudinous discussion from which no one would gain anything but a lack of respect for tutorials. Secondly, the more aggressive members of the group

[*]*Ibid.,* pp. 211, 304.

should not be allowed to have more than their share of the instructor's attention, nor should the less aggressive be allowed to remain passive spectators. Thirdly, and of great importance, the instructor should not turn the tutorial hour into a lecture. The temptation to do this might be very great if the students came unprepared and were neither able to answer the instructor's questions nor ready with any difficulties of their own that they wished explained. If this situation were to arise, i.e. if the students were to come unprepared, as they might early in a course of tutorials, the instructor should merely dismiss the group until its next meeting. If it were made plain in this way that the instructor was not going to expound to unprepared and passively listening students, it is unlikely that many of these hours would go by default. In short, the tutorial, to be successful, would have to be conducted by an instructor who was aware of both the potentialities and the weaknesses of this method of instruction and who was both sympathetic towards his students and, at the same time, prepared to maintain firm control over the tutorial hour.

While we are on the subject of tutorials, we would mention specifically the clinical teaching that is carried on in small groups either at the bed-side or in the outpatient department. Too often this becomes a lecture, but one that is given more or less extemporaneously, in the rather noisy environment of the ward or clinic, to students who, after standing in one place for as long as half an hour or even an hour, are more intent on relieving their aching backs or feet than on what the clinician is saying. Instead, we suggest, the bed-side teaching should concentrate on what can be learnt from interrogation and physical examination of the patient; and, just as in the preclinical subjects, the instructor's function should be to deal with the problems that a student has recognized but has not succeeded in solving and to discover and make clear to the student the weaknesses that he has not recognized in his own work. For example, a student gains far more from examining an ear drum or a chest, describing his findings, and having them checked by the instructor, than from any amount of more formal teaching on the examination of the chest or the ear. Nor is it enough that physical findings be checked in one or two cases; repeated supervision of this type is necessary. Again, a student learns little from history-taking, unless his histories, both the factual material elicited from the patient and his discussion of the diagnosis, prognosis, and management of the case, are criticized in detail. Janeway, talking of the teaching of history-taking, says, "The interview, which is the fundamental method for study of a patient, is something that has been taken too much for granted in the past. The ice is breaking, and schools are beginning to examine what it is that goes into the interview, what its techniques are, and how to use it in instruction at a far more basic level than the conventional business of making the student memorize the form he must follow in history-taking as part of a course in physical diagnosis."* The importance of this part of a student's education was most clearly illustrated by some of the very poor history-taking that we saw in the practices we visited. The practitioners' difficulties were particularly evident when they were dealing with emotional problems, for which a stereotyped approach is of the least value.

Coming now to the place of the lecture, we suggest that lectures be reduced in number, that they not cover those subjects that are well covered in the standard textbooks, and that they not be designed to cover the whole course in detail, but that they deal with those subjects that are not adequately dealt with in books, those subjects that present unusual difficulty, and those subjects that the lecturer is able to approach from a different point of view or on which he is able to cast a different light. Reduction in the *number* of lectures would leave the student more time to study actively on his own and to consolidate his newly acquired knowledge. The suggested change in the *concept* of the lecture course and the greater use of tutorials—provided that the hazards mentioned above were avoided—would shift the responsibility in the teaching-learning process from the teacher to the student and would shift the emphasis from teaching to learning. We believe that it is fatally easy to confuse these two, to believe that what has been "taught" has also been learnt. If the responsibility for learning becomes the student's, then the staff member's responsibility is to help the student to learn and to satisfy himself that the student has learnt.

Our observations of the practices that we visited provide an excellent example of the difference between being taught and learning. There can be no doubt that every one of the practitioners had been "taught" the necessity of taking a good history and how to go about taking such a history, the importance of a thorough physical examination and how to carry out such an examination, and most, if not all, of the other items that were included in the rating scale that we used in making our assessments of the practices. Yet, though these things had been "taught," it was clear in some cases that they had not really been learnt, i.e. they had not become incorporated into the physician's way of thinking and acting so as to form an integral part of his practice (see page 460 for an example). We repeat that, if these flaws in a

*C. A. Janeway: Journal of Medical Education, 34, No. 10, Part 2: 113, 1959.

medical student's knowledge and practice are not to go undetected, a clinical teacher, instead of expounding to a passively listening student, must shift his interest to listening while the student actively tells him and to watching while the student actively demonstrates to him, in order that the student's inadequacies may be exposed both to the student himself and to the teacher and that the student may be assisted to deal with them. For example, there is little point in knowing the significance of râles or rhonchi if one cannot, on auscultating the chest, distinguish these from each other or from normal breath sounds (see page 294).

It is particularly important that a student's difficulties be dealt with early, since, the longer they persist untreated, the more difficult it is to approach them. Though some of the practitioners whom we saw could profit greatly from refresher courses that went right back to the fundamentals of history-taking and physical examination, it is unlikely that practising physicians would attend these courses, since men in practice would find it hard to accept, or would be outraged at, the suggestion that they needed them. It is essential, then, that the details be learnt at the appropriate stage of a student's development, before his prestige becomes such an issue that it is impossible to point out his deficiencies. As Barzun says, in criticizing college instructors for failing to instruct in such matters as the use of a library or the writing of a sentence, "Details become more and more unmentionable as the tutorial hours grow loftier in content."[*]

That we are not alone in our opinion of lectures is shown by the words of Robert C. Dickson, Professor of Medicine at Dalhousie University, who, expounding the policy of his department, says:

The teaching in the Department of Medicine at Dalhousie is based on the view . . . that teaching time that does not involve genuine effort on the part of the student is largely wasted. . . .

and:

In the past in most medical schools on this continent, the lecture has formed the key method of providing this guidance [i.e., guidance in what to read] and at Dalhousie the lecture is still the favored form in some departments. In the department of medicine, the lectures have been cut ruthlessly in order to provide time for more bed-side teaching and for the development of what has been called the group tutorial. The reason for this is threefold. First, the lecture, as do other forms of didactic teaching, lends to the words of the teacher an authority which is rarely their due. Second, it demands

[*]Jacques Barzun: The House of Intellect (New York: Harper & Brothers, 1959), p. 120.

no contribution or effort on the part of the student beyond his ability to keep awake and perhaps write an occasional note. Third, it does not stimulate thinking, except in the rare instance where a particularly gifted lecturer is able to arouse enthusiasm and thought among his listeners.*

As we listened to the practitioners whom we visited extolling the lecture course and as we heard them saying that students would not do the necessary reading, that such value as the reading list had lay in the supplementing of lectures—rather than vice versa—and that only the "unusual" student could be left to read on his own, we could not but wonder whether these statements of the practitioners were an indication that they, as students, had taken the path of least resistance, because the system allowed them to do so. Charles G. Child, III, Professor of Surgery at the University of Michigan and Chairman of the Seventh Teaching Institute of the Association of American Medical Colleges, says, in his Introduction to the Report of the Institute:

. . . how many will agree with me if I insist that medical education today is in transition from trade school to university? Slowly we learn that lectures which pack our curricula are cheap and support students in roles of dependent and passive recipients of their education. Seminars are replacing lectures— costly to be sure but invaluable in encouraging active and responsible participation of students in their own education. We appreciate more each day that students who have not accepted early responsibility for their own learning are unlikely later to reflect responsible attitudes toward patient care.†

In the preceding few pages, we have mentioned the need of the medical student for adequate unscheduled time in which to study. To realize how precious time is, one need only glance at the student's time-table. The time-tables of the Faculty of Medicine of the University of Toronto, for the first, second, and third medical years during the academic year, 1960–61, show the total number of hours of lectures, laboratory work, and clinical work to vary between 33 hours and 39 hours per week in the different terms and to average, in each of the three years, slightly over 36 hours per week. The number of hours of lectures appears to vary between 10 and 15 per week. How restricting such a schedule is, especially when the hours of necessary reading are added, is illustrated by a comment made to us recently by a brilliant medical student, who lamented the fact that the time-table, especially in the upper years of the course, was so crowded that he never had time to browse in the library, as he had done in earlier years, or to

*R. C. Dickson: Journal of the American Medical Association, *173*: 1298 and 1299, 1960.
†C. G. Child, III: Journal of Medical Education, *36*, No. 4, Part 2: **xxiii**, 1961.

read anything except what was directly concerned with the work of the moment. We contend that a student who has as little leisure as this does not have time to consolidate his knowledge, i.e. to organize the material according to his own needs so that it becomes an integral part of himself. We come back to Cantor's admonition (see page 361) that students be left alone "to find their own way, *at their own tempo* [italics ours]." How difficult it may prove, however, to make more time available to the student was made clear recently by Irwin M. Hilliard, Professor of Medicine at the University of Saskatchewan, who said, "Recently the suggestion to loosen up the curriculum was made to our faculty. The aim was to provide more free time for projects and for library work on medical and non-medical subjects. However, nearly every department wanted to increase what was taught by their particular department rather than to cut down."*

The one subject whose laboratory work was frequently criticized by the general practitioners, especially in Ontario, was physiology (see page 351). It was said that "no one knew the object of the lab" and that the experiments seldom worked. If these criticisms were valid, then it seems that the laboratory course was not so designed as to be a means by which the students could "get rid of their dissatisfaction" with their problems or "satisfy their curiosity," to refer again to one of the conditions named by Cantor as conducive to learning (see page 363). The complaints of the practitioners find support in the physiology department of Baylor University. Writing in 1957, Hoff, Geddes, and Spencer say, "The neglect into which the student laboratory of physiology has fallen is almost without counterpart in a century that has seen unprecedented advances in almost every other sphere of human activity."† They point out that the smoked-drum kymograph "became the mediator of the great 19th century renaissance in physiology," that, "in its day, the kymograph brought physiological advances directly to the student," and that "the student laboratory and the research laboratory were in full and free communication and a wide horizon of physiological investigation opened before each student as he entered the laboratory." They go on to describe how the kymograph was supplanted, in the research laboratory, by other instruments, which did not find their way into the student laboratory. Describing the situation in this century, they say:

When the era of widespread electronic instrumentation began in the 20's, . . . the student laboratory had already been dissociated from the field

*I. M. Hilliard: Ontario Medical Review, *28*: 346, 1961.
†H. E. Hoff *et al.*: Journal of Medical Education, *32*: 181, 1957.

of electrophysiology for more than 35 years, and the tradition perforce had to be accepted that student teaching need not and could not deal directly with a main current of day-by-day advance in physiology. Thus, the student laboratory could no longer open its door to the new fields of investigation as it had in Bowditch's day with the kymograph. Students and teachers alike were not long in becoming aware of this situation. . . . To the student it meant the loss of the only place where nature could speak directly to him without the mediation of the instructor. . . . To the instructor it meant a divorcement of his own research program, almost wholly laboratory centered, where each day's experiment conditions those of the days to follow, from his teaching program in the student laboratory.

Hoff and his associates state that "To the best of our knowledge, . . . no full scale attempt has yet been made at a fundamental solution to the problem of the complete re-creation of the student laboratory in physiology," but that "it is only within very recent years that an attack on the problem of adequate instrumentation for the student laboratory could have been made." The body of their paper describes a new instrument, the physiograph, which they have introduced into their student laboratory and which, they claim, places "the student laboratory again at the frontier of physiological advances." In a later paper, they summarize their experience with the physiograph by saying, "it has served significantly to change the status of the laboratory in the teaching of Physiology, reorienting emphasis from obtaining results to understanding and interpreting them, broadening the spectrum of what the student can experience, and teaching him the recourse to experimentation. Thus, it has fostered the problem-solving approach, which leads from analysis of a problem to an effective solution."[*]

We have spent some time on the laboratory work in physiology because it serves to illustrate two points. The description, given by Hoff and his associates, of the student physiology laboratory as being removed by half a century or more from the investigation being carried on at the present time shows that the complaints of the practitioners, i.e. of the former medical students, about their education may, at least in some matters, be well grounded. Secondly, the developments described in the papers that we have quoted are an example of the type of fresh and imaginative approach that can be made to problems of medical education.

A question that comes to our mind when we hear of the student physiology laboratory, whose arrested development has caused it to lag far behind the main body of physiological research, is whether laboratory courses in other subjects are being perpetuated even though

[*]L. A. Geddes *et al.*: Journal of Medical Education, *34*: 107, 1959.

they have long since ceased to serve their original, or perhaps any useful, purpose. We do not know the answer to this question; but, as we consider the medical student's crowded time-table, the increasing amounts of material with which each successive class of students has to cope, and our own observations on the quality of practice, we do think that many of the laboratory courses could well be subjected to very close scrutiny. In this regard, we note with interest that James L. Morrill, President of the University of Minnesota and one of four university presidents or chancellors who were asked by the Association of American Medical Colleges to take part in 1958 in "a panel on medical education as a university responsibility," says:

> . . . the most interesting and significant enterprise for the improvement of instruction in which I ever had any participation at another university was in the field of the biological sciences . . . in which the method of long laboratory work had been the practice and taken for granted. That was shaken up with the full acquiescence of the biological faculties, and they went to very much more table-top demonstration, with an immediate lowering of costs, better utilization of space, and after a period of 4 years of testing, the learning was found to be considerably improved. I fancy . . . that there are opportunities for some approach of the same kind in medical instruction.*

Turning now to teachers and their ability to teach, we find Cantor making certain observations that are as applicable to medical teachers as to college teachers generally:

> It is a mistake to believe that most untrained people can engage in effective college teaching without professional teaching equipment. It is strange that . . . almost no thought has been given to the professional training of college teachers. A prospective college teacher does his graduate work in his specialty, receives his advanced degree, submits his references or recommendations, is interviewed by someone in the college administration, and, if invited to join the college, it is assumed he is ready to teach. He has no professional training in one of the most difficult and complex of all professions, the profession of teaching. He is apparently qualified to teach by having successfully demonstrated his ability as a scholar, and by reason of having a more or less agreeable "personality." He, the embryonic teacher, has little if any sense of what his function as a college teacher is, although he has been motivated by an interest—his subject, a regard for academic life, or an amorphous desire to "teach."†

The practitioners whom we visited were asked which of their teachers in medical school they remembered as particularly good or

*The Presidents' Panel, President James L. Morrill, President Deane W. Malott, and Chancellor Franklin D. Murphy (James B. Conant, Moderator): Journal of Medical Education, 34: 260, 1959.

†Cantor: Dynamics of Learning, p. 77.

particularly poor. Whereas some men were named as good teachers by one practitioner and as poor teachers by another, certain names recurred again and again in the list of good teachers and others again and again among those said to have been poor teachers. Of particular significance is the fact that the latter group included not only junior members of the staff but men who for years were full professors and heads of important departments, both preclinical and clinical. Such cases were not frequent—and other department heads were mentioned as outstanding teachers—but a few poor teachers in key appointments may have a sufficiently deleterious effect on medical education to give point to Cantor's expression of surprise that no attention is paid to a staff member's ability to *teach*.

Another factor that may well play a major part in determining the quality of teaching is the comparative standings of teaching and of research. Research is highly regarded; teaching, though paid lip-service, is largely without honour. President Morrill, to whom we referred above, talking of a meeting of vice-chancellors of British Commonwealth universities, quotes the president of one of the Canadian universities as asking, " 'Are medical schools becoming research institutes, supported by general university funds and grants-in-aid of research, rather than teaching entities with associated research activities?' "* Another speaker at the Presidents' Panel, Deane W. Malott, President of Cornell University, says, "I see some dangers . . . in the development of these great medical centers, where more and more concern is being given to research for the sake of research, and not as a part of the teaching mechanism, with teaching only as the necessary concomitant in some instances, perhaps, for the enlistment of the necessary junior research workers."† In the Third Alan Gregg Memorial Lecture on "Immediate Problems for Medical Educators," Joseph T. Wearn, formerly Dean of the Medical School of Western Reserve University, says, "the status of research is such that our young men cannot be blamed if they believe it is now the principal avenue to academic advancement."‡

It is beyond the scope of our study to discuss why research is so much more highly regarded than teaching; but we would make a plea, that the glamorous trappings of research not be confused with its essence, which is inquiry, carefully and critically conducted. We make this plea, because there appears to be a tendency for many,

*The Presidents' Panel: Journal of Medical Education, 34: 250, 1959.
†*Ibid.*, p. 252.
‡J. T. Wearn: Journal of Medical Education, 36: 113, 1961.

including persons in academic life, to be beguiled by the non-essential, to be dazzled by the visions that the word "research" conjures up, visions of laboratories, of fabulous grants of money, of equipment too complex to be comprehended by the uninitiated. There is nothing wrong with these things, in themselves—in fact, as aids to research, they are most valuable—but the aura of magic with which they have invested the word "research" does tend to nourish an image of research as something more—something bigger, more heroic, and, especially, more mysterious—than what it actually is, namely, careful and critical inquiry, for the conduct of which *the* essential instrument is, not money or laboratory equipment, but an inquiring mind.

We have felt it desirable to point out the magic connotations of the word "research" because, if teaching is not to seem the ugly duckling by comparison and is not to be treated as such, it is necessary to see research for what it is. If careful, critical inquiry be accepted as the essence of research, and the inquiring mind as the one instrument essential to the carrying on of research, then surely, whether that mind engages in formal and elaborate research projects or whether it ponders over problems of teaching and learning and attempts to work out ways of bringing students to a clearer understanding of a difficult subject, such a mind and its possessor, in either case, are equally worthy of admiration, academic honour, and monetary reward. In fact, in such an institution as a medical school, whose primary function is not research but teaching, we hold that the teacher who is interested in teaching, who brings an active, inquiring mind to his teaching, and who stimulates his students should be honoured, and rewarded, more highly than the research worker, however famous he may be for his research, whose heart is not in teaching, whose perfunctory attempts to teach are an imposition on successive classes of students, and whose place is not in a teaching institution but in a research institute.

We have dealt with two matters that may affect the quality of medical school teaching, namely, whether any attention has been given to a staff member's ability to teach and the greater prestige of research than of teaching. Also of importance is the atmosphere in which a student's learning goes on. Cantor points out that "One of the important characteristics of skilled teaching is the creation of an atmosphere which encourages pupils to question, challenge, and contribute to one another's and to the teacher's growth" and that "To a professional teacher, ridiculing or being sarcastic to pupils is . . . *the* cardinal sin in teacher-pupil relations."* These points might be thought

*Cantor: The Teaching-Learning Process, pp. 79, 274.

to be so obvious as not to require stating. Yet certain teachers, all of whom were in the clinical departments, were said by the general practitioners to have "bullied," "frightened," and "sneered."

Finally, there is an economic factor that may well have an effect on the quality of teaching in the clinical departments of a medical school. All but a very few of the teachers of the clinical subjects, medicine, surgery, paediatrics, obstetrics, and the other clinical branches, are paid either nothing at all or a small honorarium which is quite disproportionate to the importance of the work for which it is given. James S. Thompson, Secretary of the Association of Canadian Medical Colleges, speaking of the part-time teachers in the clinical departments, says:

These part-time teachers are the bulwark on which medical schools depend for the major portion of the teaching to the medical students, and their importance increases over the years, instead of decreasing, as many doctors, and many part-time teachers, seem to fear. This part-time group makes up between 85 and 90% of the staff of clinical departments, and almost one-third of them receive no remuneration at all from the universities for their teaching duties. The other two-thirds receive small (often just token) honoraria for their part in the education of our students. Whether they lend their talents for so little monetary gain because of the prestige of being members of university staffs, or for the more altruistic traditions of the Hippocratic oath, or just because they like to teach is a question no man can answer.*

It would be interesting to know how much time is given by these part-time teachers. We do not know of any figures dealing with this, but undoubtedly there is great variation. Some part-time teachers give only a few hours per week. On the other hand, we were told recently by one of our colleagues that he spent thirty hours per week on teaching and looking after indigent patients in one of the hospitals. He is listed, in the directory of his university, as a clinical teacher; his remuneration, he told us, is less than $300 per year.† When we think of the forty-hour week and of labour's current hopes of an even shorter work week, a donation of thirty hours per week for virtually nothing is such as to make us pause and ask how a physician can afford to give so much time.

Is it that he makes so large an income during the rest of his time

*J. S. Thompson: Canadian Medical Association Journal, 82: 728, 1960.
†This doctor also had a position on the staff of his hospital, which he would not likely have had if he had not been willing to teach. Thus, in theory, he had a hospital to which to admit his own private patients for treatment. In practice, however, it was so rarely that he could obtain a bed, that the hospital was virtually useless to him in his own practice.

that he can well afford to give his time for nothing? In the early days of specialization in medicine, when training was much shorter and less expensive than it is today, when specialists' fees were probably higher, in relation to the cost of living, than they are today, and when income tax was low or non-existent, it is likely that the specialist *could* well afford to give his time to teaching without remuneration. Today, the situation is different in many respects. The doctor who wishes to obtain specialist qualifications must take at least five years of post-graduate training, so that he is well on towards thirty years of age, or even over thirty, before he starts his practice, which, of course, will take several years to become established. If he is married, he is likely to be heavily in debt before he starts earning. The income-tax law makes no allowance for the fact that the doctor who specializes is several years later than members of other professions in establishing a practice; and the present high rates of income tax make it exceedingly difficult for the doctor to rid himself of his indebtedness. It may be that some of the specialists are still earning such incomes that they can well afford to donate their time to teaching. For the majority, however, this is probably not true. The specialist to whom we referred above as giving thirty hours per week was earning considerably less than the median earnings that we have reported for the sample of general practitioners (see page 190) and saw no prospect of increasing his income beyond its present level, unless he gave up the teaching that he loved.

Why, then, do the medical schools perpetuate this system of using part-time, underpaid or even unpaid, teachers? Partly, it seems, because it has become traditional, and partly because it is obviously far less expensive to have men teach for little or nothing than to pay them for their time.

Yet, *does* this system reduce the cost of medical education? It is quite obvious that it does not but that it merely apportions the cost in a lop-sided way. The physician who gives, for a few hundred dollars, the amount of time that should be worth several thousand dollars is himself footing the bill for medical education to a far greater extent than any other member of the community. If he works all morning in the hospital for nothing, he must either be satisfied with what he can earn in the afternoons, which is usually inadequate, or he must extend his hours of work—i.e. his hours for routine work, not merely emergencies—to include the evenings. This leaves him little or no time for recreation or for regular medical reading; his family sees little of him; and all domestic matters, including the bringing up and disciplining of the children, must be left to his wife.

Our primary concern, however, is not with the difficulties of the part-time teacher, but with the quality of general practice and, therefore, with the adequacy of medical education. We believe that the present system has several adverse effects as far as teaching is concerned. First, the unforeseen demands of a busy practice may prevent the physician from turning up at the appointed time to give a lecture or conduct a clinic.* Secondly, the unpaid teacher is not as readily amenable to disciplinary action as the university teacher who is receiving appropriate remuneration, whose primary responsibility during the time for which he is engaged is, and is recognized to be, his university work. How important a factor this is, we do not know, but we have heard the practitioners' statements about teachers who failed to show up (see page 352), and we know of cases in which medical students, complaining that teachers have repeatedly not turned up for scheduled hours of instruction, have been told quite bluntly that they have no right to complain since the physician in question is not paid for his teaching. Thirdly, under the present system of using part-time teachers, men whose primary interest is practice are drawn into teaching because they must accept teaching responsibilities if they wish to be able to treat their own private patients in the teaching hospitals. The prestige of being on the staff of a teaching hospital, even though the beds may turn out to be difficult or impossible to obtain, probably acts as an economic inducement to some physicians to seek such an appointment even though they are little interested in teaching.

Finally—and this, we think, is perhaps the most serious disadvantage of the present system of part-time teachers of medicine—men whose primary concern is the conduct of a medical practice do not, with few exceptions, have adequate time to prepare their teaching material beforehand. To be able to deal competently with a case in one's practice demands a certain degree of familiarity with the particular type of condition: it is quite a different matter, and much more demanding, to have one's knowledge so well organized and to be so conversant with the minutiae of the subject as to be able to present it satisfactorily to students or to answer their questions. In an editorial written at the request of the Journal of the American Medical Association and entitled, "A University President Looks at Medical Education," Deane W. Malott, President of Cornell University, says:

In too many institutions, the chief members of the teaching staff are on neither a geographic nor an economic full-time basis. Hence, the individual teacher's commitment to the university is not uppermost in his way of life.

*See also, on page 418, the comment of R. A. Nelson about the tempo of medical practice.

His devotion to medical education is ancillary to medical practice, and his interest in students may therefore be more casual.*

We have dealt at some length with the system of virtually unpaid, part-time teachers, because we think that this has a direct bearing on the quality of medical teaching and, through it, on the quality of medical practice. We wish to state quite explicitly, however, that our criticism of the present system is not that physicians who are in active practice are used for teaching, but that they are used for this purpose with virtually no remuneration. We think that a considerable amount of the clinical teaching *should* be done by physicians who are having continual experience of office and home practice as well as of hospital practice; but it is our contention that these physicians should receive the same remuneration for their teaching as men of corresponding rank in other parts of the university, so that they would be able to reduce the amount of time given to their practices. Being adequately paid for their teaching and not having to extend their hours of practice in order to make up for the time given to teaching, they would have time for reading and for the preparation of their teaching and could be expected to devote the necessary time to this. To pay the teachers what their services are worth would mean a reapportionment of the costs of medical education, so that the load that is now being borne to an unfair extent by the physician-teachers themselves would be spread over the whole population. Because we think that relieving the clinical teachers of their economic handicaps would improve the quality of teaching, we suggest that now, when various governments are greatly interested in the whole problem of medical care, is the time when this hidden cost of medical education should be brought into the open and recognized and more adequate provision be made for it.

We have presented the general practitioners' criticisms of the undergraduate portion of their medical education and have discussed certain aspects of this at some length. It remains now for us to draw together the main points and to make such recommendations as we think would be likely to improve the quality of medical education. In making recommendations, we are aware that it is only too easy to say what should be done when one is not in a position to be called upon to implement one's own suggestions. We recognize, too, that medical educators are faced with many complex problems that we have not even mentioned in our discussion. Finally, the medical schools of this country have produced many extremely able doctors, some of whom

*D. W. Malott: Journal of the American Medical Association, *174*: 1532, 1960.

rank among the best in the world. Not all the graduates of Canadian medical schools, however, can be described in these terms, as is made plain by our observations on the quality of the practices that we visited. Since we have obtained a unique view of general practice and have been able, to some extent, to look back upon medical education through the eyes of the practitioners, we have felt it to be our responsibility to present our findings and our opinions, as perhaps giving a view of medical education that is not otherwise available to educators who have not been in general practice or perhaps in any type of practice.

The general practitioners' criticisms of the medical course dealt with subject-matter and with the quality of the teaching. The clinical work was repeatedly criticized on the ground that there was not enough practical work. This criticism applied to obstetrics, in which there was felt to be a need for more practical experience; to surgery, in which the practitioners thought that there was a need for more practical work in minor surgery; to medicine and paediatrics, about which they complained that too much emphasis was put on the rare and obscure conditions, while too little attention was paid to the common conditions and the less serious ones; to the minor clinical subjects; and to psychiatry, which was regarded by the Ontario practitioners as quite unpractical. The dissatisfaction that was expressed about the teaching in psychiatry is particularly interesting in view of the impression that we gained that the practitioners' work in this field was based, not on professional preparation, but on personal qualities (see page 306). About the preclinical subjects, the major complaints were that there was too much material or that it was covered in too much detail; that, in some cases, the material was poorly organized; and that certain laboratory courses were unsatisfactory.

We would recommend that the medical curriculum be subjected to a critical, detailed examination. In order that such an examination might be effective, however, it would be essential that the person or persons carrying out the examination should have clearly in mind what the objective of the undergraduate medical course is. To this question there are at least two parts. First, to what level of proficiency should the course bring the man who is going to engage in general practice? Dickson says, "It has . . . become the acknowledged aim of most medical schools to produce what has been variously termed the basic doctor or the undifferentiated doctor. The aim of undergraduate education has come to be the provision of the broad knowledge which will permit the graduate to become, with further training, a good general practitioner, specialist, research worker, or teacher. The aim is clear and not controversial."\* It appears from this—and later we shall cite other similar statements (see pages 483–484)—that it is not the objective of the medical schools to bring the student to the point where he is ready to function as a general practitioner. We shall deal with the implications of this in chapter 25.

Secondly, should the preclinical part of the medical course be designed to provide for the needs of the general practitioner only or to provide for the needs of the specialists in various branches of medicine? For example, most of the gross anatomy that every medical student learns in meticulous detail is never put to use except by those who go on to undertake surgical work. Should all medical students—including those who will become internists and paediatricians, and some who will be general practitioners but who will not do surgery—be required to master the details of anatomy—during several hundred hours of scheduled instruction and an undetermined number of unscheduled hours—simply because those who will need this knowledge and those who will not need it cannot be distinguished at the time when instruction in anatomy is given? Or would it be preferable that all students should be given a basic training in anatomy, i.e. enough anatomy to meet the needs of those who will not be doing surgery, and that those who do go on into surgical work be required later to study anatomy in the great detail that surgery requires? We have asked this question, to which we do not presume to give an answer, in order to illustrate the type of question that we think must be faced in any effective examination of curriculum and in order to make clear how essential it is that the objectives of the course be determined beforehand and be kept clearly in mind.

With the objectives of the whole medical course clearly determined, it should be easier to consider the objectives of the various parts of the course. An illustration might be the laboratory work in various courses. In anatomy, there can be no doubt that the student can more readily understand the relationships of the various structures when he sees them and handles them than when he merely sees pictures of them or has to try to visualize them from the description that he reads. In other words, it is quite clear that the laboratory is a very good place in which to learn anatomy. The *amount* of laboratory work, however, must depend on how much anatomy the student is to learn in detail, i.e. on the objective of the medical course as a whole. Similarly, pathological specimens, both gross and microscopic, serve to illustrate the subject-matter of pathology excellently; but, again, the material to be

\*R. C. Dickson: Journal of the American Medical Association, *173*: 1297, 1960.

covered must depend on the objective of the medical course as a whole. Is every student to learn to distinguish, on microscopic examination, between different types of malignant tumour, though the majority of the class will never make use of this? Or is the undergraduate work to be confined to illustrating those characteristics of malignancy which it is essential for all physicians to know, while the details that are essential to the practising surgical pathologist are omitted from the medical course and incorporated into the postgraduate training of those who choose pathology as their specialty?

We would suggest that a re-examination of the medical course might well include, not only the curriculum, but also the teaching methods. In the preceding paragraph, we pointed out that, though the learning of certain subjects is undoubtedly expedited by laboratory work, the *amount* of the laboratory work might be reconsidered. There are other subjects, however, in which the *effectiveness* of laboratory work as a teaching method might be questioned. In this regard, we have already quoted Hoff and his associates on the physiology laboratory and Morrill on the use of "table-top demonstration" as contrasted with "the method of long laboratory work." We would ask whether all the laboratory exercises in such subjects as biochemistry, pathological chemistry, and bacteriology are effective enough as aids to learning to justify the expenditure of the time that is allotted to them.

We have discussed lectures and tutorials in some detail. It is unnecessary to repeat except to say, in summary, that we recommend that the student be made to accept a greater amount of responsibility for his own education. To this end, we have suggested that lectures be reduced in number and be used, not to cover the entire course, but for certain specific purposes; that greater emphasis be put on a student's reading and that adequate time be made available for this; and that greater use be made of tutorials, in which the difficulties encountered by a student in his reading and in his practical clinical work could be resolved and in which the instructors would keep track of the progress being made by the student.

Before we leave the subject of methods of instruction, we would say a few words about books. We mentioned earlier the student's need for guidance in what to read (page 363). How much guidance he needs depends upon how adequately the subject is covered in the readily available books. In this connection, we would suggest that attention might be given to what types of book best meet the needs of the medical student. The standard textbook not infrequently contains a thousand or even fifteen hundred pages. In the prefaces to some of these works, one finds statements indicating that the particular book is intended for both medical students and physicians and that it has been the authors' purpose to cover a major field of medicine as nearly completely as is possible in one volume. Without wishing to appear to depreciate these books, many of which we consider to be of outstanding merit for certain purposes, we do question whether such books are suitable for a medical student's routine use. Is it reasonable to suppose that paediatrics or adult medicine or any other subject can be presented in a way that will meet the needs both of the student who is just beginning his study of that subject and of the physician who has had six or seven or more years of experience and is preparing for specialist examinations? There are a few books that have clearly been written specifically to meet the needs of students, but it appears that more needs to be done along this line. Is it possible, for example, that some of the clinical subjects might be more satisfactorily presented in two or three volumes, the division of the material being based, not on systems or regions of the body, but on difficulty of diagnosis and management and frequency of occurrence? Such books would be designed to meet the needs of students at various levels—perhaps elementary, intermediate, and advanced—rather than to serve as reference works; and the authors, in selecting the subjects to be covered in each volume, in deciding where to place the emphasis, and in choosing their illustrative material, would be able to bear in mind the specific needs of the more homogeneous group for whom they were writing.

Whether the suggestion that we have just made is feasible and whether the effort necessary to produce such books would be worthwhile, we do not know; but, before dismissing the suggestion, we might consider it further. If books were available that covered the subject-matter in a manner *appropriate* to a student's needs, then it should not be necessary for an instructor to reiterate the material in the form of a lecture. If he had written the book himself and had expressed himself to the best of his ability, then, in theory at any rate, there would be only two circumstances that would necessitate his lecturing on that subject again, namely, that new advances had been made or that his own thinking on the subject had rendered his writing obsolete, i.e. that he had recognized new relationships or had developed more effective ways of presenting the material. Except as one or other of these circumstances necessitated the giving of lectures, a student would be left to read the textbook, in which the instructor had said just what he thought should be said at this stage of the student's development and had said it in what he regarded as the clearest and most satisfactory way. The tutorials of which we have spoken earlier would give the student the opportunity to ask questions and would indicate to the instructor how well the student was coping with the subject. The more the textbook, whether written by someone else or by the lecturer himself, falls short of the need of the particular class of students, the greater is the need for lectures. When the available books fall so far short of the existing need that most of the material has to be covered by lectures, it is apparent that a new book is required that will meet the need.

We have spoken earlier of the relative standings of research and of teaching. From what we have said, it must be apparent that we should hope that the choice of teaching staff would be determined by teaching ability rather than by research ability. There should be no place, in medicine or in any other academic field, for the lecture that is given with little or no preparation or for the lecture that is read at high speed or in a monotone. Such lectures—and they do occur—show either that the man delivering them is unaware of his own inability to teach or that his attitude towards his students is basically one of disregard, if not of contempt. It would hardly be realistic to suggest that the man who is highly trained in a medical subject should also undertake extensive training in pedagogy. It does not seem unreasonable, however, to suggest that it should be a responsibility of senior staff members to give guidance to junior members in the methods of teaching and that the junior members might have a *limited* amount of formal instruction in the principles of pedagogy. How greatly some instructors need guidance in their teaching is illustrated by a lecture that we attended, which was given as part of a refresher course for general practitioners. The lecturer, who was a member of a university staff, was to speak on the handling of emergencies having to do with a certain portion of the body. Instead of bearing in mind the needs of his audience and choosing the three or four extremely important conditions—conditions that occur fairly commonly and may result in death in a short time—he had catalogued almost every condition relating to the part of the body under consideration, he read the catalogue in a monotone, and he made no attempt to make the important conditions stand out from those that were either rare or unimportant. Returning to the selection of teaching staff, we suggest, finally, that the writing of books that are suitable for students at various levels should be at least as highly regarded as the publishing of original research.

Our suggestions so far have had to do with the curriculum and the teaching. Finally, we believe that much could be learnt from the medical students themselves. In the preceding chapter, we pointed out the need for counselling before a student enters medical school and during his course; in chapter 5, we described the changes of plans that occurred during the training of the practitioners whom we visited; in the present chapter, we have reported that the preclinical work was enjoyed "very much" by only one-fifth of the practitioners, both in Ontario and in Nova Scotia, and less than "moderately" by almost one-quarter in Ontario and by more than one-quarter in Nova Scotia (page 357) and that more than half of the doctors in each province had felt that they were not given enough direction in what to emphasize in their studying (page 360); and, in chapter 15, we noted how much less enthusiasm the practitioners had for some types of problem than for others and how much distaste they expressed for certain things, especially emotional problems (pages 232–235). These items serve to illustrate the need for studies to be made of medical students—of their reasons for entering medicine, of their attitudes towards their work throughout the course, of their particular interests and the changes that these undergo, and of the factors that determine the various choices that they make in regard to optional subjects, interneships, and choice of ultimate career. These matters, as part of the field of health (in the broad sense of the word), we believe to be fit subjects for study either by a medical school or by a school of public health. From the purely practical point of view, it seems reasonable to suppose that the quality of medical practice might be improved if more were known about the relationships between medicine and the persons who are making medicine their career, especially those whose practices are of unsatisfactory quality. For example, if a student does not enjoy his preclinical work—and an appreciable percentage of the practitioners interviewed by us made clear that they had not enjoyed it—is he in the wrong type of work and should he be encouraged to consider some other career? Or is his dislike of the work due to factors that can be corrected—to attitudes of his own that can be modified, to inadequacies in the teaching, or to inadequate organization of the medical course as a whole—and is it possible that corrective measures might improve, not only his liking of the work at hand, but perhaps also the outlook as far as the quality of his future practice is concerned? Again, what are the attitudes of medical students towards the paediatric, medical, and psychiatric problems about which some of the general practitioners showed little enthusiasm? If medical students show no greater enthusiasm than these practitioners, then why is this, what can be done about it, and what advice should be given about going into general practice, in which these branches of medicine play so large a part?

A problem of major importance in medical education is the development of a student's diagnostic ability, since treatment depends upon diagnosis (see pages 273–275). We have given examples, in earlier chapters, of inadequate investigation of patients' complaints by some of the practitioners whom we visited. In some cases, it appeared that the physician's failure resulted from lack of interest or lack of conscientiousness. Some men, however, were obviously very conscientious but just did not know how to proceed in order to reach a diagnosis. As we have pondered over this and have looked through various books dealing with diagnosis, we have been impressed by the fact that the individual symptoms and signs, such as cough, headache, or fever, are discussed in detail and that the various complexes of signs and symptoms that we recognize as disease entities, such as pneumonia or rheumatic fever, are fully described, but that little is said that is helpful in a practical way to the student or physician who is trying to learn *how* to bridge the gap between the group of symptoms that the patient presents and the diagnosis that the physician must reach if his patient is to benefit. It may be said that this is learnt by practice. Perhaps it *is* practice that accounts for the great success of some physicians as diagnosticians. But what of those who are poor diagnosticians? It is unlikely that continued practice by itself will enable them to overcome their difficulties. Can they be helped by more detailed supervision of the way in which they work through a series of diagnostic problems? Or can more systematic methods be evolved for dealing with problems of diagnosis? Or is it possible that some people are capable of the type of mental activity that is necessary in the diagnosis of medical conditions, but that others, though of equal general intelligence, lack this particular faculty to such an extent as to be handicapped as far as medical practice is concerned? Because diagnostic ability is essential to the successful practice of medicine, further attention might well be given to the causes of some students' difficulties in dealing with diagnostic problems and to the development of effective methods of coping with these difficulties.

By whom should the various studies that we have suggested be made? We are of the opinion that they should not be the responsibility of non-medical persons primarily, since it is virtually impossible for a non-medical person, however interested and well informed he may be, to comprehend the problems that are involved in a type of education and of life of which he has had no experience. Nor do we think that such studies should be left, on a part-time basis, to faculty members whose major interests and whose major responsibilities lie in their own particular disciplines. Rather, we suggest that such studies should be carried out by physicians whose primary interest is the study of medical students and medical education, and that such studies could be based either in the dean's office or in a division of research on medical education. We should hope, however, that the other members of the medical school staff would be encouraged to take an interest and to contribute, if possible, to these studies. Finally, we suggest that workers in such academic disciplines as psychology, sociology, pedagogy, and economics may have much to contribute and that, to some of the problems, a multi-discipline approach might be taken.*

One of three problems discussed by Wearn in a recent address on "Immediate Problems for Medical Educators" is "The adaptation of medical education to expanding scientific knowledge." In dealing with this, he says:

... more research in medical education is greatly needed. It is already under way in some schools, and, in at least two, Divisions of Research in Medical Education have been set up. . . . The investigative road in medical education will not be a smooth one, because methods must be devised, controls are difficult, and medical faculties have long enjoyed the reputation of being resistant to change. However, the factual presentation of the results of studies in medical education will stimulate others to investigate, and eventually we may even hope for objective and constructive criticism in this field, which is not altogether common to-day. Some of our best pre-clinical and clinical scientists, whose objectivity is unquestioned in the laboratory and in their presentations of their work, lose all trace of that objectivity when they discuss educational problems. . . .†

*The reader is referred to two most interesting books published shortly after this chapter was written: (1) G. E. Miller (Editor): *Teaching and Learning in Medical School* (Cambridge, Mass.: Harvard University Press, 1961) and (2) Howard S. Becker *et al.*: *Boys in White: Student Culture in Medical School* (Chicago: University of Chicago Press, 1961). In the former, many of the problems of medical education are discussed at greater length than has been possible in this chapter. The latter reports what was found in a recent sociological study of medical students at the University of Kansas and contains material about the attitudes of students that is relevant to some of the questions that we have raised. Of particular interest is the statement, in the concluding chapter (p. 439): "Medical education is now in a state of ferment. Medical educators are trying in many ways to improve the quality of the education they give their students. Our analysis suggests that reforms in medical education will be most effective when they take into account the collective character of student behavior and recognize the fact that students, as a subordinate echelon in the medical school, have a certain degree of autonomy with respect to these issues."

†J. T. Wearn: Journal of Medical Education, *36*: 115, 1961.

The need for a thorough reappraisal of medical education has recently been pointed out also by two educators, one from this continent, the other from Europe. Franklin D. Murphy, a physician, a former dean of medicine, and now Chancellor of the University of Kansas, speaking at the Presidents' Panel, says:

I would like to suggest that . . . we re-examine the whole pedagogy of medicine with candor and honesty and objectivity. There are a lot of clichés in this whole business, not exclusively in medicine but in other aspects of higher education, or so I believe. . . . I would like to suggest that, in a variety of esoteric and complex fields, under a variety of pressures, this hard thinking has been done, and done effectively. The mathematicians have now concluded that it is possible, in the twentieth century, to stop teaching exclusively Newtonian mathematics. . . . There is now . . . a vast and I think ultimately effective movement under foot to rework the whole concept of teaching twentieth-century mathematics to twentieth-century youngsters who are going to be dealing with twentieth-century phenomena.

It has abutted against the kind of thing you would predict: self-interest, professional self-interest, professional pride, and a great deal of intellectual lethargy always, of course.*

Schaefer, writing about the Second World Conference on Medical Education, which was held in Chicago in September, 1959, emphasizes the urgency of the situation:

The impression . . . was that what was brought forward, even here [i.e., at the Conference], was mainly information on the existing order of things and that its validity was only seldom radically questioned. Only occasionally did it become evident that we are in the middle of an almost catastrophic expansion of scientific knowledge and that the situation calls for extra-special efforts on our part. We must investigate all that we possess and have grown to accept to see to what extent it still applies and to assess its effects. Unless we think "radically" and act accordingly, the development will pass over our heads.†

*The Presidents' Panel: Journal of Medical Education, 34: 255–256, 1959.
†Hans Schaefer: Journal of Medical Education, 35: 563, 1960.

Medical Education as Preparation
for General Practice

*Postgraduate Education*

In this chapter, we shall consider the postgraduate phase of a general practitioner's education. As in the preceding chapter, the practitioner's opinions will be reported, and certain problems will be discussed. Before proceeding, though, we must make clear what we mean by the word, "postgraduate." For the sake of uniformity, as we pointed out earlier (page 42), we have regarded as *post*graduate training all hospital house-staff appointments* that followed the completion of the formal university courses, even though, in some cases, the medical degree was not granted until the interneship was completed.

Each of the practitioners was asked, "Did you enjoy your interneship(s) very much? Moderately? Or not very much?" and, "How much responsibility were you given in the diagnosis and care of patients? Too little? About the right amount? Or too much?" Of those house-staff appointments that had *followed* the first year of internship, all but the occasional one were said to have been enjoyed very much and to have entailed about the right amount of responsibility. The answers dealing with the *first* year of postgraduate training, which was usually a rotating internship, showed that 88 per cent of the Ontario practitioners had enjoyed it very much, 10 per cent moderately, and only

*Other types of postgraduate training, such as experience in a non-clinical department, were reported so rarely that they contributed nothing to our knowledge of the problems of the postgraduate stage of the practitioner's education.

2 per cent not very much. All the interneships that the Ontario practitioners enjoyed only moderately or not very much were served in major teaching hospitals located in three Ontario cities. Most of the Nova Scotia practitioners had spent time in several hospitals during their junior interneship. Fifty-nine per cent had enjoyed their time in each hospital very much and 2 per cent moderately; the remaining 39 per cent enjoyed at least one hospital very much and enjoyed one or more hospitals moderately, not very much, or both. The hospitals that were enjoyed only moderately or not very much included both teaching and non-teaching hospitals. The amount of responsibility that the interne was given during the first year of interneship was said by 24 per cent of the Ontario doctors to have been too little and by 73 per cent to have been about right. In Nova Scotia, 56 per cent of the physicians said that the amount of responsibility had been about right in each hospital and 39 per cent that it had been about right in some hospitals but too little in others. There was no significant relationship, either in Ontario or in Nova Scotia, between the physicians' scores* and their statements about their enjoyment of their interneships or about the amount of responsibility that they were allowed to assume.

When the physicians were compared by age groups, we found that, in Ontario,† only 12 per cent of the doctors over thirty-five years of age, but 55 per cent of those up to thirty-five years of age, said that they had been allowed too little responsibility ($p < 0.05$).‡ This is of particular interest, in view of a recent report of Gee and Schumacher, who sent a questionnaire to a 50 per cent random sample of the 1958–1959 internes in the United States and received answers from 2,616 internes (83 per cent of the sample). In answer to a question asking in what ways (of a number of listed possibilities) "the internship had failed to contribute to the intern's professional development," 16 per cent of the respondents said that the interneship had failed to provide "sufficient responsibility for patient care."§ Though this figure (16 per cent) does not differ markedly from our figure (24 per cent) for our entire Ontario sample, it does differ significantly ($p < 0.01$) from our

*The physicians' scores, as a measure of quality of practice, have been discussed in chapters 16 and 17.

†The answers of the Nova Scotia physicians are not comparable, since these men answered for the several parts of their internship instead of giving an over-all answer for the entire year. It is interesting to note, however, that 75 per cent of those up to thirty-five years of age said that, in at least one hospital, they had not been given enough responsibility.

‡The meaning of this is explained on pages 32–33.

§H. H. Gee and C. F. Schumacher: Journal of Medical Education, *36*, No. 4, Part 2: 52, 1961.

figure (55 per cent) for those Ontario physicians who were thirty-five years of age or younger.

There are several possible explanations of this difference. First, either sample—but more likely ours, since it is so much smaller—may be atypical in regard to the physicians' opinions about the amount of responsibility that they were allowed to assume. Secondly, though Gee and Schumacher do not make clear when their questionnaire to the 1958–1959 internes was answered, the material had been analysed and made available prior to the Seventh Teaching Institute of the Association of American Medical Colleges, which was held in October, 1959. Presumably, then, the questionnaire was answered while the 1958–1959 internes were still interning or very shortly afterwards. It may be that these doctors, having had no experience of practice on their own, were not in an adequate position to assess their interneship in respect of the amount of responsibility allowed them. In other words, were they to be questioned again after a few years of practice, a higher percentage might answer that they had not had sufficient responsibility. Thirdly, only 21 per cent of the sample of United States internes planned to be general practitioners, whereas 77 per cent planned to do specialty practice, teaching, research, or some combination of these three.* Gee and Schumacher do not state what percentage of those who planned to do general practice—who would probably take less training, and be faced with the responsibilities of practice sooner, than the remaining internes—considered the amount of responsibility insufficient. Fourthly, it may be that the United States internes answered differently from our sample because of changes that have taken place in the internship during the decade that has passed since our youngest group of Ontario practitioners was interning. Fifthly, the difference between the answers of the two groups may reflect a difference between interneships in Canada, especially Ontario, and in the United States. Because it is of great importance to know whether the physicians who are planning to enter general practice are having adequate opportunity, during their hospital training, to learn to accept responsibility, the adequacy of such opportunity should be investigated further. It would be interesting, for example, to know how Canadian internes would reply to the question that was asked by Gee and Schumacher and how the United States internes would reply if they were asked the same question again after a few years in general practice.

In order to give the physicians an opportunity to talk about their

*Ibid.*, p. 35.

postgraduate hospital training, we asked each of them, "What were the good features in your interneship(s) and what were the bad features?" We shall deal first with what the Ontario doctors said about the teaching hospitals, in which 29 of them had had at least part, if not all, of their postgraduate training. Their comments may be grouped under four headings: the work, the instruction, the working conditions, and miscellaneous. About the work, 90 per cent of the Ontario doctors had one or more things to say. Twenty-eight per cent pointed out only good features of the work, 21 per cent only bad features, and 41 per cent included both good and bad features. The good feature of the work that was most frequently mentioned, by about one-quarter of the doctors who had had postgraduate training in teaching hospitals, was the responsibility that they had been allowed to assume as members of the house staff. Yet, of those who named this as a good feature of their training, a number qualified their statements in various ways. One doctor, for example, emphasized that he and his fellow members of the house staff had been allowed to take responsibility on the medical service, but that, on all the other services, they had been allowed no responsibility and just did "the scut work." Another said that it was during the *senior* interneship, i.e. during the *second* year of postgraduate training, that they had been given responsibility. Still another said that he and his colleagues had been allowed as junior internes to assume responsibility because the war had caused a shortage of senior internes. Several other men referred to the fact that they were not allowed to assume responsibility as one of the bad features of their interneship and did not suggest that this was better on one service than on another.

Just as the amount of responsibility called forth both adverse and favourable comments, so also did the content of the interne's work. The practical experience gained and the opportunity to see a large number of cases were considered to be good features of the training, one or other of these being mentioned by almost 40 per cent of the Ontario doctors. On the other hand, almost half of the practitioners were critical of the work of the internship either because of the amount of "scut work" or because of deficiencies in the training in specific clinical subjects. By "scut work" was meant such things as the setting up of intravenous infusions, the taking of blood samples for laboratory tests, and the doing of laboratory work, which could have been done by technicians and much of which was demanded by the hospital for the sake of the completeness of its records rather than because of the needs of the particular patient. It was apparent that the complaint about "scut work" had to do with the fact that most of this work served no useful purpose as far as the interne's education was concerned. He was not being required to do laboratory work and to set up "intravenouses" in order that, and until, he should learn to do them proficiently; he was being required to do them throughout the whole year of his service as an interne, so that, in effect, he was being used as a technician. (In passing, we might speculate whether the general practitioners' manifest lack of interest in doing laboratory work themselves, which we reported earlier (page 299), possibly had its origin in a negative attitude developed during the period of hospital training.) The purely technical nature of the scut work and the physician's dislike of it were most obvious when he contrasted the scut work he had had to do with his image of the interneship as he thought it should have been. One man said, "There was an uncommonly large amount of menial work to do, with uncommonly little responsibility"; another said that the ear, nose, and throat rotation was useless, since the internes were not allowed to do anything except scut work; and another commented, "There was too much scut work and not enough time to think." It is interesting that all of these comments were made, not by men who trained long ago, but by men who were less than thirty-five years of age.

We turn now from the practitioners' complaints about what the work of the interneship included to their complaints about what it omitted. One young doctor said that, during his interneship, he had no paediatrics—a situation that he described as "ridiculous"—;* that he had not enough obstetrical experience; that, during his time on the surgical service, he was treated as a laboratory technician and a ward and operating room assistant and learned very little so that the time was "a waste of 4 months"; and that the medical service was much better but that he should have had experience in the outpatient department instead of just on the wards. Another man, one of the most recent graduates, who served his interneship in another hospital, had no time on obstetrics or gynaecology and no time on the public medical wards. His sole contact with medical cases was one month spent looking after private patients, for whom he was allowed to take little or no responsi-

---

*It is of interest that J. A. MacFarlane, reporting as Dean of the Faculty of Medicine of the University of Toronto for the year ended June, 1957, said, "The Professor of Paediatrics has already advised that for good teaching, both at the undergraduate level and particularly in the rotating interneship year, each general teaching hospital should have a children's ward staffed by members of the University Department of Paediatrics." University of Toronto, President's Report for the Year Ended June 1957, p. 56.

bility. The remainder of his interneship comprised three months of surgery, three months of anaesthesia, three months of emergency and admitting, and two months of infectious diseases in an outlying hospital. The complaints that were made by other practitioners were much the same: lack of outpatient department experience, lack of time on the paediatric service, on dermatology, etc.

The occasional doctor commented favourably on the high standards of the teaching hospitals, on the "brand new knowledge" that was available there, on the fact that the interne's contact with his patients was long enough to enable him to study the natural history of diseases, and on the opportunity to learn the personal aspects of the care of patients. There were occasional adverse comments about senior internes "taking over too much," so that the juniors were deprived of the opportunities to learn and to assume responsibility.

Having dealt with the comments that were made about the *work* of the interneship, we pass on to what was said about the *instruction* given during this part of the physician's training. About 35 per cent of those Ontario physicians who had taken postgraduate training in teaching hospitals spoke of the instruction in complimentary terms. The comments had to do with the "good ward rounds," the "good teachers," the "good supervision," and the willingness both of the members of the attending staff and of more senior members of the house staff to instruct and assist. On the other hand, about one-quarter of the Ontario practitioners made unfavourable comments about the teaching, such as that the ward rounds were poor, that there was no time for reading, and that there was not enough teaching. The most disturbing and thought-provoking comment was made by one of the younger practitioners, who said that there was a tendency for the junior internes to be classified, early in their interneship, into those who were planning to take specialty training and "the also-rans." These latter, who made up the majority of the internes, were said to be given too little personal attention by the attending staff, in fact to be "neglected."

Four of the 29 doctors who had trained in teaching hospitals referred to the working conditions—the quarters, the food, the hours of work, or the fellowship of the house staff—as good features of the interneship; 13 referred to various working conditions as bad features. The conditions that gave rise to the most frequent complaint were the overwork and the inadequate rest. One younger doctor, who had interned in the principal teaching hospital associated with the medical school from which he had graduated, said that they had had "up to thirty-six consecutive hours on duty without a chance to rest." The terms that he used to express his opinion of this situation were "absolute barbarism" and "exploitation." The next most frequent cause of complaint was the poor pay during the interneship (see pages 179–181). Other matters that were less frequently mentioned were the poor food, the lack of exercise, the autocratic and unfriendly atmosphere in certain hospitals, and the living quarters of the house staff. How extremely unsatisfactory the quarters may be is illustrated by the description that one doctor gave of a hospital in which he served, in the 1950's. He told us that there were thirty doctors sleeping in one room, with one toilet and two basins. When they made a complaint, the reply that came back was, "If you want a bath, there's the ——— River." If this story is true—and other similar incidents of which we have personal knowledge in other hospitals lead us to believe that it is—one can only marvel at the attitude of the persons in charge of that hospital and at the failure of the senior members of the profession—both the attending staff of the particular hospital and the Canadian Medical Association or the particular provincial division—to intervene and to demand that the members of the house staff be treated in accordance with their status as members of a respected profession. Other hospitals have provided quarters in which the unmarried members of their house staffs can live with comfort, dignity, and the privacy that is necessary both for rest and for study.

Miscellaneous points that were each mentioned once as good features of teaching hospital internships were the "inspiration" that was derived from the spirit of service that the doctor saw all around him, the "confidence" that the doctor developed, the fact that the interneship was "a lot of fun" (without further elaboration), and, more specifically, "fun with the nurses."

In reference to the non-teaching hospitals, in which 16 of the Ontario doctors had either all or part of their postgraduate training, the practitioners' remarks again had to do chiefly with the work, the instruction, and the working conditions. The work drew the most frequent comments, from about three-fifths of those who had served in non-teaching hospitals. All but a few of these comments were favourable. They referred to the facts that the internes had been given "lots of responsibility," that they had gained practical experience, and that they had seen many patients and a variety of cases. The occasional unfavourable comments about the work concerned the small volume of cases on certain services and the fact that the interne had had little responsibility because the patients in hospital were all private patients of practising physicians.

Instruction was mentioned as a good feature of the non-teaching hospital postgraduate training by 25 per cent and as a bad feature by 25 per cent; the remainder made no mention of instruction in discussing this part of their training. Those who made adverse comments said that there had been no teaching programme or that what teaching there had been had been insufficient or inadequately organized. One man's opinion of the inadequacy of the instruction that he had had is apparent from the comment that he made about himself as a junior interne: "I was the top man on the totem pole."

The working conditions in the non-teaching hospitals were commented on favourably and adversely by equal numbers of the Ontario doctors. The favourable comments referred to the hours, the food, the fact that there was some pay for the work, the lack of interference, and the pleasant treatment by the attending physicians. One remark that referred to a Department of Veterans Affairs hospital was interesting. The doctor said that, because there was enough clerical and non-medical personnel, the histories were dictated instead of being written by hand, and that, as a result, the internes were able to devote their time to "actual medical work."

The bad working conditions of some non-teaching hospital interneships were said to be the hours, the fact that in certain hospitals the lay administrators overruled the internes on medical matters and that the staff physicians did not make any attempt to back up the internes, and the red tape in a Department of Veterans Affairs hospital, though this was only mentioned once and was regarded as a "mild drawback."

When we compared the remarks that were made by the Ontario doctors who had had postgraduate training in teaching hospitals and those made by men who had had training in the non-teaching hospitals, we found that the two groups did not differ significantly in the proportions that made adverse comments or favourable comments about the instruction or the working conditions; nor did they differ in the proportions that mentioned good features of the work itself. Bad features of the work, however, were pointed out by 62 per cent of those who had served in teaching hospitals but by only 12.5 per cent of those who had served in non-teaching hospitals. Whether the difference, which is significant ($p < 0.01$), reflects a difference between the work of the interne in the non-teaching hospital and that required of his counterpart in the teaching hospital or whether the latter is more critical than the former, we have no way of knowing. The finding does suggest, however, that the teaching hospitals might well look critically at the work that they require their internes to do and might consider whether certain changes would be advisable.

Because most of the Nova Scotia practitioners had had internships that were divided between several hospitals, teaching and non-teaching, it was not possible to separate their comments about the two types of hospital. The large amount of clinical material that was seen was the good feature that was mentioned most frequently, by almost 60 per cent of the doctors. Other good features were said to be the opportunity of taking responsibility, of learning to associate with patients, of increasing one's self-confidence, and of becoming better acquainted with the attending staff. Instruction was mentioned as a good feature rather infrequently, though some practitioners referred to the willingness of the attending staff to help the interne; and it was stated explicitly that there was a lack of instruction in some hospitals, especially certain non-teaching hospitals. Some doctors complained of the lack of opportunity to assume responsibility. The most frequent criticism, given expression by about 40 per cent of the Nova Scotia doctors, was that too much of their time was taken up with trivial tasks and routine laboratory work. As in Ontario, there were some complaints also about the long hours, the lack of sleep, the lack of remuneration, lack of time for study, and discourteous treatment by members of the hospital staff. In brief, the remarks of the Nova Scotia doctors did not differ greatly from those of the Ontario doctors.

In answer to a specific question regarding the effect of their hospital training on their health, one-sixth of the Ontario doctors said that their health had been affected adversely. The various age groups did not differ appreciably in this. The effects mentioned were of various sorts, both physical and mental, but did not include tuberculosis. The doctors attributed them to overwork. In only an occasional case had the disorder persisted and become permanent. Rarely did a Nova Scotia doctor say that his health had been affected by his internship.

Of the 1958–1959 internes in the United States who were questioned about their internships (see page 387), 133 (5 per cent) said that their internships had been either of little, or of no, value.* Hutchins has reviewed the comments made by this group of internes and has grouped them into fourteen categories. The four most frequent types of complaint, in decreasing order of frequency, are "Too much scut work," "Very little or poor teaching," "Little or no responsibility for patients," and "Attendings [i.e., attending physicians] have no desire to teach or lack the time." Hutchins says, "Although the comments summarized here are from those respondents who indicated that their internships had been of little or no value to them, comments made by

*H. H. Gee and C. F. Schumacher: Journal of Medical Education, *36*, No. 4, Part 2: 47, 1961.

respondents who generally felt their internships had been of value were nevertheless largely negative in character and fell roughly into the same categories."* It is interesting to note that the United States internes' complaints were much the same as those made by the practitioners whom we visited.

After being questioned about the good and bad features of their interneships, the practitioners were asked, "How could interneship be improved as a method of teaching medicine?" A few of the physicians referred to the need for better hours, which would give the interne adequate time for rest and for medical reading. Between one-quarter and one-third of the doctors in each of the two provinces thought that there should be more instruction of various sorts. They suggested that there be more frequent case presentations, that the senior members of the house staff take more interest in instructing the junior internes, that there be more lectures, that the internes should be given an outline of the reading that they should do, that there should be more full-time staff members who could devote themselves to the teaching that men in private practice do not have time to do, and that the staff members give more time to criticizing the internes' histories and physical examinations in order that errors might be detected early and be corrected. In Nova Scotia, several doctors said that the interneship, or a large portion of it, should be spent in small, non-teaching hospitals, whereas several others urged that the internes be kept in the large teaching centres.

The remaining group of suggestions, to which almost half of the practitioners in each province contributed, appeared to be of particular importance in that the suggestions all attempted, in one way or another, to relate the interneship to the future needs of the doctor. Thus it was said that an interne should be allowed to take more responsibility and that his time should not be taken up with work that would be of no value to him in practice. This latter suggestion referred, not only to the "scut work" mentioned above, but to other things also. It was suggested that paper work could be reduced by the use of dictaphones and more clerical help. (The use of stenographers to reduce an interne's load of record-keeping was suggested in an editorial in the *Journal of the American Medical Association* as much as forty years ago.†) One physician claimed that so much time had to be given to writing by hand the extensive histories required on admission of patients to hospital that little time was left to an interne in which to

*E. B. Hutchins: Journal of Medical Education, 36, No. 4, Part 2: 61, 1961.
†Editorial: Journal of the American Medical Association, 75: 418, 1920.

give thought to the diagnosis and treatment of the case. Several physicians were of the opinion that to require an interne who was never going to do surgery to assist at a long operation where he saw almost nothing and did nothing except hold retractors was a waste of his time. One said that if a man intended to carry on a practice that would not include surgery and anaesthesia, he should not be required to spend time on these services but should have more time on the services that would be of value to him, especially adult medicine. An occasional man mentioned the need for more experience in obstetrics and paediatrics; but more often mentioned was the need for training in the techniques of minor surgery and for more experience and teaching in the outpatient department.

It was said that there was a need for more emphasis to be put on the common ailments. One doctor said that the internes should be warned to pay attention to the things that they would require in practice, such as plaster technique, rather than such glamorous things as gastrectomy. Another said that there should be more practical demonstrations relating to problems that would occur in practice, e.g. how to inject haemorrhoids instead of how to operate for mitral stenosis. Because some men thought that much of what a future practitioner would see in practice did not enter the wards, or even the outpatient department, of the hospital, they urged that an interne should spend some time with a general practitioner in the course of his interneship. One doctor, himself on the staff of a teaching hospital, commented that most physicians are "thrown into practice without a background of how to handle people and their families" and thought that members of the attending staff should take their internes to see, and to assist in the treatment of, their private patients. This same doctor, who marvelled at how little practical instruction is given in the handling of small problems that occur daily in office practice, believed that there should be a professor, or at least an assistant professor, of general practice. Finally, one doctor suggested that men going into practice should be taught about the organization of an office and that this might be done more satisfactorily during the interneship than in medical school.

Only the occasional doctor made reference spontaneously to the need for more time to study; but, in answer to the specific question, "Did you have enough time for medical reading and studying during your interneship?" which was put to 37 Ontario doctors and to 41 Nova Scotia doctors who had interned, 57 per cent of those in Ontario and 51 per cent of those in Nova Scotia replied in the affirmative, the remainder in the negative. Of the latter group, one doctor said that he had had no time for reading as he was usually short of sleep, another that "my medical reading was confined almost completely to subjects dealing with diseases which my patients on the ward had." Of those Ontario doctors who said that they had had enough time for reading and studying, about 20 per cent said that they had done little or no reading during their interneships, that they had asked questions instead, either of the attending staff or of the more senior members of the house staff. One practitioner who said that he had done no reading added, "When I have a problem I can't handle, I prefer to ask someone. I was never strong on reading." One of the older Nova Scotia doctors said, "It was rare that any interne had time to read; if you had time off, you didn't have the inclination or energy to read." One of the younger ones said, "A reduction in routine laboratory procedures would enable the interne to devote more time to reading."

To determine the adequacy of library facilities in the hospitals, we asked the doctors, "Was a good selection of medical books and journals *readily* available to you while you were interning?" This question, addressed to 37 Ontario doctors and 41 Nova Scotia doctors, was answered in the affirmative by 70 per cent of those in Ontario and by 56 per cent of those in Nova Scotia, and in the negative by 27 per cent and 44 per cent in the two provinces respectively; the one remaining Ontario doctor described the selection of books and journals as "fair." These figures, we think, give a somewhat more favourable picture than the facts warranted, since some Ontario doctors gave affirmative answers about hospitals whose library facilities we knew to be either non-existent or so inaccessible as to be all but useless. Some of those who said that books and journals were not readily available were the men who preferred to ask questions rather than to read, and they said that they did not feel the lack of books. Others, however, referred to the library facilities as poor and said that they had had to depend on their own textbooks or else obtain books from libraries outside their hospitals.

The different age groups did not differ significantly, either in Ontario or in Nova Scotia, in the answers that they gave either about the adequacy of the time that they had had for reading and studying or about the books and journals that had been readily available to them. Nor did the comments that the Ontario practitioners made about the teaching hospitals differ significantly in either of these matters from those that they made about the non-teaching hospitals. Though one might have supposed that the teaching hospitals would have recognized the need for time for reading and for adequate reading material, the practitioners' adverse comments included references to several of the best known teaching hospitals in Canada. Of the Ontario doctors who had interned in teaching hospitals, approximately 11 per cent expressed dissatisfaction with both the time available for study and the library facilities, 36 per cent were satisfied with both, and 54 per cent were satisfied with one and dissatisfied with the other.

Because it became apparent, early in the Nova Scotia study, that the Nova Scotia practitioners had not had as great freedom of choice of hospitals to which to apply for their junior internship as had their counterparts in Ontario, the remaining Nova Scotia physicians were questioned about this limitation. Of the 36 who were questioned, 1 said that he had not been limited, 26 that they had been free to choose among a limited number of hospitals, and 9 that they had been given no choice but had been told by the medical school where they were to interne. Of the 26 whose choice had been limited but who had been given some choice, 17, if given the same alternatives, would have made the same choice again, whereas 8 would have made a different choice, most of them a teaching hospital instead of a non-teaching hospital; and 1 doctor was uncertain. Of the 17 who would have made the same choice from the same alternatives, 7, if they had not been limited to choosing among a limited number of hospitals, would have applied for internships elsewhere, 1 in a Nova Scotia teaching hospital, the other 6 in large teaching hospitals in Toronto, Montreal, the United States, and the United Kingdom. Of the 9 who had had no choice, 2, if they had had unlimited choice, would have gone to the same hospital in which they actually did interne, 6 would have chosen Nova Scotia internships but internships with better rotations than they actually had had, and the 1 remaining doctor was uncertain what his choice would have been.

After the practitioners had been questioned about their undergraduate medical education and about their postgraduate hospital training, they were asked a question designed to discover what they thought of the adequacy of present-day medical education, undergraduate and postgraduate taken as a whole, as a preparation for general practice. The question was, "Do you think that the present medical school training plus one year of rotating internship prepare a doctor adequately for general practice as regards (1) physical illness? (2) emotional problems? and (3) social problems of patients?" All of the 86 doctors answered each of the subdivisions of the question.

For the handling of physical illness, the training was regarded as adequate by approximately 60 per cent of the doctors in Ontario and in Nova Scotia, and as inadequate by approximately 40 per cent in each province. For emotional problems, the training was considered adequate by 18 per cent of the Ontario, and by 43 per cent of the Nova Scotia, physicians, and inadequate by 82 per cent and 55 per cent in Ontario and Nova Scotia respectively; 1 Nova Scotia physician replied that he did not know whether the training was adequate. For social problems, 20 per cent of the Ontario doctors and 31 per cent of the Nova Scotia doctors said that they considered the training adequate, the remaining 80 per cent in Ontario and 69 per cent in Nova Scotia that they considered it inadequate. The different age groups did not differ significantly in their answers either in Ontario or in Nova Scotia. The present training was considered adequate for all three types of problem by 11 per cent of the Ontario doctors and by 19 per cent of those in Nova Scotia, whereas 36 per cent in Ontario and 24 per cent in Nova Scotia regarded the present medical school training plus one year of rotating interneship as inadequate preparation for all of the three types of problem with which the practitioner would be confronted in practice. The opinions expressed by the younger practitioners, who, having been trained the most recently, might be expected to be well prepared for practice but yet did not differ significantly from the older physicians in their answers, suggest strongly that there is a wide divergence between the training that they had received and the needs that they recognized when they were carrying on their own practices. (In passing, we might recall also that a considerable percentage of the men in each province did not think that a doctor's education prepared him adequately to take an active part in the non-medical activities of the community (see page 170).)

In answering the question about the adequacy of the present training as preparation for general practice, a number of the Ontario doctors added comments. The one comment that was made repeatedly was that the handling of emotional problems and social problems could not be taught in medical school but had to be learned in practice. Very occasionally we heard it suggested that more teaching of how to take a history from a patient whose problem was emotional, or more outpatient department experience, would be of value. The fact that the great majority of those who commented regarding the handling of social problems and emotional problems as something to "learn on your own in practice" is in keeping with the impression that we gained from observing the physicians' practices, namely, that their handling of these problems was based on personal, rather than on professional, qualifications (see page 306).

The practitioners were asked which of a number of changes they thought would help to remedy the defect in the present training. The replies are shown in Tables 93 and 94, where the items have been arranged in decreasing order of the frequency with which they were listed by the Ontario and the Nova Scotia doctors, respectively. A longer period of postgraduate hospital training was recommended by 55 per cent of the Ontario practitioners and by 33 per cent of those in Nova Scotia. Most of these men were in favour of two years, and a few in favour even of three years, of postgraduate training. One man who thought that the postgraduate training should be of two years' duration said that he regarded the present rotating internship as a waste of time for prospective general practitioners, and he suggested, instead, that there be four months of obstetrical experience and that,

TABLE 93

OPINIONS OF ONTARIO PHYSICIANS ABOUT MEASURES TO REMEDY THE INADEQUACY THEY THOUGHT EXISTED IN THE PRESENT MEDICAL SCHOOL TRAINING PLUS ONE YEAR OF ROTATING INTERNESHIP AS PREPARATION FOR GENERAL PRACTICE

| Measure to remedy defects of preparation for general practice | Stage of training | Physicians | |
|---|---|---|---|
| | | Number | % |
| Preceptorship with a general practitioner | * | 40 | 90.9 |
| A longer period of hospital training | After graduation | 24 | 54.5 |
| More obstetrical experience | "          " | 22 | 50.0 |
| More time in the medical outpatient department† | "          " | 19 | 43.2 |
| More time in the paediatric outpatient department‡ | "          " | 19 | 43.2 |
| More time on the medical wards† | "          " | 16 | 36.4 |
| More time on anaesthesia | "          " | 15 | 34.1 |
| More time on the paediatric wards‡ | "          " | 14 | 31.8 |
| Caring for one indigent family under the supervision of a member of the medical school staff during one academic year | Before graduation | 13 | 29.5 |
| More time on the surgical wards | After graduation | 10 | 22.7 |
| More operative surgical experience | "          " | 10 | 22.7 |
| More time on radiology | "          " | 5 | 11.4 |
| More laboratory experience | "          " | 2 | 4.5 |

*Preceptorship was recommended at the undergraduate level only by 15.9 per cent of the physicians, at the postgraduate level only by 36.4 per cent, and at both levels by 38.6 per cent.

†More time on medicine was recommended by 50.0 per cent of the physicians. More time on the wards only was recommended by 6.8 per cent, in the outpatient department only by 13.6 per cent, and in both places by 29.6 per cent.

‡More time on paediatrics was recommended by 47.7 per cent of the physicians. More time on the wards only was recommended by 4.5 per cent, in the outpatient department only by 15.9 per cent, and in both places by 27.3 per cent.

TABLE 94

OPINIONS OF NOVA SCOTIA PHYSICIANS ABOUT MEASURES TO
REMEDY THE INADEQUACY THEY THOUGHT EXISTED IN THE
PRESENT MEDICAL SCHOOL TRAINING PLUS ONE YEAR OF ROTAT-
ING INTERNSHIP AS PREPARATION FOR GENERAL PRACTICE

| Measure to remedy defects of preparation for general practice | Stage of training | Physicians | |
|---|---|---|---|
| | | Number | % |
| Preceptorship with a general practitioner | * | 38 | 90.5 |
| More time in the medical outpatient department† | After graduation | 30 | 71.4 |
| More time in the paediatric outpatient department‡ | ,, ,, | 25 | 59.5 |
| More obstetrical experience | ,, ,, | 21 | 50.0 |
| More operative surgical experience | ,, ,, | 18 | 42.9 |
| More time on the medical wards† | ,, ,, | 17 | 40.5 |
| More time on anaesthesia | ,, ,, | 16 | 38.1 |
| More time on the paediatric wards‡ | ,, ,, | 15 | 35.7 |
| A longer period of hospital training | ,, ,, | 14 | 33.3 |
| More time on the surgical wards | ,, ,, | 11 | 26.2 |
| More time on radiology | ,, ,, | 8 | 19.0 |
| More laboratory experience | ,, ,, | 7 | 16.7 |
| Caring for one indigent family under the supervision of a member of the medical school staff during one academic year | Before graduation | 3 | 7.1 |

*Preceptorship was recommended at the undergraduate level only by 7.1 per cent of the physicians, at the postgraduate level only by 21.4 per cent, and at both levels by 61.9 per cent.

†More time on medicine was recommended by 73.8 per cent of the physicians. More time on the wards only was recommended by 2.4 per cent, in the outpatient department only by 33.3 per cent, and in both places by 38.1 per cent.

‡More time on paediatrics was recommended by 64.3 per cent of the physicians. More time on the wards only was recommended by 4.8 per cent, in the outpatient department only by 28.6 per cent, and in both places by 31.0 per cent.

of the remaining twenty months, one-third be given to medical and paediatric outpatient department work and the other two-thirds to work on the medical and paediatric wards. Another doctor emphasized the importance of allowing a physician to assume more responsibility during the second year of his postgraduate training. Yet another, on being asked whether he favoured a longer period of postgraduate training than one year, said, "It depends on whether you are being *trained* or not." He went on to explain that he made a sharp distinction between "real training," which he thought occurred on certain services of certain teaching hospitals, and being merely a "writer of histories" for the hospitals and a "holder of retractors" for the surgeons.

More postgraduate training in obstetrics was advocated by 50 per cent of the practitioners in each province, more training in adult medicine by 50 per cent of the Ontario physicians and by 74 per cent of those in Nova Scotia, and more training in paediatrics by 48 per cent and 64 per cent of the Ontario and the Nova Scotia physicians, respectively. Many of those who favoured more training in medicine and in paediatrics would increase both the time on the wards and the time in the outpatient department, though some mentioned only the one place and some only the other. In view of the much greater emphasis that most training centres place on ward work than on outpatient department work during the undergraduate and the postgraduate stages of the physician's education, it is of particular significance that, in Ontario and in Nova Scotia, the practitioners who called for more outpatient department experience, both in paediatrics and in adult medicine, outnumbered those who thought that the time spent on the wards should be increased (Tables 93 and 94). The occasional doctor stressed, however, that to be of value, the outpatient department would have to be better organized than are the outpatient departments in some of the teaching hospitals. The different age groups did not differ significantly, in either province, in the percentages that called for longer postgraduate training in obstetrics, in medicine (on the wards or in the outpatient department), or in paediatrics (on the wards or in the outpatient department).

In contrast with the percentages of doctors who would increase the length of training in medicine, paediatrics, and obstetrics, only 23 per cent of the Ontario practitioners called for more operative surgical experience and the same percentage for more time on the surgical wards; and, whereas 44 per cent of the Ontario doctors over forty-five years of age favoured more surgical training, both on the wards and in the operating room, only 8 per cent of those up to forty-five years of age were of this opinion ($p < 0.05$). Those who favoured more training in operative surgery constituted almost exactly the same percentage of the Ontario doctors in towns of over 10,000 and in towns of under 10,000. Only an occasional doctor added comments to explain what type of operative surgical experience he had in mind. One man indicated that this should include appendectomy, tonsillectomy, and hernial repair. Another man said, "The junior interne should have more opportunity to learn to use the surgical instruments himself rather than act as assistant ... otherwise the weeks spent on surgery are excess baggage to the G.P."

In Nova Scotia, 26 per cent of the practitioners recommended that more time should be spent on the surgical wards, and 43 per cent that a young doctor's training should include more operative surgical experience. There was no significant difference between the percentages of the doctors in the various age groups, or between the percentages of those in communities of over 10,000 and of those in communities of under 10,000, that made these recommendations.

Thirty-four per cent of the Ontario practitioners and 38 per cent of those in Nova Scotia said that the time given to anaesthesia during the period of postgraduate training should be increased. In Ontario, they made up only 18 per cent and 20 per cent, respectively, of the doctors up to thirty-five years of age and between thirty-six and forty-five, but 56 per cent of the doctors over forty-five years of age ($p < 0.05$). In Nova Scotia, the age groups did not differ significantly in this respect.

Of all the items listed in Tables 93 and 94, however, the one about which the practitioners were most enthusiastic was a preceptorship with a general practitioner. Approximately 90 per cent of the doctors, both in Ontario and in Nova Scotia, thought that preparation for general practice should include the spending of some time with a general practitioner who would act as a preceptor. This was more often advocated as part of the postgraduate, than as part of the undergraduate, experience. The few comments that were made in support of a preceptorship during the undergraduate part of the training were to the effect that it was at this time that students were trying to decide what type of medical career to choose and that many students chose a specialty because their lack of familiarity with general practice made them afraid of it. Those who favoured a preceptorship as part of the postgraduate training varied greatly in what they had in mind. Some physicians thought that the preceptorship should be of one or two months' duration in the course of the junior interneship, one that it should be of a year's duration and follow two years of postgraduate hospital experience, and some of those who commented seemed to think in terms of six months or a year, after the junior interneship. One physician, who said that he would advise every doctor to spend at least a year with a good general practitioner, emphasized that it was important that the preceptor be "really good."

In recent years there has been a good deal of discussion of the preceptorship. Some medical educators appear to favour it; others oppose it. John Z. Bowers, Dean of Medicine at the University of Wisconsin, where a preceptorship programme has been in operation for more than a quarter of a century, says of it:

. . . it is claimed that the preceptor programmes will guide increased numbers of students into rural general practice. It is my impression that those students who are assigned to a first-rate general practitioner may enter general practice. They always return from such preceptorships more interested in general practice. As a corollary, many of our students come away from the preceptorships convinced that specialty practice in a clinic is ideal.

and:

It is difficult to change a preceptor programme—more difficult than to alter the curriculum in the medical school.

In some preceptor programmes medical students may carry too much of a work load. They may not receive sufficient guidance. They may function as interns in small, poorly organized hospitals.

A well-controlled, carefully selected preceptor programme may be a distinct contribution to medical education.*

Somewhat less cautious in its opinion is an excerpt from a letter in which Bowers discusses the advantages and disadvantages of the programme at the University of Wisconsin and concludes by saying, "The study of our Preceptor Program supports the sentiment that Medical Schools vary considerably in their problems and their needs. There is general agreement that the Preceptor Program is a valuable part of medical education at Wisconsin."†

This excerpt from Bowers's letter is one of more than a dozen opinions of the preceptorship that are included in the Report of the Fifth Teaching Institute of the Association of American Medical Colleges. One of the most outspoken critics of the preceptorship is George G. Reader, Professor of Medicine at Cornell University, who says:

There is no question that some subjects might be taught particularly well by the preceptorship method. A close relationship develops between student and teacher in a preceptorship, and the preceptor is able to determine areas of deficiency in the student as a result of observing him under the stress of practice and give him needed help. But there is one great obstacle to this form of teaching—lack of adequate supervision and direction of the preceptors. . . . Rarely, if ever, have preceptors been recruited with the same care exercised in selecting other members of the faculty. . . . Supervision has been dependent upon student reports or very occasionally on circuit riding by some member of the faculty. Lacking clearcut criteria for performance, the student and supervising faculty member alike must be at a loss to determine anything but the grossest deviation from good teaching practices. A notable part of the supervisory problem is the lack of definite goals for preceptor teaching. Some preceptors believe it is their mission to

*J. Z. Bowers: Medicine: A Lifelong Study, Proceedings of Second World Conference on Medical Education, Chicago 1959 (New York: World Medical Association, 1961), pp. 221, 222.
†J. Z. Bowers: Journal of Medical Education, 33, No. 10, Part 2: 207, 1958.

teach physical diagnosis or "something out of the book"; others consider that they must show students it isn't necessary to do things as they are taught in the medical school, that "you can get away with a lot less."

Presumably an extramural preceptorship that was organized within a department under the supervision and discipline of a full-time department head could be a useful adjunct to clinical teaching. It would require frequent meetings within the school to set realistic teaching goals and definite teaching aims, and it would require constant review of the practices of the preceptors themselves. This has never been done to my knowledge. . . .

Until it has been demonstrated that extramural preceptorships can accomplish maintenance of high standards in teaching, I believe that any school that uses them must be considered to be providing its students with second-rate teaching, and that extramural preceptorships presently in existence should be abolished or reorganized.*

A somewhat similar opinion was expressed by J. H. F. Brotherston, Professor of Public Health and Social Medicine at the University of Edinburgh, in a talk entitled, "Preceptorships and Comprehensive Care." Referring to the current "interest . . . in developing short-term experiences for medical students of apprenticeship or attachment to general practitioners," he said:

It seems to me that if such attachments are limited to an opportunity for permitting the student to see something of the workings of general practice and the work of the general practitioner they are useful, but only to a very limited extent. A very short experience, perhaps a week or two, is all that is necessary, because it is neither timely nor appropriate for medical students at this stage in their education to try to master the art of general practice. . . . There are certain dangers too; the number of general practitioners able to do this kind of work really well is very limited. Willing and enthusiastic helpers are far more numerous than those really competent to do the job, and there is always the possibility that the unexplained contrast in the methods, and sometimes in the quality, of care which the student sees may lead him to draw the wrong conclusions. If the objective of this kind of attachment is not so much to learn about general practice as to learn about "comprehensive care," then let us remember that the kind of teaching required for this is an extremely sophisticated business if the right things are to be shown to the student and he is to draw correct conclusions from them. It cannot be expected that any but the quite exceptional general practitioner will be able to do this sort of teaching well without a good deal of guidance. It is so easy and, in a sense, also so inexpensive simply to farm out students to willing general practitioners and to believe that all is well.†

In the Report of the Sixth Teaching Institute of the Association of

*G. G. Reader: Journal of Medical Education, 33, No. 10, Part 2: 210, 1958.
†J. H. F. Brotherston: Medicine: A Lifelong Study, Proceedings of Second World Conference on Medical Education, Chicago 1959 (New York: World Medical Association, 1961), p. 207.

American Medical Colleges, Charles A. Janeway, Professor of Pediatrics at Harvard University, says, "Preceptorships were the subject of considerable institute discussion which, of course, ended up with the conclusion that these are as useful as the preceptors. One problem is how to select the preceptors, but one of the worst problems is how to get rid of a preceptor once selected if he turns out to be a bad one."* This Report, which includes information obtained by means of a pre-Institute questionnaire, shows that only 10 per cent of medical deans in the United States consider the preceptorship to be of "much value," that 50 per cent consider it to be of "some value," that 35 per cent regard it as of "little or no value," and that 4 per cent think that it is "harmful."† The heads of departments are shown as differing little from the deans in their opinions of the preceptorship.

It is apparent from the quotations that we have given that, though there may be some merits in the preceptorship, it has such serious drawbacks, at least as far as undergraduate medical students are concerned, that medical educators tend to look very much askance at it. Possibly this might be a fruitful area for careful field study.

Some of the practitioners visited by us made suggestions of their own about ways in which a young doctor might be prepared more effectively for general practice. Several said that there should be more experience in the outpatient department during the undergraduate years and that, during the postgraduate training, more time should be spent in the emergency department. The need for more psychiatry and for more dermatology was mentioned. Several doctors suggested that the medical students should be given lectures by general practitioners on "problems of general practice," but these men did not specify what problems they had in mind. Now and then, it was recommended that a young doctor work with another practitioner or with a group, in order to gain experience under supervision, before going into practice by himself; but one of those who suggested such experience said that "in clinics, junior men are exploited" and that, to be of value, this type of experience would have to be arranged in such a way as to minimize the risk of exploitation. Other men emphasized the need for a young doctor to assume responsibility himself, and one said, "I don't know of any way to qualify a person except for him to *do* general practice himself. It takes a considerable period of time *in* general practice to become experienced." We shall return

*C. A. Janeway: Journal of Medical Education, 34, No. 10, Part 2: 111, 1959.
†Journal of Medical Education, 34, No. 10, Part 2: 111, 1959.

to these matters of experience, responsibility, and supervision in chapters 25 and 26.

When asked how well their medical training had prepared them to do the laboratory work necessary in general practice, all of the Ontario practitioners said that it had prepared them very well. Some, however, said that they did little laboratory work themselves, and one doctor said that he tended to let this slide and that, in more than twenty years of practice, he had never made a blood film. The Nova Scotia practitioners were not questioned about the adequacy of their training for laboratory work.

One of the needs of any physician who has direct contact with patients is to be able to deal with them as individuals. W. V. Johnston, Executive Director of the College of General Practice of Canada, has said, "It is becoming increasingly clear that a majority of people want a personalized type of medical care.... They want it to be warmly human as well as scientific.... They want their physician to bring the best technical knowledge as well as the priceless remedy of a personal interest in them as people."* A general practitioner, dealing with a great variety of persons in an endless variety of situations, probably has greater need of ability to handle patients as persons than has any of the specialists, with the possible exception of the psychiatrist. In order to find out how adequately prepared they were, we asked each of the practitioners whom we visited several questions about this aspect of his medical education. The first question was, "How well did your instructors in medical school prepare you for the kinds of problem that you might meet in handling patients themselves as persons? Very well? Fairly well? Not especially well? Or not at all well?" In Ontario, 25 per cent answered, "very well," or, "fairly well," 73 per cent, "not especially well," or, "not at all well," and one doctor did not answer. In Nova Scotia, 45 per cent replied, "very well," or, "fairly well," and 55 per cent, "not especially well," or, "not at all well" (Table 95). The difference between the two provinces was not statistically significant. The different age groups did not differ significantly in their replies, in either province.

Next, the practitioners were asked, "By and large, in medical school and during your hospital training, were patients generally discussed with you as individual persons or as disease entities?" Eighty-two per cent in Ontario and 74 per cent in Nova Scotia answered, "as disease entities," and only 16 per cent and 26 per cent in the two

*Editorial Comment: College of General Practice (Medicine) of Canada, Bulletin, 7: 2, 9, 1960.

TABLE 95

OPINIONS OF ONTARIO AND NOVA SCOTIA PHYSICIANS ON
PREPARATION FOR HANDLING PATIENTS
(How well their instructors in medical school prepared them for
the kinds of problem that they might meet in handling patients
themselves as persons)

| Physician's opinion on how well he was prepared | Ontario physicians | | Nova Scotia physicians | |
|---|---|---|---|---|
| | Number | % | Number | % |
| Very well | 7 | 16.3 | 3 | 7.1 |
| Fairly well | 4 | 9.3 | 16 | 38.1 |
| Not especially well | 16 | 37.2 | 16 | 38.1 |
| Not at all well | 16 | 37.2 | 7 | 16.7 |
| Total physicians | 43* | 100 | 42 | 100 |

*One other physician did not answer. He believed that, before one reached university, one should have learnt from one's parents how to deal with people.

provinces respectively, "as individuals." Again, the different age groups did not differ significantly in their replies, in either province. A few of those who answered, "as disease entities," attributed this to "the busy hospital routine." One practitioner said that the specialists had discussed patients as disease entities, whereas the general practitioners had discussed them as individual persons, but that the general practitioners at his medical school had not been very good teachers as they did not know enough of the minutiae. It is interesting that similar answers were obtained recently from United States medical students to whom a questionnaire was sent. Reader reports that, of a sample of 1,322 students at fifteen medical schools, 32 per cent said that their faculty members, in discussing patients with them, presented the patients as individual persons, whereas 64 per cent of the students said that patients were presented as disease entities. Reader states, also, that there was "considerable variation from school to school."*

The final question bearing on the handling of patients as persons was, "Generally speaking, were your instructors in medical school more skilled in the realm of physical diagnosis and treatment or more skilled in handling the social and psychological aspects of patients' problems or were they equally skilled in both?" In Ontario, 36 per cent of the practitioners thought that their instructors were more skilled in physical diagnosis and treatment, 57 per cent said that they were equally skilled in both, and the remaining 7 per cent could not answer. In Nova Scotia, 81 per cent thought that they were more

*G. G. Reader: Journal of Medical Education, 33, No. 10, Part 2: 166 and 173, 1958.

skilled in physical diagnosis and treatment, and 19 per cent that they were equally skilled in both. It is of interest that, in Ontario, the instructors were considered equally skilled in both aspects of medicine by 82 per cent of the practitioners over forty-five years of age, by 54 per cent of those between thirty-six and forty-five years, and by 36 per cent of the doctors up to thirty-five years of age. This trend is statistically significant ($p < 0.05$). There was no evidence of a similar trend in Nova Scotia.

Schumacher and Gee sent a questionnaire to a 50 per cent random sample of the physicians who graduated in the United States in 1950 in order "to explore how and during what period in his medical education today's young physician learned to handle the physician-patient relationship." On the basis of the replies received from 1,953 physicians (75 per cent of the sample), they discovered:

Our physicians tended to learn by observation during medical school and by trial and error after graduation. Since the majority rated their post-graduate learning opportunities higher than they did their opportunities during medical school, we are led to believe that these physicians are more satisfied with their trial-and-error experiences than with what they learned by observation. That this state of affairs is not considered desirable, however, is demonstrated by the extent to which practical instruction in the physician-patient relationship is cited as having been the most deficient of several areas of medical school instruction by those physicians who emphasize medical practice in their present careers.[*]

In this connection, it is interesting to note that Richard Christie, Adjunct Professor of Psychology at Columbia University, in discussing sociological studies in medical education carried out in several medical schools, has said, "The clinical faculty usually do not know how the student actually handles the patient. They base their evaluation on ward records, the student's work-up of the case, the way he presents the material in case seminar, and the like. . . . As an outside observer, I am struck by how little most faculty know about the interaction of students and patients."[†]

Since it was conceivable that practitioners located in communities of different sizes or in different parts of Ontario or of Nova Scotia might differ in their training needs, all the doctors were asked, "Do you think that a doctor entering general practice in *your* community

[*] C. F. Schumacher and H. H. Gee: Journal of Medical Education, *36*, No. 4, Part 2: 162, 1961.
[†] R. Christie: Journal of Medical Education, *33*, No. 10, Part 2: 161, 1958.

or *your* area of the country requires any special training that would not be necessary for the average general practitioner in Canada?" Seven Ontario physicians (16 per cent of the sample) answered in the affirmative. They were not concentrated in any particular part of the province or in communities of any particular size. Three of these men gave answers that were not really relevant but that were interesting comments on the profession and its relationship to society. One said that, because medical politics were bad in a large city, there was a need for "tolerance and spiritual understanding." Another, practising close to a large city, said that the doctor must have "better than average culture and manners," which he thought would be less necessary in a more remote district. The third doctor, who was practising in a city that has a medical school, said that in his city a general practitioner had to maintain a fairly high level of practice, because, in a teaching centre, there could not be too great a discrepancy between a general practitioner and a specialist. This remark illustrates the beneficial effect that a teaching hospital may have on the standard of practice in its own community. Yet this remark and the one preceding it are somewhat disturbing in the suggestion, which is implicit in them, that a doctor's standard need not be as high in communities that are more remote from the large medical centres.

Only 4 doctors, 9 per cent of the entire Ontario sample, said that a physician doing general practice in their communities would need extra training in specific subjects. Geriatrics, paediatrics, psychiatry, and anaesthesia were each named once, and surgery three times, as subjects in which extra training was required. Only 1 doctor related the need for extra training to the distance of his community from consultants.

In Nova Scotia, 5 physicians (12 per cent of the sample) said that special training would be needed by a doctor doing general practice in their communities. One said that a training in "practical dispensing" was needed because of the remoteness of drugstores, and another that it was necessary to have experience in dental extractions because the nearest dentist was located forty-five miles away. Of the remaining three physicians, one spoke of the need for more training in anaesthesia, because there was no certificated anaesthetist in his city, and the other two spoke of the need for training in traumatic surgery, because of the concentration of heavy industry in the region. It was interesting to note that there was a qualified surgeon in the area and that the community was large enough to support a full-time anaesthetist, but that, as our informants made clear to us, the general practitioners were unwilling to refer their traumatic surgery to the surgeon who was there or to encourage an anaesthetist to settle in the area.

We must now consider the meaning of what the general practitioners told us. The present medical school training plus one year of rotating internship were considered by four-fifths of the Ontario practitioners and by between one-half and three-quarters of the Nova Scotia practitioners to be inadequate preparation for handling patients' social and psychological problems, and were considered by two-fifths of the practitioners in each province to be inadequate preparation for dealing with physical illness. Nor was there any significant difference between the percentages of younger and older physicians who expressed these opinions. From this, it is quite obvious that this training is not meeting the needs of the young man who wishes to make general practice his career, unless such great changes have occurred in the past few years that the opinions of the most recent graduates whom we visited must be discounted. This is unlikely, however, especially in view of the statements received by Gee and Schumacher in reply to the questionnaire that they sent to the 1958–1959 internes in the United States (see page 387). Of 2,130 doctors who served rotating internships, 50 per cent said that the internship failed to provide "sufficient review and criticism" of their work with individual patients, 38 per cent that it failed to provide "Adequate instruction in the application of scientific knowledge to patient care," 24 per cent that it failed to provide "Sufficient opportunity to treat patients adequately (too many patients)," and 22 per cent that the internship failed to provide "Educational experiences that were more than mere duplications of clerkship experiences." Gee and Schumacher sum up their findings in these words:

Although high-ability graduates of financially secure medical schools serving internships in good major teaching hospitals are inclined to view their internship experience favourably, we cannot conclude that the present-day internship is serving its function well. The individuals just described are very unlikely to be planning to go directly into practice. They have before them several years of residency training and, likely as not, the internship year serves them as something of a breather. The intern who faces imminently the responsibilities of a career in general practice, however,—and who is not unusually well endowed intellectually, whose medical school struggled with problems of inadequate finances, and who is serving an internship in a non-teaching hospital—is far less complacent, and evidently with reason. This is not to say that all individuals who fit the latter description are inadequately prepared to launch into their medical careers. . . . What we can say, however, is that each of these factors represents the less favorable end of a continuum with respect to judgments made by recent medical school graduates about the values of their clerkship and internship experiences. Lack of the kind of attention needed to produce constructive review and criticism of one's work, lack of instruction in clinical applications of the basic sciences, and a surfeit of low-level practical experience emerge as the most notable inadequacies of present-day internships.*

The practitioners whom we visited suggested a number of ways in which the preparation for general practice could be made more effective. The suggestion that was voiced most often, by approximately 90 per cent of the practitioners in each province, namely, that, at some stage in the training, there should be a period of preceptorship with a general practitioner, emphasizes, more than anything else that they said, how strongly they felt that the undergraduate medical course and the hospital training were not enough by themselves. Yet, in spite of the fact that the practitioners themselves were so much in favour of the preceptorship, we are not justified in concluding that this is the solution to the problem. Quite apart from the difficulties that would be involved in finding enough general practitioners who would be willing to act as preceptors, in determining that their own practices were of good enough quality for them to be examples to others, and in ensuring that the student's or interne's experience was worthwhile and that he was not exploited, we do not think that the preceptorship goes to the root of the difficulty that the young physician has in bridging the gulf between his hospital experience and the very different conditions obtaining in practice. We shall deal with this problem of the transition from internship to the acceptance of full responsibility in chapters 25 and 26.

The one example of home-care experience about which we asked the practitioners' opinions, namely, a medical student's caring for one indigent family under the supervision of a member of the medical staff during one academic year, found favour with only 30 per cent of those in Ontario and with only 7 per cent in Nova Scotia (Tables 93 and 94, page 400). Janeway, however, in the Report of the Sixth Teaching Institute of the Association of American Medical Colleges, in 1958, says, "I hope very much that they [i.e., home-care programmes] will come in for more study at future Institutes, because I think everyone who did consider them agreed they have much to offer. In terms of a natural opportunity for giving a student maximum responsibility and continuity in the care of an individual patient, and

*H. H. Gee and C. F. Schumacher: Journal of Medical Education, 36, No. 4, Part 2: 53, 59, 1961.

perhaps maximum opportunity to see in operation those forces with which the behavioral scientist is particularly intrigued, these programs have much to recommend them."[*]

More than half of the Ontario practitioners and one-third of those in Nova Scotia recommended that there be at least two years of postgraduate hospital training. The three clinical subjects on which they placed the emphasis were obstetrics, adult medicine, and paediatrics. A point to which those who are responsible for planning house-staff programmes might pay particular attention is that, in Ontario and in Nova Scotia, those who called for increased time in the outpatient department, both medical and paediatric, exceeded in number those who would increase the time on the wards, though many believed that ward experience and outpatient department experience should both be increased. We know of some hospitals in which the members of the house staff have no outpatient department experience or, at best, spend an hour or two on one or two days each week in the general medical clinic or in one or another special clinic. In such a situation as this, it is impossible for an interne to see the number of patients and to have the continuity of experience that are necessary if he is to develop facility in dealing with this type of practice, which resembles, far more closely than do the ward cases, what he will see in his own office and home practice. Again, when, as happens in some hospitals, the acutely ill patient is treated in the emergency department at night by an interne, but is told to report back in a day or two, for further treatment, to a regular clinic where he is seen, not by the interne, but by a member of the attending staff, the interne has lost the opportunity to find out whether his diagnosis and treatment were correct—to find out, for example, that what appeared initially to be a case of nasopharyngitis was really a case of measles in the pre-eruptive stage.

We suggest that, if the outpatient department experience is to be a worthwhile one, certain conditions must be fulfilled. First, the work in the outpatient department must be, not a part-time, and minor, responsibility additional to a heavy load of ward work, but a full-time responsibility, to which an interne can give his full attention. Secondly, the term of service must be long enough to allow an interne to gain sufficient experience. In view of the fact that a general practitioner's office and home practice far exceeds his hospital work in volume, it hardly seems unreasonable to suggest that the work in the outpatient department should be of several months' duration. In this connection,

[*]C. A. Janeway: Journal of Medical Education, *34*, No. 10, Part 2: 112, 1959.

it is interesting to hear what was said by Janeway at a special session on paediatric education that was held at the time of the Ninth International Congress of Pediatrics, in Montreal, in 1959. Wegman, who reported on this session from the verbatim recording that was made, says, "it seemed to him [i.e., Janeway] that beds are not the end of the pediatric line; rather, it is the outpatient department which is the heart of a hospital or university medical center, just as the heart of practice is the office of the doctor. One ought to talk more about how many outpatient visits there are per year."*

Thirdly, as we have already indicated, each time a particular patient returns, he must be seen by the same member of the house staff. This, quite apart from being in the patient's interest, is necessary for the interne's learning.

Fourthly, there must be adequate supervision of an interne's work. If his work is not supervised, he can make mistakes without ever being aware that he is making them. In fact, it is perhaps not too much to say that, if he is not supervised, he might almost as well be practising in his own private office, as far as the educational value of the experience is concerned. As an example of the type of supervision that is possible but not, we think, common, we would describe the supervision that we were fortunate enough to have in one hospital in the course of our own training. The outpatient department was in the charge of a fully qualified paediatrician who had not yet started his own private practice. Because he was not required to see any particular number of patients himself, he was available, in a few minutes, to any of the internes who might wish to ask him a question or who might wish him to see one of their patients. He was interested in teaching and made the internes feel that he was there to help them and was glad to be called upon. In addition, he insisted that the internes keep adequate records on every patient, and each evening he read the charts of every one of the patients seen in the clinic during that day, usually more than a hundred in number. When he came across things that had been missed and needed attention urgently, he would have the patient called back to the clinic. For less urgent matters, he would put a note on the chart, such as, "Have you thought of the possibility of ——?" or "How about a chest film?" or "Call me when this patient comes in next." This type of supervision calls for someone whose heart is in teaching. Also, it is expensive; but is it, in the long run, as expensive as sending out into practice men who, if we may judge both from our own observations and from the practitioners' statements, are inadequately prepared for practice?

*M. E. Wegman: Journal of Medical Education, *36:* 50, 1961.

Finally, if the outpatient department experience (or the ward experience) is to be a satisfactory one, an interne must not be over-whelmed by the volume of work. We know of one clinic, in a teaching hospital, in which the work load was so disproportionate to the facilities of the clinic that patients who had come at eight o'clock in the morning were still being seen at four in the afternoon. Under these conditions, the case that demanded something unusual and time-consuming—the baby with possible pyloric stenosis whom one wished to feed and watch for twenty minutes, or the child that required a lumbar puncture—was a misfortune; and the educational opportunity presented by the patient whose disorder was a difficult diagnostic or therapeutic problem was lost in the service demands of the clinic (see also page 440). The number of patients that an interne can see in a given time probably varies with the interne. It is obvious —yet perhaps it is worth stating, because so often we think in terms of averages instead of in terms of individuals with their great variation —that the satisfactory number of patients for any given interne is the number that *he* can see satisfactorily, a number that probably can be determined only by the adequate supervision of which we have spoken. To impose upon an interne a load that exceeds his capacity is to teach him a bad lesson, as far as his future practice is concerned. A single case of a particular disease—if it is thoroughly investigated, if the disease processes underlying the signs and symptoms are under-stood, and if the treatment, not only its details, but also its rationale, are learnt—a single case, if dealt with in this way, is worth, from the educational point of view, any number of cases that are managed hastily, superficially, and with inadequate understanding.

What we have been saying about one situation, the outpatient department experience, is what the general practitioners in many of their remarks said about the entire postgraduate training, namely, that it should be designed to meet the educational needs of those who are undergoing the training. We have heard the practitioners' complaints that, as internes, they were required to do "scut work" in large amounts, that they were required to serve in the operating room where they learnt little but provided the physical strength necessary to hold the incision open for the surgeon, that they were required to work long hours and had little time for rest or for study, that they were treated as the "also-rans" and were "neglected." In addition to this, 24 per cent of all the Ontario* doctors whom we visited, and 55 per cent of those up to thirty-five years of age, had not been allowed

---

*As has been pointed out on page 387 (footnote), the answers of the Nova Scotia physicians are not comparable.

to assume the responsibility in the care of patients which they regarded as necessary if they were to be adequately prepared to practise on their own.

If the training does not meet the needs of those who are "being trained," then there is little justification for calling it "training." This seems too obvious to need stating. Yet it does need to be stated. Repeatedly, we have seen evidence that the educational needs of internes have been forgotten or ignored. A few years ago, we were told by one interne after another in a certain hospital that he regarded his year of rotating internship in that hospital as a wasted year. Yet, at the same time, a senior member of the hospital's attending staff boasted to us that that hospital was a wonderful centre for training, and the staff of the hospital was loud in its demands that the hospital be recognized for specialty training, not only at the junior interne level, but right up to the level of resident. Again, in the course of the Survey, we were introduced to a hospital administrator who expressed the hope that the Survey would be instrumental in providing him with more internes to meet the needs of his hospital, but who showed no awareness of, or interest in, the educational needs of the internes. These were both non-teaching hospitals; but in the teaching hospitals, also, this situation obtains, at least to some degree. The doctor who said that those internes who were not going to specialize were regarded as "also-rans" and were "neglected" was speaking of his own fairly recent experience in the principal teaching hospital of a medical school in Ontario. In view of the findings of Gee and Schumacher (see pages 411–412), it appears that the situation has not changed in the few years that have elapsed since the general practitioners whom we visited were undergoing their postgraduate training. Janeway, who participated in the Sixth Teaching Institute of the Association of American Medical Colleges, in 1958, made a remark that, though dealing with medical students rather than house staff, bears out our practitioner's contention that there is a tendency to give the attention to some men and neglect others. Janeway said:

It intrigued me that in one Institute discussion group there was very strong feeling that the teacher should focus his efforts on the top portion of the class who present the opportunity to develop outstanding people for medicine and perhaps for academic careers. The proponents of this idea thought the teacher should accept the fact that the bottom group had to go through the mechanics of education and, if they got through the exams, all right.

Another group took exactly the opposite point of view and felt that it didn't matter what the faculty did for the top group; they would go through school successfully and make opportunities for themselves. The major share of faculty time should be devoted to the bottom third of the class for whom teaching efforts can be most effective and from whom many more people could be salvaged for careers in medicine that would be helpful at some level.°

The information that we obtained from the practitioners, much of which has been corroborated by the recent work of Gee and Schumacher, suggests that the postgraduate hospital training should be thoroughly studied. Recently, Payson and his associates have studied the way in which each of two internes in the Grace–New Haven Hospital used their time during a period of ten days. They say, "The finding that concerned us most was the small amount of time spent with patients ... there was a remarkably rapid decrease in time spent with all patients after their first hospital day and . . . an old patient was seen less than ten minutes a day unless there were acute medical complications. The doctor spent barely enough time with his patient to establish an acquaintance, much less a relation." They go on to ask such questions as "do attending physicians sufficiently encourage interns to broaden their experience of patient-doctor contact? Are teachers making rounds more likely to emphasize differential diagnosis and tangible therapeutic matters? Do they leave problems of interpersonal relations to house staff, or do they demonstrate how to conduct a professional relation with a patient or how to approach some understanding of factors that can influence such a relation?"† These questions are particularly apt in view of the fact that only 1 doctor, out of the many in our sample who had had teaching hospital postgraduate training, mentioned, as a good feature of the training, that he had learnt the personal aspects of patient care.

We have referred to Payson's study because it indicates that an interest is beginning to be taken in what actually goes on in the period of postgraduate training. We think that there should be much more intensive studies. There are many things that should be known about this stage of the training, of which we shall mention only a few. How adequately does the formal instruction that is offered during an internship meet the interne's educational needs? What type of experience does the interne obtain during his period of training? What types of case does he see and what does he not see? At the end of his internship, has he seen the major portion of what he will encounter in practice? Is it certain that the procedures that need to be learnt are

°C. A. Janeway: Journal of Medical Education, *34*, No. 10, Part 2: 107, 1959.
†H. E. Payson *et al.*: New England Journal of Medicine, *264*: 442, 1961.

learnt before he goes forth from his interneship—that he knows, not only how to set up intravenous infusions, but how to bandage and do other minor surgical procedures? The complaints of the practitioners are disturbingly suggestive that internes do not learn these things. How adequate really is the supervision during the interneship? In view of some of the basic mistakes, in history-taking and examination, that we encountered in the practitioners' offices, one may wonder whether the supervision *is* adequate or whether internes are making mistakes without having them drawn to their attention. In this regard, we would quote Russell A. Nelson, Director of The Johns Hopkins Hospital, who says, "The tempo of medical practice makes it increasingly difficult for the active practitioner to devote sufficient time to supervision of interns and residents. More and more hospitals must make it possible for the appointment of at least a few staff members who can limit work to the individual hospital and take greater responsibility for the medical education."[*]

Again, what are an interne's habits of study and of reading? A library is regarded by Sir George Pickering, Regius Professor of Medicine at Oxford University, as one of three things necessary for proper training in a hospital;[†] and to this, Julius H. Comroe, Jr., Director of the Cardiovascular Research Unit of the University of California Medical Center in San Francisco, would add "that the hospital should also provide time for the resident to make use of the library."[‡] These, and especially the latter, would seem to be such obvious requirements of any programme claiming to be primarily and seriously educational that we should have hesitated to quote such authorities were it not for the statements that the general practitioners made about these matters, and especially the fact that between 40 and 50 per cent of those questioned in each of the two provinces said that they had not had enough time for reading and studying during their internships (see pages 396–397). It would be interesting, further, to know whether the example set by the attending staff is one that fosters study[§] and reflection or whether it pictures practice as a perpetual rush and perhaps even represents active, visible busyness as a virtue.

Another major problem is whether the man who is going to be a specialist and the man who is going to be a general practitioner should interne in the same hospital. We have heard complaints of being

*R. A. Nelson: Medicine: A Lifelong Study, Proceedings of Second World Conference on Medical Education, Chicago 1959 (New York: World Medical Association, 1961), p. 454.

†Sir G. Pickering: *ibid.*, p. 466.

‡J. H. Comroe, Jr.: *ibid.*, p. 467.

§The reading habits of the general practitioners will be discussed in chapter 24.

"neglected," of being treated as the "also-rans." It was said, too, that more senior members of the house staff sometimes took over, so that the junior internes lost the opportunities to do various things. This complaint is echoed in the words of Deitrick and Berson, who made a survey of the medical schools in the United States between 1949 and 1951. Speaking of the clinical material available, they say, "in these major teaching hospitals, the intern was caught between the clinical clerkship for the undergraduate medical student and the marked increase in the number of residents who were also seeking work with patients."* This raises the question whether some teaching units, either certain wards or even entire hospitals, should be reserved, as far as *post*graduate education is concerned, for the teaching of those who are not going to be specialists. We suggest this merely as a possibility. We do feel strongly, however, that the level at which the individual clinician teaches should be determined by his interests and his abilities. Some men, in medicine as in other fields, are interested in teaching the novice, because it is a challenge to them to bring him along. Others, perhaps through lack of interest or through inability to see the difficulties in things that they grasp easily themselves, are not suited to teaching at this level but may be excellent for more advanced students.

Bearing in mind the statements made by one-quarter of the Ontario practitioners that as internes they were not allowed to assume responsibility to a sufficient extent,† we may well ask whether, at the end of his internship, the interne is adequately prepared to bear the load of responsibility that will be his as soon as he steps into practice. It is the opinion of Stanley E. Dorst, Dean of Medicine at the University of Cincinnati, that "A one-year internship following the undergraduate programme does not provide the training he [i.e., the general practitioner] needs to-day to meet the responsibility for medical care. In the United States most attempts to develop a longer and more adequate training have not been very successful."‡ Because we regard the problem of responsibility in medicine as one of the major problems relating to quality of practice, we shall discuss this in more detail in chapter 25.

In considering some of the aspects of the internship about which more information is needed, it has, of course, to be remembered that

*J. E. Deitrick and R. C. Berson: Medical Schools in the United States at Mid-Century (New York: McGraw-Hill, 1953), p. 272.
†Regarding the Nova Scotia practitioners, see page 387 (footnote).
‡S. E. Dorst: Medicine: A Lifelong Study, Proceedings of Second World Conference on Medical Education, Chicago 1959 (New York: World Medical Association, 1961), p. 419.

there is great variation among internes, just as we found that there was among the general practitioners. More should be known about this variation, since training must take into account, not only the needs of the "average" interne, but the needs of each individual interne. Schumacher and Gee, on the basis of the information received from those physicians who graduated in the United States in 1950 (see page 409) say, "the results of this questionnaire point up . . . the need for flexibility in medical school curricula. Even among physicians following similar careers expressions of needs differ."* What Schumacher and Gee say about the medical school curriculum, we believe to be quite as applicable to the period of postgraduate hospital experience, namely, that the physicians taking the training differ in their needs. Only when more is known of these needs can changes be effected to provide for them. Moreover, because of the differences between individuals, it is a matter of necessity that there be some way of evaluating the adequacy of the postgraduate training of each individual. McClaughry, in a talk given to the Association of Hospital Directors of Medical Education on the "Responsibility of Hospitals in Graduate Medical Education," has pointed out that "Each hospital approved for internship or residency represents itself to physician applicants as an educational institution" and that, of the "two real services which an educational establishment can offer," one is "to evaluate the accomplishment of the learner so that unsatisfactory progress in any area of work leads either to correction of the deficiency or to the timely elimination of the student unsuited to the task selected."†

In summary, there is evidence that the interneship, as experienced by many of the general practitioners whom we visited, was not a satisfactory preparation for general practice. In view of our findings on the deficient quality of some of the practices we visited, this evidence is of more than academic interest. We suggest that the postgraduate hospital training be subjected to intensive study.

In addition to the problems that we have discussed so far, there is yet another, which, we believe, transcends in importance all that we have said up to this point. We refer to the conflict that exists between the educational needs of the interne and the service needs of the hospital. This, which appears to be the fundamental problem, we shall discuss in the next chapter.

*C. F. Schumacher and H. H. Gee: Journal of Medical Education, *36*, No. 4, Part 2: 163, 1961.

†R. I. McClaughry: Journal of the American Medical Association, *167*: 531, 533, 1958.

# 23 / Postgraduate Hospital Training
*Education or Service?*

Is the interne or resident* in the hospital primarily to learn or primarily to meet the service needs of the hospital? This we regard as a question that needs urgently to be faced, not only by those who are responsible for postgraduate medical education, but also by the medical profession as a whole and by society in general, which, as recipient of the benefits of medical education, has an obligation to give thoughtful consideration to its problems.

That this question is pertinent becomes quite plain as one reads what has been said in recent years. We cite first some of those who have stressed the educational aspect of the internship. Charles G. Child, III, Professor of Surgery at the University of Michigan, has said, "Men and women seeking to become doctors . . . continue to be formal students of medicine and surgery until they complete their internships and residencies."† M. R. Marshall, writing from the University of Alberta on "Graduate Medical Training: Its Organization and Administration," makes the same point:

Graduate training may be defined as well-organized and planned training in the different medical specialties. In many ways this is similar to undergraduate training in that it is planned and organized beforehand as regards time, place, and content, and has a definite aim. Graduate training consists in, or should consist in, the supervised study of the basic sciences and clinical

*In the United States, the internship usually refers to the first year of experience as a house doctor, subsequent years being referred to as assistant-residencies and residencies. What is called an assistant-residency in the United States may be called either an assistant-residency or a senior interneship in Canada.

†C. G. Child, III: Journal of Medical Education, 34, No. 10, Part 2: 35, 1959.

subjects . . . according to a curriculum specially designed for each graduate student; the aim is to qualify him for the examination leading to a certificate or degree in a medical specialty.

and:

The director [i.e., the director of graduate training] will plan the orderly exchange of residents between hospitals. . . . It is the director's responsibility that the graduate student be not exploited by the hospital or by any of its departments. Graduate students should not be moved, for example, from one hospital to another solely because of manpower shortage.*

The Canadian Medical Association, in a booklet produced in 1960 and entitled *Basis of Approval of Hospitals for the Training of Junior Interns in Canada,* repeatedly emphasizes the educational nature of the junior interneship in such statements as, "It has long been recognized that the initial internship taken by the medical graduate constitutes a crucial phase in the education of a physician," and "The junior internship is considered to be primarily an educational experience for the intern rather than the provision of an added service in a hospital." This booklet asserts, also, that "The recent requirement of the Medical Council of Canada that a pre-registration internship be served" at an approved hospital is "evidence that the junior internship is regarded as a continuing educational experience."†

Except for Marshall's limitation of his definition of graduate training to those doctors who are working towards qualifying as specialists, the statements that we have quoted make it quite clear that a major purpose of house-staff positions is said to be education. In addition, more than one hospital administrator, seeking to justify the fact that his internes were not paid, has even gone so far as to say that the members of the house staff were in the hospital *only* to learn and that they were of no value at all to the hospital. Yet, in spite of these statements, there is a conflict between the educational needs of the interne or resident and the service needs of the hospital. Julius H. Comroe, Jr., Director of the Cardiovascular Research Institute of the University of California Medical Center in San Francisco, describes this conflict:

The internship and residency, with possibly a few exceptions unknown to me, have never been designed wholly or even in large part as an experience in graduate medical education. The hospitals "approved for residency training" are not, and never have been, part of our total structure of medical education. . . .

*M. R. Marshall: Canadian Medical Association Journal, *84*: 695, 696, 1961.
†Basis of Approval of Hospitals for the Training of Junior Interns in Canada (Toronto: Canadian Medical Association, 1960), p. 4.

. . . True, today all hospitals in the United States, whether they so wish or not, must provide an educational programme to be accredited for specialty training, even though some of this is purely a programme "on paper." However, because the service of the intern and resident to the hospital comes first and the educational obligation of the hospital to the intern-resident comes second, the internship-residency is not primarily a graduate educational experience. It is service-oriented and not education-oriented.

Expediency, he goes on to point out, dictates that service rather than education shall have first claim on the time of the interne or resident:

There is no time for graduate medical education. The care of the patient comes first. Even when a hospital plans courses, the resident can attend only when clinical duties permit; he can benefit only when not exhausted from performances of technical procedures of the previous twelve to twenty-four hours. Even though his learning process was complete after the twenty-fifth intravenous infusion, the resident must perform another 500 or 1,000 of these.° The problem is simply one of expediency: who will give the infusions for the attending physician if the residency becomes a period designed more for learning and less for doing simple mechanical tasks over and over again? The resident must, of course, do many mechanical tasks, but not beyond the point of educational gain. Ideally, a residency should be a planned educational experience which continues the previous medical education in such a way that both the art and science of the specialty are learned without big gaps in either aspect. It is not expedient to do this at present. However, I am convinced that a five-year specialty residency would shrink to four or even three years if the residency were a planned learning experience stripped of everything which contributes more to the efficient management of a hospital or to the convenience of the attending staff than to the graduate education of a resident.†

Similarly, Russell A. Nelson, Director of the Johns Hopkins Hospital, speaks of the tendency to view internes as help rather than as students:

Most of our hospitals do not have employed physicians on the staff, and the larger institutions have depended on interns and residents for routine service, with the practitioners attending only a few hours each day. . . . All too frequently hospitals and their medical staffs view intern-residents as help, not students, and all too frequently hospitals feel there is no other way to give the 24-hour care.‡

We have discussed this matter privately with professors of clinical subjects in Canada and have heard the occasional one say quite

°For the general practitioners' comments on intravenous infusions and other "scut work," see pages 389–390.
†J. H. Comroe, Jr.: Medicine: A Lifelong Study, Proceedings of Second World Conference on Medical Education, Chicago 1959 (New York: World Medical Association, 1961), pp. 382, 383.
‡R. A. Nelson: *ibid.*, p. 454.

unequivocally that there is no doubt that, when a conflict occurs between the educational needs of an interne and the service needs of the hospital in which he is located, the service needs take précedence. This statement is illustrated by two episodes that have come to our attention very recently. These involve two doctors, each taking training in a different specialty and in a different hospital, which, in each case, is a major teaching hospital of a medical school. One of these young doctors was told by his professor that he was being sent, for the following year, to a certain hospital. This hospital was recognized by the young man as so inferior, from the point of view of medical education, that he declined the appointment and chose, instead, to see what he could find for himself in some other medical centre. It was his impression that his professor, rather than being interested in his training, was merely making use of him to fill a vacant position. The other young physician, who wished to spend time in certain subdivisions of his specialty in which he was weak and which would be of importance to him in his practice, was compelled, instead, to spend the time in another department of his hospital, where he assisted with work of a highly technical nature with which he would never be concerned in his own future practice. He was required to do this because the hospital was short of internes in the department to which he was assigned. In other words, the service needs of the hospital took precedence over the educational needs of the interne.

Deitrick and Berson, who made a survey of medical education in the United States between 1949 and 1951, concluded, "Interns and residents are frequently exploited. They perform valuable service functions for the hospitals and their staffs but receive far from adequate compensation in the form either of educational opportunity or of financial remuneration."*

Before we can consider solutions to this problem of conflicting interests, we must make sure that the present situation is clearly understood. This may best be achieved if we outline the development of postgraduate hospital training. Deitrick and Berson describe its origin in these words:

The term "intern" came into use in the United States approximately 100 years ago, to identify those young physicians who served in a hospital or almshouse for the purpose of gaining practical training under the guidance of a senior physician on the staff of the hospital. Frequently the young doctor paid a fee for this privilege. There was a real need for such practical

*J. E. Deitrick and R. C. Berson: Medical Schools in the United States at Mid-Century (New York: McGraw-Hill, 1953), p. 285.

experience because medical school instruction was chiefly didactic and students had little opportunity to examine patients and study them carefully.

In the late nineteenth and early twentieth centuries as hospitals became more closely associated with medical schools, internship training gradually became accepted as a routine part of a young physician's training. . . . After the turn of the century many hospitals found young physicians useful in the care of their charity or ward patients and developed internship programs. The intern lived in the hospital and could be called upon to render patient care both day and night. °

It is clear from this account that an arrangement that began merely as a means of meeting the educational needs of the young physician came to be recognized, early in this century, as being of some value to the hospitals concerned. Discussing the conflict of interests that developed, Deitrick and Berson say:

Since the establishment by the Council on Medical Education [of the American Medical Association] of standards for hospitals offering internships, there has been a constant and continuing effort on the part of educational bodies to make the internship a truly educational experience. At the same time, the demand by the hospitals for the services of interns has continuously increased. . . .

and

as far back as 1920 there was a definite conflict between the desire of the hospitals on the one hand to obtain interns because of the value of their services and the ideal of educational organizations on the other hand to make the internship predominately [sic] an educational experience. †

How valuable the services of internes were really considered to be is indicated by the efforts that hospitals in the United States made to obtain them. Deitrick and Berson report:

. . . the hospital-intern problem continued to grow. Interns became so valuable that many more hospitals sought approval by the Council on Medical Education and Hospitals. In their competition for the medical school graduates, the hospitals began to offer appointments to the students before they had completed their third year of medical school, with the understanding that the student would intern in the hospital upon graduation. Those hospitals encountering difficulty in obtaining interns frequently offered $100 to $200 per month plus board and room. In large teaching hospitals the intern rarely received more than $25 to $50 per month. In many instances he received no stipend whatever.

They conclude the story by saying:

Except for a matching plan which deals only with the mechanics of

°*Ibid.*, p. 265.
†*Ibid.*, pp. 267, 268.

appointing the interns, little progress has been made in the solution of this problem in the last 25 years.*

Deitrick and Berson were writing in 1953; but a statement made in 1959 by E. B. Hutchins, Research Associate of the Association of American Medical Colleges, that "Today there are two internships available for every student ready to intern,"† shows that the demand for internes has not abated since Deitrick and Berson published their report.

Essentially the picture is the same in Canada. That internes are similarly sought after in this country is made quite plain in the Canadian Medical Association's booklet on approval of hospitals for junior interneship:

> It is currently evident that the number of available junior interns from the graduating classes of Canadian medical schools falls short of the number of internship positions which Canadian hospitals would desire to establish. This situation imposes the obligation on the Committee on Approval of Hospitals for the Training of Interns to select for approval those hospitals which are qualified . . . to provide a well integrated programme. . . .

The booklet also says:

> One of the problems of intern placement has been the growing discrepancy between the number of internships offered by hospitals and the number of applicants available to fill them. This shortage of interns has created a hardship chiefly among smaller hospitals which, by their size, usually have a small intern quota. . . . Where the intern staff is below the recognized quota, the available interns may be called upon to give an excessive amount of time in providing hospital services at the expense of their intern training. . . . Some hospitals have aggravated the intern problem by offering excessive stipends as a means of attracting interns.‡

We began this chapter with the question, "Is the interne or resident in the hospital primarily to learn or primarily to meet the service needs of the hospital?" The conflicting statements that we have quoted make clear that this question has not been squarely faced, except in isolated instances. Failure to face the question is particularly plain in the booklet of the Canadian Medical Association, which states that "The junior internship is considered to be primarily an educational experience" (see page 422, above), but which also states that the "shortage of interns has created a hardship" (see above) for certain hospitals. The "hardship" obviously has nothing to do with the fact

---

*Ibid.*, pp. 269, 270.

†E. B. Hutchins: Journal of Medical Education, 36, No. 4, Part 2: 66, 1961.

‡Basis of Approval of Hospitals for the Training of Junior Interns in Canada (Toronto: Canadian Medical Association, 1960), pp. 3, 5.

that there is a shortage of internes to educate; the "hardship" derives from the fact that there is a shortage of internes to give service to the hospital.

We have traced the development of the present conflict between the educational needs of the interne and the service needs of the hospital. We must now consider why this conflict persists. The clue is contained in the statement of Deitrick and Berson (see page 424, above) that, "Interns and residents are frequently exploited. They perform valuable service functions . . . but receive far from adequate compensation in the form *either of educational opportunity or of financial remuneration* [our italics]." If education really took first place, it would be necessary for many hospitals to arrange a vastly different programme from that existing at present and, more important to the hospitals, they would have to forego much of the valuable service that is at present rendered by the house staff. If, on the other hand, it were generally admitted that the service needs of the hospital have the first claim on the interne's time and energy and that only in his remaining time, if any, is he permitted to satisfy his own educational needs, the hospitals would no longer have any justification for paying the grossly inadequate salaries that many pay their internes at present. Thus, in either case—whether the hospitals put education first and lose much of the service that they are at present obtaining or whether they admit that service comes first and pay their internes accordingly—the hospitals would lose economically.

Since we are maintaining that economic considerations are at the root of the conflict between the educational needs of the internes and residents and the service demands of the hospitals, it is appropriate that we hear what others have to say about the remuneration of hospital house staffs. Child, speaking at the Sixth Teaching Institute of the Association of American Medical Colleges in 1958, pointed to the inadequacies of salaries at this level:

In any consideration of medical service plans as they relate to professional staff, recognition must be given the forgotten men of our teaching hospitals —the interns, assistant residents, and residents . . . these individuals constitute the backbone of medical care in most of our university hospitals. . . . That their significant and essential positions in the organization of teaching hospitals be accorded the dignity of careful attention is only just. . . . I am reminded of an editorial which appeared recently in a large city newspaper. Under the title of "Thirty Cents an Hour," this editorial reads in part:

"At the shameful bottom of the totem pole among New York City's employees are the full-time interns and residents of our city hospitals. No teen-age baby sitter would deign to sit before the television set for what these people are getting to care for the sick. They know nothing of the minimum-wage law, or extra pay for overtime. They are on active duty from 105 hours a week to over 150 hours, including nights and week-ends. . . .

"For this niggardly wage these doctors dispense the bulk of the daily medical care given to the patients of the municipal hospitals under a city administration that prides itself on labor relations enlightenment . . . Here is certainly a 'shame of the city' that should be recognized by prompt modification of the budget."

Medical teachers have it within their power to change this "shame of the city," not only in municipal and voluntary teaching hospitals, but in university hospitals as well.*

Again, Owen H. Wangensteen, Professor of Surgery at the University of Minnesota, talking on the "Education of a Surgeon," brings up the matter of adequate remuneration:

Perhaps what is needed most of all is an adequate fee for service for the trainee in the surgery program. He should be paid a living wage. In 1960, a beginning salary of $3,600 may be a bit out of line with what is the current going wage for trainees, but it is in effect a low estimate of the value of such a person to the hospital and the department he serves. From there on to completion of his training, he should, I feel, be given annual increases of $600 to $900. . . .

An experience toward the end of World War II made an important and indelible impress upon my mind. I recall discussing his work with a very able second-year house officer, some years ago, late in December. Through a fortunate circumstance, I told him it was going to be possible to increase his pay from $1,800 to $3,600 a year. For a moment, he looked at me somewhat incredulously. Then tears began to roll down his cheeks. He said, "Now I can buy my wife a Christmas present." This surprise remark suggested the need of terminating our discussion somewhat abruptly lest my feelings find similar expression.†

Seymour I. Schwartz and W. J. Merle Scott, Assistant Professor and Professor, respectively, of Surgery at the University of Rochester, in their report on the inaugural meeting of the Conference of University Surgical Residents, speak also of the implications of low salaries:

It was impressive that a frank discussion brought out the fact that over 80 per cent of the residents were in significant debt at the termination of their residency. It was proposed that a $400 to $450 per month stipend should be the minimal salary, since this would avoid debt and allow for the maintenance of a necessary term insurance policy program. It was also of interest that many hospitals held the individual resident responsible for

*C. G. Child, III: Journal of Medical Education, *34,* No. 10, Part 2: 44, 1959. The subquotation is from an Editorial, New York Times, March 23, 1958, p. 22.
†O. H. Wangensteen: Journal of Medical Education, *35:* 968, 1960.

his malpractice insurance. This should certainly be provided by the hospital or university.*

Daniel H. Funkenstein, of the Department of Psychiatry of Harvard University, referring to the "pressing problems of the married interns and residents," says, "In many cases the financial plight of the young resident's family has resulted in extremely strained relationships between him and his wife, with deleterious effects on their children."†

We referred in the preceding chapter (see pages 387, 394, 411–412) to the information collected by Gee and Schumacher from 2,616 internes in the United States in the year 1958–1959. These two workers, who are the Director of Research and the Assistant Director of Research, respectively, of the Association of American Medical Colleges, conclude their report of this study by raising a question of ethics:

> The data in this study tend to support the popular view of the internship as a period of indentured servitude for many young physicians. Where such conditions exist, one is forced to inquire as to the inadequacy of mechanisms for approving internships and to inquire as well into the ethics of demands for service in the guise of fulfilling an educational requirement made by the medical profession.‡

Finally, it is important to note what the Canadian Medical Association says in its booklet on the approval of hospitals for junior interneship. Under the heading, "The Junior Intern's Duties," is the statement, "The conscientious intern, although requiring a reasonable amount of free time, should give his patient's welfare his first consideration in thought and deed on a ROUND-THE-CLOCK basis."§ Under the heading, "The Junior Intern's Welfare," remuneration is discussed as follows:

> The internship has traditionally been considered an extension of the medical student's education. Emphasis, therefore, should be placed on the training of the intern rather than service to the hospital. However, the intern should recognize that the hospital does pay out a considerable amount of money on his behalf and, therefore, it is reasonable to expect that interns will provide services to the hospital in recompense for the highly valuable experience and training that they receive through their hospital practice.
> Because of the increased costs of medical education and additional financial obligations that are placed on many graduates, most hospitals now

*S. I. Schwartz and W. J. M. Scott: Journal of Medical Education, *35*: 276, 1960.

†D. H. Funkenstein: Journal of Medical Education, *33*, No. 10, Part 2: 50, 1958.

‡H. H. Gee and C. F. Schumacher: Journal of Medical Education, *36*, No. 4, Part 2: 60, 1961.

§Basis of Approval of Hospitals for the Training of Junior Interns in Canada (Toronto: Canadian Medical Association, 1960), p. 13. The capitals occur in the booklet from which the quotation is taken.

provide interns with a reasonable stipend for their services. However, payment of excessive stipends, bonuses or other forms of remuneration as a means of attracting interns, may place undue emphasis on service to the hospital to the disadvantage of the intern's education. If excessive payments are necessary to attract interns, there may be reason to question the adequacy of the intern training programme.*

One other statement having to do with remuneration occurs in the section on "The Junior Intern's Duties," namely, "Since the intern is a full-time student, he should devote all of his time to his professional education and may not accept outside remunerative positions."†

The Canadian Medical Association has thus stated its belief that the interne is a student and its concern lest his studies be jeopardized if the financial remuneration‡ from the hospital is too great or if he attempts to earn money in any other way; and it calls for "a reasonable amount of free time" for the interne. Yet the Association does not indicate in any way what it regards as a reasonable amount of free time but does make quite plain, to the extent of using capital letters, that the patient's welfare is to be the first consideration "on a ROUND-THE-CLOCK basis." The Association says that "interns should be encouraged to spend a substantial amount of time in the study and review of current medical literature pertaining to the service to which they are assigned,"§ but makes no mention of the necessity for the hospital to see that the interne has adequate time for study.‖ A library

*Ibid.*, p. 14.

†*Ibid.*

‡The amounts currently being paid to internes in Canadian hospitals have been discussed at some length in chapter 13 (pages 179–181 and 184 and Table 33). In summary, we found that the salaries paid to junior internes varied greatly but that the mean salary for junior internes in hospitals having university affiliations was $121 per month. This was exclusive of room and board, which we estimated would bring the unmarried interne's remuneration to $2,492 per annum and the married interne's remuneration to less than this amount (page 182). If we assume a twelve-hour day, on the average, for 300 days in the year—and these figures are a conservative estimate—the interne's pay works out to be higher than the *New York Times'*s 30 cents an hour (page 427); it is probably about 70 cents an hour on the average.

§Basis of Approval of Hospitals for the Training of Junior Interns in Canada (Toronto: Canadian Medical Association, 1960), p. 10.

‖How unsympathetic hospital administrators may be towards the requirements of education is illustrated by an episode that occurred a few years ago in a major teaching hospital. An extremely conscientious interne was called before the administrator and reprimanded for being out of the hospital before five o'clock in the afternoon. The reason given by the interne, that he was returning medical books to a library, did not appease the administrative wrath, though it was at the instance of the administrator, himself a physician, that the books had been borrowed. Whether this is typical of administrators, we do not know. This occurrence does illustrate, however, what can happen when the demands for service and the needs of education come into conflict.

is listed as a "Desirable Feature," but not as one of the "Essential Requirements," of a "Fully Approved Hospital."* Finally, in a section on the "Intern's Health," no mention is made of the need for adequate rest, exercise, or other recreation or of the need for making time available for these. When all of these facts are added together, it is hard to escape the conclusion either that the Canadian Medical Association has not *really* faced the question whether the interneship is primarily for education or primarily for service or that the Association is willing to allow the interneship to persist, in the words of Gee and Schumacher, "as a period of indentured servitude" (see page 429, above). At this point, we wish to make quite clear that we are not suggesting that, in an emergency, the interne or resident should put his educational needs first, to the detriment of a patient. Such conduct would be unthinkable. If, however, a constant series of service demands, whether emergent or routine, is interfering with the interne's educational efforts, then are those who demand, in the name of ethical behaviour, that the interne put service to others before his own needs themselves acting ethically?

From the evidence that we have presented—the statements of eminent medical educators on the value of internes' and residents' services, the findings of Deitrick and Berson, the more recent report of Gee and Schumacher, and the current salaries offered in Canadian hospitals—it is apparent that, in general, members of hospital house staffs are inadequately paid for the work that they do. It is easy to understand, from the description given by Deitrick and Berson (see pages 424–426, above), how this situation developed. Its persistence, we have pointed out (page 427), is fundamentally a matter of economics. Because hospitals for many years have had a notoriously difficult time financially, they have not wished to increase their financial burden by paying their house staff any more than they absolutely had to. Some hospital administrators have attempted to make this treatment of their house staff appear respectable by maintaining that the internes were in the hospital entirely for their own good and that they were of no value to the hospital. This, which was true, perhaps, a hundred years ago, is no longer true and has not been for many years. The truth is, as the quotations that we have given make amply clear, that the services rendered to the hospitals by their house staffs are of very great value. In fact, it can be said, without exaggeration, that if the first-rate hospitals were left without house staff, they would cease to be first-rate hospitals within a matter of

*Basis of Approval of Hospitals for the Training of Junior Interns in Canada (Toronto: Canadian Medical Association, 1960), p. 17.

days, unless the attending staff were willing to abandon their non-hospital work and to devote themselves on a full-time basis to maintaining the standard of care in the hospital. As Child has said (see page 427, above), the internes and residents "constitute the backbone of medical care in most of our university hospitals." The proof of the value attached to the interne lies in the description that we have quoted from Deitrick and Berson (see page 425) of the eagerness with which the hospitals compete for internes; and the booklet of the Canadian Medical Association indicates that hospitals in this country are just as eager to have internes as are those in the United States (see page 426, and also 416 for the comment of a hospital administrator).

There are at least two factors that assist the hospitals in maintaining the present unsatisfactory situation. First, the licensing regulations insist upon a year of interneship. As a result of this, there is, each year, a supply of internes available, in the persons of the newly graduated physicians.*

Secondly, though there have been isolated attempts for at least forty years to ensure that internes were not exploited, the medical profession as a whole has shown a remarkable lack of interest in the problem. There appear to be several reasons for this. Among the practising physicians, as we have already reported (see pages 186–188), there is great variation of opinion regarding both the value of internes' services and whether the internes should be paid even what their services are acknowledged to be worth. Some men appear to be indifferent to the problem; others say, as one of our general practitioners said, "I wasn't paid as an interne; why should these young fellows be paid?" When these men have their attention directed to the longer training required today, the earlier marriages, and the indebtedness of some of the men in house-staff positions (see page 428), they tend to shrug their shoulders, to say that the young physicians should not marry until they are older, or to dismiss their indebtedness as of no importance, without apparently recognizing the precarious situation of a young doctor's family if he should die prematurely.

Another reason why some members of the profession are not willing to take a stand against the exploitation of internes and residents is a fear that to do so will give government an excuse to nationalize the practice of medicine. The argument given is that, since the hospitals can barely make ends meet as it is, the money necessary to pay internes

*Three Canadian medical schools require that the interneship be served prior to the granting of the degree.

adequately would have to come from government and that, as government would then be paying for postgraduate medical education, it would establish a right to a young physician's services for the rest of his working life. This argument, if it could be considered valid at all—and this strikes us as highly doubtful—would be valid only if an interne's salary could be regarded as a grant in aid of his education. In the event that the period of postgraduate training were to be reorganized so that an interne's educational needs received first consideration, his salary, if paid on a full-time basis, *could* be so regarded. (But, in the event of such a reorganization, he would have no more and no less reason than postgraduate students in other fields to expect a salary or any other form of financial aid.) The interneship as it exists at present, however, is, in the words of Comroe (see page 423), "service-oriented and not education-oriented." So long as its orientation remains as it is, whatever the interne is paid is *not* an educational grant but is payment for services rendered. We do not know what percentage of the practising physicians have the fear—which, with the present orientation of the interneship and residency, is illogical—that payment of adequate salaries to house staff would give government an excuse to nationalize the practice of medicine; but the very fact that we have encountered this fear at all indicates, in itself, the need to face the question whether the interneship and residency exist primarily to meet the interne's educational needs or primarily to satisfy the hospital's service needs.

Finally, as Deitrick and Berson have pointed out, "It would be impossible for many senior staff members to care for more than a fraction of the number of their private patients were it not for the work of the interns and residents. This is especially true of the surgeon. . . ."* To use Comroe's word, it is a matter of "expediency" (see page 423). If the interneship and residency were so arranged that medical education took precedence over the service needs of the hospital, who would give the intravenous infusions and do all the other things that contribute "more . . . to the convenience of the attending staff than to the graduate education of a resident?" This question we shall try to answer later (see pages 441–443). At present, we are merely pointing out that it is likely, and understandable, that this problem of expediency is one of the factors accounting for the practising profession's failure to insist that the period of postgraduate training be made truly and primarily educational. It is in this regard,

*J. E. Deitrick and R. C. Berson: Medical Schools in the United States at Mid-Century (New York: McGraw-Hill, 1953), p. 283.

of course, that the query of Gee and Schumacher about "the ethics of demands for service in the guise of fulfilling an educational requirement made by the medical profession" (see page 429) is particularly pertinent.

We have indicated several reasons why the medical profession as a whole has not demanded either that the educational needs of the interne take precedence over the hospital's service needs or else that the interne be adequately paid for his services. Every one of these reasons we have encountered at various times; but what the relative importance of each one is, we can only surmise. The important point, however, is that the profession, except in isolated instances, has remained silent or has shown itself actively opposed to change. It is not surprising, then, that hospital trustees, having to depend on the advice of their attending staff in professional matters, have remained deaf to the demands of their internes when they have seen that the senior members of the profession are not in favour of making changes.

We have described the development of the present situation, in which internes and residents do not receive adequate compensation for their services "in the form either of educational opportunity or of financial remuneration" (see page 424), and we have discussed several factors that operate to maintain the present system, namely, the financial difficulties of the hospitals, the licensing regulations, and the attitude, of apathy and sometimes of hostility, of members of the profession towards any change. Our concern in this study, however, is not primarily with the financial difficulties of house staff, but with the *quality of practice*. How is the situation that we have just pictured related to the quality of practice?

It is related in several ways. For the sake of simplicity, we shall consider the effects of inadequate educational opportunity and the effects of inadequate financial remuneration separately, though, as will soon be seen, they are related. First of all, what is the effect of inadequate financial remuneration? Unless an interne's salary, including room and board, is at least as great, per unit of time worked, as the remuneration of such employees as secretaries and laboratory technicians, it is obviously to a hospital's advantage to require internes to write out their histories instead of dictating them for typing and to make use of internes instead of technicians for much routine laboratory work. In short, there is a great temptation for a hospital to use its internes for the wrong *type* of work, whereas, if an interne's remuneration, per unit of time worked, were greater than that of the less highly trained personnel, the hospital would find it an indefensible extravagance to use an interne to do the work of a secretary or of a technician. In addition, because non-medical personnel work a limited number of hours whereas there is no limit to what may be demanded of an interne, the hospital and the medical staff are strongly tempted to impose too great a *volume* of work on the interne. Lest the reader suppose that hospitals do not *really* make such demands, we recall to his attention the comments of the general practitioners about "scut work" (pages 389, 395) and about being overworked (pages 391, 394), the statements, made by 43 per cent of the Ontario doctors and by 49 per cent of those in Nova Scotia, that they had not had adequate time for reading and studying during their interneships (page 396), and Comroe's statement that "There is no time for graduate medical education" (page 423). In this regard, it is interesting and encouraging to note the concern that was expressed at the Presidents' Panel (see page 370) by Deane W. Malott, President of Cornell University, who said:

. . . there is the pressure which I know I find of concern in common with our medical faculty that in these centers [i.e., "these great medical centers" of which he had been speaking] there is an ever-increasing tendency to use the students in a variety of ways, serving the purposes of the total organization, because warm, strong bodies of reasonable maturity and great vigor and strength are useful in a great variety of ways having little, if anything, to do with the educational processes for which those warm bodies are present.*

We have said that the fact that internes receive inadequate financial remuneration leads to their being required to do too great a *volume* of work and the wrong *type* of work. There is another factor that acts in conjunction with inadequate financial remuneration to produce these two effects. That other factor is the failure of the profession to state *unequivocally,* and of the hospitals to acknowledge, that an interne is in a hospital primarily to satisfy his educational needs. The Canadian Medical Association, for example, though recognizing that "Overburdening an intern with responsibility for an excessive number of patients lowers the educational value of the internship and is just as damaging as a limited experience with too few patients," nevertheless says, "it is reasonable to expect that interns will provide services to the hospital in recompense for the highly valuable experience and training that they receive,"† and does not indicate how an interne is to be

*The Presidents' Panel: Journal of Medical Education, 34: 252, 1959.
†Basis of Approval of Hospitals for the Training of Junior Interns in Canada (Toronto: Canadian Medical Association, 1960), pp. 6, 14.

protected from exploitation. If the profession were to state unequivocally that education was the reason for an interne's being in the
hospital and that service needs must be met in some other way, then,
even though an interne were paid very little, it would be more difficult
for a hospital to ignore his educational requirements.

We have considered the effects of inadequate financial remuneration.
Closely related to this are the effects of inadequate educational opportunity in the interneship or residency. If any significant proportion of
an interne's time is being spent on tasks that have nothing to do with
his education, then it is obvious that the amount of time available to
him for educational purposes is reduced by that amount and that his
postgraduate training must be correspondingly prolonged. Comroe
has stated his conviction (see page 423) "that a five-year specialty
residency would shrink to four or even three years if the residency
were a planned learning experience stripped of everything which contributes more to the efficient management of a hospital or to the
convenience of the attending staff than to the graduate education of
a resident." The unnecessary prolongation of training may have any
one of several effects. Some physicians who wish to be general practitioners may not be able to take as much training as they wish. Such
was the case with 11 per cent of the Ontario practitioners and 26 per
cent of the Nova Scotia practitioners whom we visited, who said that,
if it had not been for their financial situation, they would have taken
further training, but with the intention of engaging in general practice.
Other physicians are forced to be general practitioners because they
cannot afford the prolonged training that is required for specialty
qualifications. Thirty-six per cent of our Ontario sample and 19 per
cent of our Nova Scotia sample would have chosen a specialty as their
career instead of general practice, if it had not been for their financial
difficulties. Thus almost half of the practitioners in each province had
been directly affected by the financial situation obtaining during the
period of postgraduate hospital experience (see pages 185–186).

Physicians who *are* able to complete the postgraduate training they
wish are, nonetheless, being put to an unnecessary expense if the
training is unnecessarily prolonged. John G. Darley, Professor of Psychology and, at that time, Associate Dean of the Graduate School of
the University of Minnesota, issued a warning at the Fourth Teaching
Institute of the Association of American Medical Colleges, when he
spoke about the ill effects of holding medical trainees in economic
dependence over a prolonged period:

At the point of admission you are dealing with a group, . . . who for the
first 18 years lived in urban communities in homes that would probably be

in the upper 2, 3, or 4 per cent of the income standards of the entire United States; they had comfortable homes. . . . You put these students in a highly rigorous and competitive situation in the medical school. They were originally to a considerable extent economically motivated to medicine, and now you put them into an internship, followed sometimes by residencies. You hold over their heads now the concept of a specialty board. You use them as residents and fellows, as a form of Chinese cheap labor, to render wonderful service in your teaching institutions. You pay them at the prevailing low hospital rate. . . . Ultimately these people are boarded members of the profession and they have had it. You have held them in a state of high economic dependence for a long time and they are now going to catch up with the world.[*]

At the Seventh Teaching Institute, Darley repeated his suggestion that "one cannot take a young man from the upper socioeconomic classes into the long grind of medical education, withhold economic rewards for a long period, and then expect him to be indifferent to making up economically for the lost years."[†]

Funkenstein, speaking at the Fifth Teaching Institute of the Association of American Medical Colleges, also pointed to the problems arising from the length of medical education and from the failure of medical faculties to keep up with social changes:

The rapidly ongoing changes in our society are having their effect on the psychosocial development of medical students. In considering the problems created thereby, it must be borne in mind continually that medical education has become so lengthy that it is out of step with the student's development, and students, unwilling to postpone the satisfactions of adulthood until their thirties, are marrying and having children. Concomitantly, the students develop an increased preoccupation with vocationalism and the necessity for earning a living, concerns that do not leave time for the cultivation of certain areas of importance in education. The situation is further complicated by the fact that many medical school faculties are lagging behind these social changes under the influence of their outdated stereotype of the student.

He has warned:

The price for failure to facilitate in every way the mature development of the doctor is paid in the quality of patient care.[‡]

Deitrick and Berson, who concluded that "Insufficient thought has been given to the effect on the young physician as a person of long training periods with low income and rather rigid regimentation,"[§]

[*]J. G. Darley: Journal of Medical Education, 32, No. 10, Part 2: 180, 1957.
[†]J. G. Darley: Journal of Medical Education, 36, No. 4, Part 2: 92, 1961.
[‡]D. H. Funkenstein: Journal of Medical Education, 33, No. 10, Part 2: 52, 53, 1958.
[§]J. E. Deitrick and R. C. Berson: Medical Schools in the United States at Mid-Century (New York: McGraw-Hill, 1953), p. 286.

discerned several attitudes that tend to develop as a result of such training. Of one of these attitudes, which relates to fees, they give the following description:

The third attitude is one which should be decried in the practice of medicine: that is, that the charging of high fees is justified. One is reluctantly forced to the conclusion that some aspects of the system of medical education and hospital training are conducive to this point of view. The young man who has paid a fairly high tuition for four years of medical schooling and has then spent another three to five years in residency training with a low salary is generally twenty-eight to thirty years of age when he has obtained his board certification. During this period his maximum earnings have not averaged more than $1,200 or $2,500 per year, and in many instances he has either delayed marriage or has required financial assistance. When he enters the practice of medicine, he can usually anticipate a maximum of 30 to 35 years of real earning capacity. In the first few years he may have difficulty in establishing his practice and a reputation. Thus, when patients do seek his services, he feels justified, on a logical basis, in charging high fees in order to make up for his earlier lack of earning capacity.[*]

To what Deitrick and Berson have said, we would add that the alternative to charging high fees, if it is necessary to make up for the lack of earnings of so many years, is to see a larger number of patients, which a doctor may accomplish either by shortening the time given each patient and doing superficial work or by extending his hours of work excessively. In the former case, quality suffers at once; in the latter, quality will probably deteriorate over a longer period owing to lack of time for reading and study and to chronic fatigue on the part of the physician. In interrogating the doctors whom we visited, we did not ask their opinions of any possible relationship between internes' salaries and the practitioners' subsequent fees, but one doctor, speaking in favour of adequate salaries for internes, added the comment, "Then, later, fees need not be as high."

These effects of inadequate educational opportunity—unnecessary prolongation of training, resulting in inability of some men to obtain the desired training and the tendency of others to make up the financial loss by charging high fees in practice—would be avoided if it were acknowledged that the service demands of a hospital take precedence over an interne's educational needs and the interne were paid a salary that was commensurate with the value of his services.

Thus, whether we consider the effects of inadequate financial remuneration of an interne or whether we consider the effects of inadequate educational opportunity, we come to the same conclusion: that

[*]*Ibid.*, p. 284.

it is essential to decide which takes priority, the educational requirements of an interne or the service needs of a hospital. That these are
at present in conflict with each other and that this conflict is detrimental to medical education needs general *recognition* and *acknowl-
edgement*. It is not enough that these facts be recognized by medical
educators. They must be recognized, also, both by the profession as a
whole, so that the profession will support, rather than oppose, the
necessary corrective measures, and by the hospitals, so that those
hospitals that are not prepared to make the interneship *truly* educational will stop trying to obtain internes. Until it is generally recognized
that the present situation is unsatisfactory and that changes are needed,
there can be little hope of proceeding further. It is for this reason that
we have devoted so much of this chapter to demonstrating that an
unsatisfactory situation exists. If service is to take priority, as it does
at present, then it is essential that there be remuneration commensurate
with the value of the services rendered. If education is to take priority,
then it is essential that it take priority, not merely in word, but in fact.
At present, the hospitals are able to pay their internes and residents
grossly inadequate salaries, under the pretext that the interneship or
residency is merely education, and are able, to a large extent, to
negate the educational value of the experience because an interne has
no way of preventing a hospital from imposing on him excessively long
hours, an undue volume of work, and work of a type that has no
educational value.

We must now consider what should be done about the present
unsatisfactory situation; and, in proposing remedies, we must bring
forward the question that we ignored earlier, namely, who would look
after the service needs of the hospitals if the interneship and the
residency were so arranged that medical education took precedence.

It will be necessary to determine what the optimal course of postgraduate training would comprise. Since we are considering the
conflicting demands of service and of education on an interne's or
resident's time, we might consider that his time would be divided
between more or less formal instruction (in the shape of lectures,
seminars, and bedside or outpatient-department teaching), reading and
other forms of individual study dictated by the student's educational
needs rather than by the hospital's service needs, and clinical experience (i.e., the development of the ability to put into practice what
has been learnt in theory). What proportion of an interne's or resident's
time should be devoted to each of these three types of activity could
be ascertained only by experimentation, which would have to include
evaluation of the educational results of the various programmes tried.

At present, however, the amount of time devoted to practical clinical work is determined, not by an interne's educational needs, but by a hospital's service needs. The results of this are that often far too little time is left for formal instruction or for individual study and that even the practical experience itself may be stripped of much of its educational value if pressure of other work that *must* be done prevents an interne from exploring the avenues of speculation or of investigation that are opened by the case in hand. McClaughry has pointed out that "With an increasingly rapid turnover of patients, a significantly greater portion of the time of the house staff is taken up by the initial examination of patients. . . . A too frequent result . . . is that the physician is overwhelmed, and so a routine and slipshod job is done of all aspects of the study of the patient."*

In listing the activities between which an interne's or resident's time would be divided in the optimal course of postgraduate training, we omitted one group of activities: his non-professional activities, including sleep, exercise and other types of recreation, and attention to whatever domestic or other personal responsibilities he may have. The importance of adequate rest and recreation to the effectiveness of an interne's study, let alone his service to the hospital, is so obvious as to need no explanation, and is mentioned only because the practitioners' comments to us and some of the quotations cited above make clear that too often these needs of an interne are forgotten or ignored by a hospital. That an interne have adequate time to discharge his domestic responsibilities we regard as equally important. In our own practice, we have looked after the children of physicians who were serving as internes or residents and have seen some of the unfortunate situations that can develop when the father is seldom able to get home so that the whole burden of disciplining and rearing the children is thrust upon the mother. We ask how a man can be expected to understand his patients and *their* problems and responsibilities, when his very training requires him to ignore primary responsibilities of his own. If this postgraduate period is to be education, and not merely vocational training, it must take a wider view of a physician's life than that mere technical competence, or even the practice of medicine, is all that matters. In this connection, we recall with pleasure an episode that came to our notice a few years ago. A young doctor, taking postgraduate training, was offered the residency on a major service of an internationally famous hospital. When he learnt that the

*R. I. McClaughry: Journal of the American Medical Association, *167*: 534, 1958.

chief of the service expected him to make rounds each evening between six and seven o'clock, he said that he would have to decline the appointment unless that hour could be free, since it was the one hour out of the whole day that he saved for his two-year-old son. His professor replied that, in that case, rounds would be at seven o'clock.

When experiment has shown what the optimal, i.e. the *educationally* optimal, amount of clinical work is for the average interne at various stages of his postgraduate education, it will then be possible to calculate how far the work done by him, now that he is truly treated as a graduate student, will fall short of satisfying a hospital's service needs. This deficit of service is a matter of first importance, since a hospital's primary responsibility is to provide adequate care for its patients. How is this deficit to be made up? Russell A. Nelson, Director of the Johns Hopkins Hospital, in answer to the question how hospitals can provide twenty-four-hour service to patients, without internes or residents, says, "Thousands of our institutions do a good job without any interns or residents. They do it through good organization of the attending staff and greater use of nursing and technical assistance."* We would suggest, in addition, that, in hospitals in which the service demands are heavy, especially the teaching hospitals, there should be some full-time salaried physicians. They might be of two kinds: permanent and temporary. Some hospitals already have a few permanent, full-time positions in which the physicians' time is entirely occupied by teaching, research, and clinical service within the hospital. These men are too few, however, to provide the extra service that would be needed if the internes' and residents' load of clinical service were reduced as we have recommended. Therefore, besides these full-time, permanent, salaried physicians, we suggest that there be a certain number—the number being determined by a hospital's service needs—of full-time physicians employed by the hospital for periods of three, six, nine, or twelve months. These positions would be *service* positions; they would *not* be *educational* positions, except in the sense that one is bound to learn something from any experience. These positions should not be open to those enrolled as graduate students. Finally, those appointed to these service positions should be paid according to the prevailing rates of remuneration for the type of service rendered.

Who would be interested in holding such positions? We think,

*R. A. Nelson: Medicine: A Lifelong Study, Proceedings of the Second World Conference on Medical Education, Chicago 1959 (New York: World Medical Association, 1961), p. 454.

though we have no proof, that they might well be of interest to two groups of physicians: to some of those who had just completed their postgraduate education and wished to earn some money before going into practice on their own and, secondly, to men who had been in practice, either general or specialty practice, for some years and who wished to return to a teaching hospital for a limited period to refresh themselves and become familiar with recent advances. At the present time, for the latter group to return to a hospital is difficult for at least three reasons, because they must compete with the recent graduates for the interneships, because they find it difficult to leave their practices for a year, and because they find it economically crippling to work for an interne's pittance. The positions that we have suggested would provide a reasonable income, since they would be service rather than educational positions; and the shorter appointments, those of three or six months' duration, would enable a practitioner to leave his practice with less difficulty.

We have said (page 439) that it is necessary that the hospitals recognize the conflict between their own service needs and the educational needs of internes and residents, so that those hospitals that are not prepared to provide a truly educational experience will not continue to try to obtain internes. It is the non-teaching hospital, whose connection with a university is either non-existent or, at most, tenuous, that is least prepared to take responsibility for postgraduate medical education. Gee and Schumacher, on the basis of the information obtained from the 2,616 United States internes (see page 387), say, "It is disquieting ... to see ... that very few rotating interns in nonaffiliated hospitals receive adequate instruction in the application of scientific knowledge to patient care." Comparing teaching and non-teaching hospitals, they say:

Considering the intern's over-all evaluation of his internship in terms of the type of hospital in which it took place, it is apparent that hospitals having some teaching affiliation with a medical school are rated higher than nonteaching hospitals, and that an internship in a major teaching hospital is generally considered more valuable than one in a minor hospital. This same trend occurs with respect to the balance between theory and practice in the internship and with respect to the specific ways in which the internship contributed or failed to contribute to the intern's professional development. Thus, the major teaching hospital was apt to provide better opportunity than others in terms of responsibility for patient care, breadth of experience with varieties of disease, instruction in the application of the basic sciences to patient care, and constructive review and criticism of work with patients.*

*H. H. Gee and C. F. Schumacher: Journal of Medical Education, *36*, No. 4, Part 2: 53, 58, 1961.

Though it is doubtful whether many of the non-teaching hospitals are able to provide the educational experience that a graduate student of medicine should have, there is no reason, if Nelson's suggestion (see page 441) does not meet the needs of these hospitals, why they should not have a number of the short-term *service* positions that we have just described, which, again, might be expected to appeal, for a period of six to twelve months, to a man who had just completed his postgraduate education and wished to earn some money before establishing his own practice.

In connection with the suggestions that we have made, we must say a few words about the matter of authority. At present, internes and residents, being employees of their hospitals, are subject to the orders of the hospital administrators and of the attending staff of the services to which they are assigned. It is because a member of the house staff is an employee of the hospital that his own educational needs have to take second place to the hospital's service needs. If the suggestions that we have made were to be implemented, those physicians who were appointed to the non-educational, salaried, service positions would be hospital employees, of course, but the graduate students, who would be in the hospitals primarily for education and who would be giving only a limited amount of service, should be enrolled in the graduate school of a university and should be under the control of the university. Child, who was Chairman of the Seventh Teaching Institute of the Association of American Medical Colleges, after pointing out that "University trustees seem to avoid responsibility for care of patients and hospital boards shun concern for education," has put the question, "Is it too much to ask that universities accept responsibility for continuing house officer education in hospitals legitimately coming within their regional jurisdiction?"*

It is interesting to find that, in recent years, a good deal has been written about the conflicting demands of education and of service in the case of the student nurse who is enrolled in a hospital nursing school;† and the economic basis of this is suggested in the statement made by Edith K. Russell that "Unfortunately, the hospital nursing school appears to be an economic asset for the hospital and provides

---

*C. G. Child, III: Journal of Medical Education, 36, No. 4, Part 2: xxii, 1961.

†(1) J. M. Geister: Modern Hospital, 89: 64, 1957. (2) M. J. Stephenson: Canadian Hospital, 36: 57, 1959. (3) H. K. Mussallem: Spotlight on Nursing Education: The Report of the Pilot Project for the Evaluation of Schools of Nursing in Canada (Ottawa: Canadian Nurses' Association, 1960), pp. 75, 84. (4) W. S. Wallace: Report on the Experiment in Nursing Education of the Atkinson School of Nursing, The Toronto Western Hospital, 1950–1955 (University of Toronto Press), p. 5.

often its main source of nursing labour; thus the reason for its persistence."* Certain experiments have been carried out in which nurses have been trained in schools that were independent of the hospital nursing service. The results of these experiments are interesting and worth noting. Lord, who directed the Evaluation of the Metropolitan School of Nursing in Windsor, Ontario, writes, "The conclusion is inescapable. When the school has complete control of students, nurses can be trained at least as satisfactorily in two years as in three, and under better conditions, but the training must be paid for in money instead of in services."† Wallace, writing of the experiment at the Toronto Western Hospital, says:

... the experiment in nursing education conducted at the Toronto Western Hospital since 1950 . . . has demonstrated that, once a school of nursing is given control of the student's time, it is possible to prepare a nurse as satisfactorily in two years as in three.

It is also my opinion that if a third year of internship is added, the graduate nurse is likely to be much better equipped than under the old system. . . . I should explain here that, while the student in her third year comes under Nursing Service, she still remains a member of the School of Nursing. Her schedule is planned by the Director of Nursing Service . . . the length of time spent by the internes in the various departments of the Hospital is jointly agreed upon by the Directors of Nursing Service and Nursing Education, and assignment to night and evening duty is also controlled.‡

Miss Russell, in her report, makes mention of the two-year courses with a third year of "interneship" but warns: "This [i.e., the interneship] could provide an excellent preparation for nursing practice, but not necessarily so ... the interneship might develop into just another form of cheap nursing labour without educational value."§ Among her recommendations having to do with the hospital schools of nursing, she includes "each school to have its own administrative board, prepared to accept educational responsibility, and quite apart from the governing board of the hospital," "each school to have full control over the use of the student's time when in hospital," "That hospital

*E. K. Russell: The Report of a Study of Nursing Education in New Brunswick (Fredericton: University Press of New Brunswick, 1956), p. 18.

†A. R. Lord: Report of the Evaluation of the Metropolitan School of Nursing, Windsor, Ontario (Ottawa: Canadian Nurses' Association, 1952), p. 54.

‡W. S. Wallace: Report on the Experiment in Nursing Education of the Atkinson School of Nursing, The Toronto Western Hospital, 1950–1955 (University of Toronto Press), p. 14.

§E. K. Russell: Report of a Study of Nursing Education in New Brunswick (Fredericton: University Press of New Brunswick, 1956), p. 19.

schools have no primary responsibility for servicing the hospitals," and "That a student's life be secured fully for every student."*

Thus, some nursing educators, having recognized the conflict between education and service, have shown that, when education takes priority, the training can be shortened significantly; and these educators have recognized that, if there is a year of "interneship" for the nurse, they must be on their guard lest what should be an educational experience become merely the provision of cheap labour. Whether the same successful results could be obtained if our suggestions for postgraduate medical education were carried out could only be determined by experimentation. We have quoted Comroe's opinion (page 423) that a five-year residency might be reduced to four, or even three, years if it were stripped of those things that have no educational value. He calls for the creation of "one truly graduate school of medicine" in the United States.†

The changes that we have suggested raise certain economic problems about which we must say a few words. If the present interne or resident became a graduate student in fact, and not merely in word, he could be expected to pay fees to his university as other graduate students do. On the other hand, for the service that he would render his hospital, even though that service would be more limited than at present, he should be paid.

As far as the hospitals are concerned, there is no doubt that, if their services were reorganized as we have suggested, they would cost more than they do at present, because some of the service, which at present is supplied as cheap labour by the internes and residents, would have to be paid for at the rates prevailing in medical practice. This means, in effect, that, whereas at present the internes and residents are subsidizing the care of hospital patients to a greater extent than any other members of society—in fact, to the extent of some hundreds or thousands of dollars each per year—the cost would be spread over the whole of our society. Yet surely it is not necessary for a society whose affluence is visible on every side to allow a young physician to mortgage his own and his family's future in order to balance the hospital's books. Indeed, if the extra cost to the hospitals be urged as a reason for maintaining the present system, this very argument becomes proof of the degree to which internes and residents are being exploited.

*Ibid., p. 58.
†J. H. Comroe, Jr.: Medicine: A Lifelong Study, Proceedings of Second World Conference on Medical Education, Chicago 1959 (New York: World Medical Association, 1961), p. 384.

Furthermore, from the purely practical point of view, it would be interesting to know—and, we think, important in view of the statements that have been made (see pages 342–343) about inadequate numbers of suitable applicants for medicine—how many potential doctors are deterred from entering medicine by what they hear of the circumstances of the postgraduate period.

Lee A. DuBridge, President of the California Institute of Technology, who spoke at the Seventh Teaching Institute of the Association of American Medical Colleges on the subject, "Physicians, Scientists, and Engineers," compared the position of young graduate doctors and engineers:

> The question of how the budding young technologist, be he engineer or physician, is to acquire this experience with practical problems is, of course, the most baffling problem in all technical education. There are two extreme positions that are sometimes defended.
>
> The first of these states that needed experience cannot be acquired at the university at all but must be acquired on the job. The other extreme is that to a very large degree this experience must be acquired in the university before any private practice at all is allowed. Actually, of course, some compromise between these extremes is nearly always followed. Some type of apprentice training is always required of both the engineer and the physician. The chief difference seems to be that the engineer—fresh from his Ph.D., let us say—gets well paid for his apprenticeship while the fledgling M.D. gets almost no pay at all during his four, five, or six years of apprentice training. This, I think, is thoroughly wrong and I wish it could be remedied at the earliest possible moment.[*]

DuBridge has pointed out that both the physician and the engineer obtain practical experience on the job, but that the engineer is adequately paid whereas the physician is not. Various medical educators, including Wangensteen and Child whom we have already quoted, have called for more adequate remuneration for internes and residents. There are two other differences, however, between an engineer gaining experience in a job and a physician gaining experience as a hospital house doctor. First, an engineer's job is more or less permanent, whereas a house doctor's position is temporary. This means that it is to a company's advantage to see that the experience and training of its young engineer are sound, whereas a hospital, having no stake in its house officer's future, is more easily tempted to exploit him. Secondly, the engineer's activities and responsibilities over a long period of years will be supervised and controlled by his company. Since the young doctor is likely to enter private practice, where he

[*]L. A. DuBridge: Journal of Medical Education, *36*, No. 4, Part 2: 177, 1961.

will be subject to little or no control, within a few years of graduation from medical school, he must be brought much more rapidly to the point where he can accept the necessary responsibility. This, we believe, makes it more necessary that his practical experience be determined by educational, rather than service, needs. That education take precedence over service is even more imperative in the case of a man whose hospital postgraduate experience is likely to be limited to one year, or possibly two, i.e. a general practitioner, than in the case of a specialist who will have five or more years of such experience before being on his own.

If postgraduate medical education is not to be reorganized so that it becomes truly educational, then the alternative is to acknowledge that service comes first and pay an interne or resident accordingly. Then, at least, he will be able to afford to prolong this experience instead of either going into general practice with less training than he thinks he should have or going into general practice when his real interest is a specialty.

Whose is the responsibility to bring about the necessary changes? In the first instance, the responsibility appears to rest with the medical educators, to recognize the problem and to spare no effort to make it widely known. The necessary changes will require the co-operation of the professional organizations (including the licensing bodies), of the profession as a whole, and of hospital administrators and trustees. The ultimate sanction, however, must come from society, of which the medical profession is a part. If society truly wishes the high quality of medical care for which it calls, then it must recognize that it has a responsibility and that it must make a sacrifice. The responsibility of society is to ensure that the important stage of postgraduate medical education is really educational; and, to this end, society must be prepared to pay for the services that at present are being rendered for virtually nothing by the postgraduate student, to the detriment of his learning and of the care that he will be able to give in his own practice.

# 24 / Some Problems of General Medical Practice

In the past several chapters, we have dealt with problems relating to the period of formal medical education. The end of this period, however, does not bring the end of a physician's educational problems. Rather, they are complicated, and perhaps intensified, by the different conditions obtaining in practice, some of which are inimical to continuing education. These we shall consider presently, but first we must ensure that the reader understands the importance of the problem of continuing education. Ellis has described medical education as "the vital link between medicine and medical practice. It is responsible for passing the advances of medicine on to professional practice."* Suppose that this vital link were broken when a physician passed from his postgraduate training into practice, i.e. that there were no continuing education. In times past, it would have made little practical difference, because major advances were infrequent; but the breaking of this vital link in recent years would have meant that physicians who are at present over fifty years of age would be practising the medicine of more than twenty-five years ago, when there were no sulphonamides, no antibiotics, no antihistamines, no ACTH or cortisone, and no antihypertensive drugs. So rapidly is medicine advancing in this present era that, if a physician is to maintain the quality of his practice, he must continue his education as long as he continues to practise.

The practitioners visited by us were asked a number of questions having to do with the problem of keeping up with recent advances.

*J. R. Ellis: Journal of Medical Education, 33, No. 10, Part 2: 224, 1958.

## TABLE 96
MEDICAL JOURNALS TO WHICH THE PHYSICIANS SUBSCRIBED

### A. *Ontario*

| Title of journal* | Physicians Number | % |
|---|---|---|
| Canadian Medical Association Journal | 43 | 97.7 |
| Medical Clinics of North America | 18 | 40.9 |
| Postgraduate Medicine | 16 | 36.4 |
| New England Journal of Medicine | 9 | 20.5 |
| Surgical Clinics of North America | 7 | 15.9 |
| American Practitioner and Digest of Treatment | 3 | 6.8 |
| Journal of the American Medical Association | 3 | 6.8 |
| Practitioner | 3 | 6.8 |
| Canadian Anaesthetists' Society Journal | 3 | 6.8 |
| DM; Disease-A-Month | 2 | 4.5 |
| Geriatrics | 2 | 4.5 |
| Lancet | 2 | 4.5 |
| Obstetrics and Gynecology | 2 | 4.5 |
| Pediatric Clinics of North America | 2 | 4.5 |

### B. *Nova Scotia*

| Title of journal† | Physicians Number | % |
|---|---|---|
| Canadian Medical Association Journal | 37‡ | 88.1 |
| Postgraduate Medicine | 15 | 35.7 |
| Medical Clinics of North America | 12 | 28.6 |
| Surgical Clinics of North America | 10 | 23.8 |
| Practitioner | 9 | 21.4 |
| American Practitioner and Digest of Treatment | 5 | 11.9 |
| Geriatrics | 5 | 11.9 |
| New England Journal of Medicine | 4 | 9.5 |
| Pediatric Clinics of North America | 3 | 7.1 |
| DM; Disease-A-Month | 2 | 4.8 |
| Obstetrics and Gynecology | 2 | 4.8 |

*Each of the following journals was named by 1 physician: (1) Anesthesiology, (2) Anesthesia and Analgesia; Current Researches, (3) Annals of Internal Medicine, (4) Annals of Surgery, (5) British Journal of Clinical Practice, (6) British Journal of Surgery, (7) Canadian Journal of Surgery, (8) Medical Services Journal, Canada, (9) Circulation; Journal of the American Heart Association, (10) GP, (11) International Journal of Anesthesia, (12) Journal of Gerontology, (13) Journal of Pediatrics, (14) Proceedings of the Staff Meetings of the Mayo Clinic, (15) Union Médicale du Canada, (16) University of Toronto Medical Journal, and (17) University of Western Ontario Medical Journal.

†Each of the following journals was named by 1 physician: (1) American Journal of Psychiatry, (2) Annals of Surgery, (3) British Journal of Clinical Practice, (4) British Journal of Surgery, (5) Canadian Journal of Public Health, (6) Canadian Journal of Surgery, (7) Clinical Obstetrics and Gynecology, (8) GP, (9) Industrial Medicine and Surgery, (10) Journal of the American Medical Association (17 other physicians said that they received this journal without subscribing for it—they said that the publishers had "selected" them to receive the journal at no cost for one year), (11) The Lancet, (12) University of Ottawa Medical Journal, (13) a journal devoted to anaesthesia (title unknown), and (14) a journal devoted to occupational medicine (title unknown).

‡As 39 physicians stated that they belonged to the Canadian Medical Association, it appears that 2 physicians forgot to list the Canadian Medical Association Journal.

First, each physician was asked to list the medical journals to which he was subscribing at the time of our visit. Thirty-one journals were named by the Ontario physicians, and 25 by those in Nova Scotia; but only a few of these were purchased by 10 per cent or more of the doctors (Table 96). Apart from the *Canadian Medical Association Journal*,* which is sent to every doctor who is a member of the Association, the two most popular journals, in each province, were the *Medical Clinics of North America* and *Postgraduate Medicine*, one or other or both of which were bought by 57 per cent of the Ontario, and by 50 per cent of the Nova Scotia, doctors.

Approximately one-third of the Ontario, and one-fifth of the Nova Scotia, physicians subscribed to no journals other than the *Canadian Medical Association Journal* and the journal of their provincial medical society. Almost one-fifth of the doctors in Ontario and one-third of those in Nova Scotia subscribed to 1 other journal, and the remaining physicians to 2 or more other journals. There was no apparent relationship, in either province, between the number of journals purchased and the quality of the physician's practice. This is in contrast with Peterson's finding in North Carolina that "journal purchases seem to vary, on an average, directly with the qualitative assessments which have been made."†

When the physicians were listing the journals to which they subscribed, they were invited to comment on any of these. Repeatedly, the *Medical Clinics of North America* and *Postgraduate Medicine* were described as "good" or "excellent." Peterson also lists these two journals among the three that "were most frequently commended" by the general practitioners of North Carolina (see his page 89). Of the doctors who received the *Canadian Medical Association Journal*, some did not comment. Several of these men said that they had little time for reading, that they did not read the *Journal* much, or that they would "only glance at it." The remaining doctors, more than 80 per cent of those in each province who received the *Journal*, were divided fairly evenly into those who made remarks that were at least predominantly, and in many cases entirely, favourable and those whose criticisms were unfavourable. Unfortunately, those who described the *Journal* as "excellent" or "good" did not amplify their

*Since all those who were members of the Canadian Medical Association were members also of their provincial association, they would have received either the *Ontario Medical Review* or the *Nova Scotia Medical Bulletin*. Many of the doctors, however, did not mention their provincial journal.

†O. L. Peterson *et al.*: Journal of Medical Education, *31*, No. 12, Part 2: 1–165, 1956; see page 88.

statements. On the other hand, the adverse criticisms were quite specific. One physician said that the editorial standards were not high enough. All the rest of those who commented unfavourably said that the *Journal* contained too much research, too much "rare stuff," too much "theory," too much "tripe and padding," that it was "too technical" or "too scientific," that it was hard to read, or that it contained too little that was of interest or of practical use to a general practitioner. One man said, "It's interesting for the obituaries, but much too abstruse, not much use for the G.P." When asked to elaborate, he said, "The editor's trying, but he has a difficult job. The universities put the emphasis on papers on bizarre conditions." Another practitioner glanced at an issue of the *Journal* lying on his table, noted that it contained an article on carbon tetrachloride poisoning, and said, "Now, when would I ever see that?" Those who were dissatisfied with the *Journal* made clear that what they wished was more articles on "down-to-earth subjects," frequent reviews, and "more practical stuff."

The practitioners were questioned about medical conventions and postgraduate courses that they had attended during the previous year. So many, however, could not remember the dates, the durations, or the sponsoring bodies of the courses or conventions that we are unable to deal with the data beyond saying that there was a wide variation, from those who attended courses and conventions frequently to those (at least one-fifth of the doctors whom we visited in each province) who had not attended a convention or course during the preceding year.

Eighty-six per cent of the Ontario practitioners and 88 per cent of the Nova Scotia practitioners said that their hospitals held regular staff meetings, some at monthly intervals, others as often as every week. Some physicians indicated that there were several series of meetings that they might attend. Eighty-one per cent of the Ontario doctors and 83 per cent of those in Nova Scotia named one or more local medical societies, whose meetings varied in frequency from one a year to one every other week. One-quarter of the Ontario men belonged to journal clubs. In Nova Scotia, none of the doctors mentioned journal clubs, but 60 per cent spoke of the lectures that were arranged by Dalhousie University and given, in various towns throughout the province, by lecturers from this and other medical centres.

In order to obtain an over-all picture of the importance of various possible sources of medical information in the general practitioner's life, we questioned each physician about twelve sources, which are

TABLE 97

FREQUENCY WITH WHICH ONTARIO PHYSICIANS USED VARIOUS SOURCES
OF INFORMATION AND VALUE ASSIGNED TO EACH SOURCE

| Sources of information | Number* of physicians using | | | Number* of physicians rating value as | | | |
|---|---|---|---|---|---|---|---|
| | Regularly | Occasion- ally | Never | Great | Moderate | Slight | Nil |
| Medical journals | 28† | 16 | 0 | 16† | 19 | 8 | 1 |
| Medical textbooks | 21 | 21 | 2 | 20 | 17 | 5 | 1 |
| Medical digests | 24 | 15 | 5 | 7 | 24 | 6 | 5 |
| Publications of pharmaceutical companies | 14 | 25 | 4 | 4 | 16 | 17 | 5 |
| Formal consultations | 41 | 3 | 0 | 30 | 9 | 3 | 2 |
| Informal discussions with colleagues | 42 | 2 | 0 | 31 | 11 | 2 | 0 |
| Hospital staff meetings | 35 | 3 | 6 | 15 | 14 | 6 | 4 |
| Local medical society meetings | 28 | 8 | 8 | 16 | 12 | 7 | 2 |
| Ontario Medical Association convention | 16 | 10 | 18 | 7 | 13 | 5 | 2 |
| Canadian Medical Association convention | 1 | 22 | 21 | 4 | 13 | 5 | 2 |
| Other conventions | 5 | 5 | 30 | 6 | 3 | 1 | 0 |
| Postgraduate courses | 18 | 14 | 12 | 27 | 4 | 1 | 0 |

*When the numbers total less than 44, it is because the remaining physicians either gave indefinite answers or did not answer at all.

†These numbers include 1 physician who specified that he read 1 journal regularly and found it of great value but that he read other journals only occasionally and found them of moderate value.

TABLE 98

FREQUENCY WITH WHICH NOVA SCOTIA PHYSICIANS USED VARIOUS
SOURCES OF INFORMATION AND VALUE ASSIGNED TO EACH SOURCE

| Sources of information | Number* of physicians using | | | Number* of physicians rating value as | | | |
|---|---|---|---|---|---|---|---|
| | Regularly | Occasion- ally | Never | Great | Moderate | Slight | Nil |
| Medical journals | 27 | 15 | 0 | 16 | 24 | 2 | 0 |
| Medical textbooks | 15 | 25 | 0 | 16 | 21 | 3 | 0 |
| Medical digests | 27 | 13 | 2 | 4 | 20 | 16 | 2 |
| Publications of pharmaceutical companies | 10 | 29 | 3 | 6 | 3 | 25 | 8 |
| Formal consultations | 27 | 15 | 0 | 32 | 9 | 1 | 0 |
| Informal discussions with colleagues | 34 | 8 | 0 | 25 | 15 | 2 | 0 |
| Hospital staff meetings | 29 | 9 | 4 | 2 | 22 | 13 | 3 |
| Local medical society meetings | 24 | 11 | 7 | 0 | 20 | 14 | 4 |
| Convention of Medical Society of Nova Scotia | 10 | 27 | 5 | 1 | 15 | 19 | 4 |
| Canadian Medical Association convention | 1 | 28 | 13 | 3 | 14 | 9 | 13 |
| Other conventions | 4 | 7 | 31 | 5 | 5 | 1 | 6 |
| Postgraduate courses | 16 | 11 | 15 | 15 | 11 | 0 | 7 |

*When the numbers total less than 42, it is because the remaining physicians either gave indefinite answers or did not answer at all.

TABLE 99

DISTRIBUTION OF PHYSICIANS ACCORDING TO THE FREQUENCY WITH
WHICH THEY USED MEDICAL JOURNALS AND MEDICAL TEXTBOOKS

| Number of physicians using textbooks | Number of physicians using journals | | Total number of physicians |
|---|---|---|---|
| | Regularly | Occasionally | |
| A. *Ontario* | | | |
| Regularly | 17 | 4 | 21 |
| Occasionally | 10* | 11 | 21 |
| Never | 1 | 1 | 2 |
| Total number of physicians | 28 | 16 | 44 |
| B. *Nova Scotia* | | | |
| Regularly | 9 | 6 | 15 |
| Occasionally | 16 | 9 | 25 |
| No answer | 2 | — | 2 |
| Total number of physicians | 27 | 15 | 42 |

*One of these physicians specified that he read 1 journal regularly but other journals only occasionally.

listed in Tables 97 and 98. About each of these, we asked whether the doctor used it regularly, occasionally, or never, as a source of information, and whether he regarded its value as great, moderate, slight, or nil. The replies are shown in the tables. The item that was most frequently named as a regular source of information, by 95 per cent of the Ontario practitioners and by 81 per cent of those in Nova Scotia, was informal discussions with colleagues. Formal consultations, though the value assigned to them as a source of information did not appear to differ significantly between the two provinces, were used as a regular source of information by 93 per cent of the Ontario doctors, but by only 64 per cent of those in Nova Scotia. The difference is significant ($p < 0.01$).* Postgraduate courses were said to be attended regularly by 41 per cent of the Ontario doctors and by 38 per cent of the Nova Scotia doctors, and occasionally by 32 per cent and 26 per cent respectively. Of those who attended at all, 84 per cent in Ontario and 59 per cent in Nova Scotia declared that these courses were of great value. Hospital staff meetings, local medical society meetings, and the conventions of the Canadian Medical Association and of the provincial medical associations were less highly regarded.

*This is explained on pages 32–33.

Of the two important forms of medical literature, journals were used regularly by 64 per cent of the doctors in each province and occasionally by 36 per cent; and textbooks were used regularly by 48 per cent, occasionally by 48 per cent, and "never" by 4 per cent of the Ontario practitioners, and regularly by 37.5 per cent and occasionally by 62.5 per cent of the 40 Nova Scotia doctors who answered. The practitioners' reading habits, regarding textbooks and journals, are summarized in Table 99. The most surprising finding was that, according to their own statements, 27 per cent of the Ontario physicians visited by us and 21 per cent of those in Nova Scotia read neither textbooks nor journals more often than "occasionally." When the practitioners were divided into those up to thirty-five years of age, those between thirty-six and forty-five, and those over forty-five years, no significant differences were found between these groups, either in Ontario or in Nova Scotia, in the frequencies with which they used the various sources of information.

Some of the doctors, especially in Ontario, added comments about the various items. Though not numerous, the comments do cast some light on the problem of a practitioner's continuing education. Conventions were criticized as concentrating on specialists' problems and not including enough for the general practitioners, as being "too big," and as being mostly of interest socially. Speaking about local medical society meetings, a few doctors made adverse remarks to the effect that these meetings were business, rather than scientific, meetings or that they were mainly social in nature. A much more significant statement, and one that we heard frequently, was that local meetings were of value when there were visiting speakers from large medical centres. In North Carolina also, Peterson observed (see his page 83) that "the physicians were often dissatisfied with what were described as 'only local speakers.' Several doctors stated that it was their policy to attend only those medical meetings at which a speaker came from a medical school."

Each doctor was asked to name some of the books that he found "most helpful." Some of the men named a number of books, and one said, "My library is everything"; but 14 per cent of the Ontario practitioners and 10 per cent of those in Nova Scotia did not name even one book, and several others mentioned a single standard reference work but said that their use of it was "occasional" or "rare." One of these latter, who was not well informed about medicine, said that he probably learned most from talking to other doctors and to drug salesmen.

The sum total of continuing educational activities varied greatly from one practitioner to another. One older man, for example, named four journals to which he subscribed, listed nine books that he found helpful, and had attended three conventions and ten one-day post-graduate courses during the preceding two years. In contrast with him was another practitioner in the same age group who received the *Canadian Medical Association Journal* but regarded it as of no value, listed no books, and attended one local medical society meeting per year but no conventions, postgraduate courses, or hospital staff meetings. He "never" read textbooks, read journals "occasionally," and regarded both as of "no value." The yearly meeting of the local medical society consisted of business and one paper on a general medical topic. Apart from this meeting, his only "regular" sources of information were formal consultations and informal discussions with colleagues, both of which were of moderate value in his opinion. *Modern Medicine of Canada* he read occasionally and considered of moderate value. The only source of information that he considered of great value was the publications of the pharmaceutical companies, which he read occasionally.

Each practitioner was given an opportunity to name any sources of information other than the twelve about which specific inquiry was made. There was one mention of the clinical-pathological conference as being of great value, and several men referred again to visiting speakers from the various universities. One physician told us that he spent fifty dollars a month on long-distance telephone calls. Whenever he was in doubt or difficulty, he did not hesitate to call and ask the advice of one or another of a group of consultants who were members of the staff of a medical school. In addition, whenever he visited the city, he made it his habit to go around the hospitals and ask a few of the consultants such questions as, "Do you use ——?", "Is it of value?", and "What is your experience with ——?" Though, geographically, this man's practice was one of the most remote from any medical school, the observer felt that the physician was in contact with the medical world. On the other hand, other physicians, situated only a fraction of the distance from a medical school or even in the heart of a large city, gave the impression of almost complete isolation from the medical profession.

After the physicians had been questioned about the various sources of information, they were asked, "How difficult do you find it to keep up with medical advances? Very difficult? Moderately difficult? Or not particularly difficult?" In Ontario, 9 per cent found this very diffi-

TABLE 100

DEGREE OF DIFFICULTY EXPERIENCED BY ONTARIO AND NOVA SCOTIA
PHYSICIANS IN KEEPING UP WITH MEDICAL ADVANCES

| How difficult physician found keeping up | Ontario physicians | | Nova Scotia physicians | |
|---|---|---|---|---|
| | Number | % | Number | % |
| Very difficult | 4 | 9.1 | 8 | 19.0 |
| Moderately difficult | 21 | 47.7 | 25 | 59.5 |
| Not particularly difficult | 19 | 43.2 | 9 | 21.4 |
| Total physicians | 44 | 100 | 42 | 100 |

cult and 48 per cent moderately difficult. The corresponding figures
for Nova Scotia were 19 per cent and 60 per cent (Table 100). There
was no significant relationship, in either province, between the replies
given by the physicians and either their ages, the quality of their
practices, as measured by their scores, or the size of the communities
in which they were practising.

Those practitioners who stated that they found it difficult to keep
up with the advances in medicine were asked, "What are the causes of
the difficulty?" Lack of time for reading was the one cause named
repeatedly, by 50 per cent of the total sample of Ontario doctors and
67 per cent of the total sample of Nova Scotia doctors and by 80 per
cent and 85 per cent of those doctors, in Ontario and Nova Scotia
respectively, who had either moderate or great difficulty in keeping
up; and another 8 per cent and 5 per cent, in the two provinces respectively, attributed their difficulty to the rapidity with which
medicine was advancing. One physician, whose discussion of cases
made it obvious that he read a great deal and was conversant with the
recent medical literature, was asked how he managed this. He replied,
"My wife doesn't get out, and we have no recreation." One doctor
explained that the irregular hours of practice made it difficult to
organize his studying. Some men mentioned other causes in addition
to lack of time. Thus several said that they lacked the energy as well
as the time, one pointed out the necessity of devoting time to his
family, and a few others said that they did not know where to look
for the medical information that they required. Two doctors said that
they did not have a regular reading programme. Several claimed that
practice made it difficult to get away to courses or conventions. One
explained that, when he went to a course, he had to rush to get there
and get back, so that he had no time to settle down before the course
and no time to go over his notes before he had to hurry back to his

practice. One man mentioned the fact that there was no local medical society; and another, who was geographically isolated, said that, being alone and lacking stimulation, one lost one's enthusiasm.

Finally, the physicians were asked, "How do you think general practitioners can best be aided in their efforts to keep up with the new advances?" The item that occurred most frequently in the answers was postgraduate courses, listed by about half of the doctors in each province; but a few of those who spoke in favour of these courses were among those who never attended such courses and indicated that they did not have time to attend. Reading was mentioned by many of the doctors, some of whom pointed out changes that they thought would make the reading material fit their needs better. It was suggested that journal articles be more "practical." Frequent mention was made of the need for some sort of publication that would summarize the recent advances and keep a practitioner informed of those that were of value. Another suggestion for helping a practitioner to keep up was that there should be more local clinical meetings, but it was emphasized by those who advocated them that the speakers should be visitors from the large medical centres. A few men felt that there were enough meetings, courses, and reading material, and that the problem was entirely a matter of time. One middle-aged doctor attributed the lack of time to economic factors. He said, "It goes right back to finances. Doctors are not paid early enough; they have too short a time to collect an estate." (See also page 438.)

We have stated (page 456) that 58 per cent of the Ontario practitioners whom we visited and 79 per cent of those in Nova Scotia said that they were having at least moderate difficulty in keeping up with medical advances and that 9 per cent and 19 per cent in the two provinces, respectively, were having great difficulty. This is evidence that the continuing education of the general practitioner is a problem of some magnitude. It appears, from what the practitioners told us, that a number of factors contributed to the difficulty. The principal of these was claimed to be lack of time for reading. When we examined the working hours of those who were having moderate or great difficulty, we found that, in Ontario, 10 per cent were working less than 40 hours per week, 50 per cent were working between 40 and 59 hours per week, and the remaining 40 per cent were working 60 or more hours, and some even 80 or more hours, per week. In Nova Scotia, 52 per cent of those who were having moderate or great difficulty in keeping up with the advances were working between 40 and 59 hours per week, and the other 48 per cent were working 60 hours or more, several of them well over 80 hours per week. These figures, as we stated in an earlier chapter (see page 105), do not include mealtimes and do not take into account night calls made by the physician after he had completed his regular evening work. Nor do they take into account the fact that, during the remaining hours, when he was not actually working, the physician was usually on call, so that he did not know, from one moment to the next, how long he would be able to continue reading if he were to start or how long it might be before he would have another opportunity to rest if he should devote the present moment of quiet to study instead of to relaxation (see also page 85). Though one may question whether the men who were working less than 40 hours per week could legitimately claim to have insufficient time for studying, this may well be so in the cases of those working more than 40 hours and is almost certainly so in the cases of those working 60 or more hours per week. The rapidity with which medicine is advancing was mentioned by a number of the doctors as a cause of their difficulty in keeping up. This is closely related to lack of time, in that the rapidity with which advances are occurring is a major factor determining how much time will be required for study if the doctor is to remain abreast of the advances. Because of its importance, we shall defer further consideration of the practitioner's time to later pages (465 ff.), where we shall be able to consider the problem in more detail.

That other factors, also, contribute to a practitioner's difficulty in keeping up is apparent from what we have reported earlier in this chapter. Eighteen per cent of the Ontario practitioners and 17 per cent of those in Nova Scotia either had no local medical society meetings in their areas or failed to attend the meetings of the local societies; and another 20 per cent in Ontario and 36 per cent in Nova Scotia attended but considered the meetings of little or no value. Similarly, hospital staff meetings were not within reach of, or were not attended by, 14 per cent of the Ontario doctors and 10 per cent of those in Nova Scotia; and were attended, but were rated as of little or no value, by another 23 per cent and 33 per cent in Ontario and Nova Scotia respectively. The doctors who rated hospital meetings or meetings of their local medical society as of little or no value were, with a few exceptions, practising in communities in which there was no medical school. The two major defects of these local meetings were said to be an inadequate number of case presentations and inability on the part of the local members of the profession to present programmes of interest and value. In contrast, comments were made to us repeatedly about the value and the interest of the programmes when there were speakers from the large centres.

These defects of local programmes are understandable. A practitioner, working long hours, does not have the time to devote to the preparation of papers or even of case presentations; and, because he does not acquire the experience, with a particular type of case or with a particular type of treatment, which is acquired by a man in the large teaching centre who is carrying on investigative work with ample clinical material available, the local practitioner tends either to report on so small a series of cases that no conclusions can be drawn or to prepare a paper that is merely a review of the textbooks and journals. Such a review, if well prepared—and adequate preparation takes much time—can be most rewarding both for the man who prepares the review and for his audience; if poorly done, it is a dull affair, indeed. On the other hand, it is not easy, either, for the practitioner, especially in a small community, to leave his practice to attend the postgraduate courses that are held in the teaching centres.

Yet another group of causes of the practitioner's difficulty in keeping up appeared to be connected more intimately with the practitioner himself than with the conditions obtaining in his practice. Of those physicians who told us that they found it not particularly difficult to keep up, 22 per cent in Ontario and 56 per cent in Nova Scotia were considered, on the basis of the detailed observations discussed in chapters 16 and 17, to be carrying on practices of unsatisfactory quality and another 28 per cent and 11 per cent in the two provinces, respectively, to be practising medicine that, though not definitely unsatisfactory, was not clearly satisfactory (Table 101; see also pages

TABLE 101

DISTRIBUTION OF ONTARIO AND NOVA SCOTIA PHYSICIANS ACCORDING TO QUALITY OF PRACTICE AND DEGREE OF DIFFICULTY EXPERIENCED BY THEM IN KEEPING UP WITH MEDICAL ADVANCES

| Physician's score % | Number of Ontario physicians who found keeping up with advances | | Number of Nova Scotia physicians who found keeping up with advances | |
|---|---|---|---|---|
| | Very or moderately difficult | Not particularly difficult | Very or moderately difficult | Not particularly difficult |
| 0–40 | 8 | 4 | 17 | 5 |
| 41–60 | 4 | 5 | 8 | 1 |
| 61–100 | 13 | 9 | 8 | 3 |
| Total number of physicians | 25 | 18 | 33 | 9 |

313–314). That certain men could be carrying on practices of unsatis-factory quality and at the same time say that they had little or no trouble keeping up suggests strongly that one of the major problems in these practices was the physicians' inability to recognize that they were in serious difficulties. Another somewhat similar difficulty that we observed was inability to profit from such learning opportunities as presented themselves. For example, one of the practitioners and the observer attended a hospital meeting at which an internist gave a clear exposition of the principles involved in the management of a case of anaemia. By chance, within a few hours' time, the doctor had a patient whom he considered anaemic. By his failure to establish definitely that the patient was anaemic, to determine the cause of the condition, and to choose therapy that would be specific for the particular type of anaemia, he demonstrated that he had not profited in the least from what had been said in his presence such a short time earlier. This incident illustrates that neither the existence of medical meetings nor even the physician's physical attendance at such meetings necessarily results in his keeping up.*

Some of the physicians who said that it was either moderately or very difficult for them to keep up were among those who told us also that they read neither textbooks nor journals more often than occa-sionally (see page 454). In some of these cases, the physician claimed that he lacked, and quite obviously did lack, the time for reading. A few, however, who said that they were having difficulty keeping up and who said that they read only occasionally, appeared to have ample time to read if they had so wished. In other words, these men, who might have profited from reading—though this is by no means a certainty—were deterred from reading, not by the conditions of their practices, but by their own personal characteristics. (In passing, however, we should mention that there were some physicians who said that they read only occasionally but who seemed, nonetheless, to have been successful in keeping up with the advances of medicine.) Simi-larly, some men who were living in cities in which conventions and postgraduate courses take place with some regularity told us that they never attended courses or conventions and yet told us also that they had difficulty in keeping up.

It may be that, in some cases, the physician's difficulty in keeping up is due to the lack of certain necessary stimuli. As we have reported above (page 457), one man attributed his difficulty to being alone and

---

* See also page 365 regarding the difference between being "taught" and learning.

having no other doctor around to arouse his enthusiasm. In other offices, not all of which were located in small or isolated communities, we had the definite impression that the practitioner was in an isolated position as far as the world of medicine was concerned. The man who is isolated, lacking stimulation from his colleagues, must depend upon his own enthusiasm and conscience to move him to keep up to date. Furthermore, being isolated, he does not have the opportunity of comparing his own work with that of other physicians, so that, in effect, the only standard that he has before him is that gained from reading, if he does read, or from what he remembers of the teaching centres during his years of training. Though we have been speaking of the problem of keeping up with recent advances, we would digress briefly to remind the reader that our method of assessing the physicians' practices (see chapter 16) placed the emphasis, not on recent advances, but on long-established methods of diagnosis (for the reasons, see pages 273–275), and that those practices that were seriously deficient in quality were deficient, not in regard to the details of recent advances, but in regard to the fundamentals of clinical medicine (see page 315), which the physicians should have learnt as medical students. If it is possible for physicians to go into practice without adequate preparation—and the statements of the practitioners about the adequacy of medical education as preparation for practice (see pages 398–399) are further evidence that it is possible—then those of them who practise in isolation have before their eyes neither the standard that is set by colleagues nor their memory of the high standard of their training days (since they did not achieve this level themselves), but only the unsatisfactory standard that they had achieved when they left the stimulating atmosphere of the teaching centre.

William M. Arnott, Professor of Medicine at the University of Birmingham, who reviewed the proceedings of the First World Conference on Medical Education at the opening session of the Second World Conference on Medical Education, said, "In conclusion I wish to emphasize one consideration which seems to me of paramount importance in the lifelong study of medicine and which was implicit in much of the work of the First Conference. The lifelong maintenance of a high standard of informed, critical, and conscientious practice depends more than anything else on the avoidance of professional isolation."*

*W. M. Arnott: Medicine: A Lifelong Study, Proceedings of Second World Conference on Medical Education, Chicago 1959 (New York: World Medical Association, 1961), p. 14.

There does not appear to be any solution to the problem of self-imposed isolation in the large or moderate-sized community, as long as medical practice continues to be mainly an individual enterprise; but in a group practice, as we shall suggest in chapter 26, steps could be taken to prevent the individual from isolating himself. In the case of a geographically isolated practitioner, on the other hand, the ideal solution would appear to be to limit the period of practice in the remote, small community to two or three years, i.e. to end the isolation before the practitioner loses touch with what is going on in the world of medicine. Under the present system of medical practice, little could be done about this problem except to make clear to a young physician the danger of remaining too long in an isolated area. If the state takes over the control of medical practice, however, it could, and probably should, include, as a definite part of its programme, such measures as are necessary to limit the period served by those who undertake to practise in isolated areas. An alternative, but probably less effective, solution would be to break the isolation by bringing a physician back to a teaching centre for several months every two or three years.

To recapitulate, it appeared that some practitioners' difficulties in keeping up with recent advances or in making good the deficiencies of their original training were the result of lack of stimulation, which, in turn, was the result of professional isolation. This we regard as one of the strongest arguments against any system of medical practice that would exclude a general practitioner from the work of a hospital and hence tend to isolate him. In discussing this matter with *specialists* from certain northern European countries in which a general practitioner has no hospital privileges, we have been greatly interested to find these specialists critical of this particular feature of the systems existing in their countries.

We turn now to consideration of another stimulus that may well be necessary if a practitioner is to keep up. One of the younger men visited by us said, "It is frustrating to realize that you can never advance." He said that, once a man finished his training and went out into general practice, he was condemned to that for the rest of his life. In his own words, "You're through." He explained that what he meant was that one could not advance to greater measures of responsibility and authority—as could an engineer working for a company—because the only way to leave general practice was to go back into hospital training at a prohibitive cost. Another doctor, not yet middle-aged, said, "There is no opportunity in general practice to progress. When you leave a teaching centre, you are not allowed to *do* more, and there is no opportunity to learn more. This is not made clear to you until too late. There must be control, but not control that eliminates any hope of progress." He referred to general practice as a "blind end" and said that restrictions on what a general practitioner may do kill his enthusiasm. Then came the statement, "Whether you practise reasonable medicine or make a racket out of it doesn't matter a damn. You may as well make a racket out of it, unless you're very altruistic." None of our observations suggested that this doctor did make a "racket" out of medicine, but his statement was disturbing as indicating the strength of his frustration.

These doctors' complaints about the existing organization of medical practice referred to the fact that, if a general practitioner wishes to "advance," he must give up his practice and take the full training necessary to qualify as a specialist. The regulations of the Royal College of Physicians and Surgeons of Canada call for four years of postgraduate training in addition to the year of rotating interneship.* In view of the salaries paid to internes and residents (see pages 179–182, 184), it would be so crippling economically as to be practically out of the question for a man with family responsibilities to give up his practice and go back into training. In addition to virtually fixing a general practitioner in his position permanently, the present system of specialty training appeared to have another adverse effect. A number of practitioners told us that they would advise a young man contemplating a career in general practice to qualify first as a specialist. If those who are actually taking specialty training have the same attitude—and it is likely that some of them have—then specialty training is being taken by physicians who are not necessarily particularly interested in the specialty itself but who recognize that it is "now or never," i.e. that, if they are to take the training, they must do so while they have relatively few domestic responsibilities and before they become accustomed to a standard of living higher than the penurious one of the interne, because they will be unable to manage such training later.

Some of the practitioners who were critical of the Royal College for its strictness in maintaining the standards set by it for specialty qualifications thought that experience gained in one's own practice should be accepted by the College in lieu of a considerable part of the hospital training demanded and that the emphasis should be put on ability to pass the examinations rather than on the type of experience that the candidate had had in preparation for them. One difficulty with putting the emphasis on the examination was apparent in the fact

*Canadian Medical Association Journal, 82: 790, 1960.

that we encountered the occasional practitioner who talked better medicine than he practised, and who might have been able to pass the Royal College's examinations even though his own practice was unsatisfactory even at the non-specialist level. To the suggestion that the practitioner's experience in his own practice be accepted as part of his preparation for the examinations for specialist standing, the obvious reply is that such experience is unsupervised, so that the practitioner who is making mistakes without being aware of them is likely to continue to make the same mistakes, however long his experience may be.

We have pointed out that the failure of some practitioners to keep up with the advances of medicine appears to have such psychological causes as lack of stimulation and a feeling of hopelessness as far as professional advancement is concerned. If one thinks of the general practitioner as some sort of stereotype, it may be difficult to understand these factors as causes of difficulty. Indeed, in discussing with colleagues the need for advancement that some men expressed, we have sometimes encountered an impatience that has appeared to be based in the belief that a practitioner should obtain ample satisfaction from doing "a good job" and should not have any need of further recognition or advancement. As we have demonstrated in earlier chapters, however, and particularly in chapter 14, the general practitioner is not one individual, but many individuals possessing widely differing characteristics. It is not surprising, then, to find that some practitioners have, as one of their needs, the need to advance steadily and visibly in their profession. Nor should such ambition, when manifested by a general practitioner, evoke any greater impatience than the similar ambition that is probably one of the forces raising many men to high positions, including professorial positions in the various medical fields. We believe that, instead of being impatient with the ambition shown by some of the practitioners, the profession should recognize the difficulty that was expressed by those men who referred to general practice as a blind end lacking opportunities for advancement and should consider what steps might be taken to cope with this problem. We have already suggested (pages 441–442) that there should be positions in the teaching hospitals to which men in practice could return for periods of three, six, nine, or twelve months to refresh their knowledge and that these positions, being service positions, should be adequately paid, so that it would be possible for a man to leave his practice for a period without crippling himself economically. Other measures that would meet the psychological needs of the practitioners for stimulation and advancement, we outline in chapter 26.

From the number and the variety of the factors that cause the physicians' difficulty in keeping up, it must be apparent that there is no single remedy for the problem. In particular, because increasing emphasis has been put on short postgraduate courses in recent years, it should be noted that these are not a panacea. Those physicians in our samples who had attended such courses in the preceding year or two had scores* that ranged from more than 90 per cent to less than 30 per cent. Other physicians—and, in our samples, they had scores ranging from less than 30 per cent to more than 70 per cent—simply do not choose to attend postgraduate courses.

We turn our attention now to the problem of time in a doctor's life. Earlier in this chapter (page 456), we reported that between one-half and two-thirds of the entire group of practitioners whom we visited in each province, and four-fifths or more of those in each province who had either moderate or great difficulty in keeping up with medical advances, said that their difficulty in keeping up was the result of lack of time for reading. This is a problem that is new to medicine within the past few decades. Prior to this, medicine's advance was so slow that, once the physician was trained, he could absorb the changes as they appeared, one by one, at long intervals. Today, discoveries are being made and new methods evolved with a rapidity never before known. Some of these will stand; others will prove to be of no value and will pass away. A practitioner's problem is not only to keep abreast of what is going on in the world of medicine, but to distinguish the valuable from the valueless. His problem is made more acute by the overwhelming volume of material that is published, part of which is of great value, but part of which serves little or no useful purpose. To go through even a very small part of the published material in order to remain familiar with what is going on, to pick out what is of value, to weigh the opinions of conflicting authorities, to decide what should be applied in one's own practice now and what should be borne in mind but not applied until additional authoritative reports appear, and to master the details that must be learnt about what one does decide to incorporate into one's practice are not routine tasks to be disposed of casually. These are duties, the adequate performance of which demands two things, the reader's undivided attention and sufficient time.

*The physicians' scores as a measure of quality of practice have been discussed in chapters 16 and 17.

We lay emphasis on the need for time because we believe that this is not sufficiently acknowledged to be the problem that it is. The undergraduate medical student, in at least one university, as we have pointed out (page 367), has, on the average, thirty-six hours per week of scheduled work of one sort or another in three of his four years in the medical course, so that almost all of his reading must be done in the evening, when he is least fresh. More than two-fifths of the practitioners visited by us in each province complained of not having had enough time for reading during their interneships (page 396). Finally, not one of the practitioners, in giving us the details of his weekly schedule, made any mention of time set aside for reading. These facts suggest that reading is really not acknowledged as an integral part of the practice of medicine, but rather that it is regarded as something to be worked in, as best it may, when a physician's "essential" duties have been completed.

We hold that keeping up with medical advances is an essential part of the practice of medicine. It is not too much to say that, when a physician is studying how to use a new drug correctly, he is working for his patients just as certainly as when he is actually administering the drug at the bed-side. It is important that private practitioners recognize the necessity of setting aside time for study. It is even more important, however, that those governments that are thinking in terms of some type of comprehensive medical coverage should have it brought to their attention that a doctor's reading, in these days of rapid changes, is not a luxury, a self-indulgence, or a foible of the individual doctor but is a part of medical care and that the time required for this must be borne in mind when the manpower requirements and the costs of a medical service are being computed.

Besides the rapidity of medicine's advance, there have been other changes that have a bearing on the problem of a doctor's time. In certain respects, medical practice itself is probably more strenuous than it used to be, in that some of today's methods of treatment, which can accomplish a great deal of good, have also greater potentiality for harm than some of the procedures of half a century ago, which were not particularly beneficial—though they were the best available—but were not potentially harmful, either. For example, fluids given intravenously to a baby that is within minutes of death from dehydration may restore it to life in a manner that verges on the miraculous. Yet those same fluids, if administered incorrectly, can cause death. Again, a doctor's travel from one house call to another is probably more strenuous today than in years gone by. Much of the time that the doctor used to spend jogging along behind a horse was relaxing. The same cannot be said of the time spent behind a steering wheel in the city's rush-hour traffic or on the death-dealing highway.

A doctor's life must be considered, also, in relationship to certain changes that have occurred in our society in recent years. One such change is the almost complete disappearance of domestic help. In contrast with the days before World War II, when it was common for a professional man's household to contain at least one servant, we found that, of the practitioners visited by us, only the occasional one had full-time help in the house. In addition, it is our impression that it has become more difficult in recent years to obtain satisfactory help for such outside work as garden maintenance, snow removal, etc. The result of these changes is that the householder and his wife have had to do more of their own work themselves. Speaking of "those who work with their minds," Barzun says:

Though they toil longer hours than any other group, the time left by modern society for their genuine work is far less than that enjoyed by their nine-teenth-century counterparts, and their permanent output is proportionately less. One lack that hampers them more than most, since their work is domestic and not capable of mechanization, is: servants. It may make edifying reading in the biography of a Justice of the Supreme Court that he generally cooks breakfast for the whole family [Barzun quotes an authority], but the condition of self-help of which this is a symbol is regrettable—as regrettable for the college student as for the justice. Not that manual labor is degrading or "beneath" anyone; but that life is short and the moments of the talented are precious. When society says that he has no right to squander them, it is presumably not to squander them itself.*

In spite of the regret expressed by Barzun, it is a fact that the services that used to be available no longer exist and that a doctor must divert time and energy from the professional duties for which he was trained to household matters of whose existence he would, in the past, have been barely aware.

Another problem that confronts a doctor is the need of his family, both his wife and his children, for some of his time. We are referring now, not to the need for the doctor to take over some of the functions of the vanished servant, but to the need for companionship, guidance, and that participation in family activities which is so necessary if the family is to continue as the basis of our society. One of the practitioners visited by us told us that he had given up his intention of taking train-ing in a specialty because he did not wish "to leave my wife to a lonely existence." We have referred (see page 440) to other examples

*Jacques Barzun: The House of Intellect (New York: Harper, 1959), p. 260.

of domestic problems arising from the father's infrequent appearances at home during his postgraduate training. The problem of a physician's lack of time for his family is not confined, however, to the period of training. One practitioner told us that, not infrequently, he did not see his children from breakfast of one morning until the evening meal of the next day. The question in his mind was how he could take the time to investigate his patients' complaints adequately and to do the reading that was necessary if he was to keep up and yet make an adequate living without charging higher fees than those laid down in the tariff of the Ontario Medical Association. At the time of our visit, he persisted in maintaining the quality of his practice and keeping up his reading, but his annual income was grossly inadequate—his hourly remuneration was considerably less than that demanded of us recently by a twelve-year-old boy for lawn-cutting—and he had little or no time for his family. How the doctor of today compares with his predecessor in the amount of time that he is able to devote to family activities, we do not know. It is possible, however, that he may have less opportunity to be around the home, inasmuch as few doctors (only 18 per cent of our Ontario sample and 31 per cent of our Nova Scotia sample; see page 70) have their offices in their homes today.

In order to obtain information about the adequacy of the time that the practitioners had available for various activities, we asked each man whether he thought that he had "ample time, just enough time, not enough time, or little or no time" for each of seven items. These and the doctors' replies are shown in Table 102. The fact that 77 per cent of the Ontario doctors and 71 per cent of those in Nova Scotia said that they had not enough time for their families indicates how widespread this problem is. That the physicians answered as they did is not surprising when we recall that 36 per cent of the Ontario doctors and 60 per cent of those in Nova Scotia were working more than 55 hours a week (see Table 20, page 103), exclusive of mealtimes and calls during the night, and that 39 per cent in Ontario and 67 per cent in Nova Scotia had evening office hours on three or more of the five evenings between Monday and Friday (see Table 16, page 99). The magnitude of the problem of time in a physician's life is also attested to by the findings of Deisher and his associates, who have investigated certain aspects of the practice of paediatrics, which, of all the specialties, has perhaps the most in common with general practice. These workers at the University of Washington School of Medicine arranged for 91 of the state's 113 paediatricians, "excluding those in teaching or work other than practice," to answer a questionnaire. They say,

TABLE 102

OPINIONS OF ONTARIO AND NOVA SCOTIA PHYSICIANS ABOUT THE
ADEQUACY OF THE TIME THAT THEY WERE ABLE TO DEVOTE TO VARIOUS ACTIVITIES

| | Ontario physicians: Number stating that the time was | | | | Nova Scotia physicians: Number stating that the time was | | | |
|---|---|---|---|---|---|---|---|---|
| Activity | Ample | Just enough | Not enough | Little or no | Ample | Just enough | Not enough | Little or no |
| Detailed working up of patients | 4 | 13 | 27 | 0 | 10 | 12 | 20 | 0 |
| Following latest medical advances in books and journals | 3 | 12 | 26 | 3 | 4 | 9 | 28 | 1 |
| Following up own interests in field of medicine | 4 | 20 | 20 | 0 | 8 | 9 | 22 | 3 |
| Spending time with family | 5 | 5 | 32 | 2 | 7 | 5 | 21 | 9 |
| Spending time with friends | 10* | 9 | 24 | 1 | 7 | 13 | 13 | 9 |
| Reading newspapers and keeping up with current affairs | 13 | 20 | 11 | 0 | 13 | 10 | 16 | 3 |
| Following up own non-medical interests and hobbies | 4 | 11 | 27 | 2 | 4 | 7 | 25 | 6 |

*One of these 10 physicians said, "halfway between ample time and just enough."

"Each pediatrician was asked what he considered to be his greatest personal problem related to the practice of pediatrics. He was directed to avoid problems of an academic or medical nature, such as problems concerning the diagnosis or treatment of disease. The most frequent reply to this question was the lack of sufficient time for himself and his family."*

Finally, the problem of apportioning his time is complicated for a physician by his need to earn a living. The more time a doctor devotes to taking a patient's history, examining him, and carrying out whatever other procedures may be necessary, the fewer patients he is able to see in a given amount of time. If his remuneration is set, as it tends to be in some of the prepaid plans, at so much per visit rather than at so much per unit of time, it follows that, the more time a physician devotes to each patient—particularly to history-taking and physical examination—the less his remuneration per unit of time worked. To the physician who might dawdle or who might prolong a patient's visit unnecessarily, this method of remuneration, i.e. on a per-visit

*R. W. Deisher *et al.*: Pediatrics, 25: 712, 1960.

basis, may be an incentive to increase his rate of working. On the other hand, it is possible that this system of remuneration acts as a temptation to the man who gives too little time to each patient; and undoubtedly it serves to discourage the doctor who wishes to do a thorough job but finds himself inadequately paid for his time. With regard to the latter point, we reported in an earlier chapter (see pages 198–199) the complaints that were made about one prepayment plan. We refer especially to the statement that was made by several very competent physicians to the effect that the company, having set a fee for a full history and examination of a patient, would arbitrarily decide, without investigation, that the visit had been a routine office call and would cut the fee in half. These men pointed out that, if a doctor knew from previous experience that he would not be paid for the extra time that he took to investigate a case thoroughly, he would tend, through sheer economic necessity, to do the less time-consuming and less thorough work for which he was being paid. The implications of this, as far as quality of practice is concerned, are serious. We would draw attention, also, to the findings, shown in Table 102, that 61 per cent of the Ontario practitioners whom we visited and 48 per cent of those in Nova Scotia said that the time that they were able to devote to the detailed working up of patients was "not enough." Whether the reason for this was economic, they did not say.

It is not only the amount of time that a doctor devotes to each patient, but also the amount of time that he is able to give to keeping up with medical advances, that is affected by his need to earn a living. The more time he must give to earning a living, the less time remains to him in which to read or to attend postgraduate courses. If the rate of remuneration is set at too low a level, then, in order to make an adequate income without reducing the amount of time given to each patient, the physician must either limit his efforts to keep abreast of new developments or else give inadequate time to his family.

It is clear, then, that there is a relationship between the rate of remuneration of the physician and the time that he can devote to his continuing education, which, in turn, is connected with quality of practice. How great a problem exists in this area, we cannot be certain on the basis of the evidence available to us. It may be that physicians complaining of lack of time for reading really *do* lack the time; or it may be that the time is there, if only they were to organize their day or their week more satisfactorily. If they really do lack the time, i.e. if their practice as it exists at present does not leave them time for reading or keeping up in other ways, there are three possible explanations. First, it may be that the doctor is working too long hours seeing patients and is leaving himself too little time for other activities, including his professional reading, because he desires a large income. Secondly, it may be that the doctor is working too long hours and is making a large income but that the reason is that no other doctor is available to take over the excess work. Thirdly, it may be that the doctor is working too long hours because this is necessary if he is to make an *adequate* income to support his family.

In the course of our observations, we gained the impression that each one of the alternatives that we have just mentioned existed in one or another of the practices that we visited. We have not sufficient evidence, however, to arrive at any conclusions regarding the relative frequencies of the situations that we have described. Yet it disturbed us to hear one doctor say, "In general practice, you can't provide for your old age or for your dependents. You *must* have investments or business enterprises," and to be told by another, whose practice was eminently satisfactory in quality and who was not a dawdler, that he did not see how he could continue to give the individual patient the amount of time that was necessary, do the necessary reading, and still make a reasonable living, unless he included in his practice surgical work, for which he did not regard himself as qualified. Deisher and his associates, in answer to the question that they put to the 91 paediatricians (see page 468), namely, what they considered to be their greatest personal problem related to the practice of paediatrics, were told by 20 per cent that they "felt that pediatricians were not paid well enough" and by 10 per cent "that the pediatrician had to handle a large volume of practice to meet the demands of economics."[*]

We have discussed the need for a doctor to keep up with the advances of medicine and the difficulty that he has in doing this. We have pointed out that there seem to be a number of causes of this difficulty but that a major cause is thought by the doctors to be, and, in some practices, almost certainly is, lack of adequate time for reading. Further, we have suggested, and have adduced some evidence to support our suggestion, that inadequate remuneration creates a dilemma for some practitioners. The dilemma is whether to maintain the quality of their work, either by reducing to almost nothing the amount of time that they give to their families or by struggling on with an inadequate income, or whether, on the other hand, to meet the needs of their families at the cost of reducing the quality of their work to an inadequate level. This brings us to a consideration of the responsibilities of the individual physician.

A physician may be thought of as having a triple responsibility. As

[*]*Ibid.*

a physician, he has a responsibility to his patients to provide medical care of a satisfactory quality; and, if he is to remain worthy of respect, there can be no doubt that he must continue to be motivated by genuine concern for his patients' welfare. This concept was expressed in the aphorism that we remember hearing from some of the older practitioners in our student days, "You look after your patients, and the dollars will look after themselves." In carrying on his practice, however, a physician cannot justifiably confine his attention to the medical implications of his acts; he must consider, also, their social effects. We refer specifically to the cost of medical care, which is of increasing concern both to the individual patient and to governments (at various levels), which must bear part of the load and which are being subjected to pressure to make changes in the organization of medical care. Much of the cost of medical care, of course, is neither caused by, nor subject to control by, the individual physician or the medical profession as a whole, but arises from the high costs of labour and of materials. This is a point that seems too often to be unrecognized or ignored when the costs of physicians' services, nursing, drugs, and hospitalization are all lumped together and spoken of as "the cost of medical care." On the other hand, though a physician cannot accept responsibility for the high cost of the various ancillary services that we have mentioned, he does have a responsibility to his patient and to society to keep the cost of *his* services from being unduly high.

Finally, in considering the responsibilities of a physician, we must remember that, in addition to being a physician, he is also a person and that, as a person, he has both needs and responsibilities that have nothing to do with the fact that he is a physician. As a single man, his needs may be relatively simple—food, clothing, and shelter—and his personal responsibilities may be slight or non-existent. When he marries, and particularly when he has children, his responsibilities become immeasurably more complex. Apart from his responsibility to be a husband and a father in more than the mere biological sense, i.e. apart from his responsibility to enter into the lives of his wife and his children and to share himself with them, he has greatly increased financial responsibilities. He must provide for the current needs of his family; he must set aside enough to look after his own and his wife's old age—let it be remembered that he has no employer contributing to a pension fund on his behalf—; and he must face the risk of his family's being destitute if he should be incapacitated or should die prematurely.

The needs of a practising physician are determined to some extent by the economic conditions obtaining during the period of training, especially the postgraduate portion of it. These have been discussed at length in the preceding chapter, and we shall not repeat, except to recall that many young physicians must choose between not taking the training that they wish or, if they do take it, entering practice with a significant load of indebtedness (see pages 436 and 428). Another factor that must be borne in mind when a doctor's economic needs are being assessed is the expectations of society itself, because society is ambivalent in its attitude. While it criticizes a doctor if he appears to be concerned about money, society applies materialistic criteria to determine whether a doctor is a "success" or not. A community may be prepared to see a clergyman and his family look shabby or even to let them exist in outright poverty, but it regards a similar appearance on the doctor's part as evidence of lack of success.

A physician's problem, then, is to reconcile, or to find a compromise between, the conflicting needs of the patient and of society, on the one hand, for good medical care at the least possible cost and of himself, on the other hand, for money with which to support his family. Just as surely as a physician fails in his responsibility to his patients and to society when he does not give due thought to their needs, so he acts in an irresponsible way towards his family if he refuses to consider its needs.

What we have said is so self-evident that the stating of it may appear unnecessary. Yet the profession, though appearing at times to be preoccupied with financial problems, as witness the frequent discussion of fee schedules, shows a curious ambivalence in that there is also considerable embarrassment about talking in terms of money. Because medical service has to do with life and death and because it is impossible to set a monetary value upon any service, it is considered almost indecent for a physician to be interested, or at any rate to show his interest, in money. We believe that the source of the embarrassment is the fear of seeming to be eager to profit from another's misfortune. Yet a physician does not *hope* that people will be sick; but, aware that sickness is part of the lot of mankind, he does hope that those who are sick will seek his services. To hope the reverse would be absurd, if for no other reason than that it would cast doubt on his interest in medicine and would suggest that he should never have been trained as a physician.

Since a physician does not cause illness and does all that he can to prevent it, he has no reason to be embarrassed that he does in fact profit from treating what he cannot prevent. In fact, if he is to discharge his responsibilities to his patients, to society, and to his family, he must replace his present ambivalent attitude towards money with an attitude of acceptance, an attitude neither of greed nor of shame but of recognition of the fact that money is necessary to him as it is to the rest of society; and he must bring himself to acknowledge and to discuss his own needs as frankly as he does those of his patients and of society.

Society, too, has a responsibility; and, only if it measures up to its responsibility, can the dilemma that faces a physician be resolved. Society, by giving expression to its attitudes, exerts a control over a physician's rate of remuneration regardless of the method by which the physician is paid. Since this is so, it is society's responsibility to ensure that a physician *is* adequately remunerated, i.e. that he is not required either to reduce the quality of his work or to work excessively long hours in order to make an adequate living. This responsibility exists whether society is exerting its influence indirectly by frowning upon the current fee schedule of privately practising physicians or more directly by stating how much a physician is to be paid as the employee of a government-controlled medical service.

If society is to discharge its responsibility, there is one point to which its attention must be directed in particular. This is that *the rendering of good medical care takes time.* This is obvious to a patient when the item of care is the setting up of an intravenous infusion or the sewing up of a laceration, because the patient can see what is being done. When he cannot follow what is being done, however, as in the course of history-taking or physical examination, it may seem to him that the doctor is taking unnecessarily long. That the central position of the history and the physical examination in medical care is not understood by many patients is apparent both from the impatience that some of them show when an attempt is made to do these thoroughly and from their willingness to accept the diagnosis and treatment of a doctor whose investigation of the complaint has been of the scantiest order. This is vividly pictured by Taylor, to whose study of general practice in the United Kingdom we referred earlier (see pages 9–10), who reports a consultant's description of one group of general practitioners and of their patients' reaction in these words:

The third and final group were the feckless and the dangerous doctors. Often they would be charming; often, too, they would be popular with their patients. . . . Examinations would be extremely rare, yet their slap-happy attitude would appeal to many patients; their capacity to diagnose at a glance would be widely admired.*

If society is not brought to realize that medical care is time-

*Stephen Taylor: Good General Practice (London: Oxford University Press, 1954), p. 38.

consuming, and particularly if those officials of government bodies or of the insurance industry who may be more directly involved in setting rates of remuneration do not have a clear understanding of this, there is danger that they will yield to the temptation to set a physician's remuneration at so low a level as to undermine the quality of his practice. We have already heard this complaint about one prepayment plan (see page 470). There is another risk, too, namely that young people either may be discouraged from choosing medicine as their career or, having chosen it, may avoid general practice in favour of a specialty. Gee and Schumacher, of the Association of American Medical Colleges, questioned a 50 per cent random sample of the 1958–1959 United States internes about their plans for their careers and found that, of the 2,616 (83 per cent of the sample) who replied, only 21 per cent intended to enter general practice, whereas 77 per cent intended to do specialty practice, teaching, research, or some combination of these three.\* We have said (page 463) that some of the practitioners told us that they would advise a young man, even if he intended to enter general practice, to qualify himself first in a specialty. A few who said this made plain that they regarded the qualification in a specialty as a form of insurance in case the general practitioner should be badly treated in a government-controlled medical service. A few would even advise a young person against entering medicine at all, because of the uncertainty of the future of medical practice in this country. We referred earlier (page 342), also, to the concern that has been expressed by James S. Thompson, Secretary of the Association of Canadian Medical Colleges, over the number and the quality of the students who are applying for admission to the medical schools of this country. All of these facts suggest that neither general practice nor medicine itself is as attractive today as might be wished. It would be most unfortunate, then, if the attempt to minimize the cost of a medical service were to discourage suitable students from applying for entry to the medical course.

We have pointed out that society's responsibility to a physician is to ensure that he is adequately remunerated and have stressed that failure to discharge this responsibility carries with it serious risks. Before society can decide, however, how much it is willing to pay a physician on a fee-for-service basis or on a capitation basis or as a straight salary, its basic need is to know how much work can be accomplished in a given amount of time by a physician who is prac-

\*H. H. Gee and C. F. Schumacher: Journal of Medical Education, *36*, No. 4, Part 2: 35, 1961.

tising medicine of *good* quality. We have emphasized the word "good" because only those physicians who are taking the time to practise good medicine can show us how much time is needed for various procedures. Furthermore, and this seems particularly necessary if payment is on a fee-for-service basis, it is necessary to know the relationship, as far as time and remuneration are concerned, of one type of service to another. In chapter 13, we pointed out (page 205) that some of the general practitioners thought that surgical work was more remunerative than non-surgical work. Whether it really is, we do not know, but we suggested that there was a need to investigate this (page 209). Equally important, we think, is the relationship between the fees paid for history-taking and physical examination, on the one hand, and for more mechanical procedures, on the other hand. We would suggest that the taking of a good history and the doing of a thorough examination are underpaid in relation to what is paid for such mechanical procedures as giving an injection or suturing a wound. Unfortunately, so far as we are aware, no detailed studies have ever been made of the amount of work that a physician practising *good* medicine can accomplish in a given amount of time. It is to be noted, however, that neither in Ontario nor in Nova Scotia was there a significant correlation between the quality of practice observed by us and the practitioner's annual net income (Table 103). Physicians whose scores were 40 per cent or less had incomes ranging from less than $10,000 to more than $25,000. So, also, did the physicians whose scores were 61 per cent or more. When hourly rates of remuneration were calculated (see page 190), it was found that, in Ontario, the median net earnings per hour of physicians with scores of 40 per cent or less, of those with scores of between 41 and 60 per cent, and of those with scores of 61 per cent or more were $4.65, $7.10, and $5.03, respectively. The corresponding figures for the Nova Scotia practitioners were $4.56, $3.29, and $4.48. Peterson also, in his study of general practice in North Carolina, found "no linear correlation between the quality of medical care provided by a physician and his net income," and adds the comment, "Actually this is hardly surprising in view of the fact that the lay public has few valid criteria for assessing a physician's competence" (see his page 130).

We suggest that there is a need for studies to determine how much work a physician practising *good* medicine can accomplish in a given amount of time and that these studies should include an examination of the income accruing to physicians per unit of time from the various types of work undertaken by them. These would have to be field studies, since studies of records are subject to too many errors,

TABLE 103

DISTRIBUTION OF PHYSICIANS ACCORDING TO ANNUAL
NET PROFESSIONAL INCOME AND SCORE

| Income | Physician's score | | | Total number of physicians |
|---|---|---|---|---|
| | 0–40 | 41–60 | 61–100 | |
| A. *Ontario* | | | | |
| $10,000 or less | 5 | 4 | 6 | 15 |
| 10,001 to 15,000 | 2 | 1 | 7 | 10 |
| 15,001 to 20,000 | 2 | 2 | 6 | 10 |
| 20,001 to 25,000 | 2 | 1 | 1 | 4 |
| Over 25,000 | 1 | 1 | 1 | 3 |
| Total number of physicians | 12 | 9 | 21 | 42* |
| Median income | $11,650 | $13,500 | $14,000 | |
| B. *Nova Scotia* | | | | |
| $10,000 or less | 9 | 4 | 1 | 14 |
| 10,001 to 15,000 | 4 | 3 | 6 | 13 |
| 15,001 to 20,000 | 3 | 0 | 3 | 6 |
| 20,001 to 25,000 | 1 | 0 | 1 | 2 |
| Total number of physicians | 17 | 7 | 11 | 35† |
| Median income | $10,000 | $ 8,200 | $15,000 | |

*One physician did not know his income; and 1 physician was not scored.
†Of the other 7 physicians, 1 had been in practice for only the last six months of 1957, 4 declined to state either their gross or their net incomes, and 2 who gave their gross incomes as between $15,000 and $15,500 declined to state their net incomes.

especially as regards quality of practice. Probably, the studies that we suggest should be done by a physician and an accountant working as a team. They should give attention, also, to a matter that we, in the present study, have been able only to touch upon, namely the efficiency of a doctor's practice arrangements. Certainly, from the limited observations that we were able to make (see pages 79–81), it was clear that, in some practices, different arrangements would have enabled the doctor to accomplish more work per unit of time without sacrificing the quality of his work. In view of the fact that a large percentage of physicians taking postgraduate training are said to be "in significant debt at the termination of their residency" (see page 428) and in view of the effect that this is said to have on their attitude towards the economic aspects of practice (see pages 436–438), information should be obtained also about the extent of the indebtedness of physicians who have had postgraduate training of various lengths, since this must be taken into account when the rate of remuneration of physicians is being determined.

In this chapter, we have discussed certain problems that confront a practising physician. There is a physician's continuing education throughout the course of his professional career. We have considered in some detail the obstacles that stand in the way of his keeping up with medical advances. In certain cases, the difficulty appears to be professional isolation; in others, a feeling of frustration because no advancement is possible. We have made certain suggestions to cope with these difficulties. Another interesting point emerged from what the practitioners told us of the means that they used to keep up. Though some men read regularly and emphasized the value of books and journals, a little over one-quarter of the practitioners we visited in Ontario and one-fifth of those in Nova Scotia said that they read neither books nor journals more often than "occasionally." On the other hand, postgraduate courses were particularly popular, as also were visiting speakers from the large medical centres. Over all, we gained the impression that the practitioners preferred being told the facts by an authority to reading them themselves. Indeed, some men told us quite unequivocally that this was so. This raises the question whether the pattern is set during a student's years in medical school (when the teacher assumes so much of the responsibility for covering the work and when the student is left so little free time except in the evening) and during his years of postgraduate hospital experience (when, as we have seen, there is little emphasis on reading and little time available for it). If this is the case, then implementing the suggestions that we have made already, namely, that the undergraduate student be required to accept more responsibility for his work and that greater emphasis be put on reading during both the undergraduate and the postgraduate parts of the training, should serve to some extent to remedy the situation.

In the matter of reading material, the practitioners' desire appeared to be for "practical" articles and for reviews of various subjects. It may be that this need is met adequately by certain of the journals published in the United States. On the other hand, a systematic and continuing review of medicine in articles written by teachers in the Canadian medical schools might have the two advantages of coming to the notice of a greater percentage of the practitioners and of being written by men with whose ideas and teaching the practitioners are more familiar.

Because one of the most important difficulties connected with keeping up in medicine seems to be lack of time for reading, we have discussed the problem of time in some detail. Inasmuch as the present organization of medical practice, as an individual enterprise on a twenty-four-hour-a-day basis, developed before it required the detailed knowledge that it requires today, before the era of rapid advances, before the advent of the telephone, and before the disappearance of the domestic servant, we suggest that the whole problem of a doctor's time needs to be reconsidered, in the interest, not only of the doctors and their families, but of the quality of their work, which is of the greatest importance to their patients. We pointed out earlier that, though more than 90 per cent of the doctors were practising within a mile of a colleague, only an occasional doctor, among those in solo practice (see page 87), had worked out a system with colleagues whereby each had time off duty on a regular basis and, even of those who were practising in groups of two or more (see page 112), many did not have satisfactory arrangements for evenings and week-ends off duty.

We have pointed out that the problem of time is closely connected with a doctor's remuneration, and have emphasized that society, in its own interest, has the responsibility of seeing that a doctor's remuneration is high enough to allow him to give adequate time to each patient, particularly for a proper history and examination, and to set aside enough time for reading. We have suggested that rates of remuneration should be based on studies both of the amount of work that can be done in a given time by a physician who is practising *good* medicine and of the amount of indebtedness with which the physician begins his practice.

Having laid great emphasis on society's responsibility to recognize that good medical care takes time and must be paid for, we must emphasize equally that, if society is willing to pay adequately to allow a doctor to take the necessary time, the doctor has the responsibility of seeing that the care that is given *is* of satisfactory quality. Unfortunately, there are some practitioners whose poor practices appear to be determined by deficiencies within themselves rather than by any of the conditions of practice. We refer, for example, to the men who fail to recognize their own limitations or who listen to a clear exposition of the solution to a problem but are unable to see the applicability of this in their own practice. These men's practices could not be expected to improve as a result of any of the measures that we have suggested so far. The question, as far as these men are concerned, is whether they should be assuming as much responsibility as they are assuming. To this particular aspect of responsibility, we shall turn our attention in the next chapter.

# 25 / Responsibility in Medicine

A physician who is in practice by himself, as the majority of our general practitioners were, must assume complete responsibility for the medical care of the patients who come to him, except when he seeks the advice of another physician acting as a consultant. Even then, it is the physician's responsibility to decide whether or not a consultation should be requested, unless the patient demands one, and to guide the patient in his choice of consultant. Collings,* referring to general medical practice as "a unique social phenomenon," says, "The general practitioner . . . wields more power than any other citizen, unless it be the judge on his bench. In a world of ever-increasing management, the powers of even the senior managers are petty compared with the powers of the doctor to influence the physical, psychological, and economic destiny of other people. But unlike the manager, . . . the doctor . . . is largely free from the limitations which democratic principles set on the acquisition of power."† Even if allowance be made for the possibility of some exaggeration in this statement, there can be no doubt that a physician does have a tremendous amount of power. A word spoken either carelessly or in ignorance may convince a patient with an insignificant heart murmur that his heart "is ruined," as one patient described it to us, and consign him to a life of invalidism, caused, not by disease, but by his physician's inappropriate comment reinforced by the patient's own fear. On the other hand, if a physician fails to investigate a patient's complaint adequately, the result may be that a serious condition, such

*For Collings's study of general practice in the United Kingdom, see pages 8–9.
†J. S. Collings: The Lancet, 258: 555, 1950.

as cancer, tuberculosis, or meningitis, progresses to the point where cure is much more difficult, or even impossible, to achieve. These examples are enough to illustrate the enormous effect that a doctor may have on the life of his patient and the awesome responsibility that is his. Since, in his office and home practice, an independent practitioner is subject to no supervision and to no control provided he remains within the limit of the law, the factors that determine how adequately he discharges his responsibility to his patient are his professional ability and his conscience.

A most important question now to be discussed, as we consider factors affecting the quality of practice and ways in which it might be improved, is whether a physician, going forth from his training, is ready to shoulder such a load of responsibility. There is evidence that some physicians are not ready. The poor quality of practice that we found among some of the *older* physicians cannot be accepted as evidence of inadequate preparation for practice, since we cannot exclude the possibility (however unlikely in some cases) that their practices may in earlier years have been of satisfactory quality and may have deteriorated with the passage of time; but, when we find *recent* graduates practising medicine of unsatisfactory quality (see Table 82, page 319), this *is* evidence that they were not ready for independent practice. Peterson also, commenting on the "remarkable variation" that his group observed in North Carolina, states that some of the practitioners appeared to be unprepared for assuming "the responsibilities inherent in undertaking the care of a patient."[*] Again, the statements (see page 399), made by approximately 40 per cent of the doctors whom we visited in each province, that they did not regard the present medical school training plus one year of rotating interneship as adequate preparation for handling the physical illnesses of patients, and the statements made by even higher percentages in the two provinces about the inadequacy of the training as preparation for handling the social problems and the emotional problems of patients, are highly suggestive that young physicians going into general practice are taking on responsibilities for which they are not ready. We gave examples, also, in an earlier chapter (see pages 219–222), of lack of interest in medicine itself, of failure of a physician to discipline himself to take a history and do a physical examination, of disinclination to accept responsibility for sick patients, and of certain types of behaviour that could only be described as irresponsible. In each of

[*]O. L. Peterson *et al.*: Journal of Medical Education, *31*, No. 12, Part 2: 1–165, 1956; see page 47.

these cases, we are led to wonder whether the practitioner concerned should have been entrusted with the responsibility of a medical practice.

Because it appears that it is possible for a physician to undertake the responsibilities of independent practice without being ready for them, it is necessary that we consider *how* this is possible. The licensing of a physician is a provincial matter, and the regulations vary somewhat from one province to another. Since we have been concerned with the quality of practice of practitioners in Ontario and in Nova Scotia, most of whom were graduates of medical schools in their respective provinces, we shall confine our attention to the licensing regulations of these two provinces. A physician who wishes to engage in practice in Nova Scotia is required by the Medical Act of Nova Scotia* to be registered with the Provincial Medical Board. In order to be so registered, the physician, unless he is registered with the General Medical Council of the United Kingdom, either must have passed the examinations of the Provincial Medical Board or must have passed the examinations of the Medical Council of Canada. In either case, he must have served a rotating interneship in an approved hospital. For those who take their medical course at Dalhousie University, the final written examinations are held conjointly by the University, the Provincial Medical Board of Nova Scotia, and the Medical Council of Canada at the end of the fourth medical year, i.e. at the completion of the formal university courses but before the interneship.† At the end of the interneship, oral and clinical examinations are held by the University and the Provincial Medical Board conjointly, and by the Medical Council of Canada separately. In Ontario, the physician who wishes to practise medicine is required by the Medical Act of the Legislature of Ontario‡ to be registered with the College of Physicians and Surgeons of Ontario. The latter, however, does not conduct examinations but demands that the candidate have passed the examinations of the Medical Council of Canada and have served an interneship of one year's duration. In Ontario, not only are the written examinations of the Medical Council of Canada usually taken conjointly with the university's final examinations, but the clinical and oral examinations also of the Medical Council of Canada are usually taken before the interneship, i.e. immediately after the completion of the medical

*Revised Statutes of Nova Scotia, 1954, vol. 2, chapter 172, Section 15, p. 2063.
†The examination papers are read first by the examiners of the University and of the Provincial Medical Board, and the papers of the successful university candidates are then sent on to the examiners of the Medical Council of Canada.
‡Revised Statutes of Ontario, 1960, vol. 3, chapter 234, Section 19(2), p. 114.

course. Therefore, we must examine the stated objectives of undergraduate medical education in order to ascertain whether it purports to bring a student to the point at which he will be ready for general practice.

At the Second World Conference on Medical Education, Arnott, reviewing the proceedings of the First World Conference on Medical Education, spoke of the objectives of a medical school:

> There was widespread acceptance of the concept that the duty of the medical school was not to produce a general practitioner any more than a surgeon or a hygienist, etc., but the much simpler and more attainable one of advancing the education of the doctor to the point from which he can, within a reasonable period, be turned into a useful general practitioner or . . . can aspire to one or other of the more exacting specialties . . . Thus formal qualification is merely the end of the beginning, not an end in itself.*

In the course of the Second World Conference on Medical Education, the same opinion was expressed. Sir George Pickering, Regius Professor of Medicine at Oxford University, who acted as moderator of a panel discussion, is reported to have "said he thought the panel would assume that undergraduate education would be directed to training the basic doctor, and not specifically general practitioners, or specialists or research workers, or medical administrators, though it was hoped that any man trained by undergraduate curriculum would be capable of being further developed in any of those directions."† Dana W. Atchley, Emeritus Professor of Clinical Medicine at Columbia University, speaking in 1960 at the University of Kansas Medical Center Faculty Conference on Medical Education, took the same view: "It is generally accepted that the purpose of medical education on the undergraduate level is not to accomplish the training of a practitioner but to lay a scientific foundation upon which to erect a career in patient care, research, teaching, public health, or any of the various opportunities open to the recipient of the M.D. degree."‡ C. G. Child, who was Chairman of the Seventh Teaching Institute of the Association of American Medical Colleges, says in his Introduction to the report of this meeting that this Institute and the preceding one "endorsed again and again that the principal objective of medical

---

*W. M. Arnott: Medicine: A Lifelong Study, Proceedings of Second World Conference on Medical Education, Chicago, 1959 (New York: World Medical Association, 1961), p. 12.

†Sir G. Pickering: Medicine: A Lifelong Study, Proceedings of Second World Conference on Medical Education, Chicago 1959 (New York: World Medical Association, 1961), p. 463.

‡D. W. Atchley: Journal of the American Medical Association, *174*: 1414, 1960.

education is for the student to obtain a grasp of scientific method rather than any particular mass of factual knowledge."*

John R. Ellis, at that time Sub-Dean of London Hospital Medical College and now Secretary of the Association for the Study of Medical Education, has pointed out that in Britain, with the emergence of the general practitioner as "a new order in the profession," at the beginning of this century "a new form of education had been established. Its one aim, officially stated by Act of Parliament and questioned by none, was to train a man to be on graduation a 'safe general practitioner.'" After a brief description of the training, which included "a period of clinical study so arranged as to include all knowledge and all techniques considered useful" and which Ellis considers was satisfactory during the first quarter of this century, he emphasizes that the "upsurge of medical knowledge" and the obligation to "insure that the student can 'safely practise'" have together resulted in the final examination's becoming "an increasingly comprehensive test, a cumulative marathon of factual knowledge" and that, because many medical students are examined by strangers who know nothing of their records or their work, there are "failure rates of up to 50 per cent." He makes the statement, "It is clearly impossible any longer to train a man to be 'a safe general practitioner' by the time of graduation."†

From these quotations, it is clear that the medical schools do not consider themselves responsible for producing physicians who are ready to function as general practitioners. That this philosophy exists in at least one of the medical schools of Canada is plain from what Robert C. Dickson, Professor of Medicine at Dalhousie University, has said:

> The increasing complexity and scope of medical knowledge has led to general agreement that the medical student of today cannot be made proficient in even a large portion of the field of medicine. It has, therefore, become the acknowledged aim of most medical schools to produce what has been variously termed the basic doctor or the undifferentiated doctor. The aim of undergraduate education has come to be the provision of the broad knowledge which will permit the graduate to become, with further training, a good general practitioner, specialist, research worker, or teacher. The aim is clear and not controversial.‡

The medical schools, then, do not profess to train physicians for general practice, and, in fact, imply that they do not think that this can be done in the time at their disposal. We have seen that the final

---

*C. G. Child, III: Journal of Medical Education, 36, No. 4, Part 2: xxi, 1961.
†J. R. Ellis: Journal of Medical Education, 33, No. 10, Part 2: 225–227, 1958.
‡R. C. Dickson: Journal of the American Medical Association, 173: 1297, 1960.

written examinations and, in the case of the graduates of some of the medical schools in Canada, the final oral and clinical examinations required by the licensing body may be taken *before* the interneship. Who, then, accepts responsibility for seeing that a young physician, at the end of his year of interneship, is ready to assume the responsibility of independent practice? Does the hospital in which the physician internes accept this responsibility? Deitrick and Berson, who made a survey of medical education in the United States between 1949 and 1951, say, "Few if any hospitals make a careful evaluation of the intern's educational accomplishment. In fact, there are as yet no standards of accomplishment for interns to achieve by the end of their internship training."* In 1961, the National Board of Medical Examiners in the United States, whose examinations are somewhat analogous to those conducted by the Medical Council of Canada and are accepted by many of the states for licensing purposes, asked a number of hospitals for "a confidential ranking" of the candidates for the final part of the Board's examination "in terms of the top-ranking fourth and the bottom-ranking fourth of the group." They report that "a number of hospitals—even certain prominent teaching hospitals— said that they could not provide such evaluations. How was one intern to be compared with another? What criteria were to be used? . . ."†

The Canadian Medical Association, in the Introduction to its booklet on approval of hospitals for junior interneship, says, "In accepting interns, the medical staff must accept a serious responsibility not only to the medical profession as a whole and the interns during the course of their clinical teaching, but also to the communities in which these physicians will later become established."‡ Yet, further on, the booklet says: "The Committee believes that all interns are entitled to a Certificate of Service after they have completed a satisfactory training period. Under normal circumstances, hospitals are not justified in withholding Certificates of Service unless there has been gross negligence on the part of the intern in performing his duties."§

There is nothing here to suggest that an interne's work is to be carefully evaluated by the hospital or that the hospital has any responsibility for guaranteeing that an interne is ready to accept the

*J. E. Deitrick and R. C. Berson: Medical Schools in the United States at Mid-Century (New York: McGraw-Hill, 1953), p. 271.

†National Board Examiner, 9: 3, 3, 1961. Published by the National Board of Medical Examiners, Philadelphia.

‡Basis of Approval of Hospitals for the Training of Junior Interns in Canada (Toronto: Canadian Medical Association, 1960), p. 4.

§*Ibid.*, p. 14.

responsibilities of practice. In fact, it is clear that an interne's work must be very bad, indeed, before he is to be penalized by being refused a certificate of service.

We say this, not in criticism of the hospitals, but to emphasize that there is a link missing from the chain of responsibility. The medical educators state quite explicitly that the medical schools do not undertake to train physicians for general practice, but that their aim is to "produce . . . the basic doctor" or to provide "the broad knowledge which will permit the graduate to become, with further training, a good general practitioner, . . ." Yet, by many graduates, the final examinations for the licence to practise are taken before the "further training" (i.e., the internship) which is to turn the graduate into a good practitioner. This appears to be one of the circumstances accounting for the fact that it is possible, as we have found, for a physician to undertake the responsibilities of independent practice without being ready for them.

Even more serious, however, are difficulties inherent in the examination system; and these difficulties are as great in one university as in another. First of all, the correlation between academic record and quality of practice is far from perfect, as we showed earlier (see pages 322, 323n, 324). Charles A. Janeway, Professor of Pediatrics at Harvard University, speaks, in the Report of the Sixth Teaching Institute of the Association of American Medical Colleges, of the limited usefulness of examinations:

No conclusions were reached [i.e., by the Institute participants] on the subject of evaluation except: you have to know what your objectives are before you can evaluate students. When one gets to the clinical years examinations certainly have very limited usefulness, since most of our formal examination methods test knowledge solely because this is the simplest attribute to test, although knowledge per se may have little relation to the development of maturity in communication and judgment, which are so important in the actual effectiveness of the clinician.*

Another difficulty that is inherent in the examination system and that seems to us at least as important as the one just mentioned is the fact that, in the case of each candidate, an examiner must make an all-or-none decision, i.e. he must either pass the candidate or refuse to pass him. In the case of the final examinations for a licence to practise, those candidates whom an examiner passes will, after completing the year of internship, be granted a licence, whereas those whom he does not pass will not be granted a licence. This situation

*C. A. Janeway: Journal of Medical Education, 34, No. 10, Part 2: 107, 1959.

presupposes that it is possible for an examiner to divide all the candidates into two groups, those who are ready, or will after a year of internship be ready, to assume the responsibilities of practice and those who are not, and even after a year of internship will not be, ready for such responsibility. The fact that the final examinations may precede the required year of internship complicates an examiner's decision—in that it requires him to estimate how much the candidate will gain from that year—but does not affect the fundamental difficulty that confronts him, namely, that of dividing the candidates into the two groups that we have named. The root of the difficulty is the fact that the candidates form, not two discrete groups, but a continuum. Though one may arbitrarily decree that candidates obtaining, say, 50 per cent shall pass and those obtaining less than 50 per cent shall fail, there is, in fact, no appreciable difference between the candidate who obtains 49 per cent and the one who obtains 50 per cent, i.e., quite apart from the imperfect correlation between academic record and quality of practice, the one candidate cannot be said to be any more ready for practice than the other.

An examiner may have little or no difficulty in identifying a candidate who has a good grasp of a subject or one who is grossly deficient. His difficulty is with those candidates who are neither very good nor very poor, just as we, even after two or three days of observing the actual practice of each of our practitioners, found that certain practices could not be characterized unequivocally either as satisfactory or as unsatisfatcory (see page 314). Whereas we, however, could leave our evaluation of these practices in doubt, an examiner is not so fortunate. He *must* decide one way or the other. If it be suggested that perhaps the time of decision, i.e. the final examinations, should be deferred, in all cases, until after the year of internship, we must point out that this will not solve the problem, since, sooner or later, an examiner will be obliged to make the all-or-none decision. Even if it should be suggested, further, that those who are not ready for the responsibilities of practice at the end of a year of internship should be required to continue their hospital experience until they are ready, this would not furnish a solution, either, since this would mean that the hospitals' internship system would become clogged with men of unsatisfactory calibre so that the flow of those of satisfactory calibre would be impeded. Clearly, then, at some point, an examiner must make his all-or-none decision: he must permit the physician to go out and assume full responsibility in practice or he must tell him that all his years of toil have been in vain, since there is no other practical use to which the student of medicine can put his training. It is worth noting, at this point, that an examiner determining a candidate's fitness for a licence to practise is in a different position from an examiner testing candidates for specialist qualifications. Though it is true that the latter examiner must make an all-or-none decision regarding specialty practice, a decision against the candidate does not have the same overwhelming effect, since the candidate, though refused the right to call himself a specialist, is still able to carry on the practice of medicine.

Since an examiner whose decision will determine whether the candidate will be granted a licence to practise will bear a heavy load of responsibility if he fails the candidate at the end of a long and arduous course of study, and since he is more immediately conscious of the student's unhappy plight, if he fails, than of the possible risks to the man's future patients if he is allowed to pass, it is probable, and understandable, that he will give the candidate the benefit of the doubt. Ellis, talking of examiners in Britain, says, "They have without doubt (and I am one of them) done their level best to pass as many candidates as possible, especially in finals and particularly since establishment of the compulsory year of internship."[*] The National Board of Medical Examiners, to which we have referred above, has recently developed a new and more objective form of the final part of its examination, the final scoring of which is done, not on the spot by the examiner, but in the National Board's office. Hubbard, in reporting on this examination, which was used for the first time in June, 1961, says, "our examiners expressed relief at not having to make a decision as to whether a weak candidate should pass or fail the examination. In previous years, I have heard examiners say: Although I really thought this candidate was rather incompetent, I just could not bring myself to fail him at this point in his career and to jeopardize his licensure."[†] Bestor, while discussing the wide range of achievement that exists among the pupils of a public school class, points out that "The same extraordinary variation in achievement exists in the high school and college." He goes on to cite evidence that leads him to conclude that "college professors are . . . practicing 'automatic promotion' as gaily as anyone else."[‡] In view of the words of Ellis and of Hubbard, one cannot but wonder whether, in medicine also, the psychological pressures to which the examiner is subjected

[*] J. R. Ellis: Journal of Medical Education, 33, No. 10, Part 2: 232, 1958.
[†] J. P. Hubbard: National Board Examiner, 9: 3, 2, 1961.
[‡] Arthur Bestor: The Restoration of Learning (New York: Alfred A. Knopf, 1956), pp. 287, 288.

tend to force him, in some cases perhaps without his being conscious of it, towards the practice of "automatic promotion." It seems particularly pertinent to wonder this when we recall the great variation that we observed in the quality of the practices visited by us (see chapters 16 and 17) and yet learn that, in Canada, during the academic year, 1959–1960, only 2 out of 863 third-year medical students and none of 858 fourth-year students "withdrew for academic reasons."*

There are, then, two factors that make it possible for a physician to assume complete responsibility for the care of patients without being ready for such a load of responsibility: the fact that there is no educational body whose acknowledged aim is to produce a general practitioner and the fact that the system of qualification by examination demands from an examiner what is impossible in the case of some candidates, i.e. an all-or-none decision. We have said that these two factors *make it possible* for a physician to assume complete responsibility without being ready for it. This is an understatement in that a physician, once he is licensed, not only is allowed but may be virtually *compelled* to assume responsibility whether he is ready for it or not. This is so because, to a medical graduate who has not proceeded to specialized training, the only career open, except in isolated instances, is general practice. If the young man recognizes his own unreadiness for practice and seeks further postgraduate hospital experience, either he must compete for the available junior interneships with those who have graduated after him or he must compete for the more senior house-staff positions with those whose avowed interest in a specialty and perhaps better academic records make them more desirable from the hospital's point of view. In addition, for some men, further hospital training is financially impossible (see pages 185–186, 427–429). In short, some men who have graduated from medical school and obtained a licence to practise but who are not ready to assume the responsibilities of independent practice are nonetheless permitted, or even forced by circumstances, to enter general practice, in which they must assume complete responsibility, without any supervision, for the rest of their careers. This is not to suggest that all those who enter general practice are of this type. We repeat what we said in chapter 17, that we saw many satisfactory practices and some of extremely high calibre (see pages 277–278, 315); and some doctors whose practices were considered satisfactory had had only one year of interneship. On the other hand, among those whose practices were unsatisfactory were certain men who could have done much valuable

*J. S. Thompson: Canadian Medical Association Journal, 84: 689, 1961.

work under supervision but who, because of one characteristic or another, should have assumed complete responsibility for a practice only after a long period of gradually increasing responsibility or, perhaps, never. Such men, to give examples, were those who, by their actions or words, made plain that they were not comfortable accepting full responsibility, those who knew what constituted good practice but were so deficient in their concept of their responsibility to their patients that they exposed their patients to unnecessary risks by not taking a history or not carrying out an examination or not sterilizing a syringe,* and those who, though perhaps very conscientious, did not know how to practise medicine of satisfactory quality themselves and did not know when to call for assistance from more experienced colleagues.†

We have suggested that some practitioners are assuming more responsibility in practice than is warranted by their professional ability or other qualities. How much responsibility should any given physician be assuming? We believe that the answer to that question is that he should be assuming only as much responsibility as he is able and willing to discharge satisfactorily. This amount will vary from one individual to another. We regard it as highly doubtful whether it is possible for a strange examiner, examining for the Medical Council of Canada, to decide, on the basis of five written three-hour examinations and the same number of oral or clinical examinations of fifteen to thirty minutes' duration, how much responsibility a young physician should assume. Whether a university examiner, who knows more about the student, can assess this before the internship, i.e. before a student has assumed any responsibility for patient care, is almost as doubtful. Those who are responsible for the man's work during his internship would be in a better position to make such an assessment, were it not for the fact that often the hospital hierarchy interposes so many more senior members of the house staff between the junior interne and the attending staff member that the latter knows little or nothing about the interne's work save what he hears at second hand. Furthermore, medicine today is so vast and so complex that it is probably only a minority—and a minority that will decrease with the ever increasing complexity of medicine—who can be ready for the responsibilities of independent practice after a single year of interne-ship. Stanley E. Dorst, Dean of Medicine at the University of Cincinnati, has stated that "Progressive responsibility and its mirror image, progressive authority over patient care under critical supervision, are

*See page 283 regarding certain physicians' attitude towards the risk of transmitting the serum hepatitis virus.

†See pages 308–313 for discussion of the adequacy of referrals and for examples of cases that should have been, but were not, referred.

the two basic fundamentals of training implicit in the residency system as it has developed in the U.S.A.," but has pointed out that "one cannot honestly consider . . . training programmes of progressive responsibility for patient care without saying quite frankly that we must improve our methods and our techniques in the area of graduate training of the general physician."* Joseph T. Wearn, Dean of Medicine at Western Reserve University, speaks of the inadequacy of "only one year of a rotating interneship":

This usually means three months of internal medicine or surgery and then practice involving advanced problems in internal medicine or major surgery . . . Practice after such hopelessly inadequate training—both in time and educational content—is inexcusable, for by no stretch of the imagination does such training qualify one for practice in a single discipline —much less several—where his decision may result in the loss of a human life.†

At this point, it is appropriate to consider briefly certain measures that have either been tried, or at least suggested, as likely to improve the quality of practice. On the matter of longer postgraduate training, some pertinent comments have been made by Paul Fuchsig, Head of the Department of Surgery at the University of Vienna. While taking part in a panel discussion at the Second World Conference on Medical Education, he pointed out that increasing the length of postgraduate training did not in itself guarantee the desired effect. To quote the Proceedings:

Dr. Paul Fuchsig (Austria) said that up to about fourteen years ago in Austria a doctor could practise as soon as he got his degree, without any post-graduate training, but now, however, a three-year period of postgraduate intern and residency training for general practitioners had been established. This included nine months each in a medical and a surgical department, and three- or two-month periods in other departments. How did this work out? So far as he could see, this was not regarded by young graduates as a time for serious study. If they happened on a department where the chief was not a good teacher they did not learn very much. They were apt to regard the specified period of study merely as an obligation to be fulfilled. He therefore thought it would be better to return to the principle of freedom of teaching and of learning without setting time limits, making the acquisition of knowledge a matter of individual responsibility.‡

*S. E. Dorst: Medicine: A Lifelong Study, Proceedings of Second World Conference on Medical Education, Chicago 1959 (New York: World Medical Association, 1961), pp. 418, 419.
†J. T. Wearn: Medical Clinics of North America, *41*: 907, 1957.
‡P. Fuchsig: Medicine: A Lifelong Study, Proceedings of Second World Conference on Medical Education, Chicago 1959 (New York: World Medical Association, 1961), p. 464.

From time to time we have heard it said, and indeed one of the practitioners in our sample said (see page 173), that another way of coping with the problem of unsatisfactory practice would be to demand that a general practitioner be re-examined every few years. This we consider either unpractical or undesirable for a number of reasons. First, it would be a tremendous undertaking, because of the number of physicians. Secondly, who should do the periodic examining? It would be an odious task for specialists to have to undertake, especially in view of the fact that over half of the physicians whom we visited in each province felt that general practitioners did not have as much prestige as they should have with the specialists (see page 156). If the re-examination were done by general practitioners, who would determine that the examiners were qualified for the task, and who would re-examine *them* periodically, or would they be exempt? Thirdly, a system of periodic re-examination might well divert a physician's attention from carrying on a first-rate practice, which should be his objective, to passing examinations. One is constantly on trial in the practice of medicine, but we question whether being repeatedly subject to the *artificial* type of trial that an examination constitutes is wholesome either for a physician or for his practice. Fourthly, we have pointed out above how difficult it is for an examiner to fail a medical student who is in the zone that lies between the definitely satisfactory and the definitely unsatisfactory. To fail a practising physician would be well-nigh impossible because of the devastating effect both economically and psychologically. Finally, there is at present no mechanism for rehabilitating the doctor who might fail upon being re-examined. This would influence an examiner in his all-or-none decision. It would mean, also, that, if a doctor failed and presumably lost his licence, his abilities, which, though not adequate for independent practice, could nevertheless be of benefit in the total medical picture, would be completely lost. For these reasons, the suggestion of periodic re-examination of doctors seems to us to be quite unpractical.

For several years, the College of General Practice of Canada has been considering the advisability of establishing a higher qualification in general practice in the form either of certification or of fellowship, such as exist in the specialties at the present time. Recently the College polled its members by means of a questionnaire. Forty-five per cent (946 members) answered the question, "Do you favour establishing a Fellowship as an additional category of membership?" Of these, "69% were in favour of Fellowship." The Board of Representatives of the College at its meeting in March, 1961, directed "the Committee on Fellowship to proceed with setting up the mechanics of implementation of the plan."*

It is beyond the scope of our study to discuss the advantages and disadvantages of such a higher qualification, except as they are related to the quality of practice. From this point of view we would make one comment. In the explanatory letter that was sent with the questionnaire to the members of the College, the Chairman of the Fellowship Committee, talking of "the pros and cons of a Fellowship Plan," said, "Those who favour its implementation, reason that such a category of membership will raise the standards of general practice."† This may well be so. Those to whom this programme will appeal, however, and those on whose practices it will have an effect are likely to be the practitioners who are least in need of such a stimulus, namely, those whose practices are already of excellent, or at least of satisfactory, quality. The major problem is left untouched by this programme, in that it does not ensure that those whose practices are of unsatisfactory quality are brought up to a satisfactory level.

In this chapter, we have pointed out that the medical schools do not profess to bring the student to the point at which he will be ready to function as an independent general practitioner. The medical field is now so vast that it is thought to be impossible to accomplish this by the time of graduation, or perhaps even by the end of a year of interneship. We have emphasized, also, that, because of the defects inherent in the examination system and especially the all-or-none decision that the system requires of the examiners, it is impossible for this system to ensure that those who go out into practice are ready to assume the full responsibilities of practice. Nor do we consider that making the final examination follow the interneship would solve the problem, since the all-or-none decision would still face the examiners. Our criticisms of the examination system, however, are not to be interpreted as indicating that we favour the abolition of this system, since we believe that this, in spite of its defects, is probably necessary to give some indication of a student's progress in those areas in which it is possible to measure his progress; but we must bear in mind Janeway's warning that, in the clinical years, "examinations . . . have very limited usefulness" (see page 486).

Since it appears impossible, either by means of changes in the

---

*Canadian Medical Association Journal, *84*: 1155, 1156, and 1160, 1961.

†College of General Practice of Canada: A Special Survey Regarding Fellowship, November 8, 1960, p. 1.

training or by means of examinations, to guarantee that a young physician is ready to assume the full responsibilities of an independent practice, we have reached the conclusion that what is required is a change in the organization of medical practice. Today a doctor who goes out into practice on his own accepts, save in the hospital where he may be subject to some measure of control, complete responsibility for his patients from the day when he begins his practice. If he does not recognize the need to have the opinion of someone more skilled than he,* a patient will not be referred unless he asks the doctor to refer him. In an earlier chapter, we pointed out, also (see page 160), that some men indicated to us that they made it difficult for their patients to ask for a more expert opinion or to have certain parts of their care rendered by a specialist. It is probable, in addition, that the amount of responsibility that is assumed by a doctor starting in practice is determined to a great extent by what he thinks is expected of him by his professional colleagues. The very fact that he is *allowed* to assume complete responsibility for a practice tends to suggest to him that he is ready, or at any rate that he should be ready, for such responsibility. This being so, it may seem to him that to ask for advice about clinical problems (as distinct from matters of office organization) may involve too much loss of face, especially if the need for advice recurs with any degree of frequency. We do not think that a young physician should be placed in this position. In fact, we suggest—and we refer the reader back to what Ellis has said of the changes that have occurred in the past half-century (see page 484)— that there is no more justification today for expecting a young doctor to take complete responsiblity, or even a large measure of responsibility, at the beginning of his practice than there would be for putting a newly graduated engineer, or one who had had only a year of practical experience, in charge of a major engineering project. We recommend that the profession give thought to organizing practice in such a way that a young physician would begin with a minimum of responsibility and a maximum of supervision and would work up over a period of time, longer or shorter depending on his individual ability, through positions of increasing responsibility. We suggest further that it should be recognized that different men would vary in their rates of progress and that some might never reach the stage of being ready to accept complete responsibility for a practice but could yet render valuable service in subordinate positions. This recommendation will be elaborated upon in the following chapter.

*See pages 308–313 for our observations on the adequacy of referrals.

# 26 / The Future

One of the major challenges in the field of medical care at the present time has been put succinctly by Joseph T. Wearn:

Our greatest challenge is to develop educational programs and health service mechanisms which will assure that the products of our expanding scientific research will be applied promptly and effectively, in comprehensive care of patients in every community, not just in our most elaborate university medical centers.

This is the concept of Great Medicine with which Alan Gregg challenged this Association . . . in 1952. The challenge is still before us, the need to meet it is urgent, but our time is running out.[*]

With these words, Wearn concluded the Third Alan Gregg Memorial Lecture to the Association of American Medical Colleges in 1960. That a gap exists between the type of medical care possible with our present knowledge and the type of medicine practised by the less proficient members of the profession is abundantly evident from the observations we made of the work being done by the practitioners whom we visited in Ontario and in Nova Scotia. That this problem is widespread is quite clear from what Peterson reported of general practice in North Carolina[†] and from the reports of Collings[‡] and of Taylor[§] about general practice in Britain.

The problem with which we are concerned is how the gap between the best practice and the poorest may be narrowed. We have already suggested steps that might be taken in the matter of medical educa-

[*] J. T. Wearn: Journal of Medical Education, 36: 118, 1961.
[†] O. L. Peterson et al.: Journal of Medical Education, 31, No. 12, Part 2: chapter 3.
[‡] J. S. Collings: The Lancet, 258: 557–568, 1950.
[§] Stephen Taylor: Good General Practice (London: Oxford University Press, 1954), pp. 7–8, 37–38.

tion; of these we shall say no more. In the preceding chapter, we showed that it was probably inevitable that a certain number of candidates would be passed by the examiners and licensed to practise even though they were not ready to assume full responsibility for a practice; and we said, further, that not only would they be permitted to engage in general practice, but they would be virtually forced by circumstances to do so. We suggested that practice should be so organized that a practitioner would begin by assuming a minimum of responsibility under maximum supervision and would progress to greater and greater degrees of responsibility in accordance with his own individual ability. Before considering how practice could be so organized or the advantages that would accrue, we would say that the suggestion that we have made appears to us to be the only way of circumventing the difficulty of the all-or-none decision (this has been discussed at length in chapter 25) that an examiner must make at the present time. By this we mean that, instead of a candidate's either being allowed to go out and take full responsibility for an independent practice (for which he may not be ready) or not being allowed to practise at all (which may not do justice to his readiness to do productive work and to take *some* responsibility), he would assume as much, but only as much, responsibility as he could discharge adequately and would progress in a step-like fashion. In other words, the present single promotion from being allowed no responsibility (or almost none) as a final-year student to being allowed full responsibility as a physician would be replaced by a series of promotions of lesser magnitude. This would apply, not only to his hospital work, but to all of his work.

What we envisage is group practice. When we say this, however, we have in mind something that would be essentially different from most of the groups in existence today. The difference may most easily be made apparent if we consider the fundamental character of present group practice. In a recent book, which is the work of thirty-five contributors in various parts of the United States under the editorship of Edwin P. Jordan, Executive Director of the American Association of Medical Clinics, a "reasonable definition for group practice" is said to be "that adopted by the House of Delegates of the American Medical Association" in 1948: "Group medical practice is the application of medical service by a number of physicians working in systematic association with the joint use of equipment and technical personnel and with centralized administration and financial organization."*

*E. P. Jordan (Editor): The Physician and Group Practice (Chicago: Year Book Publishers, 1958), p. 20.

Missing from this definition, and from other similar ones that occur in the literature on group practice, is any suggestion that those members of the group who are not ready to assume complete responsibility for the care of patients should be working under close supervision and that the ultimate responsibility for care given to each individual patient should rest only with those members of the group who are of proven ability. Rather, the definition that we have quoted concerns itself, as do others, with such matters as equipment, ancillary assistance, and economics. Collings, to whose findings we referred earlier (see pages 8–9), recommended the formation of "basic group-practice units" in Britain, but made no mention of the need for supervision of the less capable members of the group.* Similarly, when each of the practitioners whom we visited was asked to name the advantages of his type of practice, i.e. solo practice or group practice, not one of the fifteen Ontario, or fourteen Nova Scotia, doctors who were practising in groups of two or more suggested that there was an opportunity in this type of practice for the supervision of the less experienced by the more experienced, though one Ontario physician listed, as a disadvantage of having a salaried assistant, the fact that the older man was responsible for the assistant's mistakes (see pages 87–90).

One project that was undertaken with a view to the improvement of the quality of medical care was the establishment of the Hunterdon Medical Center in Hunterdon, New Jersey, where "Continuity of care by the general physician, coupled with guidance of his work at the Center to the extent needed by staff specialists, is the most fascinating and the most questioned aspect of the entire Medical Center development."† Ray E. Trussell, Director of the Center during its formative period and for the first two years after its opening in 1953, in assessing "This new and untried type of medical relationship between the family doctors practicing in small rural communities and specialists practicing only at the Medical Center," says, "Integration of the general practitioner and the specialist in a new type of working relationship . . . has been remarkably successful."‡ This organization, however, while attempting to bring to the community specialist services that were not previously available and while apparently giving some degree of supervision of the work of the general practitioners in hospital, did not exercise any control beyond the confines of the Medical

*J. S. Collings: The Lancet, 258: 577, 1950.
†Ray E. Trussell: Hunterdon Medical Center (Cambridge: Published for the Commonwealth Fund by Harvard University Press, 1956), p. 174.
‡*Ibid.*, pp. 174, 216.

Center. Yet, as we have seen, the greater part of general practice is carried on in the physician's office and in his patients' homes, where inadequate history-taking and examination may have serious consequences; and some of the practitioners visited by us, though they had hospital privileges, seldom set foot in a hospital. That Trussell was well aware that such a development as Hunterdon Medical Center was not the whole answer to the problem of practice of unsatisfactory quality is apparent from his own words:

> . . . an organization such as the Hunterdon Medical Center can do little about the problem of the doctor who has no professional affiliations. The physician who practices in a community but does not belong to a local hospital staff or to the county medical society is, in effect, subject only to the standards maintained by the medical examining board of each state. As a general rule, these standards are minimal, and once a physician has a license rather extreme violations of law or professional conduct can occur before the state licensing agency becomes aware of and undertakes to review his professional conduct.*

We must now explain what we mean when we talk of supervision. We have found that the histories taken by some of the practitioners were excellent but that others ranged from being less than satisfactory to being no more than a mockery of a history. Similarly, the physical examinations that we observed varied from excellent to grossly inadequate (see chapters 16 and 17). Yet all of the practitioners whom we visited had passed the examinations of their respective medical schools, had passed the licensing examinations, and might have been assumed to be capable, and cognizant of the necessity, of carrying out these two types of investigation. Earlier (pages 318–319), we pointed out also that the difficulty of determining the quality of a physician's practice except by direct observation was illustrated by our finding that, in our samples, the mean scores† of the physicians who were members of the College of General Practice of Canada and of those who were not members did not differ significantly, in spite of the standards that the College sets for membership. In view of our findings, we should hope that the young graduate going to work for a group would *not* be assumed to be capable of investigating, and caring for, various types of illness or injury until he had demonstrated his ability to his employers. As he showed that he consistently took satisfactory histories, that he did the type of examination required in the particular case, that he recognized the various physical signs, that he could

*Ibid.*, p. 223.
†The physician's score as a measure of the quality of his practice has been discussed in chapters 16 and 17.

progress from signs and symptoms to diagnosis, and that his suggested treatment of cases was sound and thorough, he could be left more on his own. In the preceding chapter (page 491), we quoted Fuchsig as not being greatly impressed by the three-year period of postgraduate training that had been established for general practitioners in Austria and as thinking that "it would be better to return to the principle of freedom of teaching and of learning without setting time limits, making the acquisition of knowledge a matter of individual responsibility." To what Fuchsig is reported to have said, we would add that an individual's reward, as in other lines of endeavour, should be determined in accordance with his discharge of his responsibility. A young physician who demonstrated his willingness and ability to do sound work should be promoted rapidly to greater measures of responsibility, and his financial remuneration should be increased accordingly. On the other hand, the less capable or less willing should advance more slowly in accordance with the degree of readiness for advancement that they demonstrated. To anyone who might object that, after a course as long as the medical course, a man cannot be kept indefinitely in a subordinate position, we would reply that the man who has, to such an extent, failed to grasp the fundamental principles, or who is so lacking in conscientiousness, that he takes little or no history, does inadequate examinations, and does not base his practice on the scientific principles to which he has been exposed has no right to lay claim to the benefits, including independent practice, that fall to those who are willing and able to give good medical care.

Who would do the supervising of which we have spoken? In a small group, the supervising would be done by the man at the head of the group; in larger groups, the physicians taking the least responsibility would probably be supervised by men in intermediate positions, who would themselves be supervised by the men senior to them. The point of greatest importance, except for the very principle of supervision and graded responsibility, is that the supervision of the the physician who is not yet ready to assume full responsibility should be done by a physician who is both willing and able to give the necessary supervision; otherwise, the so-called "supervision" would be of no value. It would be our hope that the men supervising the work of others would reach their positions, not by virtue of age as such, but by virtue of their ability to discharge the responsibilities of the position. Some of the older men whom we visited certainly did not lack the professional ability to supervise the work of those less able; but others of the older men, as a glance at Table 82 shows (page 319), could better have been the supervised than the supervisors.

Supervision, if it were a fact and were not allowed to become merely a word, with no meaning, would take time, as a result of which the men in the senior positions would have less time available for dealing with patients directly. Yet, as the junior men demonstrated their ability to deal competently with the more common and the less complicated types of case, the senior men would be relieved of the work of a more elementary nature and would be devoting their time to the more serious or complex cases. As we said (page 308), in discussing referrals, a conservative estimate of the percentage of practitioners who were referring fewer patients than the circumstances demanded was approximately 30 per cent in Ontario and in Nova Scotia. In the practices of the poorest practitioners, patient after patient should have been seen by someone more experienced. Similarly, Peterson, speaking of the situation in North Carolina, says, "Some of the less adept physicians relied heavily on their specialist colleagues, thus partly covering their own inadequacies. This was far from common, however." Further on he says, "the inference seems warranted that, in general, specialists are not utilized in a great many situations in which they could be of real value to the patient."[*] We would question, however, whether even those practitioners whose over-all performance is satisfactory but who are not acknowledged experts with a particular type of case should be satisfied to call a case hopeless, or even to continue on with a case that is not progressing satisfactorily, without having a more expert opinion. In this regard, we were interested in the statement that one practitioner made, when we were inquiring about the prestige of the general practitioner in the community, to the effect that more and more people refused to accept a serious or incurable ailment or a prolonged illness unless they had been seen by a specialist (see page 172). The amazing developments of the past decade or two and the increasing difficulty of keeping abreast of the advances (see pages 455–456) only serve to emphasize that referrals should be more frequent than they are. We should hope that, in the type of group practice that we are trying to picture, apparently hopeless cases or cases that were not making satisfactory progress would *automatically* come to the attention of the senior physician in the group. Instead of a junior doctor's having the responsibility of deciding whether or not to ask for a more expert

[*]O. L. Peterson *et al.*: Journal of Medical Education, *31*, No. 12, Part 2: 102, 103, 1956.

opinion—which both presupposes, incorrectly in some practices, that the physician knows when to ask for assistance and probably also involves a loss of face (see page 494)—the onus should be on the senior physician to satisfy himself that those cases not being seen by him are being managed satisfactorily. In other words, the ultimate responsibility should rest with the most senior members of the group.

The group that we have described would ensure that the less capable men were adequately supervised so that they were not taking responsibility for which they were not ready. Such a group would have another advantage over solo practice and over most of the present group practices, in that the most experienced physicians in the group would be devoting the major part of their clinical effort to the patients whose problems most needed their experience, instead of, as at present, spending a great deal of their time on the trivial cases that they were able to handle competently ten, twenty, or thirty years earlier. One of the doctors visited by us said that the majority of the patients coming to his office were "screened" by his assistant, who took care of the routine things (see page 89). The other 28 doctors who were working in association with one or more colleagues gave no indication that the work was apportioned according to the individual doctor's ability.

Since this division of medical work would mean, of course, that, as the physician moved up to a position of greater seniority, the patients whose less serious problems he had looked after would now have to take these to a more junior member of the group, it may be suggested that this would interfere with the doctor-patient relationship and that the patient would resent seeing less of the doctor in whom he had come to have confidence. We doubt whether this would be a serious problem. There is no reason to suppose that a patient cannot form a reasonably close relationship with more than one doctor. It might be that, for the occasional, very delicate matter, he might prefer one of the doctors to the others; but these occasions arise infrequently enough to be handled on an individual basis. It is worth noting that some physicians, at the present time, have their calls taken on certain evenings and weekends by one or two other doctors and that their patients apparently get on satisfactorily with more than just the one doctor.

The next question is who should occupy the senior positions, i.e. assume the ultimate responsibility for the work of the group. By definition, these men must be physicians who are capable of discharging their responsibilities. Those who would be best suited for this would, in our opinion, be physicians having specialist qualifications in internal medicine or those general practitioners who had qualified, not by age or length of practice but by examination, for the Fellowship that the College of General Practice of Canada proposes to establish as a higher qualification (see page 492). It may be that some of those who are at present engaged in practice are averse either to supervising the work of others or to being supervised themselves. Yet, that a system embodying supervision is possible is amply demonstrated by the better teaching hospitals, where such a system of graded responsibility has long existed on the public wards. It may be that the attitude of independence manifested by some doctors, as far as private practice is concerned, is partly, or perhaps largely, a reflection of expectations built up in them by their instructors during their days as students and that a different picture presented in the years of training would prepare them to function well in a differently organized type of practice.

We have described, but it may be worthwhile to recapitulate, the two principal advantages of the type of group practice that we are recommending. These are, first, that, provided that the senior positions were occupied by competent physicians, adequate supervision would ensure that the less experienced physicians were not assuming more responsibility than they were capable of discharging adequately and, secondly, that the abilities of the most competent and experienced practitioners would be used more efficiently than at present, in that these men would be relieved of the burden of trivia and would be free to devote themselves to the more difficult medical problems and to developing the abilities of the men junior to them. Thus the gulf that has been shown to exist between the interneship and practice (pages 398–399, 410) would be bridged, and those physicians who feel at present that there is no possibility of advancement in general practice (see pages 462–465) would know that by their own efforts they could win recognition and could move up to positions of greater responsibility.

The type of group practice that we have described would provide solutions, also, for some of the other problems that we have uncovered in our examination of practice as it exists at present. In chapter 8, we reported our findings about the ways in which the practitioners whom we visited organized their time; in chapter 24, we discussed the problem of time in the doctor's life, including lack of time for reading and other forms of study and lack of time for family, and recommended that the whole matter of the doctor's time should be reconsidered in the light of modern conditions (see pages 457–458, 465, 467–469, 478–479). Group practice would make possible more satisfactory arrangements than can be made in solo practice.

Both from the administrative inefficiency with which some practices were carried on (see pages 76–81) and from the plea that was made by more than one-quarter of the practitioners, both in Ontario and in Nova Scotia, for instruction in medical school in "practical economics," i.e. business methods (see page 346), it was apparent that young physicians are going out unprepared to cope with the non-medical aspects of organizing and carrying on a practice. Whereas the man going into solo practice has to contend with these difficulties just at the time when he has to assume the load of full medical responsibility, his counterpart entering a group would be free to concentrate on his medical work initially and would learn the non-medical aspects of practice as he worked up in the group.

If practice were organized on the basis of the type of group that we have suggested, the sort of professional isolation that we encountered in some of the practitioners' offices (see page 461) would cease to exist. At that time, we quoted William M. Arnott, Professor of Medicine at the University of Birmingham, as emphasizing the importance of avoiding "professional isolation." In addressing the Second World Conference on Medical Education, he went on to emphasize how much a physician's practice may benefit from the criticism of colleagues:

Where doctors are continuously subject to the kindly mutual criticism and approbation of their peers it becomes difficult for them to allow their standards to slip and their minds to crystallize. The circumstance that teaching hospitals are, in general, the best hospitals and that medical teachers constitute in the main the leaders of our profession is due not only to careful initial selection, but to the fact that the teachers work constantly in the fierce light of the critical appraisal of their colleagues and even more so of their students. . . . I hope, therefore, that full attention will be paid to the promotion of professional association, which is much more important than formal refresher courses. This is particularly important for family doctors.*

Similarly, one of our practitioners mentioned, as a disadvantage of solo practice, the lack of a colleague who would be close enough to one to keep a critical eye on the quality of one's work (see page 86).

Another advantage of group practice is that it meets the need that

*W. M. Arnott: Medicine: A Lifelong Study, Proceedings of Second World Conference on Medical Education, Chicago 1959 (New York: World Medical Association, 1961), p. 15.

is felt by some practitioners of not being alone. This was mentioned by some of the practitioners whom we visited (page 88), and, "According to the University of Chicago National Opinion Research Center, three out of four of today's medical students apparently do not want to practice completely alone."* Furthermore, if men of integrity, understanding, and enthusiasm occupied the senior positions in the group, undesirable characteristics such as we observed in one or another practice—lack of self-confidence, lack of concern for patients, lack of knowledge, superficial work arising from greed, gross dishonesty (rare but not non-existent), desire to split fees, and lack of interest in medicine—could, by means of supervision and restriction of responsibility, be controlled or, at least, rendered non-detrimental to the patients.

Finally, if the conditions of general practice are improved in some of the ways that we have indicated, it is to be expected that general practice will become more attractive as a career. Gee and Schumacher, of the Association of American Medical Colleges, who sent a questionnaire to a 50 per cent random sample of the 1958–1959 internes in the United States and received answers from 2,616 internes (83 per cent of the sample), say, "Judging from the expressed intentions of 1958–59 interns, and from trends over the past two decades, the general practitioner is in some danger of becoming extinct."† They point out that 45 per cent of those physicians who graduated from United States medical schools between 1940 and 1944 became general practitioners, 31 per cent of the graduates of 1950 became general practitioners, and 21 per cent of the 1958–1959 internes planned to become general practitioners.

We must now consider briefly how a change could be effected from the present system of practice, mainly solo with some groups (but lacking the essential feature of supervision and graded responsibility), to groups of the type that we have described. If the present system of private practice continues, the formation of such groups could probably be brought about only over a prolonged period of time by means of the active encouragement of the professional societies and of the leaders in medical education. With the increasing interest, however, that the various political parties are showing in problems of medical care, it is questionable how long the present system will survive.

*G. W. Hunter: in E. P. Jordan (Editor): The Physician and Group Practice (Chicago: Year Book Publishers, 1958), p. 40.

†H. H. Gee and C. F. Schumacher: Journal of Medical Education, *36*, No. 4, Part 2: 39, 1961.

Whether the changes that may be brought about in the next few years by legislative action will result in an improvement or in a deterioration in the quality of medical care is likely to depend on the wisdom of all concerned. It is to be hoped that there will not be a struggle between the reactionary and the radical, but rather that men of moderation will arrive at decisions based on calm consideration of the relevant facts. We have emphasized already one point that would have to be borne in mind in the planning of any new system of medical care, namely, that *good* medical care takes time (see page 474). If society is not prepared to pay for the necessary time, it must not complain if the quality of the care is unsatisfactory. Another point about which we wish to say a few words, especially in reference to the group practice that we have suggested, is the fear that the profession has of a bureaucratic, highly regimented system. Having seen the frustration of some of the general practitioners who felt that no advancement was possible in general practice (see pages 462–463), we should have grave misgivings about a centrally controlled system of practice, in which an individual practitioner's fate would be in the hands of an unknown administrator. We are strongly of the belief that, *if* government decides that doctors are to be paid out of public funds, the principle of competition should be preserved in the interest of maintaining the individual doctor's incentive and of stimulating the various groups to maintain and improve the quality of their care. How can there be comprehensive medical care, paid for by the taxpayer, without a high degree of centralization? The pattern exists in the Ontario public school system. Just as each municipality employs its own teachers, so it should be left to each municipality to employ its own doctors. The competition that would exist between municipalities and between various groups within the larger municipalities would be healthy. If a doctor were not treated fairly by a municipality or by the group in which he was working,* he could seek another position. He would be free to move from an undesirable situation, without reference to any central authority, just as a teacher is able to. If the municipality or the particular group acquired a bad reputation for its treatment of its doctors, it would have difficulty obtaining replacements. Similarly, physicians whose work was unsatisfactory would lose their positions. This would tend to maintain and improve the quality of practice.

There is another point to which we would draw attention. Those who favour paying doctors a straight salary sometimes tend to com-

*Matters over which difficulties might arise have been discussed on page 89.

pare them with people in other salaried positions and to suggest that there is no more reason for a doctor's being dissatisfied with this method of payment than for dissatisfaction on the part of other people. Thus Professor John Morgan, of the School of Social Work of the University of Toronto, is quoted as saying, "I don't think there would be any harm in paying the doctor a salary. I'm paid a salary and I don't think I suffer from any lack of initiative at the university."* Similarly, Mrs. Eva Sauve, in a letter to *Maclean's*, says, "Education and health go hand in hand and if the teacher works under government control, why can't the doctor?"† The point that is not stated by either of these persons, a point that we do not remember ever having heard mentioned when salaries for doctors were being discussed, is that the university professor, the school teacher, and the civil servant are employed either to work a specified number of hours or to do a specified amount of work, which can be calculated as likely to require a certain number of hours. These persons, the rest of the time, are free of the demands of their employers, except in unusual circumstances. The fear of the doctor is that he will be subject to unceasing demands day and night. Nor should we consider this fear far-fetched when we recall the statements of some of the Nova Scotia doctors to the effect that the miners whose medical care was provided by a prepayment plan expected to be seen whenever they wished to be seen (page 74). It is one thing to be an employee, whether of government or of a university, so many hours a day and to be able to call one's soul one's own the remaining hours:‡ it is quite a different matter to be the employee of a government twenty-four hours a day. If the doctor is put on salary, it is essential that there be safeguards—perhaps by a system of day and night shifts—against his being on call both day and night or, at the very least, against his being paid an eight hours' salary for twenty-four hours' work.

One other problem with which we must deal, before we leave group practice, is how the group idea could be applied in sparsely settled areas. This is a matter to which comparatively little attention has been given. Yet a few developments are worth noting. We have seen (page 91) that, in Ontario, otolaryngologists and ophthalmologists, and, both in Ontario and in Nova Scotia, radiologists were

*Toronto Daily Star, May 3, 1961, p. 21.
†Maclean's, June 3, 1961, p. 2.
‡Even those whose hours are increased by committee work, interviews, the marking of essays or examination papers, etc., are still able to plan these activities so as to have a large measure of freedom that is not possible for a doctor who is on call continuously.

visiting certain smaller communities once or twice a week on a regular basis. The Rip Van Winkle Clinic in Hudson, New York, which "was founded in an attempt to provide a means whereby people of a relatively poor rural community could be offered the best available medical care at a cost that at least 90 per cent of the people could afford," approached the problem of covering a wide area "by the establishment of branches strategically located throughout the county served."\* The growth of one of the branches is described as follows:

Seven years ago the clinic opened the first branch in Hillsdale, a town roughly 20 miles due east of Hudson. Hillsdale is a town that for many years had three doctors, and then two; but for three years before the establishment of the Rip Van Winkle branch, Hillsdale had no doctors. Today, the branch in Hillsdale has a resident staff of two internists, a pediatrician, and a dentist. It is felt that this staff will take care of approximately 80 per cent of the needs of the surrounding community. At regular specified times during the week specialty clinics are also held at Hillsdale in surgery, obstetrics and gynecology, and psychiatry by men coming out from Hudson. . . .

Through this framework a rural hamlet which for three years had not been able to attract a doctor now has available the services of board-qualified specialists in the basic fields of medicine, surgery, pediatrics, obstetrics and gynecology, psychiatry, and dentistry.†

Another development that illustrates what can be achieved by imaginative planning is Nova Scotia's Obstetrical Emergency Team, which "is available to any doctor in Nova Scotia in any obstetrical emergency, to provide consultation or actual treatment services." After consultation by telephone, "the necessary medical personnel and materials are gathered and the Team proceeds to the local area. The Armed Services co-operate by providing air transport where necessary."‡

We reported earlier (page 455) that one of the practitioners whom we visited emphasized that he did not hesitate to use the long distance telephone to obtain advice from specialists when he needed it. The surprising thing was that, in these days, this method of obtaining expert advice was not more widely used.

There is no doubt that it would be more difficult to apply the group practice idea to some regions than to other, more densely populated, ones. Yet, in an era when men can cross the Atlantic in a few hours

\*C. B. Esselstyn: New England Journal of Medicine, *248*: 488, 493, 1953.
†C. B. Esselstyn: in E. P. Jordan (Editor): The Physician and Group Practice (Chicago: Year Book Publishers, 1958), p. 111.
‡Canada's Health and Welfare, *15*: 6, 7, 1960.

and are reaching now for the moon, it is hard to believe that thought applied to the problem could not overcome the difficulties caused by distances that in these days are greater in the imagination than in reality.

We shall not proceed further with our consideration either of the organization of practice or of its financial arrangements. To discuss these in detail would be pointless and premature both because of the uncertainty that hangs over Canadian medicine at present and because it is our hope that the plan would be flexible rather than rigidly determined. Our purpose has been to set forth the general outline of a type of group practice that, for reasons that we have already discussed, would be likely, in our opinion, to improve the quality of practice. What we have proposed differs from the present concept of group practice in that its essential element would be close supervision of the less experienced physicians and advancement to greater degrees of responsibility and less supervision only if and as the individual demonstrated his readiness for such advancement.

We turn now from organization to consider what the content of general practice should be. If we assume that the content should be what a practitioner is capable of handling satisfactorily, then the question will be answered on an individual basis in the system of group practice that we have outlined, since supervision will ensure that a doctor remains within the limits of his own capabilities. Under the present system, in which an individual physician can go out and assume full responsibility from the start, with no restrictions except those that may be set by the hospitals, it is of much greater importance to consider what general practice should encompass, especially in the matter of surgery since this is most subject to control by the hospitals.

First, we shall hear what the general practitioners themselves had to say about what general practice should include. Each one was asked specifically whether general practice in *his* community should include adult medicine, paediatrics, obstetrics, psychiatry, minor surgery, and major surgery; whether general practice should include anaesthesia was asked of each of the Nova Scotia doctors and of 25 of the 44 Ontario doctors. Every one of the 86 practitioners answered in the affirmative for adult medicine and for minor surgery. All but 1, an Ontario doctor, answered in the affirmative for obstetrics; and all but 2, one in each province, for paediatrics. Seventy-nine per cent

TABLE 104

OPINIONS OF ONTARIO AND NOVA SCOTIA PHYSICIANS ABOUT WHETHER THE *Future* GENERAL PRACTITIONER SHOULD BE TRAINED TO PERFORM VARIOUS SURGICAL PROCEDURES

| | Ontario | | | | Nova Scotia | | | |
|---|---|---|---|---|---|---|---|---|
| | Physicians who said that general practice should include major surgery: | | Physicians who said that general practice should not include major surgery:* | | Physicians who said that general practice should include major surgery: | | Physicians who said that general practice should not include major surgery: | |
| | Number of physicians answering | | Number of physicians answering | | Number of physicians answering | | Number of physicians answering | |
| Surgical procedure | Yes | No | Yes | No | Yes | No | Yes | No |
| Appendectomy | 9 | 0 | 8 | 15 | 17 | 1 | 16 | 8 |
| Cholecystectomy | 2 | 7 | 1 | 22 | 11‡ | 7 | 2‡ | 22 |
| Repair of inguinal hernia | 9 | 0 | 6 | 17 | 17 | 1 | 12 | 12 |
| Caesarean section | 8 | 1 | 3 | 20 | 14 | 4 | 14‡ | 10 |
| Dilatation and curettage of uterus | 9 | 0 | 16 | 7 | 18 | 0 | 21 | 3 |
| Haemorrhoidectomy | 8 | 1 | 12 | 11 | 17 | 1 | 16 | 8 |
| Amputation of finger or toe | 9 | 0 | 17 | 6 | 18 | 0 | 19 | 5 |
| Tendon suture† | 7 | 2 | 8 | 15 | 18 | 0 | 17 | 7 |
| Removal of embedded foreign body from cornea | 6 | 3 | 11 | 12 | 12 | 6 | 16 | 8 |
| Tonsillectomy and adenoidectomy | 9 | 0 | 16 | 7 | 16 | 2 | 18 | 6 |
| Tracheotomy | 9 | 0 | 20 | 3 | 16‡ | 2 | 21 | 3 |
| Myringotomy | 9 | 0 | 16 | 7 | 9 | 9 | 11 | 13 |
| Closure of perforated peptic ulcer | 8 | 1 | — | — | 13 | 5 | 8‡ | 16 |
| Subtotal gastrectomy | 0 | 9 | — | — | 3 | 15 | 1‡ | 23 |
| Relief of intestinal obstruction —without resection | 4 | 5 | — | — | 12‡ | 6 | 5‡ | 19 |
| Relief of intestinal obstruction —with resection | 4 | 5 | — | — | 9‡ | 9 | 1 | 23 |
| Exploratory laparotomy | 3 | 6 | — | — | 11 | 7 | 4 | 20 |
| Abdominoperineal excision | 0 | 9 | — | — | 2 | 16 | 0 | 24 |
| Hysterectomy | 4 | 5 | — | — | 10 | 8 | 2 | 22 |
| Suprapubic prostatectomy | 0 | 9 | — | — | 6 | 12 | 3 | 21 |
| Radical mastectomy | 1 | 8 | — | — | 4 | 14 | 0 | 24 |
| Amputation of lower extremity | 6 | 3 | — | — | 15‡ | 3 | 5 | 19 |
| Open reduction and fixation of long-bone fracture | 2§ | 7 | — | — | 10‡ | 8 | 2 | 22 |
| Management of fracture and dislocation of cervical spine | 1 | 8 | — | — | 6 | 12 | 4 | 20 |
| Management of depressed fracture of skull | 2 | 7 | — | — | 8 | 10 | 1 | 23 |

*Of the 35 who said that general practice should not include major surgery, only 23 were questioned about the items listed.

†Of the 50 physicians who gave affirmative answers, 7 specified "extensor" tendons.

‡In each case, 1 physician specified that the operation should be done only in an emergency.

§One of these physicians added "no big ones."

of the Nova Scotia practitioners and 98 per cent of those in Ontario said that general practice should include psychiatry, though several of the Ontario doctors said that the psychiatric work undertaken by a general practitioner should be "limited." Forty-five per cent of the Nova Scotia physicians and 48 per cent of those who were questioned in Ontario would include anaesthesia in the work of a general practitioner; but several made such remarks as that the type of anaesthetic work should be limited or that it should be done under supervision for the first year or so.

Twenty per cent of the practitioners whom we visited in Ontario and 43 per cent of those in Nova Scotia said that general practice should include major surgery. The difference is statistically significant ($p < 0.05$).* In neither province, however, did the various age groups differ significantly in their answers about major surgery. Of the 9 Ontario doctors who said that general practice should include major surgery, 4 added such qualifying comments as that the major surgery should be "limited," that it should be after a second year of postgraduate hospital training, or that it should be conditional upon the physician's satisfying the hospital administration and the department head regarding his qualifications. One older, and very competent, Ontario practitioner, who said that general practice should not include major surgery, commented that there should be more teaching of minor surgical technique but that "the day of the G.P. doing major surgery is going."

In the early stages of the Survey in Ontario, those practitioners who said that general practice should not include major surgery were not questioned further, whereas those who said that it should include major surgery were asked to indicate which operations, of those listed in Table 104, "the *future* general practitioner should be trained to perform." As time went on, however, because we began to suspect that different physicians held quite different opinions about what was major and what was minor, those who said that general practice should not include major surgery were asked whether the future general practitioner should be taught the operations that are listed in the upper portion of Table 104. Of the 35 Ontario doctors who said that general practice should not include major surgery, 23 were asked about these twelve operations. In Nova Scotia, every one of the doctors visited was asked about all of the operations listed in Table 104, regardless of whether he had said that general practice should or should not include major surgery.

*This is explained on pages 32–33.

There are a few points in Table 104 to which we wish particularly to call attention. The finding that, of all the Ontario doctors who were questioned specifically and of those up to thirty-five years of age who were questioned, approximately half believed that the future general practitioner should not be trained to repair an inguinal hernia or to remove an appendix, is strong evidence that the day of the general practitioner's doing major surgery is passing, at least in Ontario. That Nova Scotia practitioners, on the other hand, are more of the opinion that general practice should include major surgery is suggested by the finding that, when questioned about appendectomy, cholecystectomy, and Caesarean section, the percentage of Nova Scotia physicians who thought that the future general practitioner should be trained to perform each of these operations was significantly greater than the corresponding percentage of Ontario practitioners ($p < 0.05$). Finally, it is to be noted that, of the 23 Ontario doctors who said that general practice in the future should not include major surgery, 8 said that the future general practitioner should be trained to perform appendectomies and 1 that he should be trained even for cholecystectomies; and that, of the 24 Nova Scotia physicians who said that general practice should not include major surgery, 16 would have the future general practitioner trained to do appendectomies, 2 would have him trained to do cholecystectomies, and 1 would include even subtotal gastrectomy. These answers can be interpreted only as indicating that some of the general practitioners do not recognize the major nature of these operations. Indeed, one physician, when asked about cholecystectomy, commented, "That's an easy procedure"; and another, as we reported earlier (page 118), told us that this operation was not "major surgery" in the estimation of the Credentials Committee of his hospital. On the other hand, several of the physicians in each province said that one should not open the abdomen unless one were prepared to cope with any situation that one might find. One physician who said that a general practitioner should not be trained to perform appendectomies pointed out that an appendectomy may be "very simple" or may be "very difficult"; and another who was opposed to the general practitioner's doing appendectomies said that sometimes on entering the abdomen the physician finds something other than appendicitis.

Because we regard this as a matter of importance and because we have so frequently heard the appendectomy referred to as a "simple operation," which a general practitioner should be able to do himself, we think it worthwhile to tell of three cases of "acute appendicitis" that we encountered during our days in training. In the first case, which we observed as a medical student, the surgeon was so certain of his diagnosis that he opened the abdomen by a McBurney incision, which gave adequate exposure of the region of the appendix but not of the remainder of the abdomen. The abdominal cavity contained fluid, but the appendix was found to be normal. Making a mid-line incision, which allowed an adequate examination of the whole abdomen, the surgeon found that the patient had a cancer of the stomach, which had perforated. The closing of the perforation was not easy, because the surrounding cancerous tissue was so friable that the sutures tended to pull out. In this case, the surgeon was a man of sufficient skill to be able to deal with a condition that he had not expected to meet.

The second case was that of a girl in her teens with what was diagnosed as perfectly straighforward acute appendicitis. We were interning and were permitted to operate, under supervision of course, because it was unlikely that we should ever have the opportunity of beginning on a simpler case than this. We entered the abdomen without difficulty, to find that the appendix was normal but that the adjacent caecum was involved in an acute inflammatory process, which, quite understandably, had caused the same signs and symptoms as would acute appendicitis but the removal of which was a formidable task. The surgeon who had been supervising our first "simple" appendectomy took over. He completed a resection of a portion of the bowel about two hours later. The only other appendix that we were to be allowed to remove, again under close supervision, we were unable to locate. When our supervisor became impatient and took over from us, it took him the better part of half an hour to mobilize an appendix which was the cause of the patient's illness but which was firmly bound down behind the ascending colon.

Those three experiences left us with a great respect for the so-called "simple appendix" and with a conviction that a physician should not open a patient's abdomen—except when no qualified surgeon is available to handle an extreme emergency—unless he is prepared to deal with *any* condition that he may encounter. In the southern part of Ontario today, there can be few communities that are so remote as to justify a practitioner's undertaking surgery for which he is not trained.* Even in the north, areas that were once extremely inaccessible are becoming less and less so with improved methods of

---

*See pages 128–129 for a description of the extent of the practitioners' training in surgery.

transportation. In Nova Scotia, also, the fact that an Obstetrical Emergency Team has been established to deal with obstetrical emergencies (see page 507) points to the fact that remote parts of the province are no longer as isolated as they once were and suggests that it may no longer be necessary for those who are not fully qualified to undertake major surgery. Physicians who undertake to practise in really inaccessible areas should probably have fairly extensive training in surgery.

Because we have expressed quite strongly our opinion that a man who has not had extensive training in surgery should not be doing abdominal surgery, it is necessary that we state quite explicitly that this opinion is not based on observations that we made of the surgery being done by the general practitioners whom we visited. As we stated earlier (see page 305), the amount of surgery that we observed was too little to enable us to form any opinion about the quality of the general practitioners' surgery.

In the future, we believe that a physician to whom a patient goes first with his complaint—whether he is called a general practitioner or not is of little moment—should make internal medicine, adult and paediatric, the centre of his practice and should be thoroughly competent in these before he assumes full responsibility for practice. Probably there is no reason why he should not include obstetrics in his practice if he so wishes. Though we did not see enough deliveries to assess this portion of the obstetrical work of the general practitioner and though some practitioners were deficient in their handling of pre- and post-natal care, we saw enough good pre- and post-natal care to be convinced that, on the average, a general practitioner can be expected to handle uncomplicated cases satisfactorily. We have already indicated our opposition to a general practitioner's doing major surgery unless he has had much more training for it than the great majority of general practitioners have had. Minor surgery, on the other hand, by which we mean surgery of the office or outpatient-department variety, would logically be part of a general practitioner's work, though it was apparent from what the practitioners said that a physician-in-training needs much more instruction than our practitioners had in minor surgery.

In these days, much emphasis is put on "comprehensive" care, "holistic" medicine, dealing with the "whole" patient, giving attention to social and psychological factors, etc. At the risk of seeming to advise a backward step, we wish to sound a note of caution. Awareness of the importance of these new areas of action should not make us forgetful of the physical part of medicine, which should be the central area of medical practice. We say that the physical should be at the centre of medical practice because no one else but the physician is trained to deal with the physical aspects of illness, whereas there are others, including social workers, clergymen, and lawyers, who can deal with some of the other areas with which medicine is tending to concern itself. It is our impression that those physicians who talk most in terms of comprehensive medicine are those whose practices are of good quality, who perhaps do not realize that some of the practitioners, as we discovered, have not succeeded in coping with medicine's central area, let alone its periphery.

As we stated in an earlier chapter (page 462), we are strongly of the belief that a general practitioner should continue to treat his patients in hospital, primarily because to exclude him from the hospital would tend to isolate him professionally. In saying this, we are apprehensive, not only lest general practitioners might be excluded from the hospitals under a government-controlled medical plan, but lest hospital privileges should ever be refused those general practitioners who are not associated with the College of General Practice of Canada. One of the practitioners whom we visited told us that membership in the College of General Practice was required by his hospital of any general practitioner who wished to be on the staff of the hospital. Furthermore, in a "summary of the transactions of the Board of Representatives" of the College of General Practice at their meetings held in March, 1961, it is stated that the chairman of the College's Committee on Hospitals "summarized some basic standards" for departments of general practice in hospitals. Included among the standards is the statement, "members, or most of them [i.e., members of a hospital's department of general practice], should be members of the College of General Practice or have equivalent postgraduate training."* Even more recently, Irwin W. Bean, President Elect of the College, has said, "Many [i.e., many hospitals] are including in their by-laws, the requirement that senior members of the general practice department must be members of the College of General Practice of Canada."† Though such a policy is laudable from the point of view of raising the standards of hospital practice, we are concerned lest exclusion of the poorer practitioners from the hospitals would, by isolating them from the most capable members of the profession,

*Journal of the College of General Practice of Canada, 7: 7, 5, 1961.
†I. W. Bean: Journal of the College of General Practice of Canada, 8: 3, 14, 1961.

depress the quality of their work even further. Unless these practitioners are to be barred from practice completely, no step should be taken that will increase their professional isolation. Rather, every effort should be made to bring them into closer contact with the best of medical practice.

We agree with W. Victor Johnston, Executive Director of the College of General Practice of Canada, who has recently said, "The day of the 'solo' general practitioner is gone."* It is not enough, however, to replace him with a group of practitioners whose practices, in effect, continue to be "solo" as far as responsibility is concerned. We have demonstrated, in chapter 17, that a significant proportion of the present general practice is not adequate. It is unlikely that educational changes by themselves will more than partially correct this or that changes in the methods of paying for medical care, either the extension of private prepayment plans or a comprehensive government plan, will bring about improvement in quality unless attention is paid specifically to quality. We have shown, also (page 318; Table 80), that, on the average, the work of the physicians who were engaging in group practice—i.e., group practice as usually defined (see page 496), with little or no supervision or gradation of responsibility—did not differ significantly in quality from the work of the solo practitioners. The primary need, as far as practice is concerned, appears to be a change in its organization, so that a young physician who is not ready to assume the responsibilities of an independent practice would not be allowed—indeed forced—to do so but would be enabled and required to work up under supervision from a minimum of responsibility in accordance with his own abilities. We have suggested, in broad outline, how this could be achieved in a different type of group practice.

*W. V. Johnston (Editorial Comment): College of General Practice (Medicine) of Canada Bulletin, 7: 2, 9, 1960.

# CONCLUSION

# Conclusion

We have completed our examination of general practice. That the points of importance may be seen in proper perspective, however, it remains for us to take a final look back at the ground that we have covered.

The goals that we had in mind when we began our study were stated in full in chapter 1 (pages 7–8). In summary, these were to determine the content and the quality of the work of general practitioners, to study the factors that have an effect upon quality of practice, and to make such recommendations as seemed indicated by our findings. The College of General Practice of Canada, which first conceived of studying general practice in this country, and the Steering Committee, which took the steps that brought the study into being, both hoped originally that it would be possible to carry the study into all the provinces of Canada. Why this was not possible was reported in chapter 1 (page 12). We refer to it here in order to remind the reader that the statements that we have made about the practitioners and about the quality of their practices relate only to the two provinces that we were able to study, Ontario and Nova Scotia. How greatly or how little the other provinces differ from these two, we have no way of knowing. On the other hand, though our observations were limited to two provinces, we believe that much of what we have said about the problems of medical education and of medical practice is as applicable to the other provinces as to Ontario and Nova Scotia.

Though we have presented the Ontario and the Nova Scotia findings together, we have been interested in studying each of the provinces for its own sake rather than for the sake of comparison with the other.

For this reason, little space has been devoted to discussion of similarities and differences between the two groups of practitioners. There is one point, however, that we would call to the reader's attention, namely, the remarkable similarity between the two groups with respect to many of the items studied.

In chapters 3–14, in which we tried to picture in their natural setting the men who do the work of general practice, probably the most striking single finding, in each province, was the endless variation existing among them. *The* general practitioner is merely a figment; the reality is many different practitioners.

The content and the volume of the practitioners' work were examined in detail in chapter 15. All but the occasional practice included adult medicine, paediatrics, obstetrics, and minor surgery, though the volume of these varied greatly from one practice to another. Only one-third of the Ontario practitioners, but almost two-fifths of those in Nova Scotia, did abdominal surgery; many of the rest did excisions of tonsils and adenoids and uterine curettage. Anaesthesia was a particular interest of 14 per cent of the Ontario practitioners; in Nova Scotia, 33 per cent gave more than occasional anaesthetics, though only 10 per cent professed a particular interest in anaesthesia; but the remaining physicians in the two provinces gave general anaesthetics only occasionally. For reasons that have been given (page 286), it was not possible to form a clear picture of the psychiatric portion of the general practitioners' work.

The quality of the practice observed by us varied from excellent to extremely poor. The criteria upon which we based our assessments and the observations that we made have been described in detail in chapters 16 and 17 respectively. In summary, the evaluations were based upon the medical and paediatric work and the pre- and post-natal part of the obstetrical work done by the practitioners. We were unable to assess the quality of the anaesthesia, the surgery (except the diagnostic part), or the psychiatry, though we have made certain observations about the last (see pages 306–307). Our assessment of obstetrical care was limited, by force of circumstances, to pre- and post-natal care. Both in Ontario and in Nova Scotia, some of the practices that we visited were considered definitely satisfactory and some so unsatisfactory as likely to expose the patients to serious risks; the remainder could not be labelled unequivocally as either satisfactory or unsatisfactory. Though the true percentages of satisfactory and unsatisfactory practices in each of the two provinces may differ considerably from the percentages (see page 313) that we found in the relatively small samples with which we were dealing, yet the evidence is strongly suggestive that there are an appreciable number of practices of unsatisfactory quality both in Ontario and in Nova Scotia (see page 314). The deficiencies that we observed in the practices did not relate to recent discoveries or rare diseases but to the fundamentals of clinical medicine (see page 315). Pre- and post-natal care, though markedly deficient in some cases, appeared, in each province, to be handled more capably, on the average, than the rest of the general practitioners' work. In each province, in approximately 30 per cent of the practices, at a conservative estimate, patients were not referred as often as they should have been for more expert advice or treatment; and, in some practices, patient after patient should have been referred.

We have, of necessity, given more attention to the unsatisfactory than to the satisfactory. This was partly because it was our duty to discover whether practice was in need of improvement and, if so, how it could be improved rather than to attempt to establish that no improvement was needed. Also, as Becker and his associates have pointed out, in describing the procedure used by them in their very recent sociological study of medical students, "The point of concentrating on instances where things do not work well is that it helps one discover how things work when they do work well, and these are discoveries that are more difficult to make in situations of harmony because people are more likely to take them for granted and less likely to discuss them."* We too have concentrated on the unsatisfactory, but we wish to emphasize that many of the practitioners were giving good care and some of them care of a very high calibre indeed.

After examining quality of practice in relation to many of the facts known to us about the practitioners, we are unable to attribute to any one cause the unsatisfactory practice that we observed; nor is this surprising when we recollect the great diversity that we found among the physicians. Rather, it is our conclusion that the quality of a practitioner's work is the resultant of many influences, including factors in his undergraduate and postgraduate education, the conditions under which practice is carried on today, and, not least in importance, personal characteristics of the individual physician.

As we have discussed these influences in detail in earlier chapters, we have made numerous suggestions of steps that might be taken to improve the quality of practice. To recapitulate, in the realm of

*Howard S. Becker *et al.*: Boys in White: Student Culture in Medical School (University of Chicago Press, 1961), p. 21.

education, we have recommended more effective counselling of medical students (chapter 19), we have suggested that undergraduate and postgraduate medical education should be intensively studied (chapters 21, 22), and we have emphasized the pressing need to face the question whether an interne or resident is in the hospital primarily to meet his own educational needs or primarily to meet the service needs of the hospital (chapter 23). We have considered conditions obtaining in practice, especially as they relate to a doctor's attempt to keep abreast of advances in medicine, and have recommended that the whole problem of a doctor's time should be reconsidered in the light of modern conditions and that studies should be made of the economic aspects of practices of *good* quality to provide a basis for determining rates of remuneration (chapter 24). We have considered whether a young physician, on completing his training, is ready to assume the full responsibility of an independent practice, and have found that there is no guarantee that he is ready but that circumstances may force him to accept responsibilities which are beyond his capabilities (chapter 25). In view of this and of certain characteristics that we observed in one or another of the practitioners whom we visited (chapter 14), we have come, after much deliberation, to the conclusion that, in many cases, it would be in the best interests of both patient and physician that solo practice should be replaced by group practice. We have emphasized, however, that we do not mean group practice as generally defined but groups in which a young physician would start with a minimum of responsibility and a maximum of supervision and would progress to greater measures of responsibility in his own time according to his own willingness and ability or, lacking these, would remain static (chapter 26).

If the changes that we have suggested are to be implemented, there must be understanding and co-operation on the part of all those concerned, namely, the individual members of the medical profession, the professional organizations, the medical schools, the hospitals, both teaching and non-teaching, the members of the public, who are the recipients of the care rendered by the doctors and who must pay for it either directly or indirectly, and finally the various governments, which appear likely to have a greater say about the way in which medical care is to be provided and paid for. In particular, we consider it a responsibility of government to recognize two hidden costs, which are hidden because they are borne by two groups instead of being shared among all those who benefit. We refer to the fact that some practising physicians are giving a large amount of time to medical teaching for virtually nothing (see page 373) and to the fact that internes and residents, who have been described as "the backbone of medical care in most of our university hospitals" (see page 427), are paid only a fraction of what their services are worth. The special responsibilities of the medical profession, in our opinion, are to spare no pains to bring to the attention of government those situations that require government action and to consider whether the present system of practice makes the best use of the available medical man-power or whether some physicians are being overloaded with responsibility while the potentialities of others are being wasted.

In the past year or two, in discussing our findings on quality of practice with colleagues, including members of medical school staffs, whose own practices are of undoubted excellence, we have been disturbed to find that frequently these men, perhaps because they do not really know what the over-all picture of practice is, have tended to respond to our descriptions with the statement that there always has been some poor practice and that there always will be and to exhort us not to be disturbed by the poor practice that we have seen.

That practice of unsatisfactory quality has existed in the past is probably beyond doubt. Sixty years ago, Osler, when he was Professor of Medicine at Johns Hopkins University, related the following incident:

. . . a physician living within an hour's ride of the Surgeon-General's Library brought to me his little girl, aged twelve. The diagnosis of infantile myxoedema required only half a glance. In placid contentment he had been practising twenty years in "Sleepy Hollow" and not even when his own flesh and blood was touched did he rouse from an apathy deep as Rip Van Winkle's sleep. In reply to questions: No, he had never seen anything in the journals about the thyroid gland; he had seen no pictures of cretinism or myxoedema; in fact his mind was a blank on the whole subject. He had not been a reader, he said, but he was a practical man with very little time.*

Just as there has probably always been some poor practice, so we are not so naive as to imagine that there will not be some poor practice in the future. If those who should be concerned sit back, however, and say that poor care should just be accepted as part of the natural order of things and that we should not worry about it, then there will be more poor practice than there need be. Half a century ago, Abraham Flexner, by his classic study of medical schools, brought to light the shockingly poor "education" being offered by some

*Sir W. Osler: Aequanimitas with Other Addresses . . . (2nd ed.; London: H. K. Lewis & Co. Ltd., 1925), p. 221.

of the medical schools in the United States and in Canada.* It was precisely because the leaders of medicine did not accept the existing state of affairs as inevitable that the unsatisfactory conditions revealed by Flexner were brought to an end. Though our findings are not comparable to Flexner's, nonetheless the poor practice that exists is a challenge to the medical profession.

Though it is not likely that unsatisfactory practice will ever be eradicated completely, yet, unless there is an ideal towards which to strive, progress is not to be hoped for. We suggest that the ills that afflict medical education and medical practice make as legitimate a demand for study and correction as do the individual diseases that are subjected to such intensive scrutiny. In fact, it may not be too much to say that, in the long run, the recipients of medical care may benefit less from the elucidation of an obscure and rare disease than from a better organized and more thorough application of existing knowledge.

*Abraham Flexner: Medical Education in the United States and Canada (The Carnegie Foundation for the Advancement of Teaching, Bulletin Number Four, New York City, 1910).

# APPENDIX A

International Classification of Diseases, 1955 Revision: World Health Organization,
Palais des Nations, Geneva, 1957

| Three-digit numbers | Category | Number of visits in Ontario | | Number of visits in Nova Scotia | |
|---|---|---|---|---|---|
| | | Non-hospital | Hospital | Non-hospital | Hospital |
| | I. *Infective and parasitic diseases* | | | | |
| 001 | Respiratory tuberculosis with mention of occupational disease of lung | — | — | 1 | — |
| 002 | Pulmonary tuberculosis | — | — | 4 | 1 |
| 003 | Pleural tuberculosis | 2 | 1 | — | 7 |
| 008 | Tuberculosis, unspecified site | 3 | — | 3 | — |
| 012 | Tuberculosis of bones and joints, active or unspecified | 1 | — | — | — |
| 016 | Tuberculosis of genito-urinary system | — | — | 2 | — |
| 023 | Other cardiovascular syphilis | — | — | 1 | — |
| 030 | Acute or unspecified gonorrhoea | 5 | — | 4 | — |
| 044 | Brucellosis (undulant fever) | — | 1 | — | — |
| 048 | Unspecified forms of dysentery | 2 | — | — | — |
| 049 | Food poisoning (infection and intoxication) | 2 | — | 3 | — |
| 050 | Scarlet fever | 1 | — | 6 | — |
| 051 | Streptococcal sore throat | 9 | — | 32 | — |
| 055 | Diphtheria | — | — | 1 | — |
| 056 | Whooping cough | 2 | — | 13 | 2 |
| 061 | Tetanus | — | — | — | 5 |
| 064 | Other bacterial diseases | 4 | — | — | — |
| 070 | Vincent's infection | 1 | — | 2 | 6 |
| 082 | Acute infectious encephalitis | 1 | — | 1 | 4 |
| 085 | Measles | 23 | — | 7 | 2 |
| 086 | Rubella (German measles) | 3 | — | — | — |
| 087 | Chickenpox | 6 | — | 8 | — |
| 088 | Herpes zoster | 10 | 2 | 4 | 2 |
| 089 | Mumps | 9 | — | 3 | — |
| 092 | Infectious hepatitis | 4 | — | 17 | 4 |
| 093 | Glandular fever (infectious mononucleosis) | 1 | — | 1 | 3 |
| 096 | Other diseases attributable to viruses | 5 | — | 4 | — |
| 122 | Other protozoal diseases | 1 | — | 2 | — |
| 130 | Infestation with worms of other, mixed, and unspecified type | 3 | — | 6 | — |
| 131 | Dermatophytosis | 16 | — | 13 | 3 |
| 134 | Other fungus infections | 4 | — | 6 | — |
| 135 | Scabies | 1 | — | 6 | — |
| 138 | Other infective and parasitic diseases | — | — | 3 | 1 |
| | II. *Neoplasms* | | | | |
| 140 | Malignant neoplasm of lip | 1 | — | — | — |
| 142 | Malignant neoplasm of salivary gland | 1 | — | 2 | — |
| 151 | Malignant neoplasm of stomach | 1 | — | 4 | 14 |

*4,309 office, home, and other non-hospital visits made by 43 Ontario physicians during a total of 290 days; 1,124 hospital visits made by 41 Ontario physicians during a total of 275 days; and 3,583 office, home, and other non-hospital visits and 1,591 hospital visits made by 42 Nova Scotia physicians during a total of 253 days.

| Three-digit numbers | Category | Number of visits in Ontario | | Number of visits in Nova Scotia | |
|---|---|---|---|---|---|
| | | Non-hospital | Hospital | Non-hospital | Hospital |
| 153 | Malignant neoplasm of large intestine, except rectum | 3 | 6 | 3 | 6 |
| 154 | Malignant neoplasm of rectum | 3 | 2 | — | — |
| 155 | Malignant neoplasm of biliary passages and of liver (stated to be primary site) | — | — | — | 6 |
| 157 | Malignant neoplasm of pancreas | — | 6 | — | — |
| 158 | Malignant neoplasm of peritoneum | 1 | — | — | — |
| 162 | Malignant neoplasm of bronchus and trachea, and of lung specified as primary | 1 | — | — | — |
| 163 | Malignant neoplasm of lung, unspecified as to whether primary or secondary | — | — | 1 | — |
| 170 | Malignant neoplasm of breast | 4 | 4 | 4 | 7 |
| 171 | Malignant neoplasm of cervix uteri | — | — | — | 4 |
| 172 | Malignant neoplasm of corpus uteri | — | — | 1 | — |
| 174 | Malignant neoplasm of uterus, unspecified | — | — | — | 1 |
| 175 | Malignant neoplasm of ovary, Fallopian tube, and broad ligament | 1 | — | — | — |
| 176 | Malignant neoplasm of other and unspecified female genital organs | — | — | 2 | — |
| 177 | Malignant neoplasm of prostate | 1 | — | 2 | 7 |
| 181 | Malignant neoplasm of bladder and other urinary organs | 1 | — | — | — |
| 190 | Malignant melanoma of skin | — | — | — | 5 |
| 191 | Other malignant neoplasm of skin | — | — | 3 | — |
| 194 | Malignant neoplasm of thyroid gland | — | — | — | 2 |
| 196 | Malignant neoplasm of bone (including jaw bone) | 1 | — | — | 1 |
| 199 | Malignant neoplasm of other and unspecified sites | 5 | 7 | 3 | 11 |
| 200 | Lymphosarcoma and reticulosarcoma | 2 | — | — | 6 |
| 203 | Multiple myeloma (plasmocytoma) | 3 | — | 1 | 1 |
| 204 | Leukaemia and aleukaemia | 4 | 2 | 6 | 2 |
| 210 | Benign neoplasm of buccal cavity and pharynx | 1 | — | 1 | — |
| 213 | Benign neoplasm of breast | — | 1 | — | — |
| 214 | Uterine fibromyoma | 2 | 1 | 1 | — |
| 215 | Other benign neoplasm of uterus | 4 | 5 | 1 | 1 |
| 216 | Benign neoplasm of ovary | 3 | — | — | — |
| 217 | Benign neoplasm of other female genital organs | 1 | — | — | 1 |
| 220 | Benign melanoma of skin | — | — | 2 | — |
| 221 | Pilonidal cyst | — | 1 | 3 | 10 |
| 222 | Other benign neoplasm of skin | 1 | — | 1 | — |
| 225 | Benign neoplasm of bone and cartilage | 3 | — | 2 | — |
| 226 | Lipoma | 2 | — | 1 | 1 |
| 227 | Other benign neoplasm of muscular and connective tissue | 1 | — | — | — |
| 228 | Haemangioma and lymphangioma | 1 | — | 1 | — |
| 229 | Benign neoplasm of other and unspecified organs and tissues | 1 | — | 1 | — |
| 230 | Neoplasm of unspecified nature of digestive organs | 1 | 1 | — | — |
| 231 | Neoplasm of unspecified nature of respiratory organs | 2 | 1 | — | — |
| 232 | Neoplasm of unspecified nature of breast | 4 | — | — | — |

| Three-digit numbers | Category | Number of visits in Ontario | | Number of visits in Nova Scotia | |
|---|---|---|---|---|---|
| | | Non-hospital | Hospital | Non-hospital | Hospital |
| 237 | Neoplasm of unspecified nature of brain and other parts of nervous system | 2 | — | — | — |
| 238 | Neoplasm of unspecified nature of skin and musculoskeletal system | 3 | — | — | 4 |
| 239 | Neoplasm of unspecified nature of other and unspecified organs | — | 1 | — | 2 |
| | III. *Allergic, endocrine system, metabolic, and nutritional diseases* | | | | |
| 240 | Hay fever | 39 | 1 | 1 | — |
| 241 | Asthma | 63 | 19 | 30 | 14 |
| 242 | Angioneurotic oedema | 1 | — | 1 | — |
| 243 | Urticaria | 9 | 1 | 4 | — |
| 244 | Allergic eczema | 3 | — | 2 | — |
| 245 | Other allergic disorders | 35 | — | 13 | — |
| 251 | Non-toxic nodular goitre | 2 | — | — | — |
| 252 | Thyrotoxicosis with or without goitre | 11 | — | 6 | 1 |
| 253 | Myxoedema and cretinism | 15 | 2 | 5 | — |
| 254 | Other diseases of thyroid gland | 4 | — | 1 | 2 |
| 260 | Diabetes mellitus | 57 | 49 | 31 | 43 |
| 272 | Diseases of pituitary gland | — | 1 | 1 | — |
| 274 | Diseases of adrenal glands | — | — | 3 | — |
| 276 | Testicular dysfunction | 1 | — | — | — |
| 277 | Polyglandular dysfunction and other diseases of endocrine glands | — | — | 2 | — |
| 286 | Other avitaminoses and nutritional deficiency states | 8 | — | 2 | — |
| 287 | Obesity, not specified as of endocrine origin | 48 | — | 18 | 2 |
| 288 | Gout | 1 | — | 2 | — |
| 289 | Other metabolic diseases | 1 | — | 1 | — |
| | IV. *Diseases of the blood and blood-forming organs* | | | | |
| 290 | Pernicious and other hyperchromic anaemias | 40 | — | 18 | 5 |
| 291 | Iron deficiency anaemias (hypochromic anaemias) | 14 | — | 8 | — |
| 292 | Other anaemias of specified type | 2 | — | 1 | 5 |
| 293 | Anaemia of unspecified type | 58 | 1 | 44 | 3 |
| 294 | Polycythaemia | 2 | — | — | — |
| | V. *Mental, psychoneurotic, and personality disorders* | | | | |
| 300 | Schizophrenic disorders (dementia praecox) | 1 | — | 3 | 1 |
| 301 | Manic-depressive reaction | 2 | — | 4 | 5 |
| 302 | Involutional melancholia | 1 | — | — | — |
| 303 | Paranoia and paranoid states | — | — | 1 | — |
| 304 | Senile psychosis | — | — | 1 | — |
| 307 | Alcoholic psychosis | — | — | 1 | — |
| 309 | Other and unspecified psychoses | 3 | 2 | 2 | — |
| 310 | Anxiety reaction without mention of somatic symptoms | 81 | 13 | 54 | 15 |
| 311 | Hysterical reaction without mention of anxiety reaction | 2 | 1 | 9 | 2 |

| Three-digit numbers | Category | Number of visits in Ontario | | Number of visits in Nova Scotia | |
|---|---|---|---|---|---|
| | | Non-hospital | Hospital | Non-hospital | Hospital |
| 312 | Phobic reaction | — | — | 1 | — |
| 314 | Neurotic-depressive reaction | 3 | — | 2 | — |
| 315 | Psychoneurosis with somatic symptoms (somatization reaction) affecting circulatory system | 5 | — | 1 | — |
| 316 | Psychoneurosis with somatic symptoms (somatization reaction) affecting digestive system | 3 | 1 | — | — |
| 317 | Psychoneurosis with somatic symptoms (somatization reaction) affecting other systems | 2 | — | — | — |
| 318 | Psychoneurotic disorders, other, mixed, and unspecified types | 42 | 2 | 24 | 4 |
| 321 | Immature personality | 1 | — | 2 | — |
| 322 | Alcoholism | 11 | 2 | 7 | — |
| 324 | Primary childhood behaviour disorders | 2 | — | — | 4 |
| 325 | Mental deficiency | — | — | 1 | — |
| | VI. *Diseases of the nervous system and sense organs* | | | | |
| 331 | Cerebral haemorrhage | 5 | 6 | 15 | 24 |
| 332 | Cerebral embolism and thrombosis | 7 | 5 | 5 | 5 |
| 333 | Spasm of cerebral arteries | — | — | 1 | 2 |
| 334 | Other and ill-defined vascular lesions affecting central nervous system | 11 | 1 | 2 | — |
| 340 | Meningitis, except meningococcal and tuberculous | — | — | 1 | 3 |
| 343 | Encephalitis, myelitis, and encephalomyelitis (except acute infectious) | — | 1 | — | — |
| 345 | Multiple sclerosis | 6 | — | 5 | — |
| 350 | Paralysis agitans | 7 | 1 | — | 3 |
| 352 | Other cerebral paralysis | 2 | 16 | 1 | — |
| 353 | Epilepsy | 7 | — | 3 | 1 |
| 354 | Migraine | 8 | — | 1 | — |
| 355 | Other diseases of brain | 1 | 1 | — | 1 |
| 356 | Motor neurone disease and muscular atrophy | — | — | 2 | — |
| 357 | Other diseases of spinal cord | — | — | 1 | 1 |
| 360 | Facial paralysis | 8 | — | 2 | — |
| 361 | Trigeminal neuralgia | 2 | — | 3 | — |
| 362 | Brachial neuritis | 8 | — | 3 | — |
| 363 | Sciatica | 4 | 7 | 4 | — |
| 364 | Polyneuritis and polyradiculitis | 1 | — | — | — |
| 366 | Other and unspecified forms of neuralgia and neuritis | 25 | — | 22 | — |
| 368 | Other diseases of peripheral nerves except autonomic | 1 | — | 1 | — |
| 369 | Diseases of peripheral autonomic nervous system | — | 1 | — | — |
| 370 | Conjunctivitis and ophthalmia | 16 | — | 12 | — |
| 371 | Blepharitis | — | — | 3 | — |
| 372 | Hordeolum (stye) | — | — | 2 | — |
| 376 | Other inflammation of uveal tract | — | — | — | 1 |
| 377 | Inflammation of optic nerve and retina | 1 | 5 | — | — |
| 378 | Inflammation of lachrymal glands and ducts | 1 | — | — | — |
| 381 | Corneal ulcer | 1 | — | 2 | — |

| Three-digit numbers | Category | Number of visits in Ontario | | Number of visits in Nova Scotia | |
|---|---|---|---|---|---|
| | | Non-hospital | Hospital | Non-hospital | Hospital |
| 382 | Corneal opacity | 1 | — | — | — |
| 384 | Strabismus | — | — | 1 | — |
| 388 | Other diseases of eye | 6 | — | 7 | — |
| 390 | Otitis externa | 13 | — | 10 | 1 |
| 391 | Otitis media without mention of mastoiditis | 52 | 3 | 62 | 14 |
| 392 | Otitis media with mastoiditis | — | — | 1 | — |
| 393 | Mastoiditis without mention of otitis media | 5 | 12 | — | 1 |
| 394 | Other inflammatory diseases of ear | 3 | — | 3 | — |
| 395 | Ménière's disease | 7 | — | — | — |
| 396 | Other diseases of ear and mastoid process | 11 | — | 18 | — |
| | **VII.** *Diseases of the circulatory system* | | | | |
| 400 | Rheumatic fever without mention of heart involvement | 10 | 6 | 4 | — |
| 410 | Diseases of mitral valve | 4 | — | 1 | 2 |
| 415 | Other myocarditis specified as rheumatic | 1 | — | — | — |
| 416 | Other heart disease specified as rheumatic | 2 | — | 6 | — |
| 420 | Arteriosclerotic heart disease, including coronary disease | 98 | 67 | 63 | 85 |
| 421 | Chronic endocarditis not specified as rheumatic | 1 | — | — | — |
| 422 | Other myocardial degeneration | 21 | 3 | 7 | 6 |
| 430 | Acute and subacute endocarditis | — | 5 | — | — |
| 431 | Acute myocarditis not specified as rheumatic | 2 | — | — | — |
| 433 | Functional disease of heart | 6 | 1 | 9 | 4 |
| 434 | Other and unspecified diseases of heart | 26 | 13 | 19 | 25 |
| 442 | Hypertensive heart disease with arteriolar nephrosclerosis | — | — | 1 | — |
| 443 | Other and unspecified hypertensive heart disease | 8 | — | 20 | 10 |
| 444 | Essential benign hypertension | 130 | 15 | 135 | 8 |
| 445 | Essential malignant hypertension | 1 | — | 1 | 2 |
| 446 | Hypertension with arteriolar nephrosclerosis | — | 1 | — | — |
| 450 | General arteriosclerosis | 10 | 10 | 11 | 7 |
| 453 | Peripheral vascular disease | 4 | 6 | 2 | 4 |
| 455 | Gangrene of unspecified cause | — | — | 3 | — |
| 460 | Varicose veins of lower extremities | 11 | 7 | 11 | 25 |
| 461 | Haemorrhoids | 11 | 12 | 9 | 14 |
| 462 | Varicose veins of other specified sites | — | 1 | 3 | 1 |
| 463 | Phlebitis and thrombophlebitis of lower extremities | 1 | 1 | 2 | — |
| 464 | Phlebitis and thrombophlebitis of other sites | 12 | 6 | 3 | — |
| 465 | Pulmonary embolism and infarction | 1 | 5 | — | — |
| 466 | Other venous embolism and thrombosis | — | 1 | 1 | — |
| 467 | Other diseases of circulatory system | 8 | — | 5 | — |
| 468 | Certain diseases of lymph nodes and lymph channels | 10 | — | 11 | 3 |
| | **VIII.** *Diseases of the respiratory system* | | | | |
| 470 | Acute nasopharyngitis (common cold) | 34 | — | 34 | 2 |
| 471 | Acute sinusitis | 8 | 2 | 6 | 4 |
| 472 | Acute pharyngitis | 56 | 1 | 26 | 1 |
| 473 | Acute tonsillitis | 98 | 2 | 82 | 4 |
| 474 | Acute laryngitis and tracheitis | 19 | 7 | 21 | — |

| Three-digit numbers | Category | Number of visits in Ontario | | Number of visits in Nova Scotia | |
|---|---|---|---|---|---|
| | | Non-hospital | Hospital | Non-hospital | Hospital |
| 475 | Acute upper respiratory infection of multiple or unspecified sites | 64 | 9 | 42 | 2 |
| 480 | Influenza with pneumonia | — | — | 1 | — |
| 481 | Influenza with other respiratory manifestations, and influenza unqualified | 118 | 1 | 194 | 23 |
| 482 | Influenza with digestive manifestations, but without respiratory symptoms | 1 | — | 5 | — |
| 490 | Lobar pneumonia | 1 | — | 4 | 2 |
| 491 | Bronchopneumonia | 9 | 2 | 20 | 32 |
| 492 | Primary atypical pneumonia | 15 | 2 | 31 | 33 |
| 493 | Pneumonia, other and unspecified | 25 | 21 | 34 | 28 |
| 500 | Acute bronchitis | 40 | 1 | 36 | 8 |
| 501 | Bronchitis unqualified | 65 | 2 | 62 | 10 |
| 502 | Chronic bronchitis | 17 | 1 | 11 | 4 |
| 510 | Hypertrophy of tonsils and adenoids | 16 | 38 | 16 | 20 |
| 511 | Peritonsillar abscess (quinsy) | 5 | — | 3 | — |
| 512 | Chronic pharyngitis and nasopharyngitis | 11 | — | 5 | — |
| 513 | Chronic sinusitis | 9 | — | 16 | 2 |
| 515 | Nasal polyp | 2 | — | — | — |
| 517 | Other diseases of upper respiratory tract | 5 | — | 12 | 2 |
| 519 | Pleurisy | 5 | 6 | 10 | 2 |
| 520 | Spontaneous pneumothorax | — | — | 1 | — |
| 522 | Pulmonary congestion and hypostasis | 3 | — | 1 | — |
| 523 | Pneumoconiosis due to silica and silicates (occupational) | — | — | 2 | — |
| 525 | Other chronic interstitial pneumonia | 1 | — | 1 | — |
| 526 | Bronchiectasis | 7 | 2 | 6 | 6 |
| 527 | Other diseases of lung and pleural cavity | 14 | 5 | 13 | 15 |
| | IX. *Diseases of the digestive system* | | | | |
| 530 | Dental caries | 3 | — | 4 | — |
| 531 | Abscesses of supporting structures of teeth | 11 | — | 6 | 1 |
| 532 | Other inflammatory diseases of supporting structures of teeth | 4 | — | 5 | 1 |
| 533 | Disorders of occlusion, eruption, and tooth development | 2 | — | 3 | — |
| 534 | Toothache from unspecified cause | 1 | — | — | 1 |
| 535 | Other diseases of teeth and supporting structures | 1 | 5 | 28 | 4 |
| 536 | Stomatitis | 8 | — | 7 | — |
| 537 | Diseases of salivary glands | 1 | — | 1 | — |
| 538 | Other diseases of buccal cavity | 1 | — | 4 | — |
| 539 | Diseases of oesophagus | 3 | 1 | — | — |
| 540 | Ulcer of stomach | 12 | 4 | 8 | 11 |
| 541 | Ulcer of duodenum | 34 | 27 | 7 | 12 |
| 542 | Gastrojejunal ulcer | — | — | 1 | 2 |
| 543 | Gastritis and duodenitis | 16 | 6 | 14 | 11 |
| 544 | Disorders of function of stomach | 11 | 1 | 8 | — |
| 545 | Other diseases of stomach and duodenum | 5 | 1 | 6 | 12 |
| 550 | Acute appendicitis | 2 | 5 | 1 | 11 |
| 551 | Appendicitis, unqualified | 4 | 38 | 8 | 26 |
| 552 | Other appendicitis | 2 | — | 3 | 1 |
| 560 | Hernia of abdominal cavity without mention of obstruction | 21 | 29 | 12 | 15 |

| Three-digit numbers | Category | Number of visits in Ontario | | Number of visits in Nova Scotia | |
|---|---|---|---|---|---|
| | | Non-hospital | Hospital | Non-hospital | Hospital |
| 561 | Hernia of abdominal cavity with obstruction | 1 | 2 | — | 1 |
| 570 | Intestinal obstruction without mention of hernia | — | 6 | 5 | 6 |
| 571 | Gastro-enteritis and colitis, except ulcerative, age 4 weeks and over | 48 | 17 | 44 | 22 |
| 572 | Chronic enteritis and ulcerative colitis | 10 | — | 5 | 12 |
| 573 | Functional disorders of intestines | 9 | — | 10 | 3 |
| 574 | Anal fissure and fistula | 6 | 1 | 3 | — |
| 575 | Abscess of anal and rectal regions | 2 | 2 | 3 | 4 |
| 577 | Peritoneal adhesion | 2 | — | — | — |
| 578 | Other diseases of intestines and peritoneum | 3 | 8 | 2 | 19 |
| 581 | Cirrhosis of liver | 5 | — | — | — |
| 583 | Other diseases of liver | 1 | 2 | 2 | 4 |
| 584 | Cholelithiasis | 3 | — | 7 | 5 |
| 585 | Cholecystitis and cholangitis, without mention of calculi | 12 | 14 | 11 | 6 |
| 586 | Other diseases of gallbladder and biliary ducts | 4 | 5 | 7 | 40 |
| 587 | Diseases of pancreas | — | — | 1 | — |
| | X. *Diseases of the genito-urinary system* | | | | |
| 590 | Acute nephritis | 1 | 1 | — | 3 |
| 591 | Nephritis with oedema, including nephrosis | — | — | 2 | 2 |
| 592 | Chronic nephritis | 3 | — | 2 | — |
| 593 | Nephritis not specified as acute or chronic | 2 | 1 | 1 | — |
| 600 | Infections of kidney | 18 | 1 | 14 | 10 |
| 601 | Hydronephrosis | — | — | — | 1 |
| 602 | Calculi of kidney and ureter | — | — | 3 | 4 |
| 603 | Other diseases of kidney and ureter | 1 | — | — | — |
| 604 | Calculi of other parts of urinary system | — | — | 2 | — |
| 605 | Cystitis | 25 | 8 | 43 | 6 |
| 606 | Other diseases of bladder | 1 | 7 | 2 | 3 |
| 607 | Urethritis (non-venereal) | 9 | — | 1 | — |
| 608 | Stricture of urethra | 1 | — | 3 | 2 |
| 609 | Other diseases of urethra | 1 | — | 5 | 1 |
| 610 | Hyperplasia of prostate | 1 | 7 | 2 | 25 |
| 611 | Prostatitis | 15 | 2 | 2 | — |
| 612 | Other diseases of prostate | — | 1 | — | 2 |
| 613 | Hydrocele | 2 | — | 4 | 2 |
| 615 | Redundant prepuce and phimosis | — | — | 3 | 4 |
| 616 | Sterility, male | 2 | — | 1 | — |
| 617 | Other diseases of male genital organs | 2 | 2 | — | 2 |
| 620 | Chronic cystic disease of breast | 3 | 1 | 4 | — |
| 621 | Other diseases of breast | 2 | 1 | 9 | 2 |
| 622 | Acute salpingitis and oophoritis | — | — | 3 | — |
| 623 | Chronic salpingitis and oophoritis | — | — | 1 | — |
| 624 | Salpingitis and oophoritis, unqualified | 2 | — | 1 | — |
| 625 | Other diseases of ovary and Fallopian tube | 1 | 2 | — | — |
| 626 | Diseases of parametrium and pelvic peritoneum (female) | 3 | 2 | 2 | 1 |
| 630 | Infective disease of uterus, vagina, and vulva | 33 | — | 24 | 3 |
| 631 | Uterovaginal prolapse | 3 | 6 | 3 | 9 |
| 632 | Malposition of uterus | 7 | — | 1 | 1 |
| 633 | Other diseases of uterus | 3 | 40 | 2 | 34 |

| Three-digit numbers | Category | Number of visits in Ontario | | Number of visits in Nova Scotia | |
|---|---|---|---|---|---|
| | | Non-hospital | Hospital | Non-hospital | Hospital |
| 634 | Disorders of menstruation | 29 | 3 | 18 | 1 |
| 635 | Menopausal symptoms | 42 | 1 | 15 | — |
| 636 | Sterility, female | 5 | — | — | — |
| 637 | Other diseases of female genital organs | 12 | 5 | 6 | 8 |
| | **XI.** *Deliveries and complications of pregnancy, childbirth, and the puerperium* | | | | |
| 640 | Pyelitis and pyelonephritis of pregnancy | — | — | 3 | — |
| 641 | Other infections of genito-urinary tract during pregnancy | — | — | 3 | — |
| 642 | Toxaemias of pregnancy | 7 | 7 | 4 | 1 |
| 643 | Placenta praevia | — | 2 | 1 | — |
| 645 | Ectopic pregnancy | 2 | 2 | — | 3 |
| 648 | Other complications arising from pregnancy | 4 | 11 | 7 | 6 |
| 650 | Abortion without mention of sepsis or toxaemia | 6 | 11 | 13 | 7 |
| 660 | Delivery without mention of complication | 1 | 35 | — | 36 |
| 671 | Delivery complicated by retained placenta | — | 1 | — | — |
| 672 | Delivery complicated by other postpartum haemorrhage | — | 2 | 3 | — |
| 674 | Delivery complicated by disproportion or malposition of foetus | — | — | — | 4 |
| 678 | Delivery with other complications of childbirth | 1 | — | — | — |
| 681 | Sepsis of childbirth and the puerperium | 2 | — | — | — |
| 682 | Puerperal phlebitis and thrombosis | — | — | 1 | — |
| 688 | Other and unspecified complications of the puerperium | 1 | — | 1 | — |
| | **XII.** *Diseases of the skin and cellular tissue* | | | | |
| 690 | Boil and carbuncle | 50 | 7 | 17 | — |
| 691 | Cellulitis of finger and toe | 20 | 3 | 27 | — |
| 692 | Other cellulitis and abscess without mention of lymphangitis | 18 | 5 | 25 | 4 |
| 693 | Other cellulitis and abscess with lymphangitis | 1 | — | 2 | — |
| 695 | Impetigo | 19 | — | 18 | — |
| 696 | Infectious warts | 14 | — | 17 | 4 |
| 697 | Molluscum contagiosum | 1 | — | — | — |
| 698 | Other local infections of skin and subcutaneous tissue | 19 | — | 8 | — |
| 700 | Seborrhoeic dermatitis | 1 | — | 2 | — |
| 701 | Eczema | 14 | 1 | 12 | — |
| 703 | Other dermatitis | 46 | — | 34 | 2 |
| 704 | Pemphigus | — | 7 | — | — |
| 705 | Erythematous conditions | 3 | 1 | 3 | 1 |
| 706 | Psoriasis and similar disorders | 4 | — | 6 | — |
| 708 | Pruritus and related conditions | 17 | — | 5 | — |
| 709 | Corns and callosities | 2 | — | 3 | 1 |
| 712 | Diseases of nail | 6 | — | 2 | — |
| 713 | Diseases of hair and hair follicles | 1 | — | 3 | — |
| 714 | Diseases of sweat and sebaceous glands | 17 | 2 | 12 | 1 |
| 715 | Chronic ulcer of skin | 7 | — | 4 | 3 |
| 716 | Other diseases of skin | 3 | — | 4 | 1 |

| Three-digit numbers | Category | Number of visits in Ontario | | Number of visits in Nova Scotia | |
|---|---|---|---|---|---|
| | | Non-hospital | Hospital | Non-hospital | Hospital |
| | XIII. *Diseases of the bones and organs of movement* | | | | |
| 722 | Rheumatoid arthritis and allied conditions | 19 | 2 | 10 | — |
| 723 | Osteo-arthritis (arthrosis) and allied conditions | 15 | 3 | 14 | 4 |
| 724 | Other specified forms of arthritis | — | — | 2 | 2 |
| 725 | Arthritis, unspecified | 21 | — | 17 | 12 |
| 726 | Muscular rheumatism | 39 | — | 41 | 1 |
| 727 | Rheumatism, unspecified | 1 | — | 1 | — |
| 730 | Osteomyelitis and periostitis | 1 | — | 2 | 8 |
| 732 | Osteochondrosis | — | — | 1 | 1 |
| 733 | Other diseases of bone | — | — | — | 3 |
| 735 | Displacement of intervertebral disc | 8 | 11 | 17 | 10 |
| 737 | Ankylosis of joint | 1 | — | — | 1 |
| 738 | Other diseases of joint | 3 | — | 1 | 1 |
| 740 | Bunion | 2 | — | — | — |
| 741 | Synovitis, bursitis, and tenosynovitis without mention of occupational origin | 28 | 3 | 30 | 1 |
| 742 | Synovitis, bursitis, and tenosynovitis of occupational origin | 1 | — | — | — |
| 744 | Other diseases of muscle, tendon, and fascia | 6 | — | 1 | — |
| 745 | Curvature of spine | — | — | — | 1 |
| 746 | Flat foot | 1 | — | 1 | — |
| 747 | Hallux valgus and varus | — | — | 1 | — |
| 748 | Clubfoot | 1 | — | 1 | — |
| 749 | Other deformities | 1 | — | 3 | 1 |
| | XIV. *Congenital malformations* | | | | |
| 751 | Spina bifida and meningocele | — | — | — | 5 |
| 755 | Cleft palate and harelip | 2 | 6 | — | — |
| 756 | Congenital malformations of digestive system | — | — | 1 | 2 |
| 757 | Congenital malformations of genito-urinary system | 2 | — | 2 | 1 |
| 758 | Congenital malformations of bone and joint | — | — | 1 | — |
| | XV. *Certain diseases of early infancy* | | | | |
| 761 | Other birth injury | — | — | — | 1 |
| 763 | Pneumonia of newborn | — | — | — | 7 |
| 767 | Umbilical sepsis | 1 | — | — | — |
| 772 | Nutritional maladjustment | 14 | — | 6 | 5 |
| 773 | Ill-defined diseases peculiar to early infancy | 1 | 1 | — | 6 |
| 776 | Immaturity, unqualified | 1 | 9 | — | 11 |
| | XVI. *Symptoms, senility, and ill-defined conditions* | | | | |
| 780 | Certain symptoms referable to nervous system and special senses | 18 | — | 12 | 2 |
| 781 | Other symptoms referable to nervous system and special senses | 3 | — | 2 | — |
| 782 | Symptoms referable to cardiovascular and lymphatic system | 14 | 9 | 17 | 10 |
| 783 | Symptoms referable to respiratory system | 21 | 3 | 29 | 2 |
| 784 | Symptoms referable to upper gastro-intestinal tract | 15 | — | 8 | 12 |

| Three-digit numbers | Category | Number of visits in Ontario | | Number of visits in Nova Scotia | |
|---|---|---|---|---|---|
| | | Non-hospital | Hospital | Non-hospital | Hospital |
| 785 | Symptoms referable to abdomen and lower gastro-intestinal tract | 22 | 1 | 31 | 7 |
| 786 | Symptoms referable to genito-urinary system | 14 | 3 | 4 | 2 |
| 787 | Symptoms referable to limbs and back | 7 | — | 22 | 1 |
| 788 | Other general symptoms | 15 | — | 7 | — |
| 789 | Abnormal urinary constituents of unspecified cause | 7 | — | 6 | 1 |
| 790 | Nervousness and debility | 27 | — | 12 | — |
| 791 | Headache | 11 | — | 8 | — |
| 792 | Uraemia | — | — | 1 | — |
| 794 | Senility without mention of psychosis | 7 | — | 3 | 3 |
| 795 | Ill-defined and unknown causes of morbidity and mortality | 53 | 22 | 34 | 25 |
| | XVII. *Accidents, poisonings, and violence* | | | | |
| N802 | Fracture of face bones | 2 | 4 | 1 | — |
| N803 | Other and unqualified skull fractures | — | — | — | 1 |
| N805 | Fracture and fracture dislocation of vertebral column without mention of spinal cord lesion | 1 | — | 1 | 5 |
| N807 | Fracture of rib(s), sternum, and larynx | 7 | — | 12 | 3 |
| N808 | Fracture of pelvis | 2 | — | 1 | — |
| N809 | Multiple and ill-defined fractures of trunk | — | — | 1 | 2 |
| N810 | Fracture of clavicle | 2 | 3 | 2 | 2 |
| N812 | Fracture of humerus | 1 | 5 | 2 | 12 |
| N813 | Fracture of radius and ulna | 9 | 8 | 7 | 10 |
| N814 | Fracture of carpal bone(s) | 2 | 1 | 1 | 1 |
| N815 | Fracture of metacarpal bone(s) | 7 | — | 2 | 2 |
| N816 | Fracture of one or more phalanges of hand | 2 | 2 | 11 | 4 |
| N817 | Multiple fractures of hand bones | 1 | — | — | — |
| N818 | Other, multiple, and ill-defined fractures of upper limb | — | — | — | 1 |
| N819 | Multiple fractures involving both upper limbs, and upper limb with rib(s) and sternum | — | — | 1 | — |
| N820 | Fracture of neck of femur | — | 14 | — | 21 |
| N821 | Fracture of other and unspecified parts of femur | — | 9 | 1 | 12 |
| N822 | Fracture of patella | — | — | — | 8 |
| N823 | Fracture of tibia and fibula | 8 | 18 | 1 | 11 |
| N824 | Fracture of ankle | 4 | 7 | 2 | 5 |
| N825 | Fracture of one or more tarsal and metatarsal bones | 3 | — | 2 | — |
| N826 | Fracture of one or more phalanges of foot | 1 | 1 | 2 | — |
| N827 | Other, multiple, and ill-defined fractures of lower limb | — | 1 | — | — |
| N829 | Fracture of unspecified bones | 2 | 7 | — | — |
| N830 | Dislocation of jaw | — | — | 2 | — |
| N831 | Dislocation of shoulder | 1 | — | 1 | — |
| N834 | Dislocation of finger | 1 | — | 1 | 1 |
| N836 | Dislocation of knee | 3 | 1 | 1 | — |
| N837 | Dislocation of ankle | — | — | 1 | — |
| N838 | Dislocation of foot | — | — | 1 | — |
| N840 | Sprains and strains of shoulder and upper arm | 3 | — | 1 | — |
| N841 | Sprains and strains of elbow and forearm | 1 | — | 1 | — |
| N842 | Sprains and strains of wrist and hand | 5 | — | — | — |

| Three-digit numbers | Category | Number of visits in Ontario | | Number of visits in Nova Scotia | |
|---|---|---|---|---|---|
| | | Non-hospital | Hospital | Non-hospital | Hospital |
| N843 | Sprains and strains of hip and thigh | 1 | — | 3 | — |
| N844 | Sprains and strains of knee and leg | 3 | — | 5 | — |
| N845 | Sprains and strains of ankle and foot | 25 | 5 | 12 | 3 |
| N846 | Sprains and strains of sacro-iliac region | 7 | — | 8 | — |
| N847 | Sprains and strains of other and unspecified parts of back | 6 | — | 14 | 1 |
| N848 | Other and ill-defined sprains and strains | 12 | — | 2 | — |
| N850 | Open wound of scalp | 4 | 1 | 15 | 3 |
| N851 | Contusion and haematoma of scalp | 3 | — | — | — |
| N853 | Cerebral laceration and contusion | — | — | — | 4 |
| N856 | Head injury of other and unspecified nature | 5 | 5 | 2 | 1 |
| N862 | Injury to other and unspecified intrathoracic organs | 1 | 1 | — | — |
| N863 | Injury to gastro-intestinal tract | — | — | 1 | — |
| N868 | Injury to other and unspecified intra-abdominal organs | — | — | — | 2 |
| N870 | Open wound of eye and orbit | 1 | — | 2 | 1 |
| N872 | Open wound of ear | 2 | — | 1 | — |
| N873 | Other and unspecified laceration of face | 11 | 3 | 12 | 1 |
| N876 | Open wound of back | 1 | — | — | — |
| N877 | Open wound of buttock | 1 | — | — | — |
| N880 | Open wound of shoulder and upper arm | 2 | — | — | — |
| N881 | Open wound of elbow and forearm, and of wrist not involving tendons | 1 | — | 1 | — |
| N883 | Open wound of hand, except finger(s) alone | 15 | 2 | 10 | 3 |
| N884 | Open wound of finger(s) | 24 | 7 | 17 | 5 |
| N885 | Multiple and unspecified open wounds of one upper limb | 2 | 1 | 3 | — |
| N887 | Traumatic amputation of other finger(s) | — | — | 3 | — |
| N890 | Open wound of hip and thigh | 2 | — | — | — |
| N891 | Open wound of knee and leg (except thigh), and of ankle not involving tendons | 7 | 1 | 8 | 3 |
| N893 | Open wound of foot, except toe(s) alone | 9 | 1 | 5 | 5 |
| N894 | Open wound of toe | — | — | 1 | — |
| N901 | Multiple open wounds of both lower limbs | — | — | 1 | — |
| N908 | Multiple open wounds of other and unspecified location | 11 | 2 | 4 | — |
| N910 | Superficial injury of face and neck | 5 | — | 3 | — |
| N913 | Superficial injury of elbow, forearm, and wrist | — | — | 1 | — |
| N916 | Superficial injury of hip, thigh, leg, and ankle | 5 | — | 4 | — |
| N917 | Superficial injury of foot and toe(s) | 1 | — | 1 | — |
| N918 | Superficial injury of other, multiple, and unspecified sites | 8 | 1 | 3 | — |
| N920 | Contusion of face and neck, except eye(s) | 1 | — | 1 | — |
| N922 | Contusion of trunk | 8 | — | 11 | — |
| N923 | Contusion of shoulder and upper arm | 2 | — | — | 1 |
| N924 | Contusion of elbow, forearm, and wrist | 1 | — | 5 | — |
| N925 | Contusion of hand(s), except finger(s) alone | 4 | — | 3 | — |
| N926 | Contusion of finger(s) | 4 | 1 | 2 | 1 |
| N927 | Contusion of hip, thigh, leg, and ankle | 2 | — | 5 | 1 |
| N928 | Contusion of foot and toe(s) | 5 | 1 | 3 | — |
| N929 | Contusion of other, multiple, and unspecified sites | 6 | — | 3 | 4 |
| N930 | Foreign body in eye and adnexa | 11 | 1 | 7 | — |

| Three-digit numbers | Category | Number of visits in Ontario | | Number of visits in Nova Scotia | |
|---|---|---|---|---|---|
| | | Non-hospital | Hospital | Non-hospital | Hospital |
| N931 | Foreign body in ear | 1 | — | 1 | — |
| N932 | Foreign body in nose | 2 | — | — | — |
| N933 | Foreign body in pharynx and larynx | — | — | 1 | — |
| N935 | Foreign body in digestive tract | 3 | — | 1 | — |
| N940 | Burn confined to eye | — | — | 3 | — |
| N942 | Burn confined to trunk | 3 | — | — | — |
| N943 | Burn confined to upper limb(s), except wrist and hand | 1 | — | 2 | 4 |
| N944 | Burn confined to wrist(s) and hand(s) | 7 | — | — | — |
| N945 | Burn confined to lower limb(s) | 7 | — | 1 | — |
| N946 | Burn involving face, head, and neck, with limb(s) | — | — | 1 | — |
| N947 | Burn involving trunk with limb(s) | — | — | 1 | — |
| N948 | Burn involving face, head, and neck, with trunk and limb(s) | 1 | 1 | — | — |
| N949 | Burn involving other and unspecified parts | 3 | 2 | — | 11 |
| N958 | Spinal cord lesion without evidence of spinal bone injury | — | 1 | — | — |
| N963 | Poisoning by industrial solvents | 1 | — | — | — |
| N964 | Poisoning by corrosive aromatics, acids, and caustic alkalis | — | — | 1 | — |
| N969 | Poisoning by other gases and vapours | — | — | — | 1 |
| N972 | Poisoning by aspirin and salicylates | — | 1 | — | — |
| N974 | Poisoning by other analgesic and soporific drugs | — | — | 1 | — |
| N975 | Poisoning by sulfonamides | 3 | — | — | — |
| N978 | Poisoning by venom | 1 | — | 1 | — |
| N979 | Poisoning by other and unspecified substances | 1 | — | — | — |
| N980 | Effects of reduced temperature | 1 | — | 1 | — |
| N981 | Effects of heat and insolation | — | — | 1 | — |
| N989 | Motion (travel) sickness | 1 | — | — | — |
| N992 | Electrocution and nonfatal effects of electric currents | — | — | 1 | — |
| N995 | Certain early complications of trauma | — | — | 1 | 1 |
| N996 | Injury of other and unspecified nature | 59 | 14 | 37 | 7 |
| N997 | Reactions and complications due to non-therapeutic medical and surgical procedures | 2 | — | 3 | — |
| N998 | Adverse reaction to injections, infusions, and transfusions for therapeutic purposes | 1 | — | — | — |
| N999 | Adverse reaction to other therapeutic procedures | 1 | — | 2 | 1 |
| | *Special conditions and examinations without sickness* | | | | |
| Y00.0 Y00.3 | General medical examination or laboratory examination | 102 | — | 74 | 1 |
| Y00.5 | Well baby and child care | 58 | 4 | 35 | 23 |
| Y01 | Skin immunity and sensitization tests | 3 | — | 3 | — |
| Y02 | Persons receiving prophylactic inoculation and vaccination | 230 | — | 201 | — |
| Y06 | Prenatal care | 311 | 1 | 226 | 6 |
| Y07 | Postpartum observation | 43 | 82 | 23 | 119 |
| Y09 | Other person without complaint or sickness | 6 | 11 | 5 | 7 |

# APPENDIX B

RELATIONSHIPS BETWEEN POSTGRADUATE HOSPITAL TRAINING AND
QUALITY OF PRACTICE OF THE ONTARIO PHYSICIANS*

In examining the possible effect of postgraduate training upon the quality of subsequent practice, our attention was given to (1) the duration of the training, (2) the type of hospital in which the training was taken, i.e. whether it was taken entirely in non-teaching hospitals or whether at least part of it was taken in a teaching hospital,† and (3) the clinical services on which the training was taken. Because these factors are interconnected, it is not possible to discuss them entirely separately.

Two doctors had had no internship. One other doctor, who had had postgraduate hospital training, was not scored because of technical difficulties. Thus the relationship between quality of practice and duration of postgraduate training could be examined for 41 of the total sample of 44 doctors.

### DURATION OF POSTGRADUATE TRAINING VS. QUALITY OF PRACTICE

Between the 41 physicians' scores and the total duration of their postgraduate training, there was found to be a significant correlation ($p < 0.05$). Since some of the training had been taken in teaching hospitals and some in non-teaching hospitals, the relationship between each of these two components of the training and the quality of practice was examined separately. Twenty-two physicians had had some of their postgraduate training in non-teaching hospitals. No significant relationship was found between their scores and the duration of their training in non-teaching hospitals. Twenty-eight doctors had had some of their postgraduate training in teaching hospitals. Among those, 24 in number, who had had up to 24 months of postgraduate training in teaching hospitals, no significant relationship was evident between the duration of the teaching hospital training and the quality of practice. However, the mean score (60.9 per cent) of these 24 physicians and the mean score (84.5 per cent) of the remaining 4 physicians, who had had more than 24 months of postgraduate training in

*The reader should note that: (1) All hospital house-staff appointments that followed the completion of the formal university courses were regarded as *post*graduate training, even though, in some cases, the medical degree was not granted until the internship was completed. This is explained on page 42. (2) Throughout this appendix, wherever the word "training" is used, it is to be understood as equivalent to "postgraduate training."

†Teaching hospitals are defined, for the purposes of this study, as those hospitals in which medical students (i.e., undergraduates) are continually receiving instruction in general medicine, surgery, obstetrics, or paediatrics. Those hospitals whose activities are narrowly limited within the major fields (e.g., infectious diseases hospitals) are not counted as teaching hospitals, except when the physician was sent to such a hospital for a short period in order to round out the rotation of a major teaching hospital.

teaching hospitals, did differ significantly ($p < 0.05$). Since the group with the higher mean score and the longer training was about 2 years older, on the average, than those with the lower score and the shorter training, the difference between the mean scores appears to be independent of the inverse relationship that was found to exist between age of physician and quality of practice (page 319). Finally, when those physicians who had had only non-teaching hospital postgraduate training were compared with those who had had up to 24 months of postgraduate training in teaching hospitals, it was found that the mean scores of the two groups (46.3 per cent and 60.9 per cent, respectively) differed significantly ($p < 0.05$) and that the *total* duration of training of the former group was 16.2 months and of the latter group 19.8 months. Comparison of the mean ages of the two groups, however, showed that the group with only non-teaching hospital post-graduate training and with the lower mean score was a little more than 5 years older, on the average, than the other group. Although the age difference was not statistically significant, yet it was great enough to suggest that the difference between the mean scores might be merely a manifesta-tion of the inverse relationship between age and quality of practice. It appears, then, that the significant correlation that was found to exist between quality of practice and total duration of postgraduate training was really a manifestation of (1) the superior quality of practice of those few physicians who had had prolonged training in teaching hospitals and, perhaps, of (2) the better quality of practice of those who had had up to 24 months of teaching hospital training than of those who had had no postgraduate training in teaching hospitals, though the latter point is open to question because of the greater mean age of those who had had no teaching hospital postgraduate training.

Though the physicians who had had no postgraduate training in teaching hospitals had a significantly lower *mean* score than those who had had teaching hospital postgraduate training, it is to be noted that some men who had had no teaching hospital postgraduate training had high scores.

### Total Duration of Postgraduate Training in Specific Subjects vs. Quality of Practice

Next, an attempt was made to determine whether postgraduate training in any particular clinical subject or subjects affected the quality of practice. To this end, we examined the relationships between quality of practice and duration of training in each of the 4 major clinical subjects, internal medicine, surgery, obstetrics,* and paediatrics. For those doctors who had had some postgraduate training in the particular clinical subject, there was no significant correlation, in the case of any one of the 4 major subjects, between the duration of the training in that subject and score, though, in the case of medicine, the correlation coefficeint was close to the 5 per cent level of significance ($r = 0.327$, $r_{0.05} = 0.330$).

When those doctors who had had no postgraduate hospital training in

*Throughout this discussion, the term "obstetrics" is to be understood to include also gynaecology.

medicine but who had had some training in other subjects were compared with those who had had some training in medicine, the mean scores of the two groups did not differ significantly. Similarly, in the case of paediatrics and in the case of obstetrics, the mean scores of the two groups did not differ significantly. In the case of surgery, the difference between the mean scores was statistically significant ($p < 0.05$). When these groups (i.e., those who had had no postgraduate training in surgery and those who had had some) were compared as to the proportion of each group that had had some *teaching* hospital training in *any* subject, it was found that all 3 of those doctors who had had no surgical training had also had no teaching hospital training in any subject, whereas, of the 38 doctors who had had some surgical training and who exhibited a higher quality of practice on the average, 10 had had no teaching hospital training in any subject, and 28 had had at least some of their postgraduate training in teaching hospitals. Since the difference in composition of the two groups was possibly a real difference ($p = 0.0537$), the possible difference in quality of practice between those who had had some surgical training and those who had had none may well have been merely a manifestation of the difference in quality of practice that was found to exist between those who had had some teaching hospital training and those whose training had been entirely in non-teaching hospitals. Furthermore, although the difference between the mean age of the doctors who had had no surgical training and the mean age of those who had had some surgical training did not reach the 5 per cent level of significance, yet the difference between the mean ages of the two groups was great enough (over 6 years) to cast even more doubt on the significance of the difference in quality of practice that existed between those who had had some surgical training and those who had had none. For these reasons, we cannot claim to have found a relationship of definite importance between quality of practice and duration of total postgraduate training (i.e., teaching hospital plus non-teaching hospital training) in any one of the 4 major clinical subjects, including surgery.

TEACHING HOSPITAL POSTGRADUATE TRAINING IN SPECIFIC SUBJECTS VS. QUALITY OF PRACTICE

When the doctors were divided into those who had had postgraduate training in the particular subject in a *teaching* hospital and those who had had no teaching hospital postgraduate training in that same subject, in the case of each of the 4 major clinical subjects except paediatrics those who had had some teaching hospital training had a significantly higher mean score than those who had had none ($p < 0.05$ for medicine and surgery; $p < 0.01$ for obstetrics; $p = 0.08$ approximately for paediatrics). When the groups were compared in respect of mean age, it was found that those who had had teaching hospital training in medicine and those who had had teaching hospital training in surgery were significantly younger, on the average, than those who had not had teaching hospital training in medicine and in surgery respectively ($p < 0.05$ for medicine and for surgery). Those who had had teaching hospital training in obstetrics or in paediatrics were not significantly younger than those who had not had such training.

Perhaps of greater importance than the difference in mean ages was the composition of the groups that had had, or had not had, teaching hospital training in the particular subject. Earlier it was shown that the men who had had no teaching hospital postgraduate training (in any subject) had a mean score significantly lower than the men who had had some teaching hospital training. Of the 28 men who had had some teaching hospital training, only 1 had had no teaching hospital training in either medicine or surgery and 2 other men had had no teaching hospital training in obstetrics. Inasmuch as the groupings of those who had had, and of those who had not had, teaching hospital training in the particular subject were so similar for each of these three subjects, it is not too surprising that the same result was obtained in each case and that teaching hospital postgraduate training in no one of these three subjects was shown to be more conducive, than teaching hospital training in the others, to practice of superior quality. In fact, since almost all the men who had had teaching hospital postgraduate training at all had had some of it in each of medicine, surgery, and obstetrics, there is no reason to conclude that the "significant" difference that was found to exist between the mean scores of those who had had, and of those who had not had, training in one or another of these three subjects was anything more than another manifestation of the difference between the quality of practice of those who had had some teaching hospital training and the quality of practice of those who had had only non-teaching hospital training. In other words, there seems to be no reason for attributing the difference in quality of practice to teaching hospital postgraduate training, or lack of it, in any particular clinical subject.

Finally, for the doctors who had had some teaching hospital postgraduate training in a particular clinical subject, there was no significant correlation between the duration of the teaching hospital training in that subject and the physician's score, in the case of surgery, obstetrics, or paediatrics. In the case of internal medicine, the correlation between duration of teaching hospital postgraduate training and score was statistically significant ($p <$ 0.05). This association was apparently independent of the ages of the physicians.

PROLONGED TOTAL TEACHING HOSPITAL POSTGRADUATE TRAINING VS. PROLONGED TEACHING HOSPITAL POSTGRADUATE TRAINING IN INTERNAL MEDICINE

In the preceding paragraph, it was shown that the correlation between the quality of practice and the duration of teaching hospital postgraduate training in medicine was statistically significant. Earlier it was shown also that the difference between the quality of practice of those doctors who had had up to 24 months, and the quality of those doctors, 4 in number, who had had more than 24 months, of total teaching hospital postgraduate training was statistically significant. One of these 4 could not remember the duration of his training on the medical service. The other 3 doctors whose total teaching hospital postgraduate training had exceeded 24 months in length had all spent 15 or more months (between 48 and 78 per cent of their total postgraduate training time) on medicine. Since the group with

prolonged teaching hospital postgraduate training on all services combined
was almost the same as the group with prolonged teaching hospital postgraduate training in medicine, it may be (1) that the prolonged (i.e., more
than 24 months) *total* teaching hospital training was the primary determinant of quality of practice and that the association between quality of
practice and duration of teaching hospital training in medicine was merely a
reflection of this or (2) that prolonged (i.e., more than 12 months) teaching
hospital training in *internal medicine* was the factor of importance and
that the relationship between quality and total duration of teaching hospital
training was a secondary phenomenon or (3) that certain qualities within
the man himself induced him both to prolong his training and to devote the
major portion of the time to medicine. Which of these alternatives is the
correct one remains undetermined.

Since, of the 3 men who had had more than 24 months of total teaching
hospital postgraduate training, none had had prolonged teaching hospital
training in surgery, obstetrics, or paediatrics, we cannot say what the
quality of practice of the group who had had more than 24 months of total
teaching hospital training would have been if the major portion of their
training had been in any one of the three major clinical subjects other
than medicine.*

In summary, our findings about the relationships between postgraduate
hospital training and quality of practice in Ontario were as follows:

1. There was a significant correlation between *total* duration of postgraduate training (i.e., time spent in teaching hospitals plus time spent in
non-teaching hospitals) and quality of practice.

2. There was no evidence of a significant relationship between duration
of postgraduate training in *non-teaching* hospitals and quality of practice.

3. The practice of those physicians who had had at least some of their
postgraduate training in *teaching* hospitals was, on the average, of significantly higher quality than the practice of those whose postgraduate training
had been entirely in *non-teaching* hospitals. However, the difference between the mean ages of the two groups was great enough to suggest that
the difference in quality of practice might be another manifestation of the
negative correlation that was found to exist between age of physician and
quality of practice. If this was not so, then the difference between the two
groups in respect of quality of practice might be the result (*a*) of the
superiority of the teaching hospitals over the non-teaching hospitals as
postgraduate training institutions or (*b*) of the fact that the men who had
had teaching hospital postgraduate training had had a longer training, on
the average, than those who had had only non-teaching hospital postgraduate training or (*c*) of a tendency on the part of the teaching hospitals
to give house-staff appointments to the men with the better academic
records and to reject those with the poorer records or (*d*) of differences
in the qualities of the men making up the two groups, as a result of which
qualities both their choice of type of hospital and the quality of their

*For the relationship between quality of practice and duration of teaching
hospital postgraduate training in surgery in the case of the Nova Scotia doctors,
see page 326.

subsequent practice were affected. On the other hand, if the difference in quality of practice that was found to exist between those physicians who had had teaching hospital postgraduate training and those who had had only non-teaching hospital training *was* related to the negative correlation that was known to exist between age of physician and quality of practice, then the question still remains whether (*a*) age was the primary determinant of quality and the difference in quality that was found between those who had had, and those who had not had, teaching hospital postgraduate training was merely a secondary phenomenon or whether (*b*) the association between age and quality of practice was merely a manifestation of the fact that the doctors who had had postgraduate training in teaching hospitals were a younger group than those who had had only non-teaching hospital postgraduate training.

4. The doctors whose postgraduate training time in *internal medicine* in teaching hospitals and whose *total* postgraduate training time in teaching hospitals had both been prolonged showed a tendency to carry on practices of better quality than those whose postgraduate training in teaching hospitals had been of shorter duration. It was not possible, however, to discover whether the factor determining the better quality of practice was (*a*) the longer *total* duration of teaching hospital postgraduate training or (*b*) the longer duration of teaching hospital postgraduate training in *internal medicine*—the training, in either case, showing its effect after a long latent period—or (*c*) qualities possessed by the doctor that induced him to prolong either his total postgraduate training or its medical component.

5. It must be emphasized that the results stated in the preceding paragraphs are averages and that certain individual doctors, though they had had no postgraduate training in teaching hospitals, yet were practising medicine of a high quality and that certain others, who had had postgraduate training in teaching hospitals, were practising medicine of poor quality. From this we must conclude that individual qualities affect the quality of practice in other ways than through whatever effect they may have in influencing the individual in his choice of training hospital.

# GLOSSARY

ABDOMINOPERINEAL RESECTION. Removal of the lower portion of the large bowel by an operation carried out through an incision into the abdomen and an incision into the perineum (the region about the anus).

ALIMENTARY TRACT. The passage extending from the mouth (via throat, oesophagus, stomach, small intestine, and large intestine) to the anus.

ANTEPARTUM. Before child-birth.

AURICULAR FIBRILLATION. An irregularity of the rhythm of the heart.

AUSCULTATION. The act of listening to the heart, lungs, or other internal organs, usually with the stethoscope.

AUTOCLAVE. Apparatus for sterilizing surgical and other equipment by steam under pressure.

BACTERIOLOGY (MEDICAL). The study and identification of micro-organisms capable of causing disease.

BARIUM. Barium sulphate is used as a contrast medium in the radiological examination of the digestive system. It is taken by mouth (barium swallow) when the upper part of the digestive system is being investigated. For examination of the large intestine, the barium sulphate is introduced as an enema.

BIOPSY. The removal and examination, usually microscopic, of tissue from the living body for purposes of diagnosis.

BLOOD PRESSURE, SYSTOLIC. The blood pressure during contraction of the heart.

BLOOD PRESSURE, DIASTOLIC. The blood pressure during relaxation of the heart between successive beats.

CAECUM. The blind portion of the large intestine from which the appendix originates.

CEREBROVASCULAR ACCIDENT. Obstruction of an artery of the brain or haemorrhage from an artery of the brain.

CERVIX (UTERI). The lower portion or outlet of the uterus (womb).

CHOLECYSTECTOMY. Removal of the gall bladder.

CORONARY THROMBOSIS. The formation of a thrombus (a type of blood clot) in one of the arteries (coronary arteries) that convey blood to the musculature of the heart.

CURETTAGE, UTERINE. Scraping of the inside of the uterus (womb) for diagnostic or therapeutic purposes.

CYSTITIS. Inflammation of the urinary bladder.

DERMATITIS. Inflammation of the skin.

DERMATOLOGY. The branch of medicine concerned with the diagnosis and treatment of diseases of the skin.

DIASTOLIC. See BLOOD PRESSURE.

DUODENUM. The first portion of the small intestine, immediately below the stomach.

EMBOLUS. A blood clot or other plug brought by the blood from another vessel and forced into a smaller one so as to obstruct the circulation.

EPISIOTOMY. Surgical incision made at the outlet of the birth canal for obstetrical purposes.

ESSENTIAL HYPERTENSION. Abnormally high blood pressure without known cause.

FEMUR. The bone of the thigh.

GASTRECTOMY. Removal of the stomach.

GASTRO-INTESTINAL SERIES. Series of X-ray films taken in radiological examination of the stomach and small intestine.

GASTRO-INTESTINAL TRACT. The stomach and intestines.

GYNAECOLOGY. The branch of medicine concerned with diseases of the genital tract in women.

HAEMATOLOGY. The branch of medicine concerned with diseases of the blood and with changes occurring in the blood in the course of other diseases.

HYPERTENSION. Abnormally high blood pressure. *See also* ESSENTIAL HYPERTENSION.

HYSTERECTOMY. Removal of the uterus (womb).

IMMUNIZING AGENTS. Materials (vaccines, toxoids, and others) used to render patients immune to various diseases.

INFRACLAVICULAR FOSSA. The depression below the collar-bone.

INTERNAL MEDICINE. The branch of medicine that deals with the diagnosis and treatment of conditions such as diabetes, pneumonia, heart disease, etc. Such work as operative surgery and obstetrics are not part of internal medicine.

INTERNE. A physician serving on the house staff of a hospital in order to gain experience. In the United States, the word "interne" is usually applied only to a physician serving his first year as a member of a house staff; those house doctors who have had more than one year of such experience are usually called assistant residents or residents. In Canada, a physician who in the United States would be called an assistant resident may be called either an assistant resident or a senior interne. In this book, except where it is specifically indicated, the word "interne" is to be understood in the less restricted sense.

INTERNESHIP. A period of experience obtained by a physician serving as an interne (*q.v.* for the difference between Canada and the United States in the use of the word). *See also* ROTATING INTERNESHIP.

INTERNIST. A specialist in internal medicine (*q.v.*).

INTRACRANIAL. Within the skull.

LARYNX. The voice box, manifest externally as the "Adam's apple."

LEUKAEMIA. A cancerous condition involving primarily the white cells of the blood.

MEAN. The mean of a group of items is the sum of the items divided by the number of items. The mean is sometimes called the arithmetic mean or the average.

MEDIAN. The median is the value of the middle item, when the items are arranged according to size. If there is an even number of items, the arithmetic mean of the two central items is taken as the median.

MENINGITIS. Inflammation of the membranes surrounding the brain and the spinal cord.

MITRAL STENOSIS. Narrowing of the mitral valve, one of the four valves inside the heart.

MYOCARDIAL INFARCTION. Damage to the heart muscle as a result of coronary thrombosis or other process interfering with the function of the coronary arteries.

NEONATAL. Newborn.

NEONATAL DEATH. Death occurring during the first month after birth.

NEUROLOGY. The branch of medicine concerned with the nervous system.

OESOPHAGUS. The canal extending from the throat to the stomach.

OPHTHALMOLOGY. The branch of medicine concerned with the eye.

OPHTHALMOSCOPE. Instrument for inspecting the interior of the eye.

OTOLARYNGOLOGY. The branch of medicine concerned with the ear, the nose, and the throat.

OTOSCOPE. Instrument for inspecting the ear drum.

PALPATION. The act of feeling with the hand. This is a method of examination.

PATHOLOGY. The branch of medicine that has to do with the essential nature of disease. In a more restricted sense, the word is used to refer to the laboratory work that is concerned with the gross and microscope structural changes that occur in disease.

PERCUSSION. Examination carried out by tapping gently with finger or other instrument. This is used particularly in the examination of the lungs and the heart.

PHARYNX. The throat.

POSTPARTUM. After child-birth.

PLATELETS. Small particles in the blood that play an important part in the clotting of blood.

PYELONEPHRITIS. Infection of the kidney.

PYLORIC STENOSIS. Narrowing of the outlet of the stomach.

RALE. A type of abnormal sound heard in the lungs.

RHONCHUS. A type of abnormal sound heard in the lungs.

ROSEOLA INFANTUM. An acute infectious disease occurring in early childhood and somewhat resembling measles.

ROTATING INTERNESHIP. An internship during which the physician works on a number of different services in succession (medicine, surgery, paediatrics, etc.), the period spent on each service ranging from a few weeks to a few months.

SEROLOGY. The study of certain specific changes that may occur in the blood and certain other body fluids and that often make possible or facilitate exact diagnosis.

SERUM HEPATITIS. An inflammatory disease of the liver that is caused by a virus that can be transmitted from one person to another by inadequately sterilized needles and other instruments.

SIGMOIDOSCOPE. An instrument for visual examination of the lower portion of the large intestine.

SPINAL TAP. The insertion of a needle into the back and the removal, for diagnostic purposes, of a sample of the fluid present around the spinal cord (cerebrospinal fluid).

SPECULUM. An instrument for dilating passages (of the ear, nose, vagina, etc.) to allow visual examination.

STERNUM. Breast bone.

SUBMAXILLARY. Situated beneath the lower jaw.

SUBSTERNAL. Situated beneath the breast bone.

SUPRACLAVICULAR FOSSA. The depression above the collar-bone.

SUPRAPUBIC. Of the lower portion of the abdomen in the mid-line.

SYSTOLIC. *See* BLOOD PRESSURE.

TIBIA. The larger bone of the leg below the knee.

TOXAEMIA OF PREGNANCY. One of the serious possible complications of pregnancy.

TRACHEA. The windpipe.

TRANSURETHRAL RESECTION. Removal of a portion of the prostate gland by means of an instrument introduced through the penis.

TRAUMATIC. Pertaining to, or caused by, an injury.

URINARY TRACT. The organs and ducts that participate in the formation and elimination of the urine.

VALVOTOMY. A type of surgical operation on a valve of the heart.

# Index

(C.G.P. = College of General Practice of Canada; C.M.A. = Canadian Medical Association; P.S.I. = Physicians' Services Incorporated; S.G.P. = Survey of General Practice.)

Lightning Source UK Ltd.
Milton Keynes UK
UKHW010009210722
406167UK00001B/11